BENSON & PERNOLL'S
handbook *of*

OBSTETRICS & GYNECOLOGY

NOTICE

Medicine is an ever-changing science. As new research and clinical experience broaden our knowledge, changes in treatment and drug therapy are required. The authors and the publisher of this work have checked with sources believed to be reliable in their efforts to provide information that is complete and generally in accord with the standards accepted at the time of publication. However, in view of the possibility of human error or changes in medical sciences, neither the authors nor the publisher nor any other party who has been involved in the preparation or publication of this work warrants that the information contained herein is in every respect accurate or complete, and they disclaim all responsibility for any errors or omissions or for the results obtained from use of the information contained in this work. Readers are encouraged to confirm the information contained herein with other sources. For example and in particular, readers are advised to check the product information sheet included in the package of each drug they plan to administer to be certain that the information contained in this work is accurate and that changes have not been made in the recommended dose or in the contraindications for administration. This recommendation is of particular importance in connection with new or infrequently used drugs.

BENSON & PERNOLL'S
handbook *of*

OBSTETRICS & GYNECOLOGY

Tenth Edition

Martin L. Pernoll, M.D.

Formerly:
Head, Division of Perinatology,
University of Oregon Health Sciences Center,
Portland, Oregon

Chair, Department of Obstetrics and Gynecology,
Tulane University School of Medicine,
New Orleans, Louisiana

Executive Dean, Kansas University School of Medicine,
Kansas City, Kansas

McGraw-Hill
Medical Publishing Division

New York · St. Louis · San Francisco · Auckland · Bogotá · Caracas
Lisbon · London · Madrid · Mexico City · Milan · Montreal · New Delhi
San Juan · Singapore · Sydney · Tokyo · Toronto

McGraw-Hill

A Division of The **McGraw·Hill** *Companies*

Benson and Pernoll's Handbook of Obstetrics and Gynecology, Tenth Edition

Copyright © 2001 by The **McGraw-Hill Companies**, Inc. All rights reserved. Printed in the United States of America. Except as permitted under the United States Copyright Act of 1976, no part of this publication may be reproduced or distributed in any form or by any means, or stored in a data base or retrieval system, without the prior written permission of the publisher.

Previous edition copyright © 1994 by McGraw-Hill, Inc.

1 2 3 4 5 6 7 8 9 0 DOC/DOC 0 9 8 7 6 5 4 3 2 1 0

ISBN 0-07-135608-8

This book was set in Times Roman by TechBooks
The editors were Andrea Seils and Susan R. Noujaim.
The production supervisor was Minal Bopaiah.
Project management was by York Production Services.
The cover designer was Aimee Nordin.
R.R. Donnelley & Sons was printer and binder.

This book is printed on acid-free paper.

Library of Congress Cataloging in Publication Data

Pernoll, Martin L., 1939–
  Benson & Pernoll's handbook of obstetrics and gynecology / author,
    Martin L. Pernoll.—10th ed.
      p. ; cm.
  Rev. ed. of: Benson and Pernoll's handbook of obstetrics & gynecology. 9th ed. 1994.
  Includes bibliographical references and index.
  ISBN 0-07-135608-8
    1. Obstetrics—Handbooks, manuals, etc. 2. Gynecology—
  Handbooks, manuals, etc. I. Title: Benson and Pernoll's handbook of obstetrics and gynecology. II. Title: Handbook of obstetrics and gynecology. III. Benson, Ralph Criswell, 1911—Benson and Pernoll's handbook of obstetrics & gynecology. IV. Title.
    [DNLM: 1. Genital Diseases, Female—Handbooks. 2. Obstetrics—Handbooks. WP 39 P452b 2001]

RG110 .P47   2001
618—dc21   00-032909

DEDICATION

This work is dedicated to those who provided me with motivation (Zilla and Lester Elder, Lee and Martin V. Pernoll, Alta and Jess Roberts), to those who provided me with inspiration (Drs. Bernard Daly, Truman Blocker, Kermit Krantz, Warren Pearse, Marcia Pernoll, and every patient I have ever seen), and to those who reinforce that our worth is only what we can give to the future (the nursing students, medical students, residents, fellows, and graduate students with whom I have been fortunate enough to interact, Kristin Manzano, Martin W. Pernoll, and Kelsey Manzano).

CONTENTS

PREFACE

During the course of this text's ten editions, societal evolutions have materially transformed the provider-patient exchange. Each patient and each provider's perception of these alterations may vary and there are certainly differences from country to country and within different cultures; however, cumulatively these evolutions amount to a changing paradigm of provider-patient interaction. In the US the majority of these transformations are positive.

For example, as an ethical ideal, replacing patient autonomy (interdependency) for physician paternalism (dependency) places the care relationship on a much more mature and functional basis. Provider-patient interdependence is furthered by patients having nearly unlimited access to medical information (and in some cases disinformation) via the Internet. No longer is the provider the patient's only source of information. Additionally, patients today have greater freedom of choice to match their expectations and personalities to that of a provider. This has been brought about by the much welcome enhancement of sexual and racial "minorities" to what was once a very nearly homogenous provider base. Even the increasing discourse (both pro and con) concerning public health issues, such as immunizations, should result in better understanding, broader public education, and more acceptable public policies.

Other societal alterations have had more debatable impacts on the interchange necessary for care. In this category are the efforts cumulatively titled "managed care." While accomplishing their objective of cost containment, many of the methodologies are intrusive (to both providers and patients) on health care and questions of quality in such a system are rife. Another example in this category is increasingly litigious behavior. While proponents indicate this as a necessary function to protect individual rights, there is no question (in the US) that the legal process increases both direct and indirect costs of health care. Perhaps the cumulative intellect of patients, attorneys, insurers, legislators, and providers could, through a broader dialog, improve the impact of these aspects on health care.

Finally, scientific advancement has a marked impact on the provider-patient interface. While this is pervasive in all aspects of caring for women, nowhere are there greater advances than in genetics. These advances when applied to humans raise major ethical issues, for example the human genome project, the ability to detect genetic predispositions for certain conditions, and cloning. Additionally, patient, familial, and societal opinions are rapidly evolving concerning both natural and technological aspects of reproductive function. Two areas currently triggering debate are post mortem sperm acquisition for in vitro fertilization and the sale of donor eggs.

The provider-patient interface must allow the freedom for discussion of all such issues without threatening the individual beliefs, ethics, or morality of any party involved in the dialogue. True openness of discussion (listening as well as hearing) is imperative to guard against the hazard of ambiguous expectations and relationship difficulties. Moreover, the scientific, provider, legal, legislative, and patient communities must endeavor to match the free, open, nonjudgmental, and nonadversarial nature of most provider-patient exchanges.

This edition continues in the spirit of true communication started and maintained by Dr. Ralph Benson through preceding editions. We encourage the reader to provide us with their thoughts and sincerely desire that you find this edition useful.

Martin L. Pernoll, M.D.

BENSON & PERNOLL'S
handbook *of*

OBSTETRICS & GYNECOLOGY

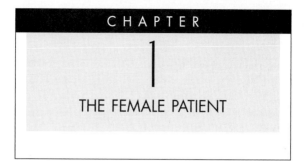

CHAPTER

1

THE FEMALE PATIENT

Most providers treasure their ability to care for patients. The joy derived from the provider–patient relationship remains intact despite additional individuals (e.g., employers, insurers, benefit managers, billing and collection specialists, utilization reviewers, etc.) and regulations interposed by the current evolution of health care.

Additionally, *providers appear to be accommodating to longer-term alterations that materially affect overall patient–provider relationships.* One feature of the changing relationship is *increasing patient autonomy.* Many factors likely have assisted this societal change, but the extraordinary *impact of readily available medical information on the Internet* certainly plays a role. Concurrently, the *paternalistic care model* (marked by the inter-action goal being determined by the provider, the provider role being motivated by being a guardian, alignment of patient values with the providers, and patient acceptance of recommendations) *is waning.*

Providers continue the search to improve the science of health care, while also seeking to improve the art of caring for patients. Indeed, during this decade there has been notable progress in both the science and art of caring for women. Included in that progress is the long overdue scientific recognition that men and women are different.

There is now *scientific recognition of both therapeutic dispari-ties attributable to gender as well as marked differences in gender inclusion in clinical trials.* Additionally, there is a renewed appre-ciation that *women frequently have different symptoms, risk factors, and drug reactions than do men.* For example, recent changes, mak-ing drug protocols more gender-specific and including women in major drug trials have reduced the disparity in treatment; however, the disparities are not yet eliminated.

Advances in the art of medicine include acknowledgment of difference in the way the two sexes approach problems. This sociolinguistic gender difference in problem solving affects the process of medical care. In general, men prefer to solve problems themselves. Male patients present problems that they expect the physician to resolve, whereas *women seek opinions or suggestions from others and then solve the problem with this consensus.* Female patients may want to discuss a problem but do not necessarily expect their doctor to resolve it. Male physicians tend to think that problems presented must be solved. *Women regard interview discussions with their physicians as opportunities to clarify problems and to obtain information about the implications of problems and treatments in their lives. This expectation can frustrate men, including male physicians.*

For some time, providers have recognized certain complexities in *communicating with female patients* (v. male patients), including: *lengthier and more detailed patient histories, more complaints expressed less succinctly in symptomatic interviews, and a greater variety of illnesses reported by* female patients. Some of the other gender difference observations concerning the provider–patient relationships are summarized as follows:

- Providers spend more time with female patients.
- More diagnostic errors are made with women patients. The most common explanation for diagnostic errors observed with female patients is the clinician's readiness to attribute women's symptoms to "overanxiousness."
- Interventions with women patients by physicians tend to be less aggressive.
- Generally, providers give more explanations to female patients.
- Providers impart more explanations rephrased from medical terms into lay terms when talking to women.
- When talking to women, providers give more responses to questions at the level of speech of the patient.
- In negotiation of treatment plans, male physicians may explain the meaning of a female patient's comments back to her and then attempt to guide her behavior through suggestions or instructions.
- Female patients may make overt attempts to share the control of the discussion by insisting on validating their symptoms with repetition, becoming more dramatic in their presentation of symptoms, switching to new symptoms, or reporting symptoms of questionable severity.

Other elements influencing the provider–patient relationship include: provider gender, the nature of the interaction, the nature of the communication, understanding the patient's perspective, communication training, and awareness of gender issues.

PROVIDER GENDER AND OTHER CHARACTERISTICS

Provider gender and other characteristics matter in shaping the provider–patient interaction. Indeed, recent studies comparing the communication of several groups of providers reveal issues useful to any provider wishing to enhance their patient communications.

- Female physicians (as well as family physicians) spend significantly more time discussing lifestyle during a first visit.
- Women physicians generally use more collaborative models of patient–physician relationship. That is, female physicians both facilitate and are more effective in developing provider–patient partnerships to enhance patient participation in the medical exchange.
- Female physicians spend more time with their patients. The National Ambulatory Medical Care Survey reported that male providers spent 18.7 minutes per patient, whereas female providers averaged 23.5 minutes.
- Female physicians spend more time communicating, specifically more time: gathering information, offering explanations, negotiating treatment, and providing emotional support. However, the additional dialogue with female physicians has not been associated with greater diagnostic or treatment accuracy. Much of the extra conversation is devoted to physicians' talking rather than information gathering. This suggests that female physicians use the time to offer explanations to patients of both genders, to negotiate treatment, and to provide emotional support.
- Male physicians tend to explain the meaning of a female patient's comments back to her and then attempt to guide her behavior through suggestions or instructions.
- Female providers (v. male providers) are more likely to: have a dialogue concerning social and psychological issues, more often explore patient's feelings and emotions, talk more positively in the encounter, focus more generally on partnership building, and give information and emotional support.
- Women, family physicians, and recent graduates are significantly more likely to have an empathetic communication style.
- Women and recent graduates are significantly less likely to have a directive, problem-oriented approach to care.
- Medical and surgical specialists are more supportive of patients' rights (than primary care providers).

- Female physicians are likely to view patient autonomy and initiative more negatively than their male colleagues, indicating again that women prefer consensual decision-making.

THE NATURE OF THE INTERACTION

The *character of a therapeutic relationship may be described by who* (patient or provider) *controls variables within the interaction.* These interactional variables include: *determination of the interaction goals, the provider's understanding of his or her role (obligations), the role of patient values in the visit, and expression of patient autonomy.* Given these variables, relationship types occur across a range from medical paternalism to patient consumerism.

At one extreme is the *paternalistic model.* Characteristically, in paternalism the *goal of the visit is determined by the provider.* The *provider's role (motivation) is that of a guardian* taking action in the patient's best interest. Patient's values are assumed to be aligned with those of the provider. Patient response to the provider's recommendations is anticipated to be agreement. The other end of the relationship spectrum is the *informative* (consumerist model). In this model, *goals are patient generated.* The *provider's role (motivation) is that of an expert who conveys technical information.* The patient selects the medical intervention deemed most appropriate from their various options. In a *total consumerist model, patient values are not explored or linked to the information provided and patient autonomy is defined as independent control over medical decision making.*

Between these two extremes are patient–provider relationships of collaboration and partnership. It is within these relationships that the exploration of patient values is most authentic and the achievement of patient autonomy is most fully insured. In these models, the following occur: *mutual goal setting, a provider's role as collaborator, mutual consideration of patient values, and ensurance of patient autonomy.* Although in all human interactions, *communication is crucial,* for providers to succeed in collaborative/partnership models requires special attention to their communication. Indeed, communication is the key to address perceived unmet needs in compassion of care in our technologically evolved medical model. Thus, a brief consideration of communication may be of assistance.

UNDERSTANDING THE
PATIENT'S PERSPECTIVE

Communication is the key to any healthcare provider in their vital role of caring for patients. Communication is defined as the *exchange of thoughts, messages, or information.* Ideally, communication leads to those involved *understanding each other's position(s).* Goals of *successful communication* include: *discerning issues and concerns from the other's point of view, identification of key issues and concerns, the determination of what would constitute an acceptable solution, and successful ascertainment of possible options to achieve those results.* To accomplish these goals requires *effective listening* to the others involved in the communication. At a minimum, *listening requires patience, openness, and the desire to understand.* More effective listening requires being an *empathic listener,* that is, *identification with, and understanding of another's situation, feelings, and motives.* Steps to empathic listening go beyond *mimicking content* to *understanding the message well enough to rephrase content, including the emotional context* of the message. Communication is influenced not just by speech, but also by behavior, body language, nonverbal signals, environment, and a host of other factors.

Certainly, *how the provider asks about symptoms* (open-ended questions are most desirable), *how the provider validates signs and/or symptoms,* and *the patient's comfort* in the atmosphere of that particular provider, influences the quality and quantity of information transmitted. This is particularly true when there are difficult issues or problems (including psychological or physical abuse) involved.

Thus, the *very success of diagnosis, treatment, and prevention often rests on the provider's cumulative communication skills.* Improved clinician–patient interpersonal communication has a positive impact on both therapeutic adherence and health outcomes. Similarly, less than desirable provider–patient communication has untoward outcomes for both patient and provider. *Crucial issues in the provider–patient interaction* frequently questioned (often through a legal or quality assurance process) include: *gathering and validating information for a correct diagnosis, informed decisions, informed consent, and motivation to a therapeutic regimen with the best outcomes.*

When providing information, it is necessary for the provider to consider other issues concerning the material they are attempting to communicate.

- Do I *cognitively understand* the information well enough to communicate it?
- Have I communicated in a *clear and unambiguous manner?* Ambiguity (naturally occurring or experimentally produced) leads to reduction in attention engagement.
- Was there something in my *behavior* that influenced the manner in which the information was received?
- *Is my communication acceptable to the patient* (given their culture, circumstances, etc.)?

- Does my communication involve making a change that is *unacceptable to the patient?*

Many times provider communication involves the desirability (or necessity) for a patient to change. These changes may be simple (e.g., one medication to another), complex (lifestyle or weight), or in conflict with established habits or addictions (smoking, drug use, alcohol, etc.). Providers may not understand, believe, or accept the logic (or thought processes) their patients employ in such situations. In these cases, providers need to recall a basic tenet of change, that is, *no one can persuade another to change. The commitment to change must come from within the individual doing the changing.*

Additionally, the provider must consider the mental status of the patient. A number of mental conditions will materially affect the patient's communication and nearly all of these are enhanced in intensity or frequency of occurrence during the internal surrounding birth.

DEPRESSION

Major depressive disorders are more prevalent in women. Although individual environmental experiences play a major role in the development of depression, these disorders are more heritable in women (as compared to men). Certainly, most providers are familiar with traditional depressive symptoms (sleep disruption, mood depression, and appetite disturbance). These traditional symptoms, however, are only a portion of the more global expression of depression. Other, and perhaps more subtle, signs of depression include nonverbal hostility, social withdrawal, and/or submissive and affiliative behaviors. Although depressed women generally express more socially interactive behaviors than men, both may demonstrate global restriction of nonverbal expression.

GUILT

Guilt contains elements of shame, aggression, and vagueness in communication. The emotion of guilt most commonly arises when a woman perceives herself a failure in her responsibilities and most commonly arises in situations when a woman lacks control over the multiple demands made on her from different life responsibilities. Guilt may also occur in situations where a woman assertively puts herself and the responsibility for her own needs above others. Frequently, such conflicts and subsequent emotions arise about her multiple responsibilities with children. Guilt is characterized by its emotional strength, repetition, and consistency.

ANGER

Gender role socialization can lead (or even teach) women to suppress anger. This may lead to denial of a sense of self as well as to somatization. Women in this circumstance may profit from assertive communication education. The outcome of teaching women assertive communication is to provide effective tools to regain control of their life experiences. Frequently, it is necessary to move from the belief that "others are responsible for meeting women's needs," to the belief that, "women are personally responsible for meeting their own needs."

PELVIC PAIN

Pelvic pain patients generally express more hostility than patients with other conditions. Attitudinal and personality factors may alter both the expression of pain as well as the patient's medical experience, but providers should be prepared to deal proactively with the hostility. Generally, poor prognostic indicators include: more severe levels of pain, a greater number of impaired functions of daily life, and endometriosis; however, therapy is beneficially influenced by the provider's success in communication. Indeed, providers' subtle attitudinal and personality factors modify patients' experience in these challenging conditions.

PATIENT COMPLAINTS

Publications concerning patient complaints, while difficult to statistically quantify and compare, reveal trends that may assist the provider in avoiding behaviors or events triggering patient dissatisfaction. Overall, nearly two thirds of complaints concern clinical care. The major dissatisfaction is with outcome. More than 20% of complaints pertain to rudeness or poor communication, and more than 10% relate to unethical or improper behavior. Women register 70% of complaints and nearly half of complaints are on behalf of another person. Over half of complaints arise from events occurring in doctors' consulting rooms.

PATIENT–DOCTOR COMMUNICATION SURROUNDING CRUCIAL LIFE EVENTS

Clearly, communication about end-of-life care both improves the perception of quality of that care as well as beneficially influencing advanced directives. Equal benefits occur for thoughtful communication with patients who have complications, untoward outcomes, or multiple disease states. As noted previously, all too frequently these patients have a variety of care providers, all well intentioned, but none assuming the important task of communication.

COMPLEMENTARY OR ALTERNATIVE THERAPIES

Currently, patients may not fully disclose their use of complementary or alternative therapy to their traditional medical provider(s). This is the case in even those who welcome an open discussion and in those with serious problems. For example, in breast cancer patients, nearly three fourths of patients initially use (and by 6 months approximately two thirds) at least one complementary or alternative therapy. Only slightly more than one half, however, disclose this use to their medical provider. By contrast, over 90% discuss details of their biomedical treatments with their alternative practitioner. In sum, if the health provider does not initiate or encourage discussion concerning complementary or alternative therapy, it may be an important area not communicated.

MULTIDISCIPLINARY TEAMS

Special attention to communication is mandatory in team care situations. Multidisciplinary teams require *theoretical, clinical, and professional consistency.* Indeed, consumer ambiguities may be expected if the entire team does not share *common missions, objectives, and language.* Consistency is easier to obtain in team care models planned for specific purposes than it is in situations where the team comes together for only that patient, or that particular problem (e.g., crucial events in patient care).

COMMUNICATION TRAINING

Provider communication difficulties can be overcome by communication training. Providers of both genders can be effectively trained to use more patient-centered skills. Once trained, these skills become evident in their practices. Moreover, female patients report greater involvement with male and female physicians who received communication training. Other provider opportunities in gender specific communication include: reducing gender bias by being aware that it exists and being aware of the implications posed by potential gender differences in both verbal and nonverbal behavior.

THE UNIQUENESS OF THE PATIENT–PROVIDER INTERACTION

Each female patient presents a unique set of circumstances, beliefs, and expectations. Her sexual and reproductive experiences and organ function are quite individual. She may be fearful of the gynecologic examination or may be uncomfortable confiding things that she considers private or embarrassing. Alternatively, she may be totally matter of fact about her body and its problems. Each patient at every visit is a whole person. *She should not be regarded as an assemblage of parts,* some of which are more interesting—pregnant or more apt to become cystic or cancerous—than others.

To assist in establishing rapport early in the doctor–patient relationship, ascertain how *the patient prefers to be addressed.* Some women prefer the use of their first name, whereas others prefer to be addressed using the formal salutation of Miss, Ms., or Mrs. Make a notation of her preference, because she will recall the inquiry and expect her response to be remembered.

In addition to possessing competence and skill, the provider must be able to *instill confidence about the privacy* of all discussions. Above all, the patient must sense that *medical personnel truly care about her.* A major step toward achieving this goal during the initial visit is to obtain the history in a quiet office with no sense of haste and with the patient fully clothed. Information not readily volunteered early may be disclosed when the patient becomes more comfortable as the interview progresses in a *nonjudgmental* fashion. Review pertinent episodes in her past medical history, family history, social history, and the review of systems, perhaps using a standardized questionnaire completed by the patient before seeing the care provider. *Focusing on details of the patient's concern early in the process may be helpful.* For example, leaving the genitourinary system discussion until last may cause her to believe that you are avoiding her problem. Information about the number of pregnancies, deliveries, abortions, contraception, sexually transmitted diseases, drug usage, sexual practices, and marital status is essential. Current medications and any allergies should be prominent in the review of past history. Ascertain whether or not she has a family doctor, since the physician providing reproductive care may be the only one to examine the patient routinely and must, therefore, provide primary care.

The patient's answers to personal questions may not coincide with the caregiver's personal moral standards, religious beliefs, sexual practices, or experience. He or she must not judge, however, but *assist with the patient's problems within her frame of reference. Nonetheless, do not neglect to give information about safe sexual practices, proper therapy, and potential consequences* of her or her partner's actions. Occasionally, one must stress that certain behaviors may affect not only the patient herself but also her offspring (e.g., drug use, infection). The caregiver must be prepared to consider marital difficulties, sexual dysfunction, and sexually transmitted diseases including AIDS.

THE PHYSICAL EXAMINATION

The initial examination should be a general physical examination, including a breast examination and the gynecologic examination. If the patient is not performing breast self-examination regularly and properly, plans should be made for her to receive instruction in the correct method.

Arrange the examining room to reassure the patient that her *privacy is not being invaded* via the doors or windows. For example, even the view of a beautiful garden can be distressing to the patient who fears that a gardener may suddenly appear during the examination.

The patient should be undressed completely and *draped for examination.* Sensitivity to the patient mandates that she not be placed in the dorsal lithotomy position to await the caregiver's arrival. This position may soon become uncomfortable and may leave her feeling vulnerable.

When performing the pelvic examination, have a *female nurse or attendant present,* if possible, for assistance and to provide a measure of comfort and reassurance to the patient. Explain the procedure before performing any maneuver, and give advance warning of any procedure that may be uncomfortable or even painful. Use instruments deftly. Warn the patient that you will be doing a vaginal or rectal examination before insertion of fingers or instruments. Warming the hands and instruments is a small act that indicates interest in the patient's comfort.

The teenage patient responds to open, honest dialogue. Parent(s), if present, should be asked to wait in the reception room unless the patient (not the parent) insists otherwise. It may be difficult to obtain an accurate history from the teenager because there may be a high degree of misinformation or misunderstanding of the function of sexual organs and the terminology. Open-ended questions, however, should provide the examiner with a fairly accurate estimate of the patient's knowledge and understanding. Never underestimate the ability of a teenager to deny reality—for example, she may not believe that she is pregnant despite amenorrhea, gross weight gain, and a protuberant abdomen.

Although the elderly patient may no longer be concerned with reproductive function, she may be faced with residual genitourinary problems as a result of pregnancies and aging. Her risk of cancer of the breast and reproductive organs is increased. She is at risk for osteoporosis and fractures. She may still enjoy an active sexual life or may have little or no interest in sexual activity. She may have lost her mate and be lonely and regard the visit to the health care provider as a social event. Alternatively, she may have financial worries that cause her to delay seeking medical help in the hope that the problem will go away. Because a higher percentage of the female population is living 20, 30, and even 40 years past menopause, the percentage of gynecologic care required by these patients has increased dramatically. Thus, it is essential to be knowledgeable about the many problems that arise in the geriatric patient.

When the health care provider recommends a particular course of therapy, she or he must be prepared to offer alternatives, to accept a second opinion, and, above all, to allow the patient the opportunity to participate in decision making. There may be instances when financial concerns dictate the best course of action under the circumstances without compromising care. Care providers must recognize, without affront, that what they would choose for themselves may be unacceptable to the patient because of her lifestyle or financial and social situation.

Thus, the patient must be respected as an individual. The expression of that respect must continue through the *development of a partnership with the patient to improve her health and well-being.*

NORMAL DEVELOPMENT OF THE UROGENITAL SYSTEM

The female generative and urinary systems develop in close association. Clarity, however, requires a description of the evolution of each system separately, with mention of important relationships and incorporations during development.

The development of the female urogenital system is well under way by the *fourth week after implantation,* following the sequence shown in Figures 1-1, 1-2, 1-3, and 1-4. The external female genitalia evolve after about the seventh week.

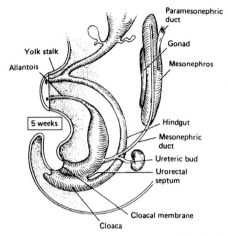

FIGURE 1-1. Left-side view of urogenital system and cloacal region before subdivision of cloaca by urorectal septum. Position of future paramesonephric duct is shown (begins in the sixth week). Gonad is in the indifferent stage (sexually undifferentiated).

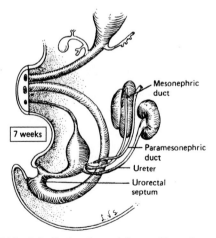

FIGURE 1-2. Left-side view of urogenital system. Urorectal septum nearly subdivides the cloaca into the urogenital sinus and the anorectal canal. Paramesonephric ducts do not reach the sinus until the ninth week. Gonad is sexually undifferentiated. Note incorporation of caudal segment of mesonephric duct into urogenital sinus (compare with Fig. 2-6).

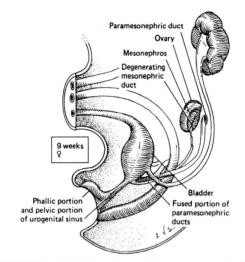

FIGURE 1-3. Left-side view of urogenital system at an early stage of female sexual differentiation. Paramesonephric (mullerian) ducts have fused caudally (to form uterovaginal primordium) and contacted the pelvic part of the urogenital sinus.

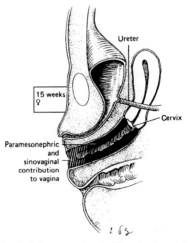

FIGURE 1-4. Sagittal cutaway view of differentiated urogenital sinus and precanalization stage of vaginal development. The drawing depicts one of several theories about the relative contributions of paramesonephric ducts and sinovaginal bulbs to the vagina (there is little consensus).

ORIGIN OF THE OVARIES

During the *fifth to sixth week,* primitive sex cells migrate from the yolk sac into the dorsal mesodermal genital ridge, destined to become the ovary. The sex cells, each likely to develop into a *primordial ovum,* then occupy the outer portion (cortex). Soon they are surrounded by smaller, moderately differentiated cells that will develop into granulosa cells. Cells just peripheral to the *granulosa cells,* which appear less differentiated but have otherwise similar stromal elements, will evolve into *theca cells.* Nondescript fibroblasts support a delicate vasculature. Coarse connective tissue and

FIGURE 1-5. Embryology of the ovary.

(From B. Pensky, *Review of Medical Embryology.* Macmillan, 1982.)

large blood vessels characterize the *medulla.* By the eighth week, the ovary is a recognizable organ (Fig. 1-5).

ORIGIN OF THE FEMALE GENERATIVE DUCTS

The *mullerian ducts* will become the uterine tubes, uterus, cervix, and upper portion of the vagina. The ducts are cordlike structures that begin to differentiate in the embryo at about *6 weeks.* The *upper ducts elongate and the lower ducts fuse.* The tract then canalizes to form *patent oviducts, the uterine cavity, the cervical canal, and the upper two thirds of the vaginal canal.* The *lower one third* of the vagina *is formed from invagination of the cloaca.* This duct development requires *4–5 months.*

ORIGIN OF THE FEMALE EXTERNAL GENITALIA

The external genitalia are pericloacal in origin, with the genital tubercle becoming the *mons pubis* and *clitoris.* The *hymen* represents the merge of the upper vaginal (mullerian) portion and the lower vaginal urogenital sinus.

Because of the intricate interdevelopment and the small size of the parts, the sex of the fetus rarely can be determined with confidence by ultrasonic scanning or even direct visualization until after the 22nd week.

ORIGIN OF THE KIDNEYS AND URETERS

Three stages mark the development of the human renal excretory apparatus.

The *pronephros* (or primordial kidney), a transitional incomplete duct with lateral vestigial tubules, develops in the posterior-lateral mesoderm during the third and fourth weeks. It may transport minimal celomic fluid. The duct alone survives to become the *mesonephric (wolffian) duct.*

The *mesonephros* (middle kidney) forms caudal to the pronephros along the mesonephric duct, which finally extends to the cloaca. Along the duct, mesonephric tubules, each with an arteriole and a venule, form primordial glomeruli. The mesonephros, developed by the seventh week, extracts waste products from celomic fluid and blood. By the ninth week, the tubules degenerate. The mesonephric

**COMPLETE BILOCULAR
UTERUS**

**BILOCULAR UNICERVICAL
UTERUS**

**BICERVICAL UTERUS
BICORNIS**

**UNICERVICAL UTERUS
BICORNIS**

UNICORNUATE UTERUS

UNILATERAL ATRESIA

FIGURE 1-6. Congenital uterine abnormalities.
(From B. Pensky, *Review of Medical Embryology.* Macmillan, 1982.)

TABLE 1-1
ADULT DERIVATIVES AND VESTIGIAL REMAINS
OF EMBRYONIC UROGENITAL STRUCTURES[a,b]

Embryonic Structure	Male	Female
Indifferent gonad	*Testis*	*Ovary*
Cortex	*Seminiferous tubules*	*Ovarian follicles*
Medulla	*Rete testis*	Rete ovarii
Gubernaculum	Gubernaculum testis	*Ovarian ligament*
		Round ligament of uterus
Mesonephric tubules	*Ductuli efferentes*	Epoophoron
	Paradidymis	Paroophoron
Mesonephric duct	Appendix of epididymis	Appendix vesiculosa
	Ductus epididymidis	Duct of epoophoron
	Ductus deferens	Duct of Gartner
	Ureter, pelvis, calyces, and *collecting tubules*	*Ureter, pelvis, calyces,* and *collecting tubules*
	Ejaculatory duct and seminal gland (vesicle)	
Paramesonephric duct	Appendix of testis	Hydatid (of Morgagni)
		Fallopian tube
		Uterus
Urogenital sinus	*Urinary bladder*	*Urinary bladder*
	Urethra (except glandular portion)	*Urethra*
	Prostatic utricle	*Vagina*
	Prostate gland	*Urethral* and *paraurethral glands*

(Continued)

TABLE 1-1
(Continued)

Embryonic Structure	Male	Female
	Bulbourethral glands	*Greater vestibular glands*
Mullerian tubercle	Seminal colliculus	Hymen
Genital tubercle	*Penis*	*Clitoris*
	Glans penis	*Glans clitoridis*
	Corpora cavernosa penis	*Corpora cavernosa clitoridis*
	Corpus spongiosum	*Bulb of the vestibule*
Urogenital folds	*Ventral (under) aspect of penis*	Labia minora
Labioscrotal swellings	*Scrotum*	*Labia majora*

[a] Modified from K. L. Moore, *The Developing Human: Clinically Oriented Embryology*, 2nd ed. W. B. Saunders Co., 1977.

[b] Functional derivatives are italicized.

duct is vestigial in the female, but it becomes the epididymis and vas deferens in the male.

The *metanephros* (true kidney) begins about the fourth week, as the mesonephric tubules develop and degenerate. The mesonephric diverticulum (ureteric bud) begins to grow out from the mesonephric duct slightly cephalad to the cloaca to become the *ureter* and the metanephros or *permanent kidney.*

During the *fifth through sixth weeks,* the ureter divides within the developing mesonephric mass to form *calices. Collecting and secretory tubules* then appear within the renal mesenchyme to connect the true vascularized *glomeruli* in the renal cortex. There is slight kidney excretion by the tenth week.

During the *second through third months,* the *bladder develops* from the widened lower wolffian ducts that merge with the allantois. The eventual bladder architecture is apparent by the tenth week, when the caudal extension, the *urethra,* finally opens into the urogenital sinus derived from the cloaca.

The *adrenal (suprarenal) glands* begin to form about the *fifth week* from mesenchymal cells, similar to those that produced the nonterminal portion of the ovary, together with nearby cells from the neural folds. A partially organized *adrenal cortex and medulla* are evident by the *ninth through tenth weeks.*

Anomalous female urogenital development, including congenital uterine abnormalities, strange anatomic inclusions, or even pelvic tumors, may represent vestigial male counterparts (Figs. 1-6 and Table 1-1).

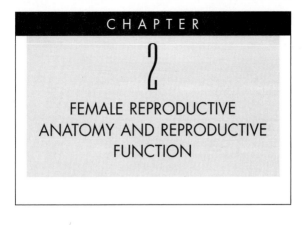

CHAPTER

2

FEMALE REPRODUCTIVE ANATOMY AND REPRODUCTIVE FUNCTION

FEMALE REPRODUCTIVE ANATOMY

The female reproductive system is composed of the external and internal genitalia. The *external genitalia* (Fig. 2-1) are collectively termed the pudendum or *vulva* and are directly visible.

The *internal genitalia* include the *vagina, cervix, uterus, uterine (fallopian) tubes, and ovaries* (Figs. 2-2 and 2-3). Special instruments are required for inspection of the internal genitalia. Simple specula or other instruments allow direct visualization of the vagina and cervix, but the intraabdominal group can be inspected only by invasive methods (laparotomy, laparoscopy, or culdoscopy) or by sophisticated imaging techniques (ultrasonography, CT scan, or magnetic resonance imaging).

EXTERNAL GENITALIA

MONS PUBIS (MONS VENERIS)

The mons veneris, a rounded pad of fatty tissue overlying the symphysis pubis, develops from the genital tubercle. It is not an organ but a region or a landmark. Coarse, dark hair normally appears over the mons early in puberty. During reproductive life, the pubic hair is abundant, but after the menopause, it becomes sparse. The normal female escutcheon is typically a triangle with the base up, in contrast to the triangle with the base down pattern in males.

The skin of the mons contains sudoriferous and sebaceous glands. The amount of subcutaneous fat is determined by heredity, age, nutritional factors, and possibly, steroid hormone factors.

21

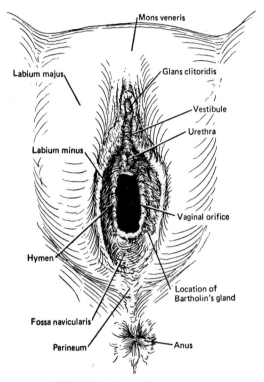

FIGURE 2-1. External female genitalia.

Innervation

The sensory nerves of the mons are the *ilioinguinal* and *genitofemoral nerves*.

Blood and Lymph Supply

The mons is supplied by the *external pudendal artery and vein*. The lymphatics merge with those from other parts of the vulva and from the lower abdomen. The crossed lymphatic circulation of the labia within the mons is clinically important because it permits metastatic spread of cancer from one side of the vulva to the inguinal glands of the opposite as well as to the affected side.

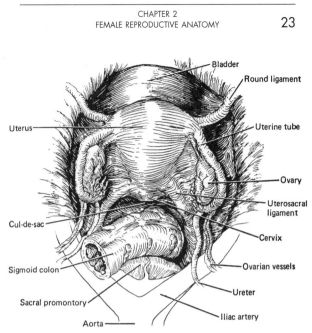

FIGURE 2-2. Internal female genitalia (superior view).

Clinical Importance

Dermatitis is common in the pubic area, and it is important to observe closely if infestation with *Phthirus pubis* (lice, crabs) is suspected. Edema can occur secondary to infections, vulvar varicosities, trauma, or carcinomatous infiltration of the lymphatics. Cancer elsewhere in the vulva also can involve the mons.

LABIA MAJORA

In the adult female, these two raised, rounded, longitudinal folds of skin are the most prominent features of the external genitalia. They are homologous to the male scrotum. They originate from the genital swellings extending posteriorly and dorsally from the genital tubercle. From the perineal body, they extend anteriorly around the *labia minora* to merge with the *mons*. The labia normally are closed in nulliparous women but later open progressively with succeeding vaginal deliveries and become thin and atrophic with sparse hair in later life.

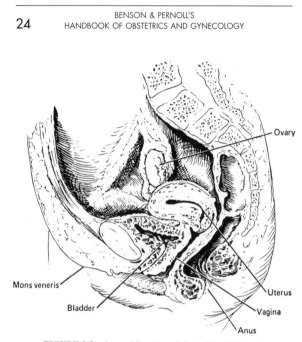

FIGURE 2-3. Internal female genitalia (midsagittal view).

The skin of the lateral surfaces of the labia majora is thick and often pigmented. It is covered with coarse hair similar to that of the mons. The skin of the inner labia majora is thin and contains no hairs. The labia majora are made up of connective and areolar tissue, with many sebaceous glands. A thin fascial layer similar to the tunica dartos of the scrotum is present within the labia just below the surface. The round ligament of the uterus passes through the inguinal canal *(canal of Nuck)* to end in a fibrous insertion in the anterior portion of the labia majora.

Small and large coiled subcutaneous sweat glands are situated all over the body except beneath mucocutaneous surfaces, that is, the labia minora or vermilion border of the lips. Normally, the fluid secretion of *small coiled (eccrine) sweat glands,* which have no relationship to hairs, has no odor. *Large coiled (apocrine) sweat glands* that open into hair follicles are found over the mons, the labia majora, and the perineum as well as the axilla. These glands, which begin to secrete an odorous fluid at puberty, are more active during menstruation and pregnancy. The sweat glands are controlled by the sympathetic nervous system.

Sebaceous glands are associated with and open into hair follicles. On the labia minora, where hairs are absent, however, sebaceous glands open on the surface. At puberty, an oily secretion with a slight odor is produced. The fluid lubricates and protects the skin from irritation by vaginal discharge. Gland secretion is mediated by hormonal and psychic stimuli. The activity of the sebaceous glands diminishes in older women.

Innervation

Anteriorly, the labia majora are supplied by the *ilioinguinal and pudendal nerves.* Laterally and posteriorly, they are innervated by the *posterior femoral cutaneous nerve.*

Blood Supply

The labia majora are supplied by the *internal pudendal artery* (derived from the anterior parietal division of the internal iliac or hypogastric artery) and by the *external pudendal artery* (from the femoral artery). Drainage is via the *internal and external pudendal veins.*

Clinical Importance

The labia majora serve no special function. *A cyst of the canal of Nuck* often is mistaken for an indirect inguinal hernia. Adherence of the labia in infants may indicate vulvitis. External force or the complications of labor can cause vulvar hematoma. *Hidradenomas are tumors that originate in aprocrine sweat glands,* but they become malignant only rarely. *Sebaceous cysts,* almost invariably benign but often infected, develop from sebaceous glands.

LABIA MINORA

The labia minora are small, narrow, elongated folds of skin between the labia majora and the vaginal introitus. They are derived from the skin folds beneath the developing *clitoris.* Normally, the labia minora are in apposition in nulliparas, concealing the *introitus.* Posteriorly, the labia minora merge at the *fourchette.* The labia are separate from the *hymen,* the structure marking the vaginal entrance, or introitus. Anteriorly, each labium merges into a median ridge that fuses with its mate to form the *clitoral frenulum,* an anterior fold that becomes the *prepuce of the clitoris.*

The lateral and anterior surfaces of the labia minora usually are pigmented. Their inner aspect is pink and moist, resembling the vaginal mucosa.

The labia minora have neither hair follicles nor sweat glands but are rich in sebaceous glands.

Innervation and Blood Supply

The innervation of the labia minora is via the *ilioinguinal, pudendal, and hemorrhoidal nerves.* The labia minora are not truly erectile, but a generous vasculature permits marked *turgescence with emotional or physical stimulation.* They are supplied by the *external and internal pudendal arteries and veins.*

Clinical Importance

The labia minora tend to close the introitus. They increase in size in response to ovarian hormonal stimulation. Indeed, without estrogen stimulation, they all but disappear. *Squamous cell carcinoma* of the vulva often originates in the labia, as do sebaceous cysts. The presence of *adherent labia minora in the infant* is usually due to inflammation. *Fusion,* however, may indicate sexual maldifferentiation.

CLITORIS

This 2–3 cm long homolog of the penis is found in the midline slightly anterior to the urethral meatus. It is composed of two small, erectile corpora, each attached to the periosteum of the symphysis pubis, and a diminutive structure *(glans clitoridis)* that is generously supplied with sensory nerve endings. The glans is partially hooded by the labia minora.

Innervation and Blood Supply

The clitoris is supplied by the *hypogastric and pudendal nerves, pelvic sympathetics,* and by the *internal pudendal artery and vein.*

Clinical Importance

Cancer of the clitoris is rare, but it is extremely serious because of problems of wide extension and early metastases. The inguinal and femoral nodes usually are involved first.

VESTIBULE AND URETHRAL MEATUS

The triangular area between the labia minora anteriorly onto which the urethra opens, bounded posteriorly by the vaginal orifice, is the *vaginal vestibule.* It is derived from the urogenital sinus and is covered by delicate stratified squamous epithelium.

The *urinary meatus* is visible as an anteroposterior slit or an inverted V. Like the urethra, it is lined by *transitional epithelium.* The vascular mucosa of the meatus often pouts or everts. This makes it appear more red than the neighboring squamous vaginal mucosa.

Innervation and Blood Supply
The vestibule and terminal urethra are supplied by the *pudendal nerve* and by the *internal pudendal artery and vein.*

Clinical Importance
Urethral caruncles, as well as *squamous cell or transitional cell carcinoma,* can develop in the urethrovestibular area.

PARAURETHRAL GLANDS (SKENE'S GLANDS)

Immediately within the *urethra,* on its posterolateral aspect, are two small orifices leading to the shallow tubular ducts or *glands of Skene,* which are wolffian duct remnants. The ducts are lined by transitional cells and are the sparse equivalent of the numerous male prostate glands.

Innervation and Blood Supply
Like the vestibule and urethral meatus, Skene's glands are supplied by the *pudendal nerve* and by the *internal pudendal artery and vein.*

Clinical Importance
Skene's glands, which supply minor amounts of mucus, are especially *susceptible to gonococcal infection,* which may be first evident here. After successful antigonorrheal therapy, nonspecific infection with other purulent organisms is common and results in *recurrent skenitis.* Destruction of the duct using electrocautery or laser may be necessary.

PARAVAGINAL OR VULVOVAGINAL GLANDS AND DUCTS (BARTHOLIN'S GLANDS AND DUCTS) AND HYMEN

Just external to the hymen are paravaginal, vulvovaginal glands, or Bartholin's glands, the counterpart of Cowper's glands in the male. On either side are two tiny apertures. A narrow duct, 1–2 cm long, connects each of these apertures with a small, flattened, mucus-producing gland that lies between the labia minora and vaginal wall. The *hymen* is a thin, moderately elastic barrier that usually partially but rarely completely occludes the vaginal canal. It is an incomplete double-faced epithelial plate covering a matrix of fibrovascular tissue.

Innervation and Blood Supply
The hymen and area of the Bartholin's glands are supplied by the *pudendal and inferior hemorrhoidal nerves, arteries, and veins.*

Clinical Importance

Bartholinitis can occur with sexually transmitted diseases, especially gonorrhea, and an abscess of Bartholin's duct can require marsupialization.

A tight hymen can result in painful intercourse *(dyspareunia)*, in which case, hymenotomy or dilatation will be required. The remnants of the lacerated hymen following intercourse or delivery are called *carunculae hymenales (myrtiformes)*. Hymenal or perineal scars also can cause dyspareunia.

PERINEAL BODY, FOURCHETTE, AND FOSSA NAVICULARIS

The perineal body includes the skin and underlying tissues between the anal orifice and the vaginal entrance. The perineal body is supported by the *transverse perineal muscle* and the lower portions of the *bulbocavernosus muscle*.

The labia minora and majora converge posteriorly to form a low ridge called the *fourchette*. Between this fold and posterior to the hymen is a shallow depression termed the *fossa navicularis*.

Innervation and Blood Supply

These structures are supplied by the *pudendal and inferior hemorrhoidal nerves, arteries, and veins*.

Clinical Importance

The perineal body or fourchette often is *lacerated during childbirth* and can require repair. Because of vascularity, an early or deep episiotomy can result in the loss of several hundred milliliters of blood. Faulty repair can be followed by *dyspareunia* or by *reduced sexual satisfaction*.

INTERNAL GENITALIA

VAGINA

The vagina (Fig. 2-3) is a thin, muscular, partially collapsed rugose canal 8–10 cm long and about 4 cm in diameter. It extends from the hymen at the urogenital cleft to the cervix and curves upward and posteriorly from the vulva. The cervix protrudes several centimeters into the upper vagina to form recesses called the *fornices*. The posterior fornix is usually deeper than the anterior fornix. The lateral fornices are similar in size. The vaginal dimensions are reduced during the climacteric, and all fornices, especially the lateral ones, become more shallow.

The vagina lies between the *urinary bladder* and the *rectum* and is supported principally by the *transverse cervical ligaments (cardinal ligaments)* and the *levator ani muscles.*

The peritoneum of the *posterior cul-de-sac (pouch of Douglas)* is closely approximated to the *posterior vaginal fornix,* a detail of surgical importance.

The vagina is lined by stratified squamous epithelium, which is thick and folded transversely in nulliparas. Many of these rugae are lost with repeated vaginal delivery and after the menopause. Normally, no glands are present in the vagina.

Innervation and Blood Supply

The nerve supply to the vagina is via the *pudendal and hemorrhoidal nerves* and the *pelvic sympathetic system* (Fig. 2-4). The blood supply is from the *vaginal artery* (a descending branch of the uterine artery) and from the *middle hemorrhoidal and internal pudendal arteries.* It is drained by the *pudendal, external hemorrhoidal, and uterine veins.*

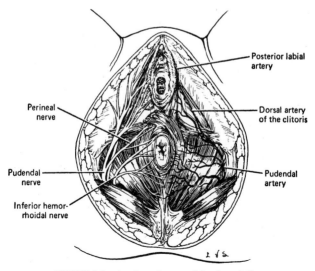

FIGURE 2-4. Arteries and nerves of female genitalia.

The lymphatic drainage of the *lower vagina* is via the *superficial inguinal nodes;* that of the *upper vagina* is to the *presacral, external iliac, and hypogastric nodes.* This is important in vulvovaginal infections and cancer spread.

Clinical Importance

Vaginal discharge is common and can be due to local or systemic disorders. Infections of the lower reproductive tract are the most common cause of leukorrhea. Estrogen depletion (senile or atrophic vaginitis) and estrogen or psychic stimulation are other causes. Primary cancer of the vagina is very rare, but secondary spread from cervical cancer is not uncommon.

CERVIX

The cervix of the nonpregnant uterus (Fig. 2-3) is a conical, moderately firm organ about 2–4 cm long and some 2.5 cm in outside diameter, with a central, spindle-shaped canal. About half the length of the cervix is supravaginal and close to the bladder anteriorly.

Childbirth lacerations account for most cervical distortions. The external os, which is initially round and only a fraction of a centimeter in diameter, may gape and be much longer as a result of these tears. Even in the absence of distortions, however, it is customary to refer to the cervix as having anterior and posterior lips.

The cervix is supported by the *uterosacral ligaments and transverse cervical ligaments (cardinal ligaments).*

The intravaginal portion of the cervix is covered by stratified squamous cells, which usually extend to approximately the external os. The cervical canal is lined by secretory columnar epithelium. The juncture of these two epithelia is variable and is subject to continual revision under the influence of infections, hormones, and trauma. The countless crevices that give the cervical canal a honeycombed appearance on transverse section are infoldings of the mucus-secreting membrane.

Excluding the epithelial covering and the cervical canal, the cervix is composed of approximately *85% connective tissue and 15% smooth muscle fibers* that join the uterine myometrium above. The anatomic structure of the cervix undergoes marked alteration during pregnancy, labor, and delivery.

Innervation and Blood Supply

Innervation of the cervix is via the *second, third, and fourth sacral nerves* and the *pelvic sympathetic plexus* (Fig. 2-4). The right and left *cervical artery and vein,* major branches of the uterine circulation, carry most of the blood to and from the cervix.

Clinical Importance

The red appearing, more friable columnar epithelium over the endocervix is responsible for *ectropion* and may contribute to *postcoital bleeding and infection.* Additionally, the squamocolumnar junction is the site of *>90% of squamous cell carcinomas* of the cervix. *Cervical cancer is the second most common female genital malignant neoplastic disease. (Endometrial cancer is the most common.) Cervical infection* may be a contributor to *infertility. Leukorrhea* often is due to *inflammation* of the mucus-secreting membrane.

UTERUS

The uterus (Figs. 2-2 and 2-3) is an inverted, pear-shaped muscular organ with a narrow central cavity situated deep in the true pelvis between bladder and rectum. The *central cavity,* which is lined by endometrium, is roughly triangular with the base up and is markedly compressed in the anterior-posterior. Each of the upper apices is connected to an oviduct, and the lower apex merges with the *cervical canal.*

The uterine tubes join the uterus, one on either side, about two thirds of the distance to the top of the uterus. That portion of the uterus above the tubal insertion is called the *fundus.* Below the insertion is the body *(corpus)* of the uterus, which is continuous with the supravaginal segment of the cervix. In contrast to the cervix, the uterine substance *(myometrium)* is 85% smooth muscle and only 15% connective tissue. Except for the anteroinferior portion of the corpus, which is invested by the bladder, the *uterus is covered by peritoneum.*

The adult nonpregnant uterus weighs about 90 g and is about 7–8 cm long and about 4 cm in its widest diameter. However, considerably larger sizes and increased weight occur with hormonal stimulation and after childbirth. During pregnancy, the uterus, which increases to weigh about 1000 g, literally balloons to accommodate the gestation.

The uterus is *supported by three paired ligaments.* Uppermost are the *round ligaments,* which pass from the uterine fundus anterior to the uterine tube to the internal inguinal canal. Laterally on each side from inferior to the uterine tube extending to the cervix and attached to the pelvic side wall are the *cardinal ligaments.* The *uterosacral ligaments* extend from each sacral attachment to the posterior uterocervical juncture.

In the nulliparous woman, the uterus and cervix usually are directed forward at almost a right angle with the long axis of the vagina. However, *25%–35% of women normally have retroverted or retroflexed uteri.*

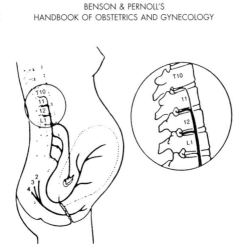

FIGURE 2-5. Parturition pain pathways. Afferent pain impulses from the cervix and uterus are carried by nerves that accompany sympathetic fibers and enter the neuraxis at T10, T11, T12, and L1. Pain pathways from the perineum travel to S2, S3, and S4 via the pudendal nerve.

(From J.J. Bonica, The nature of pain of parturition. *Clin Obstet Gynecol* 1975;2:511.)

Innervation and Blood Supply

The nerves to the uterus include the *superior hypogastric plexus,* the *inferior hypogastric plexus,* the *nervi erigentes,* the *common iliac nerves,* and the *hypogastric ganglion* (Fig. 2-5).

The *uterine artery* (a terminal branch of the hypogastric) is the primary souce of blood to the uterus, and the *ovarian artery* is a contributor. *The uterine artery passes anterior to the ureter lateral to, but near, the uterocervical junction.* This is a very important anatomical land mark! The veins draining the uterus are primarily the *uterine veins* and secondarily the *ovarian veins.*

Lymphatic drainage may be through the cervix to the *external iliac chain* or via the isthmus to the *lateral sacral nodes.* Lymph drainage within the round ligaments may extend to the *superifical inguinal nodes,* then to the *femoral,* and finally, to the *external iliac chain.* Drainage through the suspensory ligament of the ovary proceeds to the *lumbar nodes along the aorta,* above or below the kidney.

Clinical Importance

The uterus performs its reproductive function with remarkable efficiency. Although menstrual problems are common, they are not usually of uterine origin. Occasionally, *congenital* (e.g., subseptate uterus, uterus unicollis) *or acquired defects* (e.g., Asherman's syndrome) *make pregnancy difficult*. With the exception of childbirth, the uterus is infrequently subject to infection. The myometrium is rarely the site of malignancy. *Endometrial cancer,* however, *is the most common female genital cancer.* The *myometrium is very commonly the site of benign uterine leiomyomas and,* less frequently, is locally honeycombed by endometrium, resulting in *adenomyosis*.

UTERINE TUBES (FALLOPIAN TUBES)

Both uterine tubes function to *convey the ova to the uterus from the ovary*. Bilaterally, these tubes lie in the peritonealized superior border of the broad ligament termed the *mesosalpinx*. Each tube is 7–14 cm in length and generally lies horizontal near the uterus. On reaching the lower ovarian pole, it courses around the ovary to terminate by contact with the ovarian medial posterior surface.

Each tube is divided into the *isthmus, ampulla, and infundibulum*. The most medial segment is the isthmus. It is narrow in diameter, ending its uterine intramural course with an ostium of ~1 mm. More distal to the isthmus is the ampulla, which is more tortuous and wider. The ampulla terminates distally in the funnel-shaped infundibulum, which has as its most distal margin a series of fingerlike diverging processes, *the fimbriae*. The funnel-shaped mouth of the infundibulum, excluding the widely reaching fimbriae, is about 3 mm in diameter and opens into the peritoneal cavity. The infundibulum is loosely supported by the *infundibulopelvic ligament (suspensory ligament of the ovary)*.

The tubal wall consists of serous (peritoneal), subserous or adventitial (vascular and fibrous), muscular, and mucous components. The *muscular layer* is composed of outer longitudinal and inner circular smooth muscle layers. The mucosa is a ciliated columnar secretory epithelium arranged in longitudinal folds that become more complex in the ampullae. Its ciliary motion is directed toward the uterus.

Innervation and Blood Supply

The oviductal nervous supply is from the *pelvic and ovarian parasympathetic and sympathetic plexuses*. The tubal blood supply is from the *tubal branch of the uterine artery* and from the *ovarian branch of the uterine artery*. The venous drainage is through the tubal veins accompanying the arteries. The lymphatic drainage becomes retroperitoneal to the lumbar aortic nodes.

Clinical Importance

Tubal pregnancy and either intraluminal (usually gonococcal or chlamydial) or peritubal (often streptococcal) *infections* are the most common clinical concerns relative to the uterine tubes. Tubal distortion from peritubal scarring by endometriosis or infection, as well as intraluminal problems, can predispose to *infertility. Tubal cancer is very uncommon but serious.*

OVARIES

The ovaries are a pair of slightly flattened, ovoid organs that appear mottled pearly white with many surface irregularities. They lie below the pelvic brim and are supported by the *ovarian ligaments* (which extend from the uterus to the medial ovarian pole) and the *infundibulopelvic ligaments.* The ovaries rest in a fossa on the pelvic sidewall lined by peritoneum. They are *bounded above by the external iliac vessels, below by the obturator nerve and vessels, posteriorly by the ureter and uterine artery and vein, and anteriorly by the pelvic attachment of the broad ligament.* The uterine tubes are draped over the medial surface of the ovaries.

The ovaries weigh 4–8 g each and are usually 2.5−5 × 1.5−3 × 0.7−1.5 cm. They are covered by a cuboidal or low columnar epithelium and are divided into a *medulla* (consisting of numerous blood vessels, lymphatics, nerves, connective tissue, and smooth muscle) and a *cortex* (consisting of fine areolar stroma, many blood vessels, and scattered epithelial cells arranged in *follicles*).

The *graafian follicles contain the oocytes,* which with maturation (i.e., selection for ovulation) enlarge sufficiently to protrude visibly from the ovarian surface. When fully mature, the ovum is released and the follicle is transformed into a *corpus luteum.* This, in turn, is replaced by scar tissue (termed *corpus albicans*).

Innervation and Blood Supply

The ovarian nerve supply is from the *lumbosacral sympathetic chain* and passes to the ovary along the ovarian artery. The *ovarian artery* (usually a branch of the abdominal aorta, although *the left not infrequently arises from the left renal artery*) is the primary blood supply to the ovary. However, blood is also supplied from the anastomosing *ovarian branch of the uterine artery.* The veins follow the arteries to form the *pampiniform plexus* within the mesovarium. *The right ovarian vein empties into the vena cava, whereas the left ovarian vein usually enters the left renal vein.* The lymphatics drain *retroperitoneally to the aortic lumbar nodes.*

Clinical Importance

The principal functions of the ovaries include hormone production and the development of ova for the achievement of pregnancy. These functions can be interrupted by many factors. The ovaries are a *frequent site of benign and malignant ovarian tumors. Torsion* can occur, leading to vascular insufficiency and necrosis. *Ovarian infections* also occur, usually in premenopausal women.

THE PELVIC FLOOR

The pelvic floor (Figs. 2-6 and 2-7) consists of muscles, ligaments, and fascia arranged in such a manner as to support the pelvic viscera; provide sphincterlike action for the urethra, vagina, and rectum; and permit the passage of a term infant. It is composed of the *upper and lower pelvic diaphragms* and the *vesicovaginal and rectovaginal septa,* which connect the two diaphragms, the *perineal body,* and the *coccyx.* Other structures contributing to the integrity

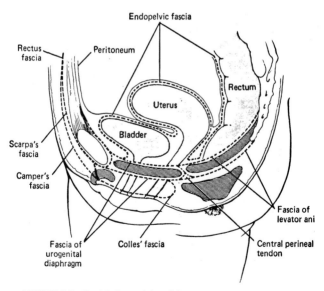

FIGURE 2-6. Fascial planes of the pelvis.
(Modified after Netter.)

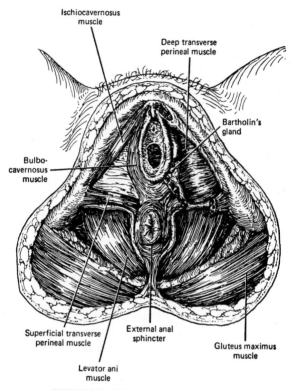

FIGURE 2-7. Pelvic musculature (inferior view).

of the pelvic floor include the *transverse cervical (cardinal or Mackerrodt's) ligaments* and the *gluteus maximus muscles.*

The *upper pelvic diaphragm* is a musculofascial structure made up of *endopelvic fascia, the uterosacral ligaments,* and the *levator ani muscles* (including the *pubococcygeus portion*). The *lower musculofascial pelvic diaphragm* includes the *urogenital diaphragm* and the *sphincter muscles at the vulvar outlet (ischiocavernosus, bulbocavernosus, and transverse perineal muscles).*

All parts of the upper and lower musculofascial diaphragms *anchor into the perineal body directly or indirectly,* like spokes into the hub of a wheel or shroud lines into the ring of a parachute. For reciprocal support, the layers of the pelvic diaphragms are interwoven and superimposed. They are not fixed but move upon one another. This makes it possible for the birth canal to dilate during passage of the fetus and to close postpartum.

The pelvic floor is perforated centrally by *three tubular structures: urethra, vagina, and rectum.* Each traverses the pelvic floor at a different angle, which enhances the sphincterlike action of the pelvic muscles.

The different tissues of the musculofascial diaphragm play an important role in providing both support and resilience. The *connective tissue* provides support but no recoil, the *fascia* gives strength but no elasticity, the *elastic tissue* has resilience but little strength, and the *voluntary and smooth muscles* provide stretch and recoil but with limited tolerances.

Weakness or relaxation of the pelvic floor can be due to a *neuropathy* or an *injury during childbirth,* or it can be of *congenital or involutional origin.*

THE BONY PELVIS

The bony pelvis is composed of *four bones, the sacrum and coccyx (posterior) and the two innominate bones laterally and anteriorly.* The *spinal column articulates* (through an arthrodial joint) with the sacrum *at L5.* Bilaterally, the *innominate bones rest on the femurs,* articulating by enarthroses (Figs. 2-8, 2-9, 2-10, and 2-11). Within the pelvis itself are two types of joints, a *synchondrosis* uniting the two pubic bones and *diarthroses* between the sacrum and ilium and between the sacrum and coccyx. The *innominate bones* have three major sections: *ilium, ischium, and pubis.*

The *ilium* is composed of the upper part *(ala or wing)* and a lower part *(body)* that forms the upper part of the *acetabulum,* uniting with the *ischium and pubis.* Medially, the ala of the ilium presents a smooth concave area that anteriorly is the *iliac fossa* and posteriorly is the *iliac tuberosity* (superior) and the *sacral articulation* (inferior). The superior border of the ilium (crest) is bounded by the *anterior and posterior superior iliac spines* and serves to attach the following muscles: *external oblique, internal oblique, transversus* (anterior two thirds), *latissimus dorsi, quadratus lumborum* (posterior), *sacrospinalis, tensor fascia latae,* and *sartorius* muscles. The lateral surface of the ilium provides attachments for the *gluteal muscles.* The posterior border of the iliac is marked by the posterior portion of the *greater sciatic notch.* Blood supply to the ilium is from the *iliolumbar, deep circumflex iliac, obturator, and gluteal arteries.*

FIGURE 2-8.   The bony pelvis (posterior view).

The ischium has a *body, superior and inferior rami,* and a *tuberosity.* The body joins with the *ilium* and *pubis to* form the *acetabulum.* The inner surface is smooth and contiguous with the body of the ilium (above), forming the posterior portion of the lateral

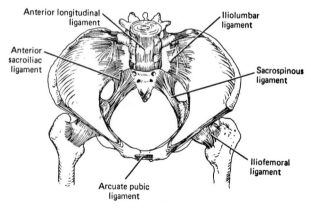

FIGURE 2-9.   The bony pelvis (superior view).

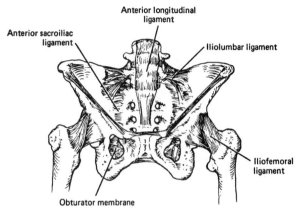

FIGURE 2-10. The bony pelvis (anterior view).

wall of the *true pelvis*. The posterior border forms the anterior portion of the *greater sciatic notch*. The *ischial tuberosity* is the most prominent portion of the bone and is the bony portion on which the human sits. The *lesser sciatic notch* occupies the posterior border

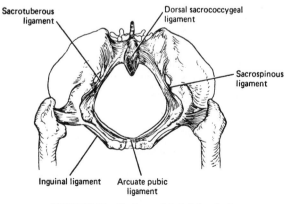

FIGURE 2-11. The bony pelvis (inferior view).

of the superior ramus. The inferior ramus joins the inferior ramus of the pubis to form the *pubic arch.* The *ischial spine* is an important obstetric landmark, being the *narrowest portion of the pelvis,* and is located along the inferior ramus. The *sacrospinous ligament* is found between the ischial spine and the sacrum. The *pudendal nerve and vessels pass under the lateral portion of this ligament.* Blood comes to the ischium from the *obturator, medial, and lateral circumflex arteries.*

The *pubis* has a body and superior and inferior rami. The body contributes to the *acetabulum.* The rami meet in the midline to form the *symphysis pubis,* and medially this is marked by the *pecten ossis pubis,* an irregular ridge. The *pubic tubercle* is found ~2 cm from the medial edge of the *superior ramus.* The inferior aspect of the superior ramus is the *obturator sulcus.* The pubis receives blood from the *obturator, medial, and lateral circumflex arteries.*

The *sacrum* is formed by union of *5–6 sacral vertebrae.* The fifth lumbar articulates (and occasionally fuses) with the first sacral vertebra. Their anterior portions form the *sacral promontory.* The posterior surface of the sacrum is convex, the midline forming the *median sacral crest* (fused spinal processes) and the fused laminae of the sacral vertebrae forming a flattened area laterally. This rough area is marked by absence of the laminae of the fifth and often, even the fourth and third sacral vertebrae. This opening of the dorsal wall of the sacral canal is the *sacral hiatus.* The lateral portions of the sacrum (from fusion of the sacral vertebrae transverse process) articulate with the ileum. The lower body of the fifth sacral vertebrae articulates with the *coccyx.* The sacrum receives its blood supply from the *middle and lateral (usually 4) sacral arteries.*

The *coccyx* is formed by 4 (occasionally 3 or 5) *coccygeal vertebrae,* which are most frequently fused into a single bone, and receives its blood supply from the *middle sacral artery.*

The bony pelvis is divided into two cavities by the iliopectineal line of the innominate bones. The *upper cavity,* which is larger and shallower, is the *false pelvis,* and the *lower,* which is smaller and deeper, is the true *pelvis.*

THE PELVIC MUSCLES, THEIR NERVES AND BLOOD SUPPLY

Muscles important to the pelvis include those of the abdomen, back, buttock, perineum, and upper extremity. Because many of the muscles have been functionally detailed in preceding portions of this chapter, Table 2-1 summarizes their nerves and blood supply.

TABLE 2-1
MOTOR NERVE AND BLOOD SUPPLY
TO ABDOMINAL AND PELVIC MUSCLES

Muscle	Motor Nerve(s)	Blood Supply
ABDOMINAL		
External oblique	T7–L4	Inferior epigastric
Internal oblique	T7–L4	Inferior epigastric, deep circumflex iliac
Transversus abdominus	T7–L1	Deep circumflex iliac
Rectus abdominus	T7–L1	Inferior epigastric
Pyramidalis	T12	Inferior epigastric
PELVIC AND LOWER EXTREMITY		
Cremasteric remnant	Genitofemoral	Inferior epigastric
Psoas minor	L1–L2	Lumbar branch of ileolumbar
Psoas major	L2–L3	Lumbar branch of ileolumbar
Iliacus	Femoral	Iliac branch of ileolumbar
Sartorius	Femoral	Muscular branch of femoral
Rectus femoris	Femoral	Lateral femoral circumflex
Vastus lateralis	Femoral	Lateral femoral circumflex
Vastus medialis	Femoral	Femoral, profunda femoris, popliteal (genicular branch)
Vastus intermedius	Femoral	Lateral femoral circumflex, obturator
Pectineus	Femoral	Medial femoral circumflex, obturator
Gracilis	Obturator	Profunda femoris, obturator, medial femoral circumflex

(Continued)

TABLE 2-1
(Continued)

Muscle	Motor Nerve(s)	Blood Supply
Abductor longus	Obturator	Medial femoral circumflex, obturator
Abductor brevis	Obturator	Medial femoral circumflex, obturator
Abductor magnus	Obturator, sciatic	Medial femoral circumflex, obturator, profunda femoris, popliteal
Biceps femoris	Sciatic	Profunda femoris, popliteal
Tensor fascia latae	Superior gluteal	Lateral femoral circumflex, superior gluteal
Gluteus maximus	Inferior gluteal	Superior and inferior gluteal, profunda femoris
Gluteus medius	Superior gluteal	Superior gluteal
Gluteus minimus	Superior gluteal	Superior gluteal
Obturator internus	Obturator internus gemellus superior	Superior gluteal
Gemellus superior	Obturator internus gemellus superior	Inferior gluteal
Gemellus inferior	Quadratus femoral gemellus inferior	Inferior gluteal
Quadratus femoris	Quadratus femoris gemellus inferior	Medial femoral circumflex
Piriformis	Superior gluteal	Superior and inferior gluteal, pudendal

TABLE 2-1
(Continued)

Muscle	Motor Nerve(s)	Blood Supply
PERINEAL		
Transverse perinaei	Perineal	Pudendal
Bulbocavernosus	Perineal	Pudendal
Sphincter urethrae	Perineal	Pudendal
Levator ani	S–4, pudendal	Inferior pudendal, inferior hemorrhoidal, inferior gluteal
Sphincter ani externus	Pudendal	Inferior hemorrhoidal, transverse perineal
Coccygeus	Pudendal	Inferior pudendal, inferior gluteal

MENSTRUATION

Menstruation, or normal periodic uterine bleeding, is a physiologic function occurring only in female primates. It is basically a catabolic process and is under the influence of pituitary and ovarian hormones. Its onset, the *menarche, usually occurs at age 8–13 years.* Its termination, the *menopause, normally ensues at age 49–50.* However, medical (e.g., gonadotropin releasing hormone agonists), radiation, or surgical intervention may cause *artificial menopause* at an earlier age.

The *interval* between menstrual periods varies according to age, physical and emotional well-being, and environment. The normal menstrual cycle is commonly stated to be 28 days, but intervals of 24 to 32 days are considered normal unless the cycles are grossly irregular. At both the beginning and the end of reproductive life, the cycle is likely to be irregular and unpredictable due to failure of ovulation. This provides a natural example of the difference between *ovulatory and anovulatory menstruation.* On reaching maturity, approximately two thirds of women maintain a reasonably regular periodicity, barring pregnancy, stress, or illness.

The *average duration of menstrual bleeding is 3–7 days,* but this also may vary.

The *average blood loss* in a normal menstrual period is approximately *35–90 mL.* About three quarters of this blood is lost during the first 2 days of the period. *Women <35 years tend to lose more blood than those >35.*

Menstrual discharge contains blood, desquamated endometrial and vaginal epithelial cells, cervical mucus, and bacteria. Prostaglandins have been recovered from menstrual blood, together with enzymes and fibrinolysins from the endometrium. The last prevent clotting of menstrual blood unless bleeding is excessive. Nonetheless, small fragile, fibrin-deficient vaginal clots may form because of the presence of mucoprotein and glucose in an alkaline moiety.

The following factors all can *influence menstrual bleeding:* (1) fluctuations in *ovarian hormones, pituitary hormones, prostaglandin, and enzyme levels;* (2) variability of the *autonomic nervous system;* (4) *vascular changes* (stasis, spasm-dilatation); and (5) *other factors* (e.g., unusual nutritional and psychologic states). (Also see p. 707)

THE TYPICAL MENSTRUAL CYCLE

The menstrual cycle is mediated by complex neuroendocrine mechanisms. A single releasing hormone, *gonadotropin-releasing hormone* (GnRH), has been identified for the gonadotropins *follicle-stimulating hormone (FSH) and luteinizing hormone (LH). GnRH is produced in the hypothalamus and transmitted to the anterior pituitary (where the gonadotropins are produced) via the periportal vascular system* (Fig. 2-12).

Normal menstrual cycles are carefully regulated by *gonadotropin secretion from the anterior pituitary into the systemic circulation.* With the onset of each cycle, *follicles ready for maturation are stimulated to develop by FSH.* One (rarely more) outstrips the others to form a prominent graafian follicle. Regression of the remaining follicles then ensues. Meanwhile, *estrogen is produced by the theca lutein cells of the follicles.* The principal ovarian estrogens are *estrone* (E1), *estradiol* (E2), and a small amount of *estriol* (E3). On the eighth and ninth days of the cycle, the estrogen level stops rising, and LH and FSH levels begin to fluctuate. On about the *14th day, a sudden LH surge triggers rupture* of the follicle and *ovulation (extrusion of the ovum).* Slight bleeding occurs, and the empty follicle soon becomes filled with blood, which clots (hemorrhagic follicle). LH and possibly, prolactin, stimulate

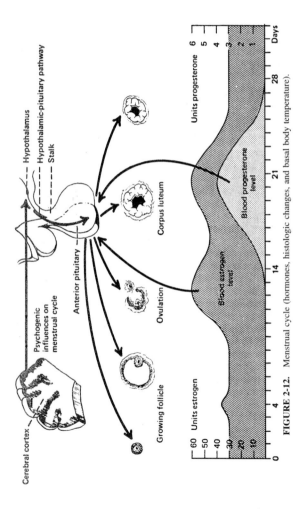

FIGURE 2-12. Menstrual cycle (hormones, histologic changes, and basal body temperature).

luteinization of the granulosa cells, and a *corpus luteum* is thus formed. The *granulosa lutein cells produce progesterone,* which *peaks on about the 23rd or 24th day.* If fertilization and nidation of the ovum (pregnancy) have not occured by this time, the *corpus luteum regresses.* The levels of progesterone and estrogen decline thereafter to reach a critical level on about the *28th day,* when endometrial bleeding (menstruation) occurs.

VASCULAR-HORMONAL INTERACTION

Blood is supplied to the endometrium by two types of arterioles: a *tortuous* (spiral) type near or surrounding the *endometrial glands* that supplies the functionalis layer or *outer two thirds* of the endometrium, and *short straight vessels* that supply only the *basalis* layer, the *inner third of the endometrium. The basalis is not shed* but remains as a reservoir of tissue for regeneration of the stroma and surface cells of the endometrial glands. Therefore, only the *superficial coiled arteries are involved directly in menstrual bleeding.*

For the first week after the onset of menstrual bleeding, the spiral arterioles are short and relatively straight. During the period of thickening of the endometrium, they lengthen. The vessels grow more rapidly than the endometrium, however, and they become coiled, particularly in the midportion of the functionalis. Blood vessels function to support the maturing endometrium under progesterone influence. Four to twenty-four hours before the onset of menstruation, periodic (every 60–90 sec) vasoconstriction alternating with relaxation of the coiled arterioles occurs. By this time, there is considerable dehydration of the endometrium. The coiled arterioles in the functionalis begin to buckle, stasis occurs in the blood within the arteriovenous channels, necrosis of the terminal arteriolar walls ensues, constriction of these arterioles within the basalis develops, and relaxation and hemorrhage from the peripheral branches begin.

Prostaglandins, largely of the PgF group, are present in considerable amounts in endometrium and menstrual blood. They also may participate in the vasoconstriction that precedes menstrual bleeding. Prostaglandins cause intense arterial spasm and smooth muscle contraction. This may assist in explaining certain types of *dysmenorrhea.*

ENDOMETRIAL CYCLES

During reproductive life, the endometrium undergoes continuous cyclic change (Fig. 2-13). Each cycle generally passes through four

FIGURE 2-13. Menstrual cycle (hormones, histologic changes, and basal body temperature).

47

FIGURE 2-14. Typical basal body temperature and plasma hormone concentration during a normal 28-day human menstrual cycle. M, menstruation; IRP-hMG, international reference standard for gonadotropins.

(From A.R. Midgley, in: E.S.E. Hafez, T.N. Evans, eds. *Human Reproduction.* Harper & Row, 1973.)

phases that correspond to ovarian hormone activity and can be identified by endometrial biopsy or multihormone assay (Fig. 2-14).

Proliferative Phase

The proliferative (estrogenic) phase can vary considerably in duration but usually is consistent with each individual. It is usually about 14 days in a 28-day cycle.

The *early proliferative phase starts on about the fourth or fifth day* of the cycle, just before the end of menstruation, and lasts 2–3 days. The end of this phase coincides with about the seventh day of the classic cycle. Surface epithelium is repaired but is thin or defective. Its thickness depends on the loss of tissue during menstrual bleeding. Glands are straight. Nuclei of epithelial cells are pseudostratified, and mitoses are frequent. Stromal cells show relatively large nuclei and little cytoplasm. There are few phagocytes.

The *midproliferative phase coincides with about the 10th day* of the cycle. It differs from the early proliferative phase only in degree. The endometrial surface is more regular, the glands are more tortuous, and glandular cells are pseudostratified. The thickness of the endometrium is increased.

The *late proliferative phase occurs on about the 14th day* of the average cycle. The epithelial surface is undulating, stromal cells are closely packed, and variable amounts of extracellular fluid are lost. Thickness is about as before, but with greater cellular concentration. The glands are increasingly tortuous and contain minimal secretion. There is no glycogen in the fluid.

Ovulatory Phase

The *ovulatory phase occurs with ovulation on about the 14th day* of a 28-day cycle. Because there is no appreciable change in the endometrium within the 24–36 h after ovulation, the 14th-day and 15th-day endometrium cannot be distinguished from each other. Distinctive changes appear in gland cells on the 16th day and thereafter, indicating corpus luteum activity and, presumably, ovulation.

Secretory Phase

The *secretory (progestational) phase technically begins with ovulation.* On the 16th day, tortuosity of the glands is increased, there are many mitotic figures, and glycogen-laden basal vacuoles appear. On the 17th day, the most pronounced vacuolization of cells occurs. Almost two thirds of the basal portion of such glands contains glycogen-laden fluid. Slight edema is noted, and mitoses are rare. On the 18th day, secretion of fluid within the glands is apparent. (This corresponds to the time when the ovum is free within the uterine cavity and must derive nourishment from uterine secretions.) On the 22nd day, the glands are more tortuous, but there is less secretory activity, and considerable mucoid secretion is seen in their lumens. Stromal edema is now at a peak. This may facilitate implantation of the ovum. The high points of secretory activity and stromal edema coincide with the period of maximal corpus luteum function.

From the 24th to the 27th day, edema regresses, and the stromal cells metamorphose into elements suggestive of decidua cells. The first change is noted in cells around the spiral arterioles, with the appearance of mitotic figures in the perivascular stroma. The glands become more and more tortuous, with serrations of their walls. Secretion of gland cells diminishes. There is infiltration by polymorphonuclear neutrophils and monocytes. Finally, necrosis and slough ensue.

If pregnancy occurs, active secretion and edema persist. The glands become more feathery and serrated; however, the predecidua is not immediately accentuated except around the ovum.

Menstrual Phase

During the menstrual phase, the endometrial edema and degenerative changes that occur at the end of the secretory phase cause tissue necrosis. This is irregularly distributed throughout all endometrial layers except the basalis. The necrosis causes blood vessels to rupture, producing scattered small hemorrhages. These enlarge and coalesce into propagating hematomas, which, in turn, cause endometrial separation and further rupture of small vessels. *Shedding of tissue fragments usually begins in a patchy fashion about 12 h after bleeding starts in ovulatory cycles.* Interestingly, an entire cast of the endometrial cavity is separated in so-called *membranous dysmenorrhea*. This painful condition results from sudden separation of the entire secretory endometrial lining, presumably because the sequence of events described is abnormally rapid and complete.

About two thirds of the endometrium is presumed to be lost with each ovulatory menstruation. By the time brisk flow ceases, tissue shrinkage and separation have occurred over the greater portion of the surface of the uterine cavity.

After a menstrual period of 4–7 days, bleeding gradually diminishes. Regional ooze is reduced by *constriction and thrombosis* of the remaining undamaged coiled arterioles, so that spotting finally ceases.

The *interval between ovulation and menstruation normally is almost exactly 14 days.* In contrast, the preovulatory period, the interval from the first day of menstruation to the day of ovulation, may vary from 7 or 8 days to more than a month. This *variability of the preovulatory period accounts for the disparity in the intervals between menstrual periods.*

CHANGES IN CERVICAL MUCUS AND VAGINAL CYTOLOGY

The *amount and consistency* of cervical mucus *vary during the menstrual cycle*. If a smear of cervical mucus is allowed to dry in air without fixation and examined under a microscope, characteristic patterns of crystalization can be identified at various stages. At the time of ovulation, the mucus dries to a striking frondlike pattern *(fern test)*. Before and after ovulation and during pregnancy, other characteristic granular patterns can be observed.

At about the time of ovulation, the cervical mucus becomes extremely clear and liquid in contrast to the yellowish, viscid mucus normally observed during the extreme preovulatory and postovulatory phases of the cycle. Just before ovulation, a drop of endocervical mucus can be stretched into a thin cobweblike strand 6 cm or longer. This quality *(Spinnerbarkeit)* is related to a high estrogen level and increased saline content.

Vaginal cytology distinctively reflects estrogen and progesterone variations (Fig. 2-15). During reproductive life, the vaginal cytology is characteristic of pregnancy or of the phase of the menstrual cycle. During the late follicular (preovulatory, proliferative) phase (days 12–15 of the menstrual cycle), a cytologic smear of vaginal fluid normally appears estrogenic, with many pyknotic epithelial cells and few white blood cells (WBC). After ovulation, the smear appears progestational, containing curled and clustered epithelial cells and occasional WBC. This is evidence of the luteal phase. A smear during normal pregnancy is marked by smaller, clumped, navicular epithelial cells with a high glycogen content and relatively few WBC.

SYSTEMIC CHANGES

During the preovulatory phase of the menstrual cycle, resting temperatures taken each morning will usually be low (<36.6°C or 98°F). Activity, infection, inadequate sleep, and alcholic beverages before retiring may cause an elevated temperature the following morning. On the day of ovulation, the temperature dips. Then, due to the *thermogenic activity of progesterone*, it *rises sharply* almost 1 degree Fahrenheit (0.5°C) and remains elevated until just before the menstrual period, when it begins to fall toward the low preovulatory levels (Fig. 2-14). This occurs only in ovulating women.

Other systemic changes after ovulation include (1) extracellular edema, which is the cause of premenstrual weight gain; (2) muscle sensitivity or hypertonicity, producing irritability and agitation (e.g., premenstrual tension syndrome); (3) vascular alteration, including pelvic hyperemia and increased capillary fragility or a tendency toward bruising; (4) mastalgia due to increased breast size and turgescence; (5) headache (e.g., menstrual migraine), which may be a hormonally mediated vascular headache.

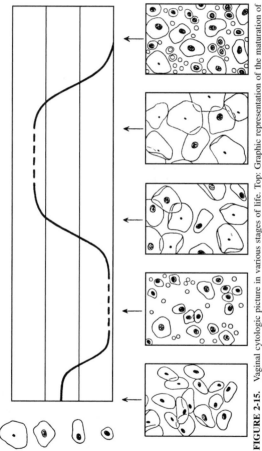

FIGURE 2-15. Vaginal cytologic picture in various stages of life. Top: Graphic representation of the maturation of vaginal epithelium. Bottom: Left to right: Epithelial maturation at birth; atrophic cell picture in childhood; beginning of estrogenic influence in puberty; complete maturation in the reproductive period; regression in old age. (From F.K. Beller et al., *Gynecology: A Textbook for Students.* Springer-Verlag, 1974.)

ANOVULATORY CYCLES

In anovulatory cycles, the maturation and differentiation of the endometrium caused by progesterone do not occur. Thus, the sequence of events is greatly altered with variable estrogen alone. *Excessive stimulation* results in a *hypertrophic endometrium,* which *leads to irregularly irregular bleeding* (i.e., irregular interval and irregular duration of bleeding). This is usually heavier in amount than normal (ovulatory) menstruation. The period is qualitatively similar to an ovulatory one, but minimal coiling of the spiral arterioles probably can cause only small fissures and no propagating hematomas. Peeling away of the functionalis layer thus takes place only imperfectly in the proliferative or hyperplastic endometrium. Bleeding from terminal arteriolar loops must occur, but tissue loss is minimal. The endometrium continues to proliferate from month to month, with the result that hemorrhage often ensues in subsequent periods from this grossly thickened tissue.

Paucity of estrogen leads to an *atrophic endometrium,* which may also lead to irregularly irregular bleeding but generally is less frequent and much lighter in the amount of blood lost.

OTHER HORMONES IMPORTANT IN FEMALE REPRODUCTION

Under the influence of releasing hormones, other tropic endocrine products are elaborated from the anterior pituitary, including thyrotropin *(TSH),* corticotropin *(ACTH),* growth hormone *(GH),* and melanocyte-stimulating hormone *(MSH).*

In contrast to the anterior lobe of the pituitary, the posterior lobe is linked with the hypothalamus by nerves. The posterior pituitary hormone *vasopressin* (antidiuretic hormone, ADH) controls plasma osmolality and is released by impulses from the supraoptic and paraventricular nuclei to be transported by nerves to the posterior pituitary. *Oxytocin,* which causes uterine muscular and myoepithelial breast ductal cell contraction to stimulate both labor and lactation, is released and stored in the posterior pituitary by similar complex neuroendocrine mechanisms.

Prolactin may be important in maintenance of the human corpus luteum, but only slight variations in the hormone occur during the menstrual period. Much higher levels are reached during pregnancy, and very high levels of prolactin are the rule during lactation.

Ovarian stromal cells normally produce small amounts of *androgen,* mainly, *androstenedione.*

3

DEVELOPMENT AND MALDEVELOPMENT

GAMETOGENESIS

The production of *ova and sperm occurs via* the process of *meiosis* (whereas somatic cells undergo division via mitosis). *Oogenesis* produces ova, and *spermatogenesis* produces sperm. One spermatogonium results in four sperm, and one oogonium results in one ovum and two polar bodies. Meiosis is a reduction division normally allowing each gamete to contain *23 chromosomes (haploid).* Thus, when fertilization occurs and the two haploid gametes unite, the resulting zygote contains *46 chromosomes (diploid)* under normal circumstances.

Two meiotic divisions occur, and each contains several stages.

FIRST MEIOTIC DIVISION

A. Prophase I has five stages.
1. *Leptotene,* wherein the chromatin condenses into individual elongated threadlike structures.
2. *Zygotene,* the migration of single threadlike chromosomes toward the nuclear equatorial plate where homologous chromosomes pair to form bivalents that exchange segments at several points (synapses).
3. *Pachytene,* where chromosomes contract and thicken, then split longitudinally into two chromatids attached at the centromere.
4. *Diplotene* is marked by crossing-over of the nonidentical chromatid constituents of homologous chromosomes at bridges or chiasms. The male sex chromatids (X and Y chromatids), however, do not cross over.
5. *Diakinesis,* the last stage, which occurs when the bivalents contract, chiasms move toward the ends of the

      chromosome, homologs pull apart, and the nuclear membrane disappears.

B. During *metaphase I,* the very short and thick bivalents are aligned along the equatorial plate of the cell spindle forms.

C. In *anaphase I,* the centromeres divide so that the homologous chromatids (rather than the identical sister chromatids) are drawn to opposite poles of the spindle.

D. *Telophase I* is marked by spindle breakage, division of cellular cytoplasm, and formation of a nuclear membrane. The cell cytoplasm is equally divided in the male but is unequally distributed in the female. In the latter, most of the cytoplasm goes to the secondary oocyte so that basically only nuclear material becomes the first polar body, which subsequently disintegrates.

SECOND MEIOTIC DIVISION

A. *Metaphase II* reveals new spindle forms, and the chromosomes align along the equatorial plate.

B. In *anaphase II,* the chromatids pull apart to opposite poles of the spindle, with complete division of the centromere.

C. *Telophase II* entails the division of the spindle and cell cytoplasm (again equally in the male and unequally in the female), forming one ovum and the second polar body.

    Secondary oocyte development arrests at metaphase II until penetration by a sperm. Then meiosis is completed, and the polar body is discarded.

FETAL MALDEVELOPMENT

TERMINOLOGY

A chromosome is the paired basic structure containing the genes in a linear arrangement. Humans have *23 pairs of chromosomes (46 total),* of which *22 pairs are autosomes* and *1 pair (either XX or XY) determine the individual's sex. A locus is a gene's specific site on a chromosome.* A gene is a sequence of chromosomal nucleotides that forms the production code for specific proteins, that is, unit of genetic information. Alleles are different genes that occupy the same position on homologous chromosomes and potentially affect a similar function. *Heterozygous refers to dissimilar members of a gene pair,* and *homozygous refers to similar members of a gene pair.* A *dominant characteristic* is recognized when the *phenotypic effect of the gene is the same in the heterozygous state as in the homozygous state.* In contrast, a *recessive characteristic* is one that is *only produced in the homozygous state.*

The *genotype* is the *genetic makeup of the individual* and is expressed with the number, then the sex chromosomes, then any specific defects (e.g., 45,XO; 46,XX; 47,XY,21+). *The phenotype is the physical appearance of the individual* with his or her various observed characteristics. The abbreviation p is used for the short arm of chromosomes and q for the long arm (as determined from the chromosome's centromere). Homologous means the same relative position and is often applied to chromosomes and genes.

A *mutagen is an agent* (e.g., physical, chemical) *that induces genetic mutation. Mutations* involve *macromolecular or micromolecular change in germ cell DNA and are a permanent transmissible alteration.* A *teratogen* is an agent (or factor) that *causes defects in the developing organism.* Teratogenic changes may be caused by mutations or by a number of other processes.

In utero development is divided into *three phases.* The *ovular phase comprises the first 4 weeks* after fertilization. This period is characterized by rapid mitotic divisions, resulting in a blastula. At *5–7 days after fertilization,* the products of conception, now characterized by development of the *blastocyst* and separation into microscopically discernible *body pole* and *preplacental zones, implant into the endometrium. Gastrulation begins,* and the organ anlagen are relatively positioned. From the *5th through the 8th weeks of pregnancy, the conceptus is termed the embryo.* This is the period of *organ differentiation.* From the *9th week until delivery,* the conceptus is termed a *fetus. Only a few new structures develop after the 8th week.* Thus, the *fetal period is principally concerned with differentiation, growth, and maturation* (Table 3-1).

Developmental age (*fetal age*) is the age of the offspring *calculated from the date of conception.* This may be important to embryologists but is rarely used by obstetricians or pediatricians, who are especially concerned with *gestational age,* that is, the calculated age of the fetus *from the first day of the LMP* (assuming a 28-day cycle). Gestational age is expressed in *completed weeks.*

CONGENITAL DEFECTS

Congenital anomalies (birth defects, malformations) are significant, usually deleterious, *deviations from normal standards of structure*

TABLE 3-1
TIME OF INSULT AND POTENTIAL MALFORMATION

Developmental Age (Weeks)	Malformation
3	Ectromelia Ectopia cordis Omphalocele Sympodia
4	Ectromelia Hemivertebra Omphalocele Tracheoesophageal fistula
5	Carpal or pedal ablation Cataract (nuclear) Facial clefts Hemivertebra Microphthalmia Tracheoesophageal fistula

6	Agnathia
	Carpal or pedal ablation
	Cataract (lenticular)
	Cleft lip
	Congenital heart disease
	  Aortic anomalies
	  Gross septal defects
	Microphthalmia

7	Brachycephaly
	Cleft palate
	Congenital heart disease
	  Ventricular septal
	    defects
	  Pulmonary stenosis
	Digital ablation
	Epicanthus
	Micrognathia

8	Brachycephaly Congenital heart disease Digital stunting Epicanthus Nasal bone ablation Persistent ostium primum

and function. In the United States, the incidence of congenital anomalies recognizable at birth is *3%–7%*. With careful longitudinal follow-up, however, the *incidence may reach 10%*. The impact of congenital defects on human life is immense. *Abnormalities are the single major cause of infant mortality* (>20% of all infant deaths). Added to the impact of these deaths is the *lost potential and expense to society* involving damaged survivors.

Practitioners are most often questioned about congenital defects arising from the following situations: the gravida exposed to a potentially fetotoxic agent, the family that has had an anomalous infant, parents with a previous abnormal offspring or pregnancy loss, or a couple with a known defect who want to reproduce. Although it is not the purpose of this text to provide all the information in detail or the skills necessary to function as a counselor in these circumstances, it is our purpose to describe certain broad principles that may be of value in caring for these patients.

CREATION OF A DEFECT

Criteria for the recognition of a defect-creating agent include the following.

- An *abruptly increased incidence* of a particular defect or association of defects (syndrome).
- A known *environmental alteration coincident with the increase* in a particular defect.
- *Evident exposure to the environmental alteration* at a stage of pregnancy (usually early) that yields characteristic defect(s).
- *Absence of other factors* that might create the same abnormality.

NATURE OF THE INSULT

Causes of some defects are known (% of total): *chromosomal aberrations or recognized genetic transmission (23%–25%), drugs and environmental agents (4%–5%), infections (2%–3%), and maternal metabolic aberration (1%–2%)*. However, the *cause remains unknown for 60%–70% of all anomalies.*

KNOWN GENETIC TRANSMISSIONS (MENDELIAN INHERITANCE DISORDERS)

Known genetic transmissions (~20%) are the largest single ascertainable contributors to mutagenic and teratogenic defects.

Roughly half of these conditions can be described by their *mendelian inheritance patterns* (i.e., autosomal dominant, autosomal recessive, or sex-linked). The chance of an offspring inheriting a characteristic can be determined by the rules of each inheritance pattern.

Autosomal Dominant

With *autosomal dominant inheritance,* a mutation in one gene of an allelic pair *results in a different phenotypic expression or characteristic.* The phenotypic expression of this characteristic (*penetrance*) can vary with environmental or other genetic influences (e.g., with recombination). Examples of autosomal dominant conditions include achondroplasia, color blindness (yellow–blue), Ehlers-Danlos syndrome, Huntington's chorea, Marfan's syndrome, mitral valve prolapse, neurofibromatosis, adult polycystic renal disease, and Von Willebrand's disease. The rules of autosomal dominant inheritance follow.

- The characteristic appears with equal frequency in both sexes.
- At least one parent must have the characteristic (unless it is a new mutation).
- Homozygous-normal mating results in all offspring having the characteristic.
- Heterozygous-normal matings result in 50% of the offspring having the characteristic.
- If it is a rare trait, most individuals demonstrating the characteristic will be heterozygous.

Autosomal Recessive

With *autosomal recessive inheritance,* one affected gene of an allelic pair is insufficient to evoke a phenotypic expression of the characteristic (i.e., different from the normal). With *homozygosity,* however, *the characteristic appears.* Environment and genetic influences may affect the expressivity of the defect in the carrier state. Examples of autosomal recessive conditions include albinism, chondrodystrophy, myotonia, color blindness (total), cystic fibrosis, dysautonomia, galactosemia, Gaucher's disease, homocystinuria, phenylketonuria, sickle cell anemia, Tay-Sachs disease, Wilson's disease, and mucopolysaccharidosis I-H, I-S, III IV, VI, and VII. The rules of autosomal recessive inheritance follow.

- The characteristic occurs with equal frequency in both sexes.
- For the characteristic to be present, both parents must be carriers.
- If both parents are homozygous, all offspring will have the characteristic.

- If both parents are heterozygous, offspring will have the characteristic in the following distribution: 25% not affected, 50% carrier (heterozygous), 25% with the characteristic (homozygous).
- Frequent occurrence of rare recessive characteristics is often related to consanguinity.

X-Linked Recessive

When *a gene on the X chromosomes is affected, but it is unable to evoke the characteristic if heterozygous, it is said to be X-linked recessive.* However, the characteristic is *expressed in males because of their single X chromosome.* Examples of X-linked recessive conditions include androgen insensitivity syndromes (both complete and incomplete), color blindness (red–green), G-6-PD deficiency, gonadal dysgenesis, hemophilia A and B, Lesch-Nyhan syndrome, and mucopolysaccharidosis II. The rules of X-linked recessive inheritance include the following.

- The characteristic occurs primarily in males.
- If both parents are unaffected but produce a male with the characteristic, the mother is a carrier.
- If the father is affected and there is an affected male offspring, the mother must be at least heterozygous for the characteristic.
- A female with the abnormal characteristic may acquire it by the following:
    Inheritance of the recessive gene from both her mother and father (father affected, mother heterozygous),
    Inheritance of the recessive gene from one of her parents and expression occurs as a result of the Lyon hypothesis (functional selection of one X chromosome for this and subsequent progeny).

X-Linked Dominant

If a *gene on the X chromosome is affected and able to produce the characteristic in the heterozygous state,* it is said to be *X-linked dominant.* Examples of X-linked dominant conditions include cervicooculoacoustic syndrome, hyperammonemia, and orofaciodigital syndrome I. The rules of X-linked dominant inheritance follow.

- The characteristic affects males and females with equal frequency.
- Affected male–normal female mating results in 50% affected offspring.
- Affected homozygous female–normal male mating results in all offspring being affected.

- Heterozygous female–normal male mating results in 50% affected offspring.
- Heterozygous females may not demonstrate the dominant characteristic (see Lyon hypothesis).

MULTIFACTORIAL INHERITANCE

Multifactorial or polygenic inheritance is the *inheritance of a characteristic as a result of the interaction of numerous genes and the environment.* Such inheritance *cannot be classified according to mendelian principles.* It is, however, extremely important in normal inheritance (e.g., human physical features) as well as many common malformations (e.g., anencephaly, cleft palate, meningomyelocele, and pyloric stenosis). That the defects are inheritable is *discerned from incidence.* That is, the defects noted occur with a frequency of *0.5–2/1000 in Caucasians but occur in 2%–5% of siblings of affected infants with normal parents.* That the abnormalities are not entirely environmental is discerned from concordance (a higher frequency of such abnormalities in monozygotic than dizygotic twins, e.g., the defects are 4–8 times more common in monozygotic twins.)

CHROMOSOME ABNORMALITIES IN NUMBER AND MORPHOLOGY

Chromosomal aberrations are *alterations in both number and morphology.* They account for *3%–5% of all human anomalies* manifest at birth. The numerical disorders probably most commonly occur *during meiosis* as a result of failure of the doubled chromosomal complement to be equally divided between the two daughter cells (*nondisjunction*). When subsequently recombined with a normal gamete, this results in one zygote having an extra chromosome (*trisomy*) and another with a missing chromosome *(monosomy).* *Autosomal monosomy is almost always lethal.* If the monosomy occurs in the sex chromosomes, however, *Turner's syndrome (45,XO)* results. Most of these individuals are spontaneously aborted, but some survive. *Autosomal trisomy* may occur with all chromosomes, but most commonly results in *trisomy 16, trisomy 21 (Down syndrome), trisomy 18, and trisomy 13.* Again, most are aborted, but a few survive through advanced pregnancy. *Sex chromosomal trisomy results in hyperploidy.*

Another etiology for chromosomal alteration of number and morphology is a *parent who has an abnormal chromosomal constituency* (e.g., balanced translocation carriers). Morphologic chromosomal defects may also relate to chromosomal breakage (e.g., Fanconi's anemia). Nondisjunction occurring in the postzygotic interval leads to *mosaicism* (cell lines with different combinations of the same basic chromosomal constituency). Mosaicism, not infrequent, must be differentiated from *chimerism* (cell lines from two different chromosomal constituencies), which rarely, if ever, occurs in humans.

Other defect etiologies (drugs and environmental agents, infections, and maternal metabolic imbalance) are discussed under "Specific Teratic Agents."

TIMING OF THE INSULT

The *stage of development when the insult occurs largely determines the potential adverse effect or malformation.* For example, the free-floating zygote is probably less influenced by deleterious agents than it might be later. An insult that affects the zygote during this interval is most likely to *result in abortion.* Injury during the *2nd–7th weeks is marked by fetal wastage, structural malformations with time-related specific defects, carcinogenesis, or severe intrauterine growth retardation* (Table 3-1). During weeks 9–40, should a defect occur the fetus may develop central nervous system anomalies, behavioral disorder, functional abnormalities, reproductive system defects, and intrauterine growth retardation.

INTENSITY OF THE INSULT

Most fetotoxic agents can be reduced to a level that is not harmful, and most relatively innocuous agents can be increased in dose to a lethal level. Thus, it is crucial to *ascertain the dosage and the time over which the exposure occurred.* Other considerations of dosage must include the *nature of the agent* and the available *information* (generally literature) *concerning the agent's mutagenic or teratogenic potential.*

HOST RESISTANCE MECHANISMS

Whether or not exposure to a fetotoxic agent creates a defect in a particular situation is *influenced by numerous factors: the interaction of the agent with the maternal organism (e.g., absorption, penetration, and elimination), transport to the fetus, interaction with the fetus (e.g., activation, inactivation, and excretion), and reparative phenomena (e.g., local host factors influencing outcome and genetic mechanisms potentially influencing outcome).*

SPECIFIC TERATIC AGENTS

PERINATAL INFECTIONS

Pregnancy results in decreased maternal resistance to infection. Thus, the potential exists for both *reactivation* of latent infections and *more severe sepsis* should infection occur. The developing embryo and fetus are at greatest risk from infective agents during the first trimester, presumably as a result of limited capability for immunologic response. Table 3-2 summarizes some specific infective agents and their potential perinatal or fetotoxicity. Additionally, the *effect of various infective agents on the mother* (e.g., fever, respiratory distress) *can adversely affect the fetus* either directly or indirectly (e.g., initiation of premature labor).

DRUGS

Despite recent attempts at reduction, the *use of multiple prescription and nonprescription drugs during pregnancy* continues. Excluding vitamins and iron, the majority of women will take at least one prescription and several nonprescription drugs at some point in pregnancy. Too frequently, this occurs at a critical time, for example, before the diagnosis of pregnancy. The FDA has established categories of potential for drugs causing birth defects to guide drug usage during pregnancy (Table 3-3).

Drug teratogenicity has such species specificity that it is *difficult to extrapolate data from one species to another.* Thus, it may be impossible to fully test human teratogenicity in laboratory animals. Indeed, few of the large number of drugs reported to be teratogenic in laboratory animals have been proven to be human teratogens. Nonetheless, there are so many fetotoxic drugs that it is beyond the purpose of this text to detail them. Every physician and nurse, however, must become familiar with each drug they administer using more complete sources. Table 3-4 includes examples of fetotoxic drugs in several categories.

IONIZING RADIATION

Ionizing radiation has long been known to have both *mutagenic and teratogenic effects.* The National Committee on Radiation Protection has stated the amount of ionizing radiation believed to be relatively safe for the embryo is *10 rads.* At >15 rads fetal exposure, there is suggestive evidence of an increased incidence of childhood leukemia by age 10. In contrast to older units, modern radiologic equipment has both vastly safer shielding and much lower exposures for imaging (e.g., a chest x-ray should not exceed 0.03 rad).

TABLE 3-2
INFECTIONS WITH KNOWN PERINATAL
OR FETAL TOXICITY

Maternal Infection	Fetotoxicity
	Viruses
Coxsackie B virus	Myocarditis
Cytomegalovirus	Microcephaly, hydrocephaly, cerebral palsy, brain calcifications, chorioretinitis, deafness, psychomotor and mental retardation, hepatosplenomegaly
Hepatitis	Hepatitis
Herpes simplex virus	Generalized or localized herpes, hydranencephaly, encephalitis, chorioretinitis, thrombocytopenia, petechiae, hemolytic anemia, death
Human immunodeficiency virus (HIV)	Growth retardation, microcephaly, boxlike forehead, flattened nasal bridge, hypertelorism, triangular philtrum, patulous lips
Human parvovirus B19	Fetal death, degenerative changes, eye defects, and congenital anomalies
Mumps	Fetal death, endocardial fibroelastosis, malformations (?)
Poliomyelitis	Spinal or bulbar poliomyelitis

(Continued)

TABLE 3-2
(Continued)

Maternal Infection	Fetotoxicity
Rubeola	Increased abortions and stillbirth
Rubella	Growth retardation, malformations (cardiac, great vessel, microcephaly), ocular aberrations (microphthalmos, cataract, glaucoma, pigmented retinopathy), newborn bleeding, hepatosplenomegaly, mental retardation, sensorineural deafness, pneumonitis, hepatitis, encephalitis
Vaccinia	Generalized vaccinia, increased abortions
Varicella zoster	Chickenpox or shingles, increased abortions and stillbirths, hydrocephalus, microcephaly, seizures, cataracts, microphthalmia, Horner's syndrome, optic nerve atrophy, nystagmus, chorioretinitis, mental retardation, skeletal hypoplasia, urogenital anomalies
Variola	Smallpox, increased abortions and stillbirths
Venezuelan equine encephalitis virus	Microcephaly, hydrocephaly microphthalmia,

TABLE 3-2
(Continued)

Maternal Infection	Fetotoxicity
	cerebral agenesis, CNS necrosis
	Spirochetes
Syphilis	Spontaneous abortion, stillbirth, congenital syphilis including hydrocephalus, frontal prominence, saddle nose, high arched palate, short maxilla, mulberry molars, notched incisors, enamel dystrophy, 8th nerve deafness, interstitial keratitis, uveitis, glaucoma, mental retardation, convulsive disorders, paralysis or paresis, cardiovascular defects
	Bacteria
Gonorrhea	Ophthalmitis
Streptococcus agalactiae (group B beta-hemolytic streptococcus)	Neonatal acute respiratory distress, septicemia, death, meningitis, infection of other organs. Possible (not conclusively proven) abortion and premature birth
Listeriosis	Abortions (including habitual), stillbirths, septicemia, meningoencephalitis
Tuberculosis	Congenital tuberculosis

(Continued)

TABLE 3-2
(Continued)

Maternal Infection	Fetotoxicity
	Protozoan
Malaria	Low birth weight, enhanced perinatal mortality
Toxoplasmosis	Microcephaly, chorioretinitis, jaundice

TABLE 3-3
FDA TERATOGENICITY DRUG LABELING

Category	Comment
A	Well-controlled human studies have not disclosed any fetal risk.
B	Animal studies have not disclosed any fetal risk or have suggested some risk not confirmed in controlled studies in women or there are not adequate studies in women.
C	Animal studies have revealed adverse fetal effects; there are no adequate controlled studies in women.
D	Some fetal risk, but benefits may outweigh risk (e.g., life-threatening illness, no safer effective drug); patient should be warned.
X	Fetal abnormalities in animal and human studies; risk not outweighed by benefit. *Contraindicated in pregnancy.*

TABLE 3-4
FETOTOXIC DRUGS

Drug	Fetotoxicity
Aminoglycosides	8th nerve defects, possible ocular damage
Androgens	Masculinization or pseudohermaphroditism
Anticonvulsant therapy	Congenital heart disease (2–3-fold increase); cleft palate (5–10-fold increase)
Antineoplastic agents	Generally potent teratogens
Antithyroid agents	Neonatal goiter, tracheal obstruction, hypospadias, aortic atresia, developmental retardation
Amphetamines	Transposition of the great vessels, withdrawal syndrome
Benzothiadiazides	Thrombocytopenia, altered carbohydrate metabolism, hyperbilirubinemia (if used in late gestation)
Chloroquine	Retinal and 8th nerve damage
Chlorpropamide	Increased anomalies generally
Cocaine	Decreased head circumference, increased CNS anomalies, increased incidence of sudden infant death syndrome
Coumarin (Warfarin)	Nasal hypoplasia, stippled epiphyses, growth retardation, mental retardation (fetal bleeding)
Diethylstilbestrol	Clear cell carcinoma of the vagina and cervix, vaginal adenosis, cervical and vaginal ridges, cervical hoods, and uterine

(Continued)

TABLE 3-4
(Continued)

Drug	Fetotoxicity
	anomalies (T-shaped uterus, constricting band, hypoplastic uterus)
Ethanol	Fetal alcohol syndrome (mental retardation, growth retardation, typical facial features, congenital heart defects, microcephaly, renal anomalies)
Isoniazid (INH)	Severe encephalopathies (may be prevented by concomitant vitamin B_6)
Isoretinoin (Accutane)	Abortion, craniofacial defects (hypoplastic nasal bridge, abnormal ears microtia, agenesis of ear canal, micrognathia, hard and soft palate clefts, etc.), CNS abnormalities (hydrocephaly, hydranencephaly, microcephaly, etc.), cardiovascular abnormalities (transposition, VSD, ASD, truncus arteriosus, PDA, tetralogy of Fallot, etc.), incomplete lobulation of lung lobes
Lithium	Cardiovascular anomalies, congenital heart disease, increased abortion rate
Narcotics (heroin, morphine, methadone)	Withdrawal syndromes (tremors, poor feeding, irritability, seizures)
Oral hypoglycemics	Increased incidence of defects (especially caudal dysplasia)

TABLE 3-4
(Continued)

Drug	Fetotoxicity
Phenothiazines	Slight increase in malformations
Phenytoin (Dilantin)	Facial anomalies, microcephaly, mental retardation, nail hypoplasia, growth retardation
Sulfonamides	Neonatal jaundice if used in third trimester
Tetracycline	Stained teeth, do not use in second or third trimester
Thalidomide	Limb reduction anomalies
Trimethadione	Developmental delay, speech difficulty, dysmorphic facies
Vitamin A	Urinary malformations
Vitamin D	Supravalvular aortic stenosis

SPECIFIC MATERNAL DISEASES WITH POTENTIAL FETAL DEFECTS

Many conditions affecting the mother will affect the fetus adversely. Some will affect fetal growth and development. Others may cause malformations or deformations.

DIABETES MELLITUS

Embryonic exposure to *hyperglycemia enhances the incidence of abortion and fetal defects* (to a threefold increase). The most commonly associated defect is cardiac (transposition of the great vessels, VSD, or coarctation of the aorta), with a fourfold increase over euglycemics. The *caudal regression syndrome* is the most specific and *rarely occurs except in diabetics.*

Fetal blood glucose levels are approximately 80% of maternal levels. Because insulin does not cross the placenta, the fetal pancreas produces insulin to attempt to regulate fetal blood glucose levels in the normal range. Thus, the fetus responds to hyperglycemia with hyperinsulinemia. Prolonged elevations in maternal blood glucose may *result in* a *macrosomic infant* with excessive glycogen storage and fat stores. This glycogen storage may cause sufficient hypertrophy of the cardiac interventricular septum to cause obstruction of outflow of blood from the ventricle and subsequent ischemia.

Excessive fetal secretion of insulin often results in hypoglycemia soon after the maternal supply of glucose is interrupted by clamping of the umbilical cord. The *hypoglycemia* is usually most pronounced in the first 1–2 h but may continue for ~48 h. *Macrosomia* may cause *dystocia and delivery complications,* especially *birth injury.* The neonate born of a noncontrolled diabetic mother also has increased incidence of *prematurity, respiratory distress syndrome, polycythemia, hyperbilirubinemia, hypomagnesemia, and hypocalcemia.*

THYROID DISORDERS

Maternal hyperthyroidism can result in *fetal goiter formation.* The *newborn can experience fatal thyrotoxicosis* if unrecognized and untreated. Symptoms usually appear 1–2 weeks after birth. Maternal antithyroid therapy can lead to perinatal goiter, tracheal obstruction, or hypothyroidism. *Maternal hypothyroidism can be associated with increased fetal wastage and postterm delivery.*

HELLP SYNDROME (HEMOLYSIS, ELEVATED LIVER ENZYMES, LOW PLATELET COUNT)

The surviving fetus (perinatal *mortality is as high as 60%*) in this condition is almost always *premature,* with *severe growth retardation.* The infant may have *pancytopenia* at birth that necessitates transfusions of platelets and packed red blood cells after birth.

SYSTEMIC LUPUS ERYTHEMATOSUS (SLE)

Maternal SLE *increases the rate of abortion* and can result in a perinate with *cardiac arrhythmia,* most notably complete heart block. There are reported cases of congenital disseminated lupus in the newborn of affected mothers. *Thrombocytopenia* may be present in the fetus and newborn of mothers with SLE.

IDIOPATHIC THROMBOCYTOPENIC PURPURA (ITP)

Maternal ITP affects the fetus by causing *thrombocytopenia* in some that can persist 1–4 months after birth. Treatment includes platelet transfusions if the platelet count is, <25,000 or active bleeding occurs.

SPECIFIC IN UTERO FETAL ANOMALIES

CONGENITAL HEART DISEASE

It is unusual for congenital heart disease (CHD) to harm the fetus in utero unless other congenital anomalies are present. Fetuses are usually carried to term and are appropriately grown. *Problems are recognized after birth,* when the lungs become the organ of respiration, supplanting the placenta. The resistance in the pulmonary vasculature normally decreases from the high level needed in fetal life to bypass the lung circuit to the low level needed to receive about half of the cardiac output for oxygenation by the lungs. If the blood is insufficiently oxygenated (>5 g unsaturated Hgb), cyanosis occurs. This can be caused by lung disease or a cardiac defect with right to left shunting of blood. A murmur and congestive heart failure can be present.

If a fetal cardiac defect is discovered and is determined to be the type likely to require repair soon after delivery, arrangements should be made to have the infant delivered in a tertiary center with neonatal cardiovascular surgery capability to avoid the delay inherent in transport of the infant after birth.

ARRHYTHMIAS

The *most common fetal arrhythmias are premature atrial or ventricular contractions.* These can be noted easily on Doppler or real-time ultrasound examinations during the second half of the gestation. Arrhythmias can be regular or irregular. The mother should be questioned about her caffeine intake (e.g., coffee, tea, chocolate or soft drinks), because excessive intake can affect the fetal heart rhythm. Decreasing the intake of these methylxanthines may improve the fetal rhythm.

Even *complete heart block* can be relatively benign for the fetus if not excessively slow; however, up to *50% will have associated congenital heart defects.* When the slow heartbeat is initially detected, the immediate concern is whether this fetus is in severe distress from asphyxia, requiring immediate delivery, or whether time is available for further evaluation and routine delivery. *Fetal echocardiography* may determine whether or not there are associated cardiac defects or signs of congestive heart failure. If *congestive heart failure* is present and the fetus is believed to be viable, cesarean section delivery should be accomplished if possible in a center where pediatric cardiology services are available to insert a pacemaker in the infant shortly after birth if necessary.

Supraventricular tachycardia (SVT) is a rhythm that must not be allowed to continue without therapy or close observation. Because the heart rate is more rapid (>220 bpm) than with other causes of fetal tachycardia (e.g., maternal fever with chorioamnionitis), this abnormality should not be confused with other conditions. Short bursts of SVT may eventually become continuous. Prolonged SVT can cause congestive heart failure and death. Treat the mother with digoxin in high therapeutic dosage to convert the fetal SVT to normal sinus rhythm and continue this drug until delivery. Occasionally, more than one drug may be required to maintain control of the rhythm. Even external electrocardioversion has been performed successfully. After birth, maintain the infant on digitalis (or other appropriate medications) for several months in an attempt to avoid recurrence.

HYDROCEPHALUS

With the increased use of sonography during pregnancy and maternal determination of AFP, hydrocephalus (frequency ~1/2000 deliveries) is often diagnosed long before delivery. When discovered, careful sonographic evaluation of the fetal spine is indicated for evidence of spina bifida, the most commonly associated anomaly. *Hydrocephalus can be a genetic defect* (X-linked recessive and autosomal dominant forms account for ~2% of cases) *or part of a genetically related syndrome.* It can be caused by *isolated aqueductal stenosis (most often Sylvius), various infections, brain tumors, lack of brain substance development, or intracranial hemorrhage.*

The location and the degree of hydrocephalus and plans for the method of delivery may be altered depending on the cause. On rare occasions, massive hydrocephalus with no chance of survival will require decompression of the fetal ventricles to allow delivery by any route. Cesarean section is required for the majority of cases. The fetus can be delivered vaginally, however, if labor is preterm or the hydrocephalus is not marked. Nonetheless, hydrocephalus should not be an indication for preterm delivery without evidence of pulmonary maturity, because surgery is very hazardous in infants with respiratory distress syndrome.

The *outlook* for the infant born with hydrocephalus varies, but it is *usually good with regard to mental development.* If *spina bifida* is present, orthopedic, urologic, and physical therapy, as well as neurosurgical follow-up are almost always necessary. The child's ability to walk will depend on the level of the neural tube defect (the higher the lesion, the less likely). An *encephalocele has a higher risk* for both mental and physical handicap than the lower lesions.

ANENCEPHALY

Anencephaly (incidence <1/2000 deliveries) is the result of *incomplete closure of the cranial portion of the neural tube.* The *upper brain never develops, the skull bone is absent, and rudimentary brain tissue is covered only by membrane* that may weep CSF. It almost always is associated with *polyhydramnios.* Moreover, the alpha-fetoprotein in the amniotic fluid and maternal serum is elevated unless there is skin covering the defect. Concomitantly, there is an *absence of adrenal cortical development.* Some will be stillborn. Others may not tolerate the stress of labor. Because there is *no effective therapy* and these *infants do not have prolonged survival,* heroic measures are contraindicated. Comfort care should be provided to the liveborn.

INTESTINAL ATRESIA

Intestinal atresia *can occur anywhere in the gastrointestinal tract* from the esophagus to the anus. Atresia proximal to the jejunum is frequently associated with *polyhydramnios* because swallowed amniotic fluid cannot pass far enough into the intestinal tract to be absorbed. *Esophageal atresia is most often associated with a tracheoesophageal fistula,* a developmental defect (the embryonic foregut is an outpouching from the trachea). Lower intestinal atresia can be secondary to a local vascular accident eliminating blood supply to an area of gut.

Intestinal atresia is *frequently associated with many anomalies.* The most common is called the VATERR syndrome (vertebral anomalies, anal atresia, tracheoesophageal fistula, renal anomalies, and radial anomalies).

Esophageal atresia, if not identified in utero, should be diagnosed in the first 24 h after birth, since the infant *cannot swallow fluids or even its own saliva* and will sputter, spit, and gag with feedings. Frothy saliva is commonly noted. If esophageal atresia is not associated with a tracheoesophageal fistula (TEF), the abdomen will show no gas on x-ray. If there is an associated TEF, respiratory distress may be evident. Radiographic evaluation should show that gas has passed into the gut (through the lower fistula into the distal esophagus), and an aspiration pattern may be evident in the chest.

Duodenal atresia can be the result of a true developmental stenosis or from obstruction by Ladd's bands or an annular pancreas. Infants with trisomy 21 (Down syndrome) have an increased incidence of duodenal atresia. One may suspect the diagnosis in utero by ultrasound examination. After birth, expect vomiting, which will be bilious if the obstruction is distal to the ampulla of Vater (where bile empties into the duodenum). Typical x-ray findings show a double bubble appearance to the stomach without gas in the bowel.

Jejunal atresia can be associated with polyhydramnios. In jejunal atresia, the infant will develop bilious vomiting. Abdominal x-ray will show an obstructive pattern. However, ileal atresia may not be diagnosed until after discharge (after a short hospital stay). Symptoms are similar to those of jejunal atresia but may appear later because more bowel length is available for distention.

Atresia of the anus is not uncommon, but *atresia of the colon is rare.* The diagnosis of anal atresia is usually made by initial physical examination. Signs of obstruction may not appear before surgery, because drainage of feces may be through a congenital fistula into the vagina, bladder, or urethra.

OLIGOHYDRAMNIOS TETRAD

The oligohydramnios tetrad, initially called Potter's syndrome, includes agenesis of the kidneys resulting in oligohydramnios, pulmonary hypoplasia, spadelike hands and feet, peculiar facies with a beaked nose, and creases under the lower eyelids. The fetus, often SGA, usually is in a breech position, does not tolerate the stress of labor, and may be stillborn. *When liveborn, the neonate has immediate respiratory distress and dies of respiratory failure* long before it could die of renal failure. Oligohydramnios is associated with fetal anuria. Renal agenesis per se is not the cause of pulmonary hypoplasia, however, which is the result of lack of amniotic fluid and thoracic constraint.

Oligohydramnios without renal agenesis also can cause pulmonary hypoplasia (e.g., prolonged rupture of membranes with continued leakage). Deformation of the face and extremities plus arthrogryposis is usual in long-standing oligohydramnios.

CHAPTER

4

MATERNAL PHYSIOLOGIC ADJUSTMENTS TO PREGNANCY

FERTILIZATION AND IMPLANTATION

THE PLACENTA

The extruded *ovum* is directed into a uterine tube by its fimbriae and the peritoneal fluid currents. Normally, a few hours after insemination, *spermatozoa* will have passed through the cervix and uterus into the fallopian tubes. *Capacitation* of the sperm (preparation for fertilization) occurs between its passage into the cervix and its reaching the midportion to outer portion of the tube. *Fertilization* occurs when a spermatozoon penetrates the ovum, usually in the outer portion of the fallopian tube. It is unusual for fertilization to occur more than 24 h after ovulation. Indeed, if this occurs, an ectopic pregnancy may result.

The *fertilized ovum* rapidly develops into an embryonic blastocyst. About 3–4 days are required for this minute, free-floating object to reach the uterus. Until implantation, the zygote is nourished by adherent granulosa cells and tubal fluids. Progress is mainly by tubal ciliary action, but peristalsis probably contributes to tubal transit. *Endometrial implantation* ensues 5–6 days after fertilization. The favored sites are the anterior and the posterior fundus. This is summarized as follows.

Last menstrual period (LMP)	Cycle days 1–7
Ovulation	Day 14 after LMP
Fertilization	Day 14–15 after LMP
Ovum transit tube to uterus	Days 15–19
Ovum free in uterus	Days 19–21
Implantation	Day 19–21 after LMP
Expected period	Missed or scanty

The early developing embryo with its tissue layers is shown in Figure 4-1.

The *chorion,* or protective covering of the fertilized developing ovum, has an outer ectodermal layer (*trophoblast*). The inner layer is mesenchyme. The trophoblast, initially a poorly defined syncytium, soon develops into two tissue types: an outer confluent but differentiated plasmotrophoblast (*syncytio-* or *syntrophoblast*) and an inner distinct *cytotrophoblast* (Langhans' striae).

The trophoblast produces proteolytic enzymes capable of rapid destruction of endometrium and even myometrium. This allows the zygote to erode quickly into the functionalis layer of the

FIGURE 4-1. Relationships of the fetus, placenta, and membranes to the uterus in early gestation. Top left, 4 weeks. Top right, 6 weeks. Bottom left, 18 weeks. Bottom right, 22 weeks.

(From K.L. Moore, *The Developing Human.* W.B. Saunders Co., 1973.)

endometrium but usually not beyond the compacta. Deeper invasion (placenta accreta) does not occur when there is formation of a layer of hyalinized fibrin (*Nitabuch's striae*).

The total products of conception reach sufficient size to appose the *decidua parietalis* and obliterate the free space in the uterine cavity by about the 12th week.

FETOPLACENTAL CIRCULATION

After implantation, small *lacunae* form in the plasmotrophoblast, and soon they become confluent. These lacunae (future intervillous spaces) fill with blood from tapped veins. An occasional maternal arteriole is also opened and, finally, a sluggish circulation becomes established (*hematotrophic phase* of the embryo).

The lacunae soon ramify and enlarge. Concomitantly, vascularized tufts grow down into the blood lakes to form villi for actual embryonic circulation. The greatest concentration of maternal sinusoids (*intervillous spaces*), as well as most of the villae, develops in the *chorion frondosum*, the site of the future placenta. As time passes, the vascularity of the decidua capsularis becomes obliterated, transforming this structure into a pale translucent membrane (*chorion*) adherent to the *amnionic membrane* within. Eventually, the fetal villous system that protrudes into the intervillous blood spaces resemble inverted trees.

The final fetal villus surface, a two-cell layer separating fetal from maternal blood, is very extensive. It may be as great as 50 m² (165 square feet), and the fetal villous capillary system may reach almost 50 km (~27 miles)—a complex but remarkably workable system.

Cotyledons (subdivisions of the placenta) can be identified early in placentation as irregular clefts. At term, one can identify six or more placental units or cotyledons.

The funis, or *umbilical cord,* usually inserts centrally. Many variants of placental development are seen (Fig. 4-2), for example, marginal insertion of the cord, bipartite (double) placenta, or succenturiate lobed placenta (with a small separate accessory lobe). If even a portion of a cotyledon (or a succenturiate lobe) is retained after delivery, serious blood loss or infection often results.

UTEROPLACENTAL CIRCULATION

Veins

Many randomly placed venous orifices can be identified over the entire *decidua basalis* (basal plate of the placenta). The human

Normal placenta.

Succenturiate placenta.

Marginal insertion or battledore placenta.

Marked circumvallate or extrachorial placenta.

Bipartite placenta.

FIGURE 4-2. Placental types.

placenta has *no peripheral venous collecting system.* Collection of venous outflow is a function frequently ascribed to a marginal sinus. However, less than one third of the blood drains from the margin of the placenta. A marginal sinus is not seen even in the early placenta, and subchorionic marginal lakes are not found commonly in the mature placenta. Dilated maternal vessels are found beneath the periphery of the placenta. These have been described as wreath veins or venous lakes. They may or may not communicate with the intervillous spaces.

Arteries

In contrast to the veins, *placental arteries are grouped closer to the decidual attachments* of the intercotyledinous septa. As the placenta matures, thrombosis decreases the number of arterial openings into the basal plate. At *term,* the ratio of *veins–arteries is 2:1,* approximately that found in other mature organs.

Even in an area beneath a well-formed placenta, some spiral arterioles empty into the intervillous spaces, although many remain coiled and compressed. Arterioles supplying the intervillous spaces appear circuitous and angulated because of fixation of the vessels and growth of the placenta. The tortuosity creates baffles, or points of deflection, that tend to slow the afferent bloodstream.

Near their entry into the intervillous spaces, the terminal maternal arterioles lose their elastic reticulum. Since the distal portions of these vessels are lost with the placenta, bleeding from this source can be controlled only by uterine contraction.

THE MATURE PLACENTA

The mature placenta (Fig. 4-3) is a blue-red, rounded, flattened, meaty organ about *15–20 cm in diameter* and *3 cm thick.* It weighs *400–600 g,* or about *one-sixth* the normal weight of the term newborn. The umbilical cord (funis) extends from the fetal surface of the placenta to the umbilicus of the fetus. Fetal membranes cover the placental fetal surface and extend from the placental margins to create the space occupied by the fetus, amniotic fluid, and umbilical cord. In *multiple pregnancy, one or more placentas may be present* depending on the number of ova implanted and the type of segmentation that occurs.

UMBILICAL CORD (FUNIS)

The umbilical cord is a gray, soft, coiled, easily compressible structure that connects the fetus with its placenta. It *averages 50 cm in* length and *2 cm in diameter (limits of 30–100 cm in length)* and is

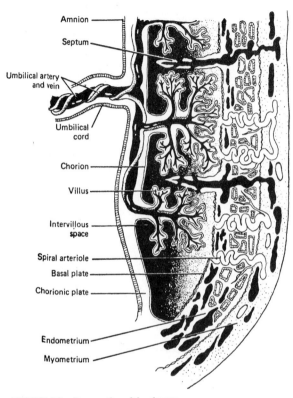

Amnion

Septum

Umbilical artery
and vein

Umbilical
cord

Chorion

Villus

Intervillous
space

Spiral arteriole

Basal plate

Chorionic plate

Endometrium

Myometrium

FIGURE 4-3. Cross section of the placenta.
(Modified after Netter.)

covered by a thin layer of stratified squamous epithelium comparable to fetal skin. The cord contains a framework of loose fibrous connective tissue and is filled with a mucoid material (*Wharton's jelly*). Normally, the cord contains two arteries that carry deoxygenated blood from the fetus and one vein to supply the fetus with oxygenated blood. As a result of aplasia or atrophy, one umbilical artery is absent in about 1% of singletons and 6% of twins. About 17% of these infants with a single umbilical artery have other multisystem structural anomalies. The cause(s) is unknown. Two-vessel cord is more common in African Americans than in others. Age and parity are unrelated factors. *Undergrowth of the fetus* is common with this anomaly, but early delivery is not attributed to two-vessel cord.

In the *common marginal insertion or battledore placenta,* the cord inserts at the periphery of the placenta. The battledore placenta poses no special problems.

In the *rare velamentous insertion of the cord,* the cord does not insert on the chorionic plate but inserts on the membranes at a point distant from the chorionic plate. The result poses a *hazard.* The unsupported umbilical vessels are at grave risk of laceration during labor and delivery, whereupon exsanguination of the fetus may occur.

True knots in the cord, generally in abnormally long cords, are observed in about *1:100* deliveries. Loose or false knots are unimportant, but tight knots may cause cord vessel occlusion, resulting in *fetal distress or death.*

FETAL MEMBRANES

The *chorion* and *amnion* join the cord, cover the placenta, and extend to envelop the fetus. They strip easily from the fetal surface of the placenta and can be separated by careful dissection.

The amnion is a double-layered translucent membrane. Its outer portion is mesodermal connective tissue, and the inner layer is ectoderm. Eventually, the amnion consists generally of stratified squamous cells with scattered patches of low cuboidal cells. Thickened squamous areas occasionally are observed, especially near the umbilical cord. The chorion is a membrane composed of an outer syncytial layer without cellular divisions and an inner cellular (Langhans') layer.

The placental membranes contain the amniotic fluid and provide *a barrier against infection* for the fetus. A *check for completeness* of the membranes at delivery is essential to avoid infection or bleeding usually associated with retained products of conception.

AMNIOTIC FLUID

At term, the fetus is submerged in *about 1 liter* of clear watery fluid (though up to 2 liters normally may be present). The amniotic fluid has a low specific gravity ($\sim$1.008) and mild alkalinity (pH $\sim$7.2). The amniotic fluid *protects the fetus* from direct injury, aids in maintaining its temperature, allows free movement of the fetus, minimizes the likelihood of adherence of the fetus to the amniotic membrane, and allows for hormonal, fluid, and electrolyte exchange. It *acts as a repository for fetal secretions and excretions.* It contains fetal squamous debris, flecks of vernix, a few leukocytes, and small quantities of albumin, urates, and other organic and inorganic salts. Hormones and alpha-fetoprotein (AFP), a protein produced by the fetus, also are found in the amniotic fluid. The *electrolyte concentration is equivalent to that of maternal plasma except for calcium,* which is lower (5.5 mg/mL).

Amniotic fluid is variously considered to be a secretion of the amnion, a vascular transudate, or fetal urine. All three sources contribute to its formation in varying amounts at different times in gestation. For example, with lengthening gestations, fetal urine becomes a more important contributor. There is *rapid amniotic fluid turnover* (~350–375 mL/h). Retention of only a few milliliters per hour soon will result in *polyhydramnios* (>2 liters of amniotic fluid), whereas excessive reabsorption or failure of production will cause *oligohydramnios* (<300 mL of amniotic fluid at term).

PLACENTAL PHYSIOLOGY

The placenta has two *principal functions:* it acts as a *transfer organ for metabolic products,* and it *produces or metabolizes* the hormones and enzymes necessary for the maintenance of pregnancy. It thus acts as a lung, a gastrointestinal tract, a kidney, and a complex of ductless glands for the conceptus.

The placenta derives most, if not all, of its *nourishment from maternal blood.* The metabolic activity of the placenta may be measured by its oxygen consumption. *Continued growth of the placenta is feasible only to a point,* and its functional capacity and oxygen consumption decline in late pregnancy.

PLACENTAL HORMONES
(FIGS. 4-4, 4-5)

With the onset of pregnancy, the pattern of circulating hormones changes abruptly from that of the normal menstrual cycle. Complete sex steroid hormone (estrogen and progesterone) production by the placenta alone is impossible because the necessary enzymes are lacking; however, the fetal and maternal adrenal cortices produce the precursors needed for placental synthesis of the hormones. This is the basis for the concept and term *maternal-fetal-placental unit.*

Estrogens are bound to serum albumin in the maternal circulation and are, therefore, metabolized slowly. *Progesterone,* on the other hand, is not bound and is metabolized rapidly. *Thyroxine* (T_4)

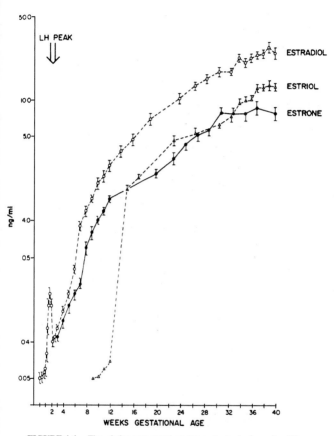

FIGURE 4-4. The relative concentrations (mean ± standard error) and the incremental patterns patterns of the three major estrogens plotted in the log scale during the course of pregnancy. (Courtesy of J. Marshall.)

(From D.N. Danforth and J.R. Scott, eds., *Obstetrics and Gynecology,* 5th ed. J.B. Lippincott Co., 1986.)

is bound to alpha-globulin and prealbumin. *Corticosteroids* are held in relatively inactive form in plasma by transcortin. Thus, the titer of hydroxycorticosteroids is high during pregnancy, although frank Cushing's syndrome is uncommon.

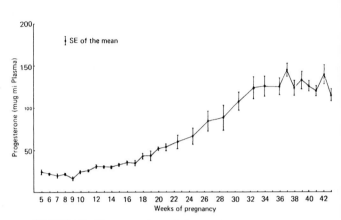

FIGURE 4-5. Plasma progesterone during pregnancy.

(From D.N. Danforth, ed., *Obstetrics and Gynecology*, 4th ed. Harper & Row, 1982.)

Estrogens

Estrogens are produced in ever-increasing amounts by the *syncytiotrophoblast.* The placenta cannot produce the required estrogen precursor but synthesizes estrogens from those supplied by the mother and the fetus. The most potent estrogen, *17β-estradiol,* is derived from dehydroepiandrosterone from both mother ovarian origin and fetus. This estrogen, like the weakest estrogen, estriol increases approximately 1000-fold from the onset of pregnancy to term. *Estrone,* metabolized principally from androstenedione (synthesized from maternal cholesterol and fetal and maternal dehydroepiandrosterone) increases only 100-fold over the nonpregnant level. Although it seems to be of minor importance, estrone together with estradiol is vital for fetal growth and development.

Estriol, the largest fraction of the total estrogens during pregnancy, is produced largely from fetal 16-hydroxydehydroepiandrosterone. Because the fetal precursors are a vitally important source of estriol, estriol determinations in maternal plasma or urine were used as measures of fetal well-being (e.g., in diabetes mellitus or preeclampsia) before more precise and cost-effective methods were available. Currently, there is interest in salivary estriol levels as a potential marker of preterm labor.

Progestogens

17α-Hydroxyprogesterone declines to very low levels after an initial (about 2 weeks after the beginning of pregnancy) mild elevation. It probably is produced by the corpus luteum, a function that is almost totally assumed by the placenta after pregnancy is well established (by at least 12 weeks).

In contrast, *progesterone,* which is produced by the placenta, increases daily after the beginning of pregnancy to more than double the prepregnancy value (Fig. 4-5). Progesterone is metabolized about equally by the maternal and the fetal liver and fetal adrenal cortex. The final metabolites are 20α-dihydroprogesterone and pregnanediol.

Progesterone is the principal *precursor of the glucocorticoids and mineralocorticoids of the fetus.* Progesterone also can be synthesized in the placenta from acetates or cholesterol (estrogens cannot.)

Human Chorionic Gonadotropin (hCG)

The placental hormone *hCG is produced by the syntrophoblast.* Its concentration rises sharply after implantation of the fertilized ovum and reaches a *peak value of ~100,000 mIU/mL about the eighth to tenth week.* Chorionic gonadotropin then falls sharply to a lower level by about the 120th day and remains at this level to term. It *disappears from the circulation at a known rate* (Fig. 4-6) of *approximately 50% per week.* hCG is secreted directly into the maternal blood, with virtually none reaching the fetal circulation.

hCG is *luteotropic* and, like LH, stimulates the production of progesterone, 17-hydroxyprogesterone, and estrogens. The physiologic role of hCG, particularly in later pregnancy, is not

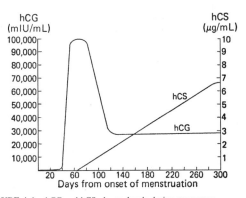

FIGURE 4-6. hCG and hCS plasma levels during pregnancy.

(From W.J. Dignam. In: R.C. Benson, ed., *Current Obstetric & Gynecologic Diagnosis & Treatment,* 4th ed. Lange, 1982.)

known. It apparently is important for maintenance of the corpus luteum in very early pregnancy, but after the first few weeks of gestation, the corpus luteum itself is no longer essential to the maintenance of pregnancy. An immunologic role for hCG (may inhibit lymphocyte response to the "foreign" placenta) has been postulated.

Tests for hCG in the urine have formed the basis for practically all pregnancy tests. This is because of its rapid rise early in pregnancy and continued high output throughout gestation. The alpha subunit of hCG is nearly identical to that of LH, but their beta subunits differ. Thus, radioimmunoassays for the beta subunit of hCG in serum have become the most sensitive tests, ensuring a very early accurate diagnosis of prenancy. hCG is not absolutely specific for pregnancy. Small amounts are secreted by a variety of gastrointestinal and other tumors in both males and females. Thus, it is measured in individuals with suspected tumors as a *tumor marker.*

Follicle-Stimulating Hormone (FSH)

FSH rapidly falls to scarcely detectable levels about 10 days after ovulation, never rising again until ovulation occurs following delivery. The activity of the anterior pituitary probably is suppressed by hCG and later by prolactin.

Human Chorionic Somatomammotropin (hCS)

Chorionic somatomammotropin (hCS), formerly known as placental lactogen (hPL), is a protein hormone produced by the syntrophoblast. It is immunologically and physiologically similar to pituitary growth hormone (hGH). Measurable amounts of hCS are detectable after the eighth week of pregnancy, with a steady increase to term, when normal values of 6–7 μg/mL are reached (Fig. 4-6).

Other Protein Hormones

The placenta also produces chorionic thyrotropin (CT) but not corticotropin.

HEMODYNAMICS

There is little short-circuiting of blood from an arterial opening to an adjacent venous outlet. This is because the arterial pressure of the maternal blood (60–70 mm Hg) actually causes it to flow quickly into the low-pressure (20 mm Hg) intervillous space. Maternal arterial blood is directed toward the chorionic plate, whereas venous blood in the placenta tends to flow along and out from the basal plate. Thus, beneficial circulation currents are established.

Maternal blood flow through the placenta at term is about 500 mL/min, whereas the fetus circulates only some 400 mL/min through the placenta. The slow rate of circulation within the placenta is off-set by the large capacity of the placenta, which exceeds that of the vessels supplying and draining it, as well as by the excess of maternal over fetal blood. Changes in maternal blood pressure, therefore, have only a gradual effect on the intervillous blood pressure in the placenta. Mechanisms to improve placental transfer are few, however. An increased rate of rhythmic uterine contractions is helpful, but strong, prolonged labor contractions are detrimental to the placental and fetal circulation. An increased fetal heart rate tends to expand the villi during systole; however, this is only a minor aid in circulatory transfer.

The pressure gradient within the fetal circulation changes slowly with the mother's posture, fetal movements, and physical stress. The pressure within the placental intervillous space is about 10 mm Hg when the gravida is lying down. After she stands for a few minutes, this pressure exceeds 30 mm Hg. In comparison, the fetal capillary pressure remains at about 20 mm Hg.

PLACENTAL TRANSFER

Transfer across the placental barrier is accomplished by at least five different processes: *simple diffusion, facilitated diffusion, active transport, pinocytosis* (engulfment of particles by cells), and *leakage* through defects.

Simple Diffusion

Substances required for the maintenance of fetal life and the elimination of its waste products are handled largely by diffusion across the placental barrier. Included in this group are *oxygen, CO_2, water, electrolytes, and urea.* Fetal blood and maternal blood have similar diffusion constants, so that passage of these substances is rapid in either direction. Large quantities of certain substances are involved, and near term, almost 4 liters of water clears the placenta each hour. The principal limiting factors are the relative anatomic inefficiency of the placenta and sluggish blood flow.

Fortunately, fetal oxygen requirements are less than those of the newborn. Oxygen tension in the intervillous space is only about one-half that in the maternal pulmonary veins. The fetus is compensated to a degree because fetal hemoglobin carries slightly more oxygen than adult hemoglobin. Moreover, fetal blood also more effectively eliminates CO_2 than adult blood.

Facilitated Diffusion

Certain substances important to the fetus (e.g., glucose) are transported across the placenta more rapidly than is possible by simple diffusion. In these instances, a carrier system functions with the chemical gradient, but the system may become saturated at high concentrations. (This mechanism differs from active transport, which operates against the gradient.)

Active Transport

This requires energy, moves against a concentration gradient, and occurs even when the system is saturated. *Amino acids, water-soluble vitamins, and large-ion substances, for example, calcium, iron, and iodine, are transported actively.* Enzymes probably are involved. *Bilirubin* is moved from fetus to mother in this manner also. Hence, it is rare for cord blood bilirubin to be >4–5 mg/dL, even with severe fetal hemolytic disease. It also explains why infants are not jaundiced even when their mothers have hepatitis.

Pinocytosis and Leakage Through Defects

The final two mechanisms both accomplish moving substances with such large molecular structures that no other means exist to move them across the placenta.

THE PLACENTAL BARRIER

The human placental barrier is represented initially by two layers of trophoblastic cells that separate the maternal and fetal blood-streams. The outer layer is the *syntrophoblast,* or plasmotrophoblast. The inner layer is the *cytotrophoblast,* or Langhans' stria. After the third month, the cytotrophoblast normally loses its continuity, and the cells become less numerous. Therefore, in late pregnancy, the only separation between maternal blood and the fetal vascular endothelium is the syntrophoblast, a single cell layer that is, in essence, a transfer membrane. This is a poor barrier, however, and only a limited number of high molecular weight substances (e.g., insulin, hCG) are blocked completely. Thus, the term *barrier is something of a misnomer.*

Nonetheless, the placenta serves as a time barrier rather than a concentration barrier in most instances. If a drug can be absorbed through the maternal gastrointestinal tract, it usually can cross the placenta. Such passage, however, takes time.

IMMUNOLOGY

Pregnancy is marked by *maternal tolerance of paternal major histocompatibility antigens while maintaining infectious immune competency.* This is accomplished by *several mechanisms,* including: fetal trophoblastic evasion of maternal immune detection (at least partially by failing to express major histocompatibility antigens class I or class II molecules); trophoblast expression of Fas ligand (causing maternal immune cells expressing Fas to undergo apoptosis at the placenta/decidua juncture); expression of complement regulatory proteins CD46, CD55, and CD59 (which exert protective effects); extravillous cytotrophoblast cells expressing nonclassic major histocompatibility gene encoding HLA-G (downregulates natural killer cell function); and uterine placental cell and decidual production of cytokines (contribute to divergence of immune response from Th1 to Th2). The alterations just noted (and probably others) effect the thymus and B cells, contributing to the suppression of autoimmune responses as well as changes in circulating and local T-cell subsets.

PLACENTAL DISORDERS

PLACENTAL INSUFFICIENCY

Placental insufficiency is an obstetric concept used to explain *reduced placental function potentially resulting in untoward fetal outcome.* The insufficiency may be *acute* (e.g., after premature partial placental separation leading to fetal distress) or *chronic* (in which there is suboptimal nutritional or gaseous exchange resulting in subnormal fetal growth, oligohydramnios, and possible passage of meconium in utero). Although a single cause of placental insufficiency may be apparent in the acute cases, all too frequently, there is not a single uteroplacental or villous lesion identifiable in chronic placental insufficiency. Certainly, it may be that current methods of determination of placental compromise are of insufficient precision. Alternatively, it may be that an accumulation of placental compromise or injury, when present for a sufficient time, leads to detectable pathologic or pathophysiologic change(s). Currently, the major endpoint determining placental insufficiency is fetal growth restriction.

The decreased fetal or neonatal growth that occurs with the chronic form of placental insufficiency is classified as abnormal when the perinate is in the *10th percentile or below.* This is a *small for gestational age (SGA)* pregnancy.

Restricted growth potential through diminished placental function may be caused by *abnormal placental anatomy* (e.g., placenta previa, circumvallate placenta, placental hemangioma, or twin-to-twin transfusion syndrome). It is associated more frequently with *abnormal placental perfusion* (e.g., cigarette smoking, chronic villitis, infarction, partial separation, and premature placental aging). Other *maternal disorders* with decreased placental perfusion include anemia (Hgb <12 g/dL), uterine or uterine vascular anomalies, diabetes mellitus, hypertension, preeclampsia, renal disease (e.g., chronic glomerulonephritis), malnutrition (e.g., inflammatory bowel disease), pancreatitis, lupus erythematosus, and cyanotic heart disease. Finally, it is possible to have restricted growth potential from the enhanced demands imposed by *multiple pregnancy.*

Care must be taken to identify SGA pregnancies with restricted growth potential (exogenous or type II) from those with decreased growth potential (endogenous or type I) because therapy modalities are very different. *Decreased growth potential may be caused by genetic disorders* (e.g., autosomal trisomies, sex chromosome disorders, neural tube defects, or dysmorphic syndromes), *fetal anomalies, congenital infections* (e.g., cytomegalovirus infection, rubella, toxoplasmosis, malaria, and listeriosis), drugs (e.g., alcohol, tobacco, warfarin, or folic acid antagonists), *radiation,* and *small maternal stature.*

Currently, therapy is not possible for the majority of those SGA pregnancies with decreased growth potential (damage), although individualized therapy of the conditions underlying restricted growth potential possibly is of benefit. With serious fetal disorders (acute or chronic), consider delivery by the easiest, least traumatic means. Avoid heavy maternal sedation, anesthesia induced hypotension, and hypoxia. Ensure proper neonatal support and treatment.

The placenta may be considerably smaller than normal or show premature aging. In addition to the *altered body proportions* (the fetal head is spared at the expense of the body), the SGA perinate has *altered body composition* (including decreased body fat, decreased total protein, decreased total body DNA and RNA, decreased glycogen) and *altered distribution of organ weights.*

The SGA fetus is at risk for *congenital malformations, hypoxia and acidosis, stillbirth, and sudden infant death syndrome (SIDS).* Neonatally, placental insufficiency can be associated with *hypoglycemia, hypocalcemia, hypothermia, hypoxia and acidosis, meconium aspiration syndrome, polycythemia, and congenital malformation.* Unfortunately, there may be *long-term sequelae,* including seizures, cerebral palsy, reduced IQ, and learning or behavior disorders.

PLACENTAL AND
MEMBRANOUS TUMORS

Amnion nodosum (small, pearly irregularities of the amnion) are composed of plaques of benign squamous cells. They may represent localized residui of disease or an incorporation of fetal extradermal derivatives. Amnion nodosum is associated with *oligohydramnios* and major fetal urinary or gastrointestinal tract *anomalies.*

With the exception of *hydatidiform mole,* trophoblastic neo-plasms (e.g., *malignant hydatidiform mole, choriocarcinoma*) are rare. *Chorioangiomas* occasionally are associated with fetal malde-velopment of one twin, probably due to shunting of placental blood by the tumor.

PLACENTAL INFARCTS

Placental infarcts, red to pale brown, firm areas, may be small to massive and located anywhere beneath the chorionic plate. In-farcts are composed of *degenerating villi and fibrin clot.* They are caused by interference with the maternal blood supply to the intervillous space, for example, thrombosis of a maternal artery to a cotyledon.

Placental infarcts are *rare in early pregnancy.* Occasional small infarcts are common in late normal placentas and may be numer-ous with preeclampsia. In postdue pregnancy, when placental ag-ing becomes evident, scattered small infarcts are common. Gross infarction occurs in partial placental separation. Extensive placen-tal infarction is associated with chronic or acute fetal distress, and even fetal death.

HEMORRHAGIC ENDOVASCULITIS

Hemorrhagic endovasculitis (HEV) probably is caused by placen-titis. In HEV, the blood vessels are injured, and fetal blood is lost into the placenta, causing temporary fetal anemia and hypoxia. Threatened abortion or fever may suggest placentitis. It probably is responsible for growth retardation and early fetal CNS injury (e.g., sensory or motor disability). Whether or not a woman with HEV in one pregnancy will have the abnormality in the next is undeter-mined.

PLACENTAL INFECTION (PLACENTITIS, CHORIOAMNIONITIS)

Bacterial or viral infection of the placenta, particularly the amnion and chorion near the cord insertion, is *common after prolonged rup-ture of the membranes.* Maternal chills, fever, uterine tenderness or hypertonicity, and malodorous amniotic fluid are suggestive signs.

Leukocytosis, with a differential shift to the left, *increased sed-imentation rate, heavy colonization* of pathogens on cervical or uter-ine culture indicates intrauterine sepsis. A *steamy or milky appear-ance of the membranes* (due to the presence of polymorphonuclear leukocytes and exudates), together with *perivascular leukocytic infiltration of the cord and fetal vessels* (funisitis), is typical. Focal villus inflammation is a late manifestation.

It is *rare for antibiotic therapy to sufficiently eradicate the infection* to allow continuation of pregnancy. Therefore, in the vast majority it is necessary to treat by prompt evacuation of the uterus, oxytocics, and massive parenteral antibiotic therapy against anaerobic and aerobic bacteria. Symptomatic therapy may be the only course in viral infections.

Parametritis, salpingitis, pelvic peritonitis, pelvic thrombophlebitis, or maternal death may ensue, as may *perinatal omphalitis, septicemia, septic pneumonia, or death.*

PHYSIOLOGIC CHANGES IN PREGNANCY

MATERNAL CARDIOVASCULAR CHANGES DURING PREGNANCY

BLOOD

Blood volume, composed of the plasma volume plus the cellular volume, increases 45%–50% during pregnancy. The plasma volume increases more and earlier in gestation than does the cellular volume, although the latter increases about 33% or ~450 mL. This creates *a declining hematocrit* (HCT) until near the 30th week of pregnancy, when the plasma volume plateaus, and is termed the *dilutional or physiologic anemia of pregnancy.* With iron supplementation, the erythrocytes increase more rapidly, and the disparity between cellular and plasma volumes is less (Fig. 4-7).

Increased plasma volume may be due to augmented plasma renin, secondary to elevated estrogen and progesterone. This encourages sodium retention by stimulating aldosterone secretion. Thus, *total body water is increased,* and there is a gradual *cumulative retention of sodium* over the course of an average pregnancy. This results in a total body water increase of 6–8 liters, of which 4–6 liters is extracellular.

The distribution of blood volume varies with changes in body position. Sitting and supine recumbency during the third trimester traps blood in the legs. This also occurs during the *supine hypotensive syndrome* (i.e., bradycardia and hypotension due to reduced

FIGURE 4-7. Blood volume changes during pregnancy and the postpartum period.

(From M.L. Pernoll and R.C. Benson, eds., *Current Obstetric & Gynecologic Diagnosis & Treatment,* 6th ed. Lange, 1987.)

blood flow to the heart), when the uterus compresses the inferior vena cava.

The success of pregnancy is correlated with the development and maintenance of a normally expanded maternal blood volume. *Hypovolemia is associated with fetal growth retardation and preterm delivery.* Women with multiple pregnancy have more of an increase in blood volume over those with a singleton. There is a finite limit, and whereas a significant increase occurs with twins, the amount is much less with each additional fetus.

Leukocytes (primarily polymorphonuclear leukocytes) *increase* from nonpregnant levels (4300–4500/mL) to 5000–12,000/mL at term. During labor, leukocytes may rise even higher (to ~25,000/mL).

There is a marked *increase (~50%) in fibrinogen* over the course of gestation. This increase is accompanied by a *general enhancement of clotting activity,* which causes a significant rise in the erythrocyte sedimentation rate (ESR). Small decreases in platelet count may occur.

CARDIAC OUTPUT

Cardiac output (CO), the *product of the heart rate (HR) and stroke volume (SV), increases ~40%* (~1.5 liters/min) during gestation. It reaches the maximum at 20–24 weeks (Fig. 4-8). SV accounts for nearly all of the increase in early pregnancy (peak of 25%–30% at 12–24 weeks). The HR increases by 15 beats/min at term but is influenced by the same variables as in the woman who is not pregnant.

Here, too, *position* of the gravida makes a significant difference—the best being the *left lateral decubitus.* During labor and delivery, contractions express blood from the uterine vascular bed. In the supine position, this increases venous return and transiently augments CO by about 25%; whereas in the lateral recumbent position, there is only a 7%–8% increase. Similarly, SV rises more in the supine vs. lateral recumbent (33% v. 7.7%), and the pulse rate falls less (15% v. 0.7%). The magnitude of these changes is modified also by the strength of the uterine contractions.

The enhanced CO is distributed primarily to certain sites. *Uterine blood flow rises steadily,* reaching ~500 mL/min at term. Early

FIGURE 4-8. Increase in cardiac output during pregnancy.

(From F. Hytten and G. Chamberlain, *Clinical Physiology and Obstetrics.* Blackwell Scientific Publications, 1980.)

in pregnancy, the *renal blood flow is increased about 30%* above the average for nonpregnant women, and the *glomerular filtration rate (GFR) increases to some 50% above nonpregnant levels.* This augmentation persists to term. *Mammary blood flow increases* considerably by term. There is no change in CNS or hepatic blood flow during pregnancy.

ARTERIAL BLOOD PRESSURE (BP)

Progesterone causes relaxation of smooth muscle. This is apparent in the venous system and results in dilated pelvic veins, increased vasculature of the uterus, and marked dilatation of the veins in the lower extremities. However, this effect also is noted in the arteries.

BP, the product of CO and peripheral resistance (PR), declines until midpregnancy. This is due to reduced vascular resistance despite the rise in CO. In later pregnancy the BP rises under the influence of factors other than progesterone. The latter diminishes peripheral resistance from ~20 weeks gestation to term.

PULMONARY ADJUSTMENTS TO PREGNANCY

Capillary dilatation throughout the respiratory tract causes voice changes and makes nose breathing difficult from early pregnancy. Radiologically, *pulmonary vascular markings are enhanced.* Uterine enlargement is accompanied by as much as 4 cm diaphragm elevation, but this altered position does not impede diaphragmatic function. Indeed, the abdominal muscles relax during pregnancy, and, thus, *respiration is more diaphragmatic.* The lower ribcage is flared outward, enhancing the subxiphoid angle and increasing the thoracic circumference by up to 6 cm.

Dead space volume increases because of conducting airway musculature relaxation. Gradual *increase in tidal volume (35%–50%)* occurs with lengthening pregnancy. *Diaphragm elevation* decreases total lung capacity by 4%–5%. *Tidal volume increases 40%. Functional residual capacity, residual volume, and expiratory reserve volume are reduced by ~20%. Alveolar ventilation is increased by ~65% by the combination of larger tidal volume and smaller residual volume. Inspiratory capacity is increased 5%–10%* by the maximum at 22–24 weeks. There is a *slight increase in respiratory rate, minute ventilation increases 50%, and by term, oxygen consumption is increased 15%–20% above the nonpregnant. Respiratory minute volume is increased ~26%* (Fig. 4-9).

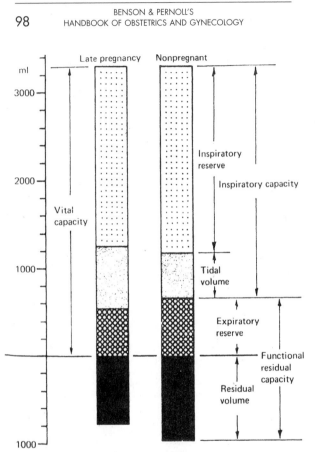

FIGURE 4-9. Lung volume changes during pregnancy.
(From F.E. Hytten and I. Leitch. *The Physiology of Human Pregnancy.* Blackwell Scientific Publications, 1964.)

Hyperventilation of pregnancy (decreased alveolar CO_2 with concomitant lower maternal blood CO_2 while maintaining normal maternal alveolar oxygen tension) occurs as a result of the alterations described. Maternal hyperventilation is *due to progesterone* action on the respiratory center mediated by peripheral chemoreceptors in the carotid body. *This allows the fetus to exchange CO_2 in the most effective manner.*

During *labor and delivery,* many patients *hyperventilate.* This may lead to *respiratory alkalosis with carpopedal spasm. Functional reserve capacity further decreases in the early phase of each contraction* (from the redistribution of blood from the uterus), and there may be more efficient gas exchange. Anesthetic administration must be altered accordingly.

RENAL ALTERATIONS

Dilatation of the renal hila, calices, and ureters occurs as early as the late first trimester but usually regresses to normal by the end of the puerperium. The right collecting system exhibits greater dilatation because of compression by the enlarged, dextrorotated uterus. Bilateral vesicoureteral reflux often occurs during pregnancy. Thus, pregnant women become more susceptible to urinary tract infection.

Renal plasma flow (RPF) increases markedly during pregnancy to attain a maximum of 60%–80% above nonpregnant levels by midgestation. Then, a gradual fall of about 25% occurs by term. *The GFR increases by ~50%* by the second trimester because of increased blood volume and renal blood flow, lowered oncotic pressure, and endocrine changes. It plateaus in the third trimester to term. The filtration fraction (FF), the ratio of GFR/RPF, decreases during early pregnancy, to rise again in the last trimester. This probably indicates hemodynamic changes within the glomerulus.

Very early in pregnancy, the *creatinine clearance (CC) increases* to ~45% over nonpregnant values. During the second trimester, the CC remains elevated, but in the third trimester, several weeks before term, it gradually falls to nonpregnant levels.

Urea and uric acid are all excreted more effectively during pregnancy, so that the blood concentrations of these substances normally are lower than in the nonpregnant state. More glucose and lactose are excreted during pregnancy. Most amino acids are eliminated more rapidly and in larger amounts during pregnancy. Ascorbic acid and folate losses in the urine occur.

Fluid volume and composition are regulated by renal control of the excretion of sodium and water. Estrogen and cortisol and the renin-angiotensin-aldosterone system contribute to the changes in sodium and water homeostasis during pregnancy. The greatly increased GFR during pregnancy causes a considerable increase in sodium filtration, but *tubular reabsorption of sodium is increased.* This results in the positive sodium balance needed to allow for fetal requirements and the increased maternal blood volume. Proportionately more water than sodium is retained during the third trimester. This contributes to the commonly observed dependent edema of late pregnancy.

GASTROINTESTINAL ALTERATIONS WITH PREGNANCY

ORAL

Salivation often increases and is more acidic. The gums may become hypertrophic and hyperemic, and epulis formation may occur in those without good oral hygiene.

GASTROINTESTINAL

During pregnancy, *both gastrointestinal motility and tone decrease* (under the influence of increased progesterone). Clinically, this leads to *delayed gastric emptying, slower transit times, and constipation.* There is more gastroesophageal reflux, which leads to *heartburn* and a very real possibility of regurgitation and aspiration if unconscious. The effect of pregnancy on gastric acidity is variable.

The *appendix is displaced superiorly and into the right flank,* and the bowel is displaced upward and laterally. This knowledge is most important when appendectomy must be performed in advanced pregnancy.

LIVER

No specific gross or microscopic changes in the liver have been noted during pregnancy. Liver function test values in pregnancy are the same as in the nonpregnant state with the following exceptions. (1) Serum albumin decreases slowly during pregnancy from about 4.2 to 3.5 g/dL, with a gradual rise to normal in 6–8 weeks after delivery. (2) Alpha and beta globulin levels increase slightly and gamma-globulin decreases very slightly in pregnancy. (3) Cephalin flocculation is elevated in 25% of pregnancies. (4) Serum alkaline phosphatase increases gradually during pregnancy; at term, average values are 6.3 Bodansky units and 19 King-Armstrong units. Tests unchanged during gestation include those for serum glutamic oxaloacetic transaminase and serum bilirubin levels. The BSP excretion test is unaffected.

GALLBLADDER

Emptying time is slowed and often is incomplete. The bile's chemical composition is not altered, but bile stasis can lead to gallstones.

MATERNAL WEIGHT GAIN
IN PREGNANCY

During the course of pregnancy, *the average weight gain will be 22–27 pounds (10–12 kg)*. At term, the components of weight gain will be distributed as indicated in Figure 4-10. Ideally, only 1.5–3 pounds are gained in the first trimester and 0.8 pounds/week during the second and third trimesters. Inadequate progressive weight gain is often associated with poor fundal growth, reflecting deficient fetal growth. Thus, inadequate progressive weight gain in pregnancy requires investigation for nutritional deficit, maternal illness, malabsorption, or an abnormal hormonal mileu (e.g., hyperthyroidism). Excessive weight gain in the latter half of pregnancy is worrisome because of the relationship to hypertensive states of pregnancy.

Individualization of maternal weight gain is key to optimal fetal growth. For example, it is recommended that underweight women gain more and obese women less. Women who are heavier at the onset of pregnancy or have excessive weight gain during pregnancy are more prone to have macrosomic babies. By contrast, underweight women and those with inadequate weight gain during pregnancy are more likely to have a fetus with intrauterine growth retardation and a small placenta.

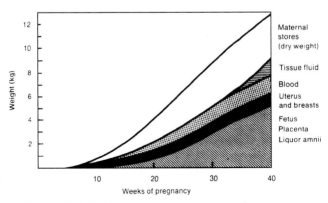

FIGURE 4-10. The components of weight gain in normal pregnancy.
(From F.E. Hytten and A.M. Thomson. Maternal physiological adjustments. In: *Maternal Nutrition and the Course of Pregnancy.* National Academy of Sciences, 1970.)

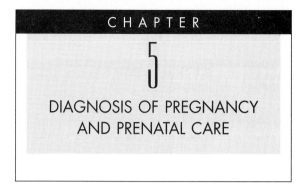

The *correct early diagnosis of pregnancy is often urgent.* For example, a diagnosis is essential to institute studies or treatment of problems that may jeopardize the life or health of mother or offspring. Today this is usually accomplished by *early beta-subunit hCG testing or ultrasonic scanning* because a definite clinical diagnosis of pregnancy before the second missed period is possible in only about two thirds of patients. However, the practitioner must be familiar with the signs and symptoms of pregnancy to properly test for and treat the early pregnancy.

CLINICAL DIAGNOSIS OF PREGNANCY

Traditionally, the clinical criteria for the diagnosis of pregnancy have been categorized into presumptive, probable, and positive (Table 5-1).

The differential diagnosis of the common signs and symptoms of pregnancy involves other conditions associated with similar complaints or alteration (Table 5-2).

PELVIC FINDINGS OF EARLY PREGNANCY

Critical to the diagnosis of pregnancy by physical examination are the pelvic findings. The presumptive indications of pregnancy include the following.

Cyanosis of the vagina (Chadwick's sign, Jacquemier's sign) is present by about 6 weeks.

TABLE 5-1
PRESUMPTIVE OR PROBABLE SIGNS AND SYMPTOMS
OF PREGNANCY*

Symptoms	Signs
Amenorrhea	Leukorrhea
Nausea, vomiting	Changes in color
Breast tingling, mastalgia	consistency, size, or
Urinary frequency, urgency	shape of cervix or
Quickening	uterus
	Temperature elevation
	(usually by BBT)
	Enlargement of abdomen
	Breasts enlarged, engorged,
	nipple discharge
	Pelvic souffle (bruit)
	Uterine contractions (with
	enlarged corpus)

*Although these may be suggestive, even ≥2 are not diagnostic of pregnancy.

Softening of the tip of the cervix (Fig. 5-1) occasionally is noted by the 4th–5th week of pregnancy. However, infection or scarring may prevent softening until late pregnancy.

Softening of the cervicouterine junction often occurs by 5–6 weeks. A soft spot may be noted anteriorly in the middle of the uterus near its junction with the cervix (Ladin's sign) (Fig. 5-2). A wider zone of softness and compressibility in the lower uterine segment (Hegar's sign) is the most valuable sign of early pregnancy and can usually be noted at ~6 weeks (Fig. 5-3). Ease in flexing the fundus on the cervix (McDonald's sign) generally appears by 7–8 weeks.

Irregular softening and slight enlargement of the fundus at the site of or on the side of implantation (Von Fernwald's sign) occur by ~5 weeks. Similarly, if implantation is in the region of a uterine cornu, a more pronounced softening and suggestive tumor like enlargement may occur (Piskacek's sign) (Fig. 5-4).

Generalized enlargement and diffuse softening of the uterine corpus usually occur ≥8 weeks of pregnancy (Fig. 5-5).

TABLE 5-2
COMPARATIVE DIFFERENTIAL DIAGNOSIS
OF PRESUMPTIVE SYMPTOMS AND SIGNS
OF PREGNANCY

	Cause(s) if Pregnant	Differential Diagnosis (Not Pregnant)
Symptoms		
Amenorrhea	hCG, etc.	Pseudocyesis or other psychoneurosis, endocrinopathies (including premature menopause), metabolic disorders (e.g., anemia, malnutrition), obliteration of the uterine cavity, systemic disease (e.g., acute or chronic infection), malignancy
Nausea, vomiting	hCG, etc.	Emotional disorders (e.g., pseudocyesis, anorexia nervosa), GI disorders (gastroenteritis, peptic ulcer, hiatal hernia, appendicitis, intestinal obstruction, food poisoning), acute infections (e.g., influenza, encephalitis)

(Continued)

TABLE 5-2
(Continued)

	Cause(s) if Pregnant	Differential Diagnosis (Not Pregnant)
Mastalgia, breast tingling	Estrogen (duct stimulation), progesterone (alveolar stimulation)	Estrogen with anovulation, fibrocystic breast disease
Urinary urgency, frequency	Estrogen (cystourethral turgescence)	Urinary tract infection (UTI), cystourethritis or cystocele, anxiety, diabetes, pelvic tumors, emotional tension
Quickening	Fetal movements >14 weeks (approx.)	Increased peristalsis, free adnexal cyst, pseudocyesis, gas, contractions
Constipation	Altered diet; hypoperistalsis	Low fluid, low fiber diet
Fatigue	Progesterone effect	Overwork
Weight gain	Gestational anabolism	Overeating
Signs		
Leukorrhea	Estrogen	Vaginitis, cervicitis, genital foreign body, tumor
Pelvic organ alterations		
Cyanosis of cervix or Chadwick's sign (>6 weeks)	Hormones of pregnancy	Vascular anomaly or tumor of cervix or uterus

TABLE 5-2
(Continued)

	Cause(s) if Pregnant	Differential Diagnosis (Not Pregnant)
Softening of cervix (>4–5 weeks)	Hormones of pregnancy	Chronic cervicitis
Softening of lower uterine segment (>5–6 weeks), Landin, Hegar's sign	Hormones of pregnancy	Vascular uterine anomaly or tumor
Irregular fundal softening, enlargement (>5 weeks)	Hormones of pregnancy	Myoma
Generalized corpus softening, enlargement (>8 weeks)	Hormones of pregnancy	Adenomyosis or myomata
Temperature elevation basal body temperature (BBT) >2 weeks	Progesterone	Infection, corpus luteum cyst, hCG or progestogen therapy, faulty thermometer
Abdominal enlargement	Uterine size	Obesity, pelvic or abdominal tumor, ascites, obesity, relaxation of abdominal muscles, pelvic and abdominal tumors, ascites, or ventral hernia

(Continued)

TABLE 5-2
(Continued)

	Cause(s) if Pregnant	Differential Diagnosis (Not Pregnant)
Breast changes		
Enlargement, engorgement, secondary areola (>6–8 weeks)	Estrogen and progesterone	Mastitis, malignancy, PMS, pseudocyesis
Colostrum (>16 weeks)	Prolactin, progesterone excess	Hypothalamic galactorrhea
Pelvic souffle (bruit)	Increased pelvic blood flow	Pelvic tumor or vascular anomaly (aneurysm)
Uterine contractions (with enlarged uterus)	Braxton-Hicks contractions	Pseudocyesis, tightening–relaxation of abdominal muscles
Skin pigmentation (chloasma, linea nigra)	Pituitary melanotropin	Ultraviolet exposure (tanning)
Epulis (>12 weeks)	Progesterone	Gingivitis

ABDOMINAL FINDINGS OF EARLY PREGNANCY

Active movements usually are palpable ≥18 weeks. By the 16th–18th week, *passive movements* of the fetus may be elucidated by abdominal and vaginal palpation. A firm tap on the uterine wall or vaginal fornix displaces the fetus as a floating body. An impulse then can be felt as a thrust as the fetus moves back to its former position (ballottement). Ascites and tumors must be excluded. After the 24th week, the *fetal outline may be palpated* in many pregnant women.

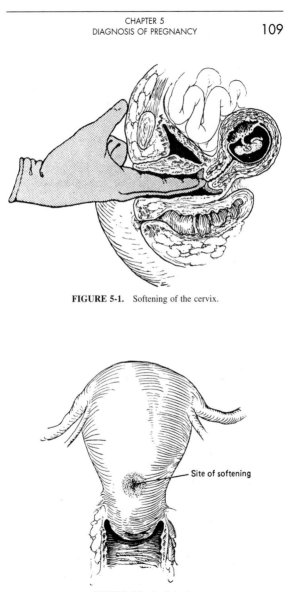

FIGURE 5-1. Softening of the cervix.

FIGURE 5-2. Ladin's sign.

Zone of softening

FIGURE 5-3. Hegar's sign.

Zone of softening

FIGURE 5-4. Piskacek's sign.

FIGURE 5-5. Bimanual pelvic examination.

No subjective evidence of pregnancy is totally diagnostic, however, and laboratory diagnosis is essential.

LABORATORY EVIDENCE OF PREGNANCY

BETA-SUBUNIT hCG

Assays for beta-subunit hCG, commonly used to diagnose pregnancy, have an admitted failure rate (~1%). Moreover, they may be positive in nongestational ovarian choriocarcinoma or in uncommon gastrointestinal or testicular tumors. Nevertheless, a positive beta-subunit hCG test may be considered reasonable proof of pregnancy. A true positive followed by a true negative pregnancy test may indicate abortion. The major methods for determining the beta-subunit hCG are as follows.

TABLE 5-3
IMMUNOLOGIC TESTS FOR PREGNANCY

Method	Materials	Results
Direct coagulation	Latex particles coated with anti-hCG + serum or urine	Coagulation if hCG is present (pregnant)
Inhibition of coagulation	Anti-hCG + serum or urine *plus* Sensitized red cells *or* Latex particles coated with hCG	Coagulation if hCG is absent (not pregnant); inhibition if hCG is present (pregnant)

IMMUNOLOGIC TESTS

Immunologic tests for pregnancy (Table 5-3) are based on hCG's antigenic potential (direct or indirect agglutination of sensitized RBC or latex particles). These tests require slides or test tubes for reagents and take from a few minutes to over an hour to complete. Test sensitivities vary widely (250–1400 mIU/mL).

Radioimmunoassay (RIA)

The hCG radioimmunoassay (RIA) requires a gamma counter for the highest sensitivity. The test, reportable in <90 min is *extremely accurate* (~20 mIU/mL.) Thus, it usually is *used when sensitivity is crucial.*

Radioreceptor Assay (RRA)

The RRA measures the biologic activity by in vitro binding of hCG to bovine corpus luteum membrane. Unfortunately, hCG and hLH cannot be separated by RRA. A commercially available RRA, Biocept G, has set its negative endpoint high to avoid false positive reports. *The accuracy does not approach that of RIA or ELISA.*

Enzyme-Linked Immunoabsorbent Assay (ELISA)

A specified monoclonal antibody produced by hybrid cell technology is used for the ELISA assay. With ELISA, the enzyme induces a color change indicating the hCG level. *ELISA is simple and rapid*

(5 min), *no isotopes are used, and it can be an office (serum) test* (e.g., Prognosis slide test, which measures to 1.5–2.5 mIU/mL). The tube, office or home test (e.g., Preco Rapid Care) measures only to 1.0 mIU/mL. Nevertheless, even ELISA home kits are at least 90% accurate within the range mentioned.

RIA, RRA, or ELISA can be used for the diagnosis of pregnancy as early as 8–12 days after ovulation. *hCH has a doubling time of 1.2–2.5 days during the first 10 weeks of pregnancy, with a slow decline to about 5000 mIU/mL thereafter.*

The latest beta-specific latex tube or slide tests that are based on agglutination or agglutination-inhibition are still adequate for the diagnosis of normal pregnancy >1–2 months. The ELISA test usually picks up earlier gestations and is more accurate, although after pregnancy, an ELISA test may require weeks to become negative. Therefore, *RIA will continue to be the method employed for serial quantitative studies in problem pregnancies, particularly trophoblastic disease.*

ULTRASONOGRAPHY

Typically, *early first trimester ultrasound has four objectives:*

- *Locate, measure, and observe the configuration of the gestational sac* (mean sac diameter, MSD = length + width + height/3),
- *Identify embryo(s), document fetal number, and record presence or absence of life* (usually determined by heartbeat),
- *Determine the extent of fetal development and measure the crown-rump length (CRL),*
- *Evaluate the uterus, cervix and adnexa.*

Currently, *endovaginal ultrasonic detection* of the implanted products of conception is possible when the *MSD is 2–3 mm.* This occurs at ~4 wk 3 d menstrual age (MA) and the hCG is characteristically *500–1500 IU/mL.* Generally, transabdominal ultrasound will detect the gestational sac at 5 mm MSD (~5 wk MA). At this time, the endometrium is markedly echogenic with prominent arcuate vessels. The sonolucent gestational sac is surrounded by trophoblastic decidual reaction that sonographically appears as a *hyperechoic rim* (or rind). In a normal early pregnancy, the *mean gestational sac diameter increases by ~1.2 mm/day.* To determine the gestational age (in days), add 30 to the mean gestational sac diameter: a mean sac diameter of 20 mm corresponds to a gestational age of 50 days.

The *yolk sac is often the first sonographic structure visualized* within the gestational sac (*from MSD 10–15 mm, 40–45 d MA*). The yolk sac is frequently visualized as a "double bleb" with the amniotic sac. The dorsal yolk sac incorporates into the primitive gut and the secondary yolk sac detaches from the midgut loop by the end of the 8th week MA. The *yolk sac increases to a maximum of ~5 mm at 11 weeks MA and disappears by 14–15 weeks MA.*

The *embryo* may be ultrasonically visualized at a *CRL of 2–3.9 mm (34–40 d MA).* There is generally *cardiac activity by 22–36 d* when the *embryo is 1.5–3 mm. An important correlation is that fetuses destined to progress will have cardiac activity by CRL of 5 mm.* At this time, the *MSD is 15–18 mm and the MA is 6.5 wk.* Generally, the early fetal heartbeat is more rapid (160 bpm) and slows with gestation. Near term, the rate is 120–140 bpm.

By *CRL of 12 mm the head should be discernable* from the thorax. *Limb buds develop by 8 weeks MA.* During the interval of 8–10 week, MA there is rapid embryonic development. *At 11 week MA (9 wk from conception), the embryo is 20–35 mm CRL and is termed a fetus.*

Early pregnancy ultrasonography may reveal findings that indicate fetal compromise or impending fetal loss. Examples of such findings include the following.

- Fetal developmental disorganization (or dissolution) and lack of a heartbeat is associated with virtually 100% fetal loss, particularly if previous development and heart activity had been sonographically determined.
- Decreased amniotic fluid (evidenced by small gestational sac size) is associated with a 94% spontaneous abortion rate.
- A MSD (mm) minus CRL (mm) of <5 is associated with an 80% spontaneous loss.
- Absence of an embryo in a gestational sac with MSD >25 mm is associated with 45% abortion rate.
- An intrauterine hematoma is associated with ~25% abortion incidence.

Ultrasonic examination is often utilized to evaluate a first trimester pregnancy complicated by vaginal bleeding. Given an embryo with satisfactory development and a heart beat, there is *roughly double the risk of spontaneous abortion when vaginal bleeding complicates a first trimester pregnancy* [e.g., <6 wk there is a 33% abortion risk with bleeding (vs. 16% without bleeding), at 7–9 wk there is a 10% abortion risk with bleeding (vs. 5%), and at 9–11 wk there is a 4% chance of bleeding (vs. 1%–2% without bleeding)].

The sonographic *differential diagnosis of early pregnancy includes: bleeding, endometritis, endometrial cysts, cervical stenosis, and the pseudogestational sacs associated with ectopic pregnancy.* Additionally, *sonographic pitfalls to be avoided* in the first trimester include: *incorrect assessment of fetal number* (somewhat obviated by fetal, not sac, visualization), *the inability to accurately determine eventual placental placement, and difficulty in assessment of morphologic abnormalities.* Examples of the latter requiring accommodation include: the early integument simulating edema, the natural extraabdominal intestinal phase, and difficulty in determining ultimate fetal cranial development that can lead to a false diagnosis of anencephaly. Although initially thought to be most accurate, caution must be exercised in sonographic gestational dating accomplished in the first trimester, for it is now apparent that *thorough second trimester assessment,* when more parameters can be measured, *may be more exact.*

DURATION OF PREGNANCY AND EXPECTED DATE OF CONFINEMENT

ESTIMATED DATE OF CONFINEMENT

After a positive diagnosis, the duration of pregnancy and the estimated date of confinement *(EDC) must be determined.* Because it is uncommon to know the exact onset of pregnancy, these calculations *start from the first day of the last menstrual period (LMP).* Pregnancy in women lasts about 10 lunar months (9 calendar months). *The average length of pregnancy is 266 days. The median duration of pregnancy is 269 days.* However, only ~6% of patients will deliver spontaneously on their EDC.* Most (60%) will deliver within 2 weeks of the EDC. Thus, as in most physiologic events, term should be regarded as a season or period of maturity, not a particular day.

A major variable in the calculated duration of pregnancy is recognized because not all women have a 28-day cycle. Hence, the physician also must *consider the length of her cycle.* A patient with a regular 40-day cycle obviously will not ovulate on day 14 but closer to or on day 26. Therefore, her EDC cannot be estimated accurately by Nagele's rule alone. Moreover, some women tend to have long or short gestations as a familial predisposition. Primiparas tend to have slightly longer gestations than multiparas. Thus, the EDC cannot be calculated precisely, although the following clinical approximations have proven useful.

NAGELE'S RULE

Add 7 days to the first day of the LMP, subtract 3 months, and add 1 year.

$$EDC = (LMP + 7 \text{ days}) - 3 \text{ months} + 1 \text{ year}$$

For example, if the first day of the LMP was June 4, the EDC will be March 11 of the following year.

Nagele's rule is based on a 28-day menstrual cycle with ovulation occurring on the 14th day. In calculating the EDC, an adjustment should be made if the patient's cycle is shorter of longer than 28 days. The discrepancies caused by 31-day months and the 29-day variation in February of leap year are not correctable by Nagele's rule. Nevertheless, it provides an acceptable estimate of the EDC.

HEIGHT OF FUNDUS AS MEASURED ABDOMINALLY

The uterus increases from a nonpregnant length ~7 cm to 35 cm at term; it increases 20 times in weight and grows in volume from 500–1000 times. Thus, the *size of the uterus should be evaluated at each prenatal visit* to determine the normality of progress. Most examinations involve an estimate of the height of the fundus uteri on the abdomen, not the length of the uterus. The superior ramus of the pubis, the umbilicus, and the xiphoid are the fixed reference points from which the height of the fundus is measured. A rough rule is provided by Table 5-4, and a more precise estimation can be made by the modified McDonald's rule.

TABLE 5-4
UTERINE HEIGHT AND STAGE OF GESTATION

Week of Pregnancy	Approximate Height of Fundus
12	Just palpable above symphysis
15	Midpoint between umbilicus and symphysis
20	At the umbilicus
28	6 cm above the umbilicus
32	6 cm below the xiphoid
36	2 cm below the xiphoid
40	4 cm below the xiphoid

Unusually *large measurements suggest* an *incorrect date of conception, multiple pregnancy, fetal macrosomia, fetal defect, or polyhydramnios.* Unexpectedly *small measurements imply fetal death, fetal undergrowth, developmental abnormality, or oligohydramnios.*

MODIFIED MCDONALD'S RULE

Measure the height of the fundus (over the curve) above the symphysis with a centimeter tape measure. The *distance in centimeters will approximate the gestational age from 16–38 weeks* ±3 weeks.

The same examiner should measure the fundus whenever possible because variations by personnel may inaccurately suggest pregnancy complications.

Additionally, a rough guide to fetal weight may be calculated from the modified McDonald's uterine measurement (Johnson's rule). However, recall that wide variations in the weights of fetuses in the third trimester may be due to the following.

- The age-weight patterns of previous infants
- An expected increase in weight of each successive infant
- Hereditary traits or acquired disorders affecting infant size, for example, race, nutrition, diabetes mellitus, preeclampsia-eclampsia.

JOHNSON'S ESTIMATE OF FETAL WEIGHT

Fetal weight (in grams) is equal to the fundal measurements (in centimeters) minus n, which is 12 if the vertex is at or above the ischial spines or 11 if the vertex is below the spines, multiplied by 155.

Example: A gravida with a fundal height of 30 cm whose vertex is at -2 station can be represented as $(30 - 12) \times 155 = 2790$ g. If the patient weighs >200 pounds, subtract 1 cm from the fundal measurement. By this calculation, an estimate within 375 g can be expected for about 70% of neonates.

QUICKENING

A rough estimate of the EDC is possible by adding 22 weeks to the date of quickening in a primigravida or 24 weeks in a multipara.

As in attempting to diagnose pregnancy, the most accurate data for EDC are provided by clinical, laboratory, and ultrasonographic studies.

EARLY hCG TESTING

Determinations of beta-subunit hCG in maternal serum compared with a scale of predetermined quantitative values provide the most accurate estimate of gestational age during the first 8–10 weeks. After this, hCG levels slowly decrease, and the method becomes inaccurate.

BIRTH DEFECT SCREENING PROGRAMS

GENERAL

The *purpose of birth defect screening is to identify birth defects as early in pregnancy as possible.* This identification allows for all options open to the parents to be available, certain conditions to be treated or their impact minimized, and birth care as well as neonatal intervention optimalization. Of course, the *technology does not currently exist to detect all birth defects,* but a vigilant search will reveal most. In many ways, birth defect screening has become a portion of standard prenatal care. For example, prenatal historical screening for those at greater risk of fetal defects has become well accepted in circumstances of advanced parental age, a specific familial history, or prior reproductive problems. Additionally, many providers now perform a patient-elected biochemical screening and ultrasound scanning.

The *age screening, prior reproductive screening, and historical screening* are generally done on the patient's first antenatal visit. Commonly, those gravidas *>32 years* of age at the time of their EDC are considered to be of *advanced maternal age (AMA).* Every patient's previous reproductive history is reviewed for *any recidive event* (including multiple spontaneous abortions) or *potentially inheritable disorder* (mendelian or multifactorial). A *three-generation family history* for mental retardation in males, previous congenital anomalies, and previous chromosomal abnormalities is performed. Many providers utilize a self-administered genetic screening questionnaire for this purpose.

Patients of *African-American ancestry are customarily offered screening for sickle cell trait or disease.* If the mother is positive for trait or disease, the father is also screened. If both have sickle cell disease or sickle cell trait, an amniocentesis is commonly offered to detect the sickle cell status of the child.

Maternal serum analyte screening for Down syndrome as well as open neural tube defects has been described as "an integral component of contemporary antenatal care." In the United States, multiple marker screening has commonly included maternal serum alpha fetoprotein (MSAFP), total human chorionic gonadotropin (hCG), and unconjugated estriol (UE$_3$). They are usually accomplished at 15–20 weeks gestation. Significant risk of Down syndrome is customarily those at >1:295 risk, whereas risk of open neural tube defect (NTD) generally are those that exceeded 2 multiples of the mean value (MOM). When abnormal multiple marker test results are obtained, reverification of gestational age (usually by ultrasound) is necessary, for a very common problem is incorrect gestational age. Multiple marker screening has proven useful for the purposes it was intended (detection of Down syndrome, detection of open NTD, and detection of trisomy 18) as well as assisting in detection of certain cases of intrauterine fetal demise, multiple gestation, and erroneous gestational dates.

Other markers are available; for example, in the United Kingdom maternal serum free beta-hCG and pregnancy-associated plasma protein-A (PAPP-A) are utilized, and allow more rapid analysis. In one study, this added an additional 16% to the detection rate accomplished by nuchal thickness and maternal age screening. Combining the four tests in screening for Down syndrome, the detection rate is reported to be 75.8%–89% with false-positive rates of ~5%.

Many authorities recommend that every gravida receive at least one *ultrasound, commonly at 16–20 weeks* gestation, geared to screen for fetal defects, ascertain multiple gestation, and determine placental location. The latter two objectives are easily met; however, there is a sizable discrepancy in reported detection of fetal malformations. This may be due to widely different levels of experience among sonographers as well as the difficulty to detect certain defects.

NUCHAL TRANSLUCENCY THICKNESS SCREENING FOR CHROMOSOMAL ANOMALIES

An important series of recent observations indicate the desirability of *sonographic screening earlier than the second trimester,* that is to say, at 10–14 weeks. These studies indicate that measuring nuchal translucency thickness is a method of screening for chromosomal anomalies (notably trisomy 21 and trisomy 18) and other disorders.

Indeed, in both high risk and low risk groups, the positive predicative value of enhanced nuchal translucency is sufficient to warrant suggesting further prenatal diagnostic testing. Because most cases are discovered after the most appropriate time for chorionic villus sampling (CVS), the majority of cases are further evaluated by amniocentesis.

The *screening is recommended at 10–14 weeks* and most authors use a nuchal thickness of >2.5–3 mm (depending on stage of gestation) as abnormal. Cumulate studies indicate a sensitivity of ~77% and a false positive rate of ~10% for aneuploidy. Selection of patients for invasive testing by this method alone allows the detection of about 80% of affected pregnancies. However, using this method for selection of patients requires about 30 invasive tests for identification of one affected fetus. Observation of a thickening that subsequently resolves is not reassuring. Fetuses with normal karotype and enhanced nuchal thickness have greater rates of spontaneous abortion related to the amount of thickness (3-fold increase with 3.0–3. 9 mm thickening and nearly seven fold increase for >4 mm).

The mechanism(s) creating enhanced nuchal thickness are not completely defined. It appears, however, that impairment of atrial contractility is involved. This has been implicated in cases of chromosomal aneuploidy as well as in cases of cardiac failure (e.g., the anemia associated with beta-thalassemia), heart, and/or great vessel defects. In the case of major congenital cardiac defects, the positive and negative predictive values have been stated to be 1.5% and 99.9% respectively. Another suggested mechanism for increased nuchal thickness is intrathoracic compression-related pulmonary hypoplasia, as seen with diaphragmatic hernia.

A potential confounder to the measurement of nuchal translucency thickness is the ~8% of fetuses having a nuchal cord at 10–14 weeks gestation. This potential bias may be reduced by use of color Doppler to confirm nuchal cord and the average 0.8 mm cord thickness subtracted.

Currently, nuchal translucency thickness sonographic screening is not a substitute for the more standard care of multiple-marker serum screening. It has not been recommended as an alternative to genetic counseling and CVS or amniocentesis in women of advanced maternal age or those with significant risk of aneuploidy. Additionally, data concerning the false negative rate (i.e., a normal nuchal translucency with aneuploidy or significant structural defect) in a risk population is not sufficient to warrant replacement of invasive testing. Indeed, it may be that combining the various modalities will prove most efficient in screening for chromosomal abnormalities.

SECOND AND THIRD TRIMESTER SONOGRAPHY

Although it is not the purpose of this text to comprehensively review ultrasonography, certain basics may assist the reader. The *objectives of later pregnancy ultrasound* include the following:

- Determine fetal life, number, and presentations.
- Estimate the amount of amniotic fluid.
- Determine the placental location, appearance (grade), and relation to the internal cervical os.
- Assess the gestational age using a variety of fetal measurements.
- Perform a fetal anatomic survey.
- Evaluate the uterus and adnexa (including documentation of size, type, and location of uterine or adnexal abnormalities).

The examination should note *abnormal heart rate and/or rhythm* as well as a *four-chamber view of the heart,* including the heart's position within the thorax. Additionally, from 16–18 weeks on, evaluation of the *cardiac outflow tracts* may be useful.

Estimation of gestational age requires several measurements. Both the biparietal diameter (*BPD*) and the head circumference (*HC*) are measured at a level including the cavum septi pellucidi and the thalamus. In cases of cephalic configuration abnormality (brachycephaly or dolichocephaly), the *cephalic index* (BPD to fronto-occipital diameter ratio) may be useful. The abdominal circumference (*AC*) is determined at the level of the *umbilical vein and portal sinus junction.* The HC/AC ratio is useful in determination of fetal growth pattern. After the 14th week of gestation, and despite considerable variation, both *femur and humerus* lengths are useful in estimation of gestational size and dates.

In addition to the previous measurements, *the fetal anatomic survey* usually includes: *cerebral ventricles, spine, stomach, urinary bladder, renal region, and the umbilical cord insertion site* on the anterior abdominal wall. Ultrasonic examination of *Multiple pregnancies* should note the *placental number, sac number, presence or absence of an interposed membrane, and comparison of fetal sizes.*

Whereas limited examinations may be useful in clinical emergencies or as a follow-up to a complete examination, *the more detailed sonography is generally more useful.* In some circumstances (e.g., potential intrauterine growth retardation, potential macrosomia) *serial interval examinations* are helpful in diagnosis and management. More specialized *(targeted) sonography* is useful in evaluation of potential fetal defects.

Early (<20 weeks) ultrasonographic measurements of the fetal BPD, AC, CRL, FL, or total uterine volume have been correlated accurately with gestational age. Fetal growth between 20 and 30 weeks is rapid and linear, and there is marked third trimester variability in fetal size (as noted previously). Hence, initial measurements should be taken and recorded as early as possible with subsequent later determinations. A comparison of these diameters with standard curves can estimate the gestational age ±11 days with 95% confidence. When only one measurement is possible or when initial measurements are obtained after the 30th week, accuracy is reduced.

PRENATAL CARE

Prenatal care, the management of pregnancy, *has numerous purposes.*

- To ensure, as far as possible, an uncomplicated pregnancy and the delivery of a live healthy infant.
- To identify and institute care for any risk state.
- To individualize the level of care necessary.
- To assist the gravida in her preparation for labor, delivery, and childrearing.
- To screen for common diseases that may affect the gravida's or child's life or health.
- To reinforce good health habits for the gravida and her family.

To achieve these, admittedly, ideal goals require an *organized and thoughtful approach.* Indeed, to be maximally effective, *prenatal care begins before conception.* Although not the only way to provide prenatal care, the following is intended as a guide or functional method that has assisted in fulfilling the stated purposes.

Standard record forms are commercially available. These, completed with explanations when indicated, will amass most of the necessary information. Thus, it is important to identify those data that should be recorded.

GENERAL INFORMATION

Record the patient's correct name, address, birth date, telephone number(s), choice of whom to call in an emergency, and special personal preferences.

TABLE 5-5
EMBRYONIC AND FETAL GROWTH AND DEVELOPMENT

Fertilization Age (Weeks)	Crown-rump Length*	Crown-heel Length*	Weight*	Gross Appearance	Internal Development
Embryonic stage					
1	0.5 mm	0.5 mm	—	Minute clone free in uterus	Early morula, no organ differentiation
2	2 mm	2 mm	—	Ovoid vesicle superficially buried in endometrium	External trophoblast, flat embryonic disk forming 2 inner vesicles (amnioectomesodermal and endodermal)
3	3 mm	3 mm	—	Early dorsal concavity changes to convexity; head, tail folds form; neural grooves close partially	Optic vesicles appear, double heart recognized, fourteen mesodermal somites present

(Continued)

123

TABLE 5-5
(*Continued*)

Fertilization Age (Weeks)	Crown-rump Length*	Crown-heel Length*	Weight*	Gross Appearance	Internal Development
4	4 mm	4 mm	0.4 g	Head is at right angle to body; limb rudiments obvious, tail prominent	Vitelline duct only communication between umbilical vesicle and intestines, initial stage of most organs has begun
8	1.7 cm	3.5 cm	2 g	Eyes, ears, nose, mouth recognizable, digits formed, tail almost gone	Sensory organ development well along, ossification beginning in occiput, mandible, humerus (diaphysis), and clavicles, small intestines coil within umbilical cord, pleural, pericardial cavities forming, gonadal development advanced without differentiation
Fetal stage 12	5.8 cm	11.5 cm	19 g	Skin pink, delicate, resembles a human	Brain configuration roughly complete, internal sex organs now

16	13.5 cm	19 cm	100 g	being, but head is disproportionately large Scalp hair appears, fetus active, arm–leg ratio now proportionate, gender determination possible	specific, uterus no longer bicornuate, blood forming in marrow, upper cervical to lower sacral arches and bodies ossify Sex organs grossly formed, myelinization, heart muscle well developed, lobulated kidneys in final situation, meconium in bowel, vagina and anus open, ischium ossified
20	18.5 cm	22 cm	300 g	Legs lengthen appreciably, distance from umbilicus to pubis increases	Sternum ossifies
24	23 cm	32 cm	600 g	Skin reddish and wrinkled, slight subcuticular fat, vernix, primitive respiratory-like movements	Os pubis (horizontal ramus) ossifies, viability possible

(Continued)

125

TABLE 5-5
(Continued)

Fertilization Age (Weeks)	Crown-rump Length*	Crown-heel Length*	Weight*	Gross Appearance	Internal Development
28	27 cm	36 cm	1100 g	Skin less wrinkled; more fat, nails appear, if delivered, may survive with optimal care	Testes at internal inguinal ring or below, astragalus ossifies
32	31 cm	41 cm	1800 g	Fetal weight increased proportionately more than length	Middle fourth phalanges ossify
36	35 cm	46 cm	2500 g (for Caucasian)	Skin pale, body rounded, lanugo disappearing, hair fuzzy or wooly, earlobes soft with little cartilage, umbilicus in center of body, scrotum small with few rugae, few sole creases	Distal femoral ossification centers present

126

| 40 | 40 cm | 52 cm | 3200+ g | Skin smooth and pink, copious vernix, moderate to profuse silky hair, lanugo hair on shoulders and upper back, earlobes stiffened by thick cartilage, nasal and alar cartilages, nails extend over tips of digits, testes in full, pendulous, rugous scrotum, or labia majora well developed, creases cover sole | Proximal tibial ossification centers present, cuboid, tibia (proximal epiphysis) ossify |

* Approximate.

HISTORY AND PHYSICAL EXAMINATION

A *complete medical history and physical examination* early in pregnancy provides the baseline for diagnosis and the treatment of disorders that may compromise pregnancy.

HISTORY OF PRESENT PREGNANCY

Obtain the last menstrual period (*LMP*) and previous menstrual period (*PMP*). Then, *calculate the EDC.* Additionally, note the following:

- Current symptoms, signs, and problems
- Any infections, medications, injuries, potential exposure to fetotoxic hazards, especially those occurring during the present pregnancy
- Menstrual history
    Age at menarche
    Interval between periods
    Duration, amount of flow, intermenstrual spotting
    Dysmenorrhea
    Leukorrhea
- Contraception: method, duration, acceptance, or reason for termination

HISTORY OF PREVIOUS PREGNANCIES

For *each gestation,* record *duration, type termination, complications, outcome, and follow-up.* In those pregnancies resulting in a *living child* (LC), determine the sex and current well being and attempt to assess the mother's attitude toward each child. The individual's reproductive history usually is recorded using the following definitions.

Gravidity (G) is the total number of pregnancies, including normal and abnormal intrauterine pregnancies, abortions, ectopic pregnancies, and hydatidiform moles. Multiple pregnancies are counted as a single experience.

Parity (P) is the birth of a >500 g infant or infants, alive or dead. When the weight is not known, use ≥24 weeks gestation. Multiple gestation is again counted as a single occurrence. A nullipara has not delivered an offspring weighing >500 g or of ≥24 weeks gestation.

Abortion (A) is pregnancy that terminates <24th gestational week or in which the fetus weighs <500 g.

Living child or children (LC) expresses the successful outcome of pregnancy.

By convention, this may be written G (number), P (number), A (number), LC (number), or further abbreviated to a series of numbers in the order given.

MEDICAL AND SURGICAL HISTORY

Record all *allergies* and *drug sensitivities, medications, important illnesses,* and *blood transfusions.*

List (with dates) all *operations* and serious *injuries* and outcomes. Detailed *fertility studies* should be included. Regarding cesarean deliveries, note the type (with particular attention to *documentation of the uterine incision*), indications, trial of labor, and special surgical problems or postoperative complications.

FAMILY HISTORY

List *medical, genetic,* and *psychiatric disorders* that may affect the patient or her offspring (e.g., diabetes mellitus, cancer, and mental disease). A three-generation pedigree is often revealing.

PATIENT'S ATTITUDES

Note *reservations or preferences as well as fears* manifested by the patient. Is this a wanted pregnancy? Exploring the following areas often will elicit information: her comfort with the pregnancy, prenatal care, early labor care, personal support during labor and delivery, analgesia, anesthesia, delivery, operative intervention, immediate postpartum care for the baby, other hospitalizations, and her response to having a baby.

Estimate the patient's maturity and general emotional stability to assist in *individualizing care.* Is she uncertain or confident?

PHYSICAL EXAMINATION

Conduct a *complete general examination* with special *emphasis on the reproductive organs and systems* most influenced by pregnancy. Examination of the head, ears, eyes, nose, and throat should be recorded. Careful *auscultation of the heart and lungs is* mandatory. Serious diseases often are first noted during an obstetric physical examination (e.g., anemia, tuberculosis, and breast tumors), thus thoroughness is important. The assessment emphasizes the following.

GENERAL EXAMINATION

Record the *vital signs* including the blood pressure (BP), pulse, and respiration. Note *weight, height, body build,* and *state of nutrition.* Assess the following.

Skin and hair. Metabolic disorders (e.g., hypothyroidism) often are first manifested by dermatologic changes.

Mouth. Evaluate oral hygiene and check for epulis. (Encourage the patient to see her dentist for prophylaxis.)

Neck. Check for abnormal masses or lymphadenopathy. Expect slight diffuse physiologic enlargement of the thyroid gland in about 60% of pregnant patients.

Breast. Conduct a careful breast examination. Special attention should be afforded the nipples. This is a good time to initiate a discussion about breastfeeding. The patient should be reminded to continue her monthly breast self-examinations.

Abdomen. Especially consider the following.

The contour, height (centimeters above the symphysis pubis), and consistency of the uterine fundus and its relationship to other organs or landmarks. Record the location of the fetal heart and its rate.

Abdominal organs that are palpable should be identified and abnormalities or extraneous masses identified. These include hernias (umbilical, inguinal, femoral, and lumbar). Hernias often become larger during pregnancy.

Extremities. Note development, deformity, and restriction of movement of legs, arms, and back. Varicosities and edema must be explained and treated if necessary.

Posture and body mechanics should be noted.

Pelvic Examination

A stepwise pelvic examination can be performed at any time before term but may be especially meaningful early (e.g., uterine size vs. calculated gestational age). Pay particular attention to the following:

Vulvar and vaginal varicosities. These may bleed at delivery.

Cervix and uterus. Examine as described in Chapter 16. Near term, it is essential to note cervical consistency, position, and degree of effacement and dilatation. Record the site and extent of previous lacerations of the cervix because tears may recur at these sites during delivery.

Pelvic masses. Distinguish between ovarian and other pelvic or retroperitoneal tumors. In many cases, ultrasonic scan will be useful.

Pelvic measurements. In most cases, clinical appraisal and recording of the pelvic configuration and major diameters by an experienced physician are adequate. If a pelvis is thought to be contracted, careful note of this should be made for a later evaluation. Clinical measurements necessary for an estimate of the pelvic outlet and inlet diameters are the following.

Biischial diameter (BI) (*normal ≥8 cm*) is the distance between the inner margins of the ischial tuberosities, and this constitutes the hypotenuse of the anterior pudendal triangle. The actual distance between the bony margins is usually >11 cm. When measured through the soft tissues, however, a normal value is ≥8 cm. This is known also as the transverse diameter of the outlet or the bituberous, intertuberous (IT), or tuberischial (TI) diameter.

Posterior sagittal diameter of the outlet (PS) (*normal 8–9.5 cm*). The PS is the distance from the midpoint of the line between the ischial tuberosities to the external surface of the tip of the sacrum (the tip of the rectal finger). This measurement is taken directly with the rectal finger touching the sacrococcygeal joint while visualizing the ischial intertuberous diameter.

Thoms's or Klein's rule: When the sum of the BI and the PS is more than 15 cm, an infant of normal size usually will pass the outlet safely.

Anteroposterior diameter of the outlet (AP) (*normal ≥11.9 cm*). This is the distance from the inferior border of the symphysis to the posterior aspect of the tip of the sacrum.

Interspinous diameter of the midpelvis (*normal ≥10.5*). *This important measurement has a lower limit of 9.5 cm for passage of an average-sized infant. A reduced interspinous diameter is the most common cause of midpelvic dystocia.*

Diagonal conjugate of the inlet (DC) (*normal >11.5 cm*) is probably the most important single measurement of the pelvis. It is from the inner inferior border of the symphysis to the midpoint of the sacral promontory (or false promontory, whichever is shorter) (Fig. 5-6). The true conjugate (conjugate vera, CV) is the distance from the anterior midpoint of the sacral or false promontory to the superior margin of the symphysis in the midline. This is calculated to be 1.5 cm shorter than the DC and represents the actual

FIGURE 5-6. Pelvic measurements.

available anteroposterior diameter of the inlet. A *DC of ≤11.5 cm or a CV of <10 cm indicates contracture of the pelvic inlet* or superior strait. The likelihood of dystocia, assuming an average-sized infant, in inversely proportional to this measurement. Significant contracture of pelvic anterior-posterior diameter often is signaled by a term gestation that has failed to engage.

Palpation

Pubic arch. Trace the pubic arch with the examining fingers. The angle formed by the pubic arch (the angle of the rami at the pubis) is *usually 110–120 degrees.* In an android pelvis, the *angle is narrow (<90 degrees),* and the BI is narrow.

Spines of the ischium. Consider the *degree of prominence, sharpness,* and extent of encroachment of the spines into the birth canal.

Sacrum. The *contour, depth, and irregularities* (e.g., false promontory) are important. Record the curvature as hollow (*deep*), average (*normally capacious*), and flat (*shallow*), and record any irregularity.

Coccyx. By grasping the coccyx between the fingers of the examining hand, with the other hand placed in the cleft between the buttocks, the direction of the coccyx, its degree of movement at the sacrococcygeal articulation, and local tenderness may be determined.

Sacrosciatic notch (*normal <3 cm*). The width of this space should be estimated and recorded in centimeters, not imprecise fingerbreadths.

Rectal Examination
Identify hemorrhoids and fissures.

DIAGNOSIS

Record the duration of pregnancy and any anticipated complications.

PROGNOSIS

Record an initial prediction of the EDC and outcome of the pregnancy (vaginal or cesarean delivery) together with the likelihood of medical or surgical complications (e.g., diabetes mellitus, inguinal hernia). The prognosis must be altered if obstetric problems develop.

PLAN AND TREATMENT

Project the care necessary for this gravida and pregnancy. A model program is noted under "Management of Normal Pregnancy."

PROCEDURES AT FIRST OBSTETRIC VISIT

After the history has been taken and the physical examination has been performed:

- Answer questions.
- Supply written prenatal care instructions, an explanatory booklet, or library references. Ask the patient and her partner to read them carefully before the next visit.

- Prescribe necessary medications.
- Arrange an appointment for the first return visit.
- Request the patient to bring a first-voided urine specimen at each subsequent visit.
- Order laboratory tests.
- Explain the costs of care.

LABORATORY TESTS

Obviously, laboratory tests must be individualized for each patient. The following is a list of commonly ordered tests for a normal gravida. They should be *done as early as possible, and certain tests (*) should be repeated* at 24–28 and 32–36 weeks gestation.

- Hemoglobin and hematocrit*, white blood cell count (WBC) with differential count.
- Serologic test for syphilis (STS or VDRL).
- Blood group and Rh factor (unsensitized Rh-negative gravidas should have another antibody determination after the 12th and after the 24th week to reveal isoimmunization).
- Antibody screening test* (a pooled series of about 29 antigens is used to detect the most common sensitizations).
- Rubella antibody test (need not repeat if immune).
- Serum alpha-fetoprotein (AFP) determination or an alternative birth defect screening (see p. 118) should be obtained at 16–18 weeks gestation when it is most accurate for detection of neural tube defects.
- Urinalysis, urine culture (if positive, obtain bacterial sensitivity to antibiotics).
- Papanicolaou (Pap) smears.
- Cervical culture for *Neisseria gonorrhoeae* (and proper screening for other suspected sexually transmitted diseases).
- All African American patients should be screened for sickle cell trait or disease (usually either a blood screening test or hemoglobin electrophoresis).

At this time, the use of certain other tests for screening remains controversial. Thus, in each case, the following should also be considered and discussed as part of the initial assessment: ultrasonic scan for screening and dating gestation (usually <20 weeks), human immunodeficiency virus (HIV) screening, hepatitis B surface antigen screening, titers for *Toxoplasma gondii,* 1 h blood glucose following 50 g glucose load, tuberculin skin testing, and culture for beta-streptococci (later in gestation).

MANAGEMENT OF NORMAL PREGNANCY

PRENATAL OFFICE VISITS AND EXAMINATIONS

Plan to see the patient once a month until the 32nd week, every 2 weeks until the 36th week, and weekly thereafter until delivery. See her more often if complications arise.

ESSENTIAL PROCEDURES AT EACH VISIT

From the initial office visit until delivery, *a continuing record of the progress of the pregnancy must be maintained.* Include symptoms, signs, habits, contacts or exposures to illnesses, medications, and laboratory test results. Additionally, the following constitute the usual structure of antenatal visits.

- Ask the patient about her general health and any complaints.
- Weigh the gravida and record her weight on the prenatal chart. Evaluate weight changes in comparison with the average curve.
- Record the patient's blood pressure.
- Examine a urine sample for protein and glucose. If significant glycosuria develops ($\geq 2+$), screen for carbohydrate intolerance. Screening consists of a 50 g oral glucose load and a 1-h blood sugar or fasting blood glucose and a 2-h postprandial blood glucose determination. If these tests are abnormal, order a glucose tolerance test (GTT).

  Repeated $>1+$ proteinuria or urinary symptoms will necessitate a clean-catch specimen for culture and microscope study. If the bacterial count is $>100,000/mL$, prescribe appropriate antibiotics. Plan a repeat urine culture 1 week after the conclusion of treatment and again if symptomatology recurs. If the count is $<100,000$ mL, obtain a 24-h urine sample for volume, creatinine clearance, and total protein determination to diagnose possible renal disease.
- Palpate the abdomen. Measure and note the height of the uterus above the symphysis. Record the fetal heartbeat and any abnormal details. After the 28th week, determine the presentation of the fetus. From the 32nd week on, in addition to these measures, record the position of the fetus, the

engagement of the presenting part, and an estimate of the weight of the fetus.

- Rectal or vaginal examinations may be done at virtually any time (in the absence of bleeding) to confirm the presenting part, establish its station, and determine the status of the cervix.

- When the EDC, calculated from the LMP, is not supported by the physical findings, employ ultrasonography for abnormal fetal development, gestational age, or growth retardation. Ultrasonography is the obstetrician's major modality in gestational age assessment. Moreover, ultrasonography can be used to evaluate patients with uncertain dates and when the fetus seems too large (due to wrong dates, multiple gestations, hydramnios, macrosomia, associated uterine, or pelvic masses) or too small (wrong dates, oligohydramnios, or IUGR). Ultrasonography can aid also in the diagnosis of patients with first trimester bleeding due to ectopic pregnancy, missed abortion, blighted ovum, subchorionic hemorrhage, or hydatidiform mole or third trimester bleeding due to placenta previa, abruptio placentae, or fetal anomalies (e.g., limb defects, neural tube anomalies).

TERM PREGNANCY

Term or fetal maturity at 37–40 weeks is that period in which *the neonate has the maximal likelihood of survival.* Term, a period rather than a day or even a week, is based on the EDC as well as other indices of fetal growth and development.

Full term (ideal maturity) is reached at 40 weeks gestation. The chance for survival then is about 99%. When there are discrepancies in the dates, other observations will be required to diagnose term, or full-term, states.

The fetus at term should weigh >2500 g, with the following approximate measurements: crown-rump 32 cm, crown-heel 47 cm, head circumference 33 cm, thoracic circumference 30 cm, occipital-frontal diameter 11.75 cm, and biparietal diameter 8.25 cm. Numerous determinants other than these measurements are required for a decision regarding age or maturity (see Chapter 8).

CLINICAL FINDINGS
AND CERVICAL CHANGES

In early pregnancy, the cervix usually is directed posteriorly in the vagina. As term approaches, the cervix becomes *soft* and *moves anteriorly* into the vaginal axis. Normally, term has been reached when this and *marked effacement and dilatation of 1–2 cm* have occurred. Cervical effacement in primigravidas begins about the 36th week and is almost complete some 2 weeks later. Multiparas rarely achieve total effacement before labor, despite dilatation.

ENGAGEMENT (LIGHTENING)

When the fetal head descends into the pelvis so that the *biparietal diameter is at or (more convincingly) slightly below the brim of the true pelvis (station 0 to 2+),* it is termed engaged. Engagement in a primigravida precedes delivery by about 2 weeks. Multiparous patients often go into labor before engagement, but if early engagement occurs, term probably has been reached.

NUTRITION IN PREGNANCY

DIETARY REQUIREMENTS

Good maternal nutrition is a major determinant of normal fetal growth and development. The daily dietary allowances recommended by the Food and Nutrition Board of the National Academy of Sciences-National Research Council are listed in Table 5-6. These should be considered approximations because adult patients who are ill or underweight, as well as adolescents who have not completed their growth, will require larger allowances.

Generally it is recommended that the pregnant patient have 36–38 cal/kg/day. A normal pregnancy diet should include the following daily components (or equivalents): 1 liter (or 1 quart) milk, one average serving of citrus fruit or tomato, a leafy green vegetable, and a yellow vegetable, and two average servings of lean meat, fish, poultry, eggs, beans, or cheese.

SUPPLEMENTAL MINERAL AND VITAMINS

Calcium must be supplemented during pregnancy to meet fetal needs and preserve maternal calcium stores. Milk is relatively inexpensive, and 1 liter (or 1 quart) of cow's milk contains 1 g of calcium, approximately the daily intake recommended during pregnancy (1.2 g) and 33 g of protein. The milk need not always be in beverage form. It can be used in the preparation of foods, such as soup, custard, or junket. If the patient cannot or will not drink whole milk,

TABLE 5-6
RECOMMENDED DAILY DIETARY ALLOWANCE FOR
WOMEN 18–50 YEARS OLD, 64 INCHES TALL, AND
WEIGHING 120 POUNDS WHEN NOT PREGNANT*

| Nutrient | Nonpregnant | Increase | |
		Pregnant	Lactating
Calories (cal)	2000	+300	+500
Protein (g)	44	+30	+20
Vitamin A (RE)[†]	800	+200	+400
Vitamin D (IU)	200	+200	+200
Vitamin E (mg α-TE)[‡]	8	+2	+3
Vitamin C (mg)	60	+20	+40
Folacin (μg)[§]	400	+400	+100
Niacin (mg NE)[‖]	14	+2	+5
Thiamine (mg)	1.1	+0.4	+0.5
Riboflavin (mg)	1.3	+0.3	+0.5
Vitamin B_6 (mg)	2	+0.6	+0.5
Vitamin B_{12} (μg)	3	+1	+1
Calcium (mg)	800	+400	+400
Phosphorus (mg)	800	+400	+400
Iodine (μg)	150	+25	+50
Iron (mg)	18	+30–60	+30–60
Magnesium (mg)	300	+150	+150
Zinc (mg)	15	+5	+10

* Food and Nutrition Board, National Academy of Science–National Research Council, Revised 1980.

† Retinol equivalents. 1 RE = 1 μg retinol or 6 μg β-carotene.

‡ α-Tocopherol equivalents. 1 α-TE = 1 mg α-tocopherol.

§ Refers to dietary sources as determined by *Lactobacillus casei* assay after treatment with enzymes to make polyglutamyl forms of the vitamin available to the test organism.

‖ Niacin equivalents. 1 NE = 1 mg niacin or 60 mg dietary tryptophan.

substitute sources of calcium (e.g., citrus juice, yogurt, and powdered milk) or prescribe a supplement (e.g., calcium carbonate).

Although ample calcium and phosphorus are required by the mother for fetal anabolism, *a relative excess of phosphorus may cause leg cramps.* Large quantities of milk, meat, cheese, and dicalcium phosphate (taken as a supplement) may impose excessive phosphorus.

Some patients, especially Native Americans, foreign-born African Americans, or certain Asians, may have a disaccharidase deficiency causing *intolerance to lactose in milk*. For these persons, *protein, calcium, and vitamins must be supplied in other forms* (e.g., fish, fruits).

Supplemental iron is needed during pregnancy for the fetus and to prevent depletion of the maternal iron stores, especially during the latter part of pregnancy. Iron is the only mineral that usually must be prescribed (i.e., *30–60 mg elemental iron* or *ferrous sulfate 300 mg bid*). Equivalents (*ferrous gluconate or fumerate*) may be better tolerated.

A pregnant woman who consumes adequate quantities of properly prepared fresh foods needs no other vitamin or mineral supplements, but many women do not eat enough vitamin-containing foods. To make certain that the vitamin intake is adequate, the common practice of *recommending prenatal vitamin supplements* is not harmful in the doses usually prescribed. *Massive doses of any vitamin or vitamin compound should be avoided.* For example, excessive ingestion of vitamins D and A may be fetotoxic.

Patients who do not eat well may benefit from folate supplements. Folic acid (folacin), 0.8 mg/day orally, may be a beneficial dietary supplement for most gravidas. Moreover, routine folate treatment will not harm a pregnant woman with unrecognized pernicious anemia.

SALT RESTRICTION

The requirement for sodium during pregnancy is increased slightly. In any case, *overemphasis on salt restriction is unjustified.*

FLUIDS

At least *2–3 quarts* of fluid should be taken daily during pregnancy to accommodate metabolic processes and aid in elimination. Limitation of fluids will neither prevent nor correct fluid retention. *Liquids containing no sodium will not contribute to edema* in the absence of renal failure. Actually, increased intake of water aids slightly in the excretion of sodium and extracellular fluid.

WEIGHT GAIN

The mother's prepregnancy weight and her weight gain during pregnancy are major determinants in the birth weight of the infant. Women of low weight (e.g., <55 kg) before pregnancy who gain a limited amount of weight (<4500 g) during pregnancy have a higher incidence of low-birth-weight neonates than heavier mothers who gain more weight during pregnancy.

FIGURE 5-7. The cumulative energy costs of pregnancy.

(From F.E. Hytten and I. Leitch. *The Physiology of Human Pregnancy,* 2nd ed. Blackwell Scientific Publications, 1971.)

Cumulative energy costs of pregnancy are shown in Figure 5-7. The gravida of average weight requires approximately *2300–2600 cal/day* during pregnancy to assure the average weight gain of *11.5–12.5 kg (25–28 pounds)* total, whereas the underweight woman, the woman with an SGA fetus, and the woman with a multiple gestation should be encouraged to gain as much weight as possible. In general, younger primigravidas should have more calories than older multiparas. How much weight should be gained during pregnancy by the obese woman is still debated. In general, there is a great variability of weight gain without apparent harm.

The *gain should be almost linear during the second and third trimesters* with an average of about 0.4 kg/week. This should equate to an approximate gain of 0.65 kg by 10 weeks, 4 kg by 20 weeks, 8.5 kg by 30 weeks, and 12.5 kg by 40 weeks. Note that the *maternal weight gain during the first trimester is small* and fetal gain is minimal. During the second trimester, maternal storage of fat, growth of the uterus and breasts, together with an expansion of the blood volume, represent the major components of the gain. During the third trimester, growth of the fetus and placenta and accumulation of amniotic fluid contribute most to the total weight gain but with little maternal weight accumulation.

Extremes are important too (i.e., patients who gain 10 kg in the first 3 months must not drastically limit future gain to, say, only 2 kg). Similarly, obese women should not attempt to reduce during pregnancy or lactation. This leads to nutritional deficiencies, poor use of protein, and excessive catabolism of fat, causing ketosis and acetonuria. Moreover, an underweight patient who is seen for the first time during the last trimester should not overeat to catch up to her "best weight" at term.

Moderate weight gain is associated with the lowest incidence of low-birth-weight infants and neonatal death. The underweight woman with a small gain in weight during pregnancy should be considered a high-risk patient. Women who gain excessive weight have the usual problems of obesity. Individualization of diet seems the best course of action. *Emphasis should be placed on good nutrition rather than on precise weight control.*

There is no convincing evidence that excessive weight gain causes preeclampsia-eclampsia, but obese gravidas are more likely to have orthopedic problems or postpartum hemorrhage, and their infants are more likely to be macrosomic. The rate of weight gain is important in the diagnosis of preeclampsia-eclampsia. An increase of ≥1814 g (4 pounds) during any 1–2 week period from 24–35 weeks gestation or ≥0.9 kg (2 lb) per week from 35 weeks to term will often presage preeclampsia-eclampsia. There has been a marked decline in the incidence of preeclampsia-eclampsia in the United States, and it seems likely that better nutrition may account for at least part of this improvement.

Vegetarians who include dairy products probably will meet their dietary need during pregnancy. However, those with major restrictions (including milk or eggs) probably will need supplements of iron, folic acid, zinc, and vitamin B_{12}.

Teenage gravidas or those with diabetes mellitus or renal disease require special diets. Dietary needs often become apparent during the initial antenatal examination of the skin, nails, hair, mouth, teeth, and musculoskeletal system.

The provider will be more successful as a nutrition counselor if emphasis is placed on *what should be eaten* rather than what should not be eaten.

MINOR DISCOMFORTS
OF NORMAL PREGNANCY

NAUSEA AND VOMITING
(MORNING SICKNESS)

About *half of all pregnant women have nausea and vomiting,* often on arising, at some time during pregnancy. This most commonly occurs during the *first 10 weeks, seemingly related to higher levels of hCG.* About 1/1000 gravidas with severe morning sickness develop intractable vomiting (hyperemesis gravidarum, pernicious vomiting of pregnancy). In such cases, a psychiatric consultation may be most useful. Hospitalization may be necessary to correct fluid and electrolyte imbalance, to remove the gravida from a stressful environment, or for study. In these severe cases, weight, nitrogen balance, liver enzymes, and fetal growth must be rigorously monitored. The addition of IV vitamins decreases the possibility of hypovitaminosis.

Usually, explanation, reassurance, and symptomatic relief are sufficient. Dietary changes are often helpful. Eating dry toast and jelly immediately on arising, before the nausea begins, helps some patients. Avoidance of disagreeable odors and rich, spicy, or greasy foods is important. Urge the gravida to drink water or other fluids between meals to avoid dehydration and acidosis, which predispose to nausea.

Antinauseants harmless for a nonpregnant woman may have unforeseen or undesirable effects on the fetus. Therefore, during pregnancy, even well-known over-the-counter drugs should be administered only when absolutely indicated and prescribed.

BACKACHE

Virtually all women suffer from at least minor degrees of lumbar backache during pregnancy. Fatigue, muscle spasm, or postural back strain most often is responsible. Relaxation of the pelvic joints from the action of steroid sex hormones or perhaps relaxin also is responsible. Backache often can be relieved by the following measures.

- *Improvement in posture* is often achieved by the wearing of low-heeled shoes. To achieve proper posture, the abdomen should be flattened, the pelvis tilted forward, and the buttocks tucked under to straighten the back.
- *Prescribe back exercises* under the supervision of a rehabilitation physician, an orthopedist, or a physical therapist.
- *Recommend sleep on a firm mattress.*
- *Apply local heat and light massage* to relax tense, taut back muscles.
- Give *acetaminophen* 0.3–0.6 g orally or equivalent.
- Obtain *orthopedic consultation* if disability results. Note neurological signs and symptoms indicative of prolapsed intervertebral disk syndrome, radiculitis.

HEARTBURN

Heartburn (pyrosis, acid indigestion) results from gastroesophageal reflux disease (GERD) in almost *10% of all gravidas.* In late pregnancy, this may be aggravated by displacement of the stomach and duodenum by the uterine fundus. Heartburn is most likely to occur when the patient is lying down or bending over. Occasional patients experience severe pyrosis during late pregnancy because of a hiatal hernia. This hernia is reduced spontaneously by parturition. *Symptomatic treatment,* not surgery, is recommended.

Hot tea and change of posture are helpful. Calcium-containing antacids (e.g., Tums) to reduce gastric irritation often are beneficial. Aluminum-based antacids are less desirable. While the histamine H_2-receptor antagonists are pregnancy category B, they may prove useful in resistant cases.

SYNCOPE AND FAINTNESS

Syncope and faintness are *common in early pregnancy because of vasomotor instability* (largely progesterone-related relaxation of vascular smooth muscle). Encourage the patient to eat six small meals a day rather than three large ones. Stimulants (spirits of ammonia, coffee, tea) are indicated for attacks due to postural hypotension.

LEUKORRHEA

A *gradual increase* in the amount of nonirritating vaginal discharge due to estrogen stimulation of cervical mucus is normal during pregnancy. Such vaginal fluid is milky, thin, and nonirritating unless infection has occurred. Persistent external moisture due to mucus may cause mild pruritus, but itching is rarely severe without infection. Reassure the patient, and suggest protective perineal pads. Excessive leukorrhea accompanied by pruritus or discoloration of the secretion may indicate bleeding or infection, requiring treatment.

URINARY SYMPTOMS

Urinary frequency, urgency, and stress incontinence in multiparas are common, especially in advanced pregnancy. These symptoms usually are due to increased intraabdominal pressure and reduced bladder capacity. Suspect urinary tract disease if dysuria or hematuria is present.

When urgency is particularly troublesome, limit caffeine, spices, and popular beverages. An 8 oz glass of cranberry juice assists in both maintaining urinary acidity as well as decreasing urinary tract infections.

BREATHLESSNESS

Breathlessness, not actual dyspnea, *is a progesterone effect.* In nonsmokers and others free of cough or allergic problems, breathlessness occurs as early as the 12th week of pregnancy, and most women have this symptom by the 30th week. There is no effective treatment.

CONSTIPATION

Constipation due to sluggish bowel function in pregnancy may be due to progesterone effect and bowel displacement. Emphasize *ample fluids and laxative foods and prescribe a stool softener* (e.g., bran or dactyl sodium sulfosuccinate). Exercise and good bowel habits are helpful. Mild laxatives (e.g., milk of magnesia) are acceptable, but purgatives should be avoided because of the possibility of inducing labor. Mineral oil is contraindicated because it absorbs fat-soluble vitamins from the bowel and leaks from the anus.

HEMORRHOIDS

Hemorrhoids, frequent in pregnancy, may cause considerable discomfort. Straining at stool often causes hemorrhoids, especially in women prone to varicosities. *Symptomatic therapy* (hemorrhoidal preparations) is usually sufficient. *Treat constipation early.* At delivery, use elective low forceps with episiotomy when feasible. Surgical treatment rarely is indicated during pregnancy. However, very recently thrombosed, painful hemorrhoids can be incised and evacuated under local anesthesia. Do not suture. Sitz baths, rectal ointments, suppositories, and mild laxatives are indicated postoperatively or postdelivery. Injection treatments to obliterate hemorrhoids during pregnancy are contraindicated. They may cause infection or thrombosis of pelvic veins and are rarely successful because of the great dilatation of many vessels.

HEADACHE

Headache in pregnancy is common and usually due to tension. Refractive errors and ocular imbalance are not caused by normal pregnancy. *Severe, persistent headache in the third trimester must be regarded as symptomatic of preeclampsia-eclampsia until proven otherwise.*

ANKLE SWELLING

Edema of the lower extremities (not associated with preeclampsia-eclampsia) *develops in at least two thirds of women* in late pregnancy. Edema is due to water retention and increased venous pressure in the legs. Generalized edema, always serious, must be investigated.

Treatment is largely preventive and symptomatic. The patient should elevate her legs frequently. Restrict excessive salt intake and provide elastic support for varicose veins. Diuretics may reduce edema temporarily but may be harmful to the mother or fetus.

VARICOSE VEINS

Varicosities can develop in the legs or in the vulva. Varices are due to smooth muscle relaxation, weakness of the vascular walls, and incompetent valves. Pressure on the venous return from the legs by the enlarging uterus also is a major factor in the development of varicosities. Large or numerous varicosities are associated with muscle aching, edema, skin ulcers, and emboli.

The patient should *elevate her legs* above the level of her body and control excessive weight gain. *Avoid forceful massage* (especially downward, i.e., against venous return) *and point-pressure* over the legs.

Patients with significant varices should be fitted with elastic stretch stockings. Large vulvar varices cause pudendal discomfort. A vulvar pad snugly held by a menstrual belt may give relief. In more severe leg or vulvar varicosities, however, a Jobst-type leotard garment may be necessary to obtain venous compression. Injection or surgical correction of varicose veins usually is not recommended during pregnancy.

LEG CRAMPS

Cramping of the muscles of the calf, thigh, or buttocks can occur suddenly after sleep or recumbency in many women after the first trimester of pregnancy. Sudden shortening of the leg muscles by stretching with the toes pointed often precipitates the cramp. Leg cramps may be due to a reduced level of diffusible serum calcium or an increased serum phosphorus level. Symptomatology follows excessive dietary intake of phosphorus in milk, cheese, meat, or calcium phosphate or diminished intake or impaired absorption of calcium. However, fatigue or diminished circulation may be contributing factors.

Treatment should include curtailment of phosphate intake (less milk and nutritional supplements containing calcium phosphate) and increased calcium intake (without phosphorus) as calcium carbonate or calcium lactate. Aluminum hydroxide gel, 8 mL orally tid before meals, absorbs phosphate. Symptomatic treatment consists of leg massage, gentle flexing of the feet, and local heat.

ABDOMINAL DISCOMFORT

Intraabdominal alterations causing distress during pregnancy include the following.

Pressure, pelvic heaviness, is caused by the weight of the uterus on the pelvic supports and the abdominal wall. The patient should rest frequently, preferably in the lateral recumbent position.

Round ligament tension, tenderness along the course of the round ligament (usually the left) during late pregnancy, is due to traction on this structure by the uterus, which is displaced by the large bowel to be rotated slightly to the right. Local heat and change of position are beneficial.

Flatulence and distention can be due to large meals, gas-forming foods, and chilled beverages. These are poorly tolerated by pregnant women. Mechanical displacement and compression of the bowel by the enlarged uterus, hypotonia of the intestines, and constipation predispose to gastrointestinal disorders. Dietary modifications often give effective relief. Regular bowel function should be maintained, and exercise is beneficial.

Uterine contractions, so-called Braxton Hicks contractions, of the uterus may be sharply painful and vexing. The onset of premature labor must always be considered when forceful, regular, extended contractions develop. If contractions remain infrequent and brief in duration, the danger of early delivery is not significant. Acetaminophen 0.3–0.6, 2–3 times daily may be of value.

Intraabdominal disorders causing pain may be due to obstruction, inflammation, and other disorders of the gastrointestinal, urinary, neurologic, or vascular system or to pathologic pregnancy or tubal or ovarian disease. These disorders must be diagnosed and treated appropriately.

FATIGUE

The pregnant patient is more subject to fatigue during the last trimester of pregnancy because of altered posture and extra weight carried. Anemia and other systemic diseases must be ruled out. *Frequent rest periods are recommended.*

COMMON PREGNANCY CONCERNS

MEDICATIONS

Discourage the use of drugs in pregnancy because of potential fetal effects. In general, give medication only when urgently required. Avoid new and experimental drugs and drugs that have been suggested as possible teratogens. Give medicaments, when needed, in the lowest dosage consistent with clinical efficacy. Record all pharmaceuticals, with doses and intervals when taken, during the pregnancy. Caution the patient about taking any preparation without first discussing it with the physician.

REST

A daily rest or nap for 1 h, preferably while lying on the side, is desirable. Eight hours of sleep at night is recommended.

SEXUAL INTERCOURSE

Sexuality continues during pregnancy, and in the normal gravida, *coitus has not been demonstrated to contribute to spontaneous abortion or premature labor.* Thus, coital restraints are neither necessary nor desirable. However, *contraindications to coitus include premature labor, rupture of the membranes, vaginal bleeding, incompetent cervix, threatened or habitual abortion, multiple pregnancy* (after the 28th week), *and genital herpes virus or other sexually transmitted infection.*

Douching is seldom necessary and may be harmful. Forceful douches, especially with a hand bulb syringe, may produce air or fluid embolism.

Provider explanation and questions and answers involving the patient and her partner are important.

EMPLOYMENT

Most women can continue to work during pregnancy. However, they should not be exposed to hazardous conditions or become seriously fatigued. Exactly how long the pregnant woman can safely remain on the job depends on the type of work, industrial hazards, the policy of the employer, and pregnancy complications. Women often work well beyond the 28th week of pregnancy without difficulty. Others whose employment requires more physical exertion may find it advisable to take maternity leave earlier. Rest periods during the day may help to avoid undue fatigue.

The capacity for work during pregnancy can be affected by weight increase, altered posture, modified physiology (e.g., cardiovascular, pulmonary, and renal), *urinary changes, or complications of pregnancy.* Fatigue may be responsible for increased tension or reduced concentration and alertness. Pregnancy complications rarely are caused by work itself, except when the gravida is exposed to trauma, toxic compounds, or laboratory pathogens. Indeed, the work site is usually safer than the home or recreational environments.

To achieve maximal care during pregnancy, the working gravida should report the pregnancy as soon as the diagnosis is made, and her obstetrician should assess (with the occupational medicine personnel) the potential impact of her employment on the pregnancy (and vice versa). This should be a part of the plan for her pregnancy. The employer should be notified of the plan and any complications or job modifications deemed necessary. The time to cease working must be individualized, but *most current U.S. guidelines recommend return to work 4–6 weeks after delivery.*

EXERCISE DURING PREGNANCY

Maintaining maternal physical fitness is most desirable during pregnancy. Women who have exercised regularly can withstand the work of labor with less alteration in fetal cord blood. However, *many variables determine how much exericise can be tolerated without fetal jeopardy* (e.g., reduced uterine blood flow, maternal hyperthermia, or fetal trauma).

During exercise, blood flow is diverted to the muscles and skin and away from the uterus. Unfortunately, the level of exercise associated with a serious decrease in uterine blood flow and how the fetus is affected is largely individually determined. For this reason, it may be useful to stress that women should train for, rather than during, pregnancy. Nonetheless, the obstetrician cannot (as yet) recommend a specific target maternal heart rate response to exercise because of great individual variation.

Before closure of the neural groove of the embryo, increased maternal core temperature augments the likelihood of neural tube defects (e.g., anencephaly, spina bifida). Later in pregnancy, thermal injuries may cause harm to the fetal thermoregulatory center. The critical levels of temperature and time have not been established. Even aerobic exercises during pregnancy can transiently raise the maternal temperature to 102°F. Moreover, dehydration increases the temperature rise during exercise. Hence, caution should be advised.

Although abdominal trauma during some exercise (e.g., aerobics) is less likely than with other contact sports, falls or other accidents may jeopardize the placenta or fetus.

In summary, the following recommendations for exercise in pregnancy seem reasonable.

- *Gravidas accustomed to moderate exercise before pregnancy may continue the program, but at a slower pace and for a shorter time* (i.e., limit exercise by one third, by term, in a linear decrease, in both rate and duration of the accustomed exercise).
- *Patients who were sedentary before pregnancy should restrict exercise to a moderate program* (e.g., walking or brief swimming).
- *Avoid fatigue.*
- *Do not initiate a new strenuous exercise program during pregnancy.*
- *Hot environments* (e.g., hot tubs or saunas) *should be avoided* during pregnancy.
- Many *pregnancy complications* (e.g., multiple gestation), *may adversely affect the ability to exercise.*

ALCOHOL

The *safe amount of alcohol intake during pregnancy is still unknown.* However, gravidas who consume >6 fluid ounces (180 mL) of whiskey or equivalent daily have at least a 20% likelihood of delivering an infant with features of the fetal alcohol syndrome. The patient who never drinks, stops drinking early in pregnancy, or reduces her alcohol intake drastically will have a much better fetal prognosis. Although >45% of all women consume alcohol during the 3 months before finding out they are pregnant, about 5% consume 6 or more drinks per week. Moreover, 60% of women consuming alcohol report not knowing they were pregnant until after the 4th week of gestation. Risk factors for alcohol consumption in the periconceptional period include the following: being unmarried, being a smoker, being white non-Hispanic, being >25 years of age, or being college educated.

SMOKING

Smoking is particularly deleterious during pregnancy. The alterations induced in the mother and fetus are summarized in Table 5-7.

Smoking is especially harmful to women >35 years or those with antepartum bleeding, poor weight gain, anemia, or hypertension. Moreover, *smoking and alcohol intake are synergistically harmful to the fetus.*

TABLE 5-7
ALTERATIONS INDUCED BY SMOKING
DURING PREGNANCY

Gravida	Fetus
Plasma volume reduced	Fetal breathing suppressed
Second trimester abortion, increased preterm delivery (associated with placenta previa, premature separation of the placenta)	Contraction of umbilical arteries diminishes fetal circulation (nicotine effect)
Cardiorespiratory problems augmented	Neonatal birthweight reduced (averages 200 g below normal—directly related to number of cigarettes smoked)
	Perinatal mortality and morbidity increased

Obstetric patients should stop smoking. If this is impossible, restrict tobacco to less than one-half pack of low-nicotine, low-tar cigarettes per day.

IMMUNIZATIONS

Generally, live virus vaccines are contraindicated during pregnancy because of the risk to the fetus. In contrast, killed virus immunization (i.e., poliomyelitis) is permitted. However, the rubella vaccine (a live virus) has, to date, not been incriminated in causing the rubella syndrome. Obviously, *all immunizations must be judged on a risk–benefit basis.*

DENTAL CARE

"For every child a tooth" is an untrue maxim. Decalcification of the mother's teeth does not occur as a result of pregnancy. Necessary dental fillings or extractions may be performed during pregnancy, preferably under local anesthesia. Routine antibiotic prophylaxis may be necessary in some patients (e.g., with a prolapsed mitral valve). Abortion or premature labor and delivery are not caused, even by extensive dental surgery.

BATHING

Bath water does not enter the vagina, and tub baths and swimming are not contraindicated during normal pregnancy. Prolonged exposure to extremely hot or very cold baths should be avoided, however. Showers may be safer than tub baths because with the awkwardness caused by pregnancy, falls in a tub may occur.

PREPARATION FOR BREASTFEEDING

Most women who breastfeed successfully do so naturally without preparation. *The advantages of nursing should be explained carefully to the patient.* If the gravida decides to nurse, institute predelivery breast and nipple care.

THE FIGURE

Pregnancy need not ruin the figure. Avoidance of excessive weight gain, continued daily exercise, and a well-fitted brassiere worn much of the time will help to preserve the figure.

TRAVEL

If a long journey is essential, air travel is best, but pregnant women should not fly at high altitudes in unpressurized aircraft unless oxygen is available. All commercial aircraft are now pressurized to 1525–2130 m (5000–7000 ft), which is safe for pregnant women. To avoid possible delivery en route, most airlines will not permit women to fly during the last month of pregnancy. With all forms of travel, it is advisable for the gravida to *walk about approximately once an hour, avoid prolonged extremity dependency, and avoid extreme fatigue.*

Travel will not cause abortion or premature labor, but the pregnant woman is jeopardized indirectly by travel, since she may be far from her obstetrician in case of an obstetric emergency. Therefore, with distant travel, she probably should *carry a copy of her antenatal record.*

DIAGNOSIS OF PREVIOUS PREGNANCY

A physician may be required because of medical or legal questions to determine if a woman has had a pregnancy. A reasonably accurate opinion often is possible, based on physical residua of pregnancy or obstetric treatment. The following are suggestive of earlier pregnancy.

Skin	Pigmentation of the nipple areola, evident linear nigra, abdominal, breast, or buttock striae
Breast	Less firm, more pendulous
Abdomen	Relaxation of abdominal wall, diastasis of rectus muscles
Vagina	Widened introitus, cystocele, rectocele
Scars	Lower abdomen (? cesarean section), cervical lacerations, perineal or episiotomy repair

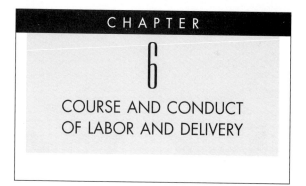

CHAPTER

6

COURSE AND CONDUCT OF LABOR AND DELIVERY

Labor is the normal process of *coordinated, effective involuntary uterine contractions that lead to progressive cervical effacement and dilatation and descent and delivery of the newborn and placenta.* Near its termination, labor may be augmented by voluntary bearing-down efforts to assist in delivery of the conceptus.

False labor is characterized by *irregular (both in interval and duration), brief contractions without fundal dominance, cervical change, or a lower station of the fetal vertex or breech.*

Dilatation of the cervix is the *diameter of the cervical os* expressed in centimeters (0–10). *Effacement is cervical thinning* that occurs before and especially during first stage labor. Effacement of the cervix is expressed as a percentage of cervical length (normally ~2.5 cm) (Figs. 6-1, 6-2). An uneffaced cervix is 0%; one about 0.25 in length is 100% effaced. Effacement and dilatation are caused by retraction (takeup) of the cervix toward the uterine corpus, not by pressure of the presenting part.

The initiation of labor in the human is poorly understood. Labor can be triggered by one or more significant endocrine or physical changes, for example, abdominal trauma. The onset of labor can occur at any time after well-established pregnancy, but the likelihood increases as term is approached. Labor can be induced or stimulated (augmented) by oxytocic agents (e.g., oxytocin or prostaglandin E_2) (Fig. 6-3).

In *~10% of gravidas, the fetal membranes rupture before the onset of labor.* This reduces the capacity of the uterus, thickens the uterine wall, and increases uterine irritability. Labor usually follows. *At term, 90% will be in labor within 24 h after membrane rupture.* If labor does not begin in 24 h, the case must be considered complicated by prolonged rupture of the membranes.

Immediately before or early in labor, a small amount of red-tinged mucus may be passed (*bloody show* or mucous plug). This is a collection of thick cervical mucus often mixed with blood and

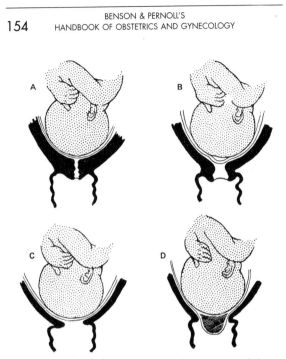

FIGURE 6-1. Dilatation and effacement of the cervix in a primipara.

is evidence of cervical dilatation and effacement and, frequently, descent of the presenting part.

The beginning of *true labor is marked by increasingly frequent, forceful, prolonged, and, finally, regular uterine contractions. Low backache* may precede or accompany the uterine contractions (pains). Each contraction starts with a gradual buildup of intensity, and a similar dissipation follows the peak. Normally, the contraction will be at its height before discomfort is felt. Dilatation of the lower birth canal almost always will cause deep pelvic or perineal pain. Nonetheless, occasional nulliparas and some multiparas may have a brief, virtually pain-free labor.

Labor entails the interaction of the so-called 4Ps.

- The *passenger* (the fetal size, presentation, position)
- The *pelvis* (size and shape)
- The *powers* (effective forces of labor, e.g., uterine contractions)
- The *placenta* (an obstruction if implanted low in the uterus)

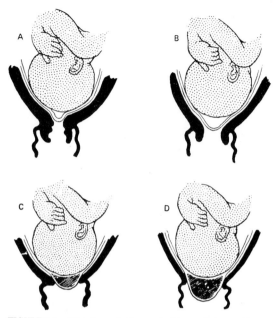

FIGURE 6-2. Dilatation and effacement of the cervix in a multipara.

FIGURE 6-3. Production of prostaglandins in human parturition.
(Modified after Liggins.) (From M.L. Pernoll and R.C. Benson, eds. *Current Obstetric & Gynecologic Diagnosis & Treatment,* 6th ed. Lange, 1987.)

Each of these factors, alone or in combination, can make for a normal or a complicated labor and delivery. For example, if the fetus is large and the pelvis is small, labor may be prolonged or progress may be impossible despite strong contractions, even with a placenta normally implanted in the fundus.

NORMAL LABOR

Since, hopefully, the end result of labor is the vaginal delivery of the fetus, membranes, and placenta, the method of judging its progress is based on assessments toward that end. The *first stage of labor begins with the onset of labor and ends with complete*

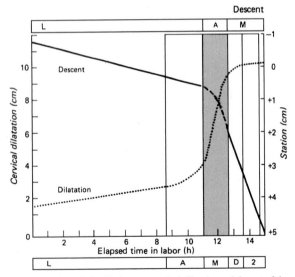

FIGURE 6-4.   Relationship between cervical dilatation and descent of the presenting part in a primipara. L, latent phase; A, acceleration phase; M, phase of maximum slope; D, deceleration phase; and 2, second stage.

(From M.L. Pernoll and R.C. Benson, eds. *Current Obstetric & Gynecologic Diagnosis & Treatment,* 6th ed. Lange, 1987.)

(10 cm) dilatation of the cervix. The first stage is the longest, averaging *8–12 h for primigravidas* or *6–8 h for multiparas.* However, the first stage of labor may be markedly shorter or longer depending on the 4Ps.

Labor is a very dynamic process, and *contractions should increase steadily in regularity, intensity, and duration.* This is not always the case, and one must set limits concerning the progress of labor (Figs. 6-4, 6-5).

It is useful to divide the first stage of labor into *two phases.* Thus, the *latent phase of labor begins with the onset of regular uterine contractions and extends to the start of the active phase of cervical dilatation* (~3–4 cm).

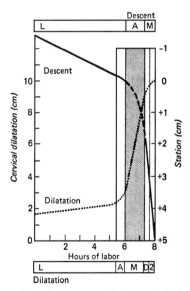

FIGURE 6-5. Composite mean curves for descent (solid line) and dilatation (broken line) for 389 multiparas. L, latent phase; A, acceleration phase; M, phase of maximum slope; D, deceleration phase; and 2, second stage. Relationship is shown between acceleration period of descent and maximum slope of dilatation (shaded area), between latent period of descent and latent plus acceleration phases of dilatation, and between maximum slope of descent and deceleration plase plus second stage.

(Redrawn from Friedman and Sachtleben. *Am J Obstet Gynecol* 1965;93:526.)

FIGURE 6-6. Major types of deviation from normal progress of labor may be detected by noting dilatation of the cervix at various intervals after labor begins.

(From K.P. Russell. In: R.C. Benson, ed. *Current Obstetric & Gynecologic Diagnosis & Treatment,* 4th ed. Lange, 1982.)

The *second stage of labor begins when the cervix becomes fully dilated and ends with the complete birth of the infant.* The second stage normally lasts *<30 min.* While one should be concerned when the second stage extends longer than 1 h (based on fetal morbidity and mortality). Safety for the fetus may be assured by thoughtful monitoring.

The *third, or placental, stage of labor* is the period from birth of the infant to 1 h after delivery of the placenta. The rapidity of separation and means of recovery of the placenta determine the duration of the third stage (Fig. 6-6).

MANAGEMENT OF THE FIRST STAGE OF LABOR

INITIAL EXAMINATION AND PROCEDURES

- Obtain a *history* of relevant medical details following the last examination.

- Record the patient's *vital signs* (temperature, pulse, and BP). Examine a clean-catch urine specimen for proteinuria and glycosuria.
- Do a brief *general physical examination.*
- Palpate the uterus to *determine the fetal presentation, position, and engagement* (Leopold's maneuvers) (Fig. 6-7). *Ausculate the fetal heartbeat,* and mark the skin where the heartbeat is

FIGURE 6-7. Leopold's maneuvers. Determining fetal presentation (A and B), position (C), and engagement (D).

loudest to note the shift and descent of the point of maximal intensity with progressive labor. This is evidence of internal rotation and descent of the fetus (the mechanism of labor).

- Note the *frequency, regularity, intensity, and duration of uterine contractions and the myometrial tone* with and between contractions. Observe the patient's reactions and her tolerance of labor. Restlessness and discomfort often develop as labor progresses.

- Check for *vaginal bleeding or leakage of amniotic fluid.* Nitrazine indicator paper will turn from green to yellow when moistened with amniotic fluid (pH 7.0). Other tests may be used in doubtful cases.

- *Examine the patient vaginally* and record both the time and results of the examination. Use a surgically clean glove.

  Identify the fetal presenting part and its station in relation to the level of the ischial spines. *Station is the level of the head or breech in the pelvis.* If the presenting part is at the spines, it is said to be at "zero station." If above the spines, the distance is stated in minus figures (−1 cm, −2 cm, −3 cm, and "floating"). If below the spines, the distance is noted in plus figures (+1 cm, +2 cm, +3 cm, and "on the perineum") (Fig. 6-8). When the most inferior

FIGURE 6-8. Stations of the fetal head.

part of the head is at the level of the ischial spines, the station is zero.

Station zero is assumed by projection to be actual engagement, that is, the biparietal diameter at the level of the inlet. However, with considerable molding, caput succedaneum, or a sincipital presentation of the head, the biparietal diameter may be a significant distance above the inlet even though the tip of the vertex is at the spines without true engagement.

Dilatation of the cervix by direct palpation is expressed as the diameter of the cervical opening in centimeters. A diameter of *10 cm constitutes full dilatation.*

Effacement of the cervix (process of thinning out) may occur before labor in the nulligravida but is less likely before the first stage of labor in the multigravida.

The position of the presenting part usually can be confirmed by internal examination.

Vertex presentations (Fig. 6-9). The fontanelles and the sagittal suture are palpated. The position is determined by the relation of the *fetal occiput* to the mother's right or left side. This is expressed as OA (occiput directly anterior), LOA (left occiput anterior), LOP (left occiput posterior), and so on.

Breech presentations are determined by the position of the *infant's sacrum* in relation to the mother's right or left side. This is expressed as SA (sacrum directly anterior), LSA (left sacrum anterior), LSP (left sacrum posterior), and so on.

Face presentation is caused by extension of the fetal head on the neck. The *chin,* a prominent and identifiable facial landmark, is used as the point of reference. As with vertex presentations, the position of the fetal chin is related to the anterior or posterior portion of the left or right side of the mother's pelvis. This is expressed as RMP (right mentum posterior) and so on.

Brow, bregma, and sinciput presentations are presentations midway between flexion and extension. These usually are temporary attitudes that convert during labor to face or occiput presentation.

Transverse presentations occur when the long axis of the fetal body is perpendicular to that of the mother. One shoulder (acromion) will occupy the superior strait, but it will be considerably to the right or left of the midline. Transverse presentations are designated by *relating the infant's inferior shoulder and back to the mother's back*

LOT

LOA

LOP

FIGURE 6-9. Vertex presentation.

or abdominal wall. Thus, LADP (left acromiodorsoposterior) means that the infant's lower shoulder is to the mother's left, and its back is toward her back.

Compound presentations, caused by prolapse of a hand, arm, foot, or leg, are complications of one of the other presentations. These unusual presentations generally are *recorded descriptively* without abbreviations.

PREPARATION OF THE PATIENT FOR LABOR

Following the initial internal examination, the following may be reasonable:

Ambulation, within reasonable limits, may add to the patient's comfort. However, keep the patient in bed after the membranes have ruptured or until the presenting part has engaged to avoid cord prolapse or compression.

Allow only *clear liquids by mouth* during labor to avoid dehydration.

Analgesia should not be given until labor is definitely established with the cervix >3 cm dilated. Analgesics and anesthesia must be ordered on an individual basis, considering each patient's obstetric problems, the quality of labor, and her desire to be alert or subdued.

FURTHER EXAMINATIONS AND PROCEDURES

Electronic fetal monitoring (EFM) is simply one of the means of assessing fetal status. It does have the advantage of being continuous. The external type is innocuous, and the internal type carries only slight risk. Although EFM is an excellent diagnostic tool, it is not a substitute for correct clinical judgment. Current retrospective and prospective data support the use of continuous internal EFM for high-risk obstetric patients. Internal EFM is preferable to external EFM because it is more precise and comprehensive in appraising fetal status. Nonetheless, electronic monitoring of low-risk obstetric patients has not demonstrated a beneficial cost–benefit ratio.

If continuous EFM is not used, auscultate and record the fetal heart tones (FHT) for 1 min following a uterine contraction at least every 30 min during the first stage, at least every 5 min during the second stage, when the membranes rupture and again within

30 min after the rupture, and every 5 min or more often as indicated if complications develop or if meconium passes in vertex presentation.

Perform external and internal examinations as often as necessary to determine the progress of the labor. Descent and internal rotation of the fetus often can be determined by external palpation alone. Too frequent vaginal or rectal examinations cause the patient discomfort and increase the incidence of intrauterine infection, particularly after rupture of the membranes.

Figure 6-6 details *normal and abnormal labor curves for both nulliparas and multiparas* as determined by measuring cervical dilatation as a function of time. The abnormal labor patterns are quantified in Chapter 7. *Encourage the patient to void frequently.* Palpate the abdomen occasionally for signs of bladder fullness. Catheterize if involuntary distention occurs or if voiding is obviously inadequate.

DELIVERY: MANAGEMENT OF THE NORMAL SECOND STAGE OF LABOR

VERTEX DELIVERY (TABLES 6-1, 6-2)

Final preparation for delivery should be completed by the time the presenting part reaches the pelvic floor, or sooner if labor is progressing very rapidly.

Spontaneous delivery of the infant presenting by the vertex is divided into *three phases: (1) delivery of the head, (2) delivery of the shoulders, and (3) delivery of the body and legs.*

Preparation for Delivery
- Place the patient in a *modified lithotomy* position for delivery. The left lateral decubitus (Sims) or squatting position may be used if a spontaneous uncomplicated birth is anticipated. Another alternative is the squatting position.
- The physician and assistants must carefully *scrub* their hands and *wear masks, eye protection, and sterile gloves.* Any delivery may become surgically complicated.
- Administer *anesthesia* if necessary (e.g., pudendal block).
- *Cleanse the pudendum* with water and surgical detergent.
- *Drape the patient* with sterile towels or sheets or both.
- Sterile instruments and necessary supplies should be arranged conveniently on a table or stand.
- *Gloves (and gown)* must be changed if contamination occurs.

TABLE 6-1
MECHANISMS OF LABOR: VERTEX PRESENTATION

Engagement	Flexion	Descent	Internal Rotation	Extension	External Rotation or Restitution
Generally occurs in late pregnancy or at onset of labor. Mode of entry into superior strait depends on pelvic configuration	Good flexion is noted in most cases. Flexion aids engagement and descent. (Extension occurs in brow and face presentations)	Depends on pelvic architecture and cephalopelvic relationships. Descent is usually slowly progressive	Takes place during descent. After engagement, vertex usually rotates to the transverse. It must next rotate to the anterior or posterior to pass the ischial spines, whereupon, when the vertex reaches the perineum, rotation from a posterior to an anterior position generally follows	Follows distention of the perineum by the vertex. Head concomitantly stems beneath the symphysis. Extension is complete with delivery of head	Following delivery, head normally rotates to the position it originally occupied at engagement. Next, the shoulders descend in a path similar to that traced by the head. The shoulders rotate anteroposteriorly for delivery. Then the head swings back to its position at birth. The body of the infant is delivered next

165

TABLE 6-2
MECHANISMS OF LABOR: FRANK BREECH PRESENTATION

Flexion	Descent	Internal Rotation	Lateral Flexion	External Rotation or Restitution
Hips: Engagement usually occurs in one of oblique diameters of pelvic inlet	Anterior hip generally descends more rapidly than posterior at both inlet and outlet	Ordinarily takes place when breech reaches levator musculature. Fetal bitrochanteric rotates to AP diameter	Occurs when anterior hip stems beneath symphysis; posterior hip is born first	After birth of breech and legs, infant's body turns toward mother's side to which its back was directed at engagement of shoulders
Shoulders: Bisacromial diameter engages in same diameter as breech	Gradual descent is the rule	Anterior shoulder rotates so as to bring shoulders into AP diameter of outlet	Anterior shoulder at symphysis, and posterior shoulder is delivered first (when body is supported)	

166

Head: Engages in the same diameter as shoulders. Flexes on entry into superior strait. Biparietal occupies oblique used by shoulders. At outlet, neck or chin arrests beneath symphysis, and head is born by gradual flexion

Follows the shoulders

Occiput (if a posterior) or face (if an occiput anterior) rotates to hollow of sacrum; this brings presenting part to AP diameter of outlet

FIGURE 6-10.   Engagement of LOA.

Delivery of the Head (Figs. 6-10 through 6-14)

- During the late second stage, the head distends toward the perineum and vulva with each uterine contraction, normally aided by voluntary efforts of the mother. A patch of scalp becomes visible. The presenting part recedes slightly during the intervals of relaxation, but it *crowns* when its widest portion (biparietal diameter) distends the vulva just before emerging.
- *Do not hasten delivery,* lest serious damage to the mother or child occur. Control the speed of delivery by pressure

FIGURE 6-11.   LOA position.

FIGURE 6-12. Anterior rotation of head.

FIGURE 6-13. Extension of head.

FIGURE 6-14. External rotation of head.

applied laterally beneath the symphysis as necessary to avoid pudendal laceration or unexpected extrusion of the infant's head. Sudden marked variations in intracranial pressure may cause intracranial hemorrhage. *As the head advances, control its progress* and maintain flexion of the head by pressure over the perineum.

Draw the perineum downward to allow the head to *clear the perineal body.* Pressure applied from the coccygeal region upward (modified *Ritgen maneuver*) will extend the head at the proper time and thereby protect the perineum from laceration.

- If *episiotomy* is elected, it should be *performed when the fetal head begins to distend the introitus.*

- In vertex presentations, the forehead soon appears, then the face and chin, and finally the neck.

- The *cord encircles the neck in about 20% of deliveries.* Note the number of loops. If the nuchal cord is tight, attempt to gently slip the loop(s) of cord over the head. If this cannot be done easily and if this is a singleton, doubly clamp the cord, cut between the forceps, and proceed with the delivery. Wipe fluid from the nose and mouth, then aspirate the nasal and oropharyngeal passages with a soft rubber suction bulb or with a small catheter attached to a deLee-type suction trap.

- Before *external rotation* (restitution), which occurs next, the head usually is drawn back toward the perineum. This movement precedes engagement of the shoulders, which are now entering the pelvic inlet.

- From this point on, *support the infant* manually and *facilitate the mechanism of labor.*

Do not hurry! If strong contractions wane, be patient—labor will resume. Once the airway is clear, the infant can breathe and is not in jeopardy.

Delivery of the Shoulders

Caution: *Never exert pressure or strong anterior or posterior traction on the head, neck, or shoulders. Do not hook a finger into the child's axilla to deliver a shoulder.* These maneuvers may result in a brachial plexus injury (Erb or Duchenne), a hematoma of the neck, or a shoulder injury.

- Delivery of the shoulders should be *deliberate.* The shoulders must rotate (or be rotated) to the anteroposterior diameter of the outlet for delivery.

- *Gently depress the head toward the mother's coccyx* until the anterior shoulder impinges against the symphysis. *Then lift the head upward.* This aids delivery of the posterior shoulder.
- The anterior shoulder is next delivered from behind the symphysis by gentle downward traction. The index and third finger should greatly exert pressure on the rami of the mandible while the opposite index and third finger exert equal and gentle pressure on the occiput. (Occasionally, it may be easier to deliver the anterior shoulder first.) Slipping several fingers into the vagina at this point to assist in delivering the posterior arm is desirable, but undue pressure must be avoided!
- In vertex presentations, a hand may present after the head. Merely sweep the infant's hand and arm over its face, draw the arm out, and deliver the other shoulder as outlined previously.

Delivery of the Body and Extremities
The infant's body and legs should be *delivered gradually by easy traction* after the shoulders have been freed.

IMMEDIATE CARE OF THE INFANT

- As soon as the infant is delivered, *hold it with the head lowered* (no more than 15 degrees) to drain fluid and mucus from the oropharynx. A *mucus trap catheter* or comparable suction device is useful in *clearing the air passages.* If the baby is below the level of the placental insertion, blood will drain from the placenta and cord to the newborn. This will amount to 30–90 mL before the cord is clamped or the placenta separates. The excess blood may benefit some neonates (e.g., isoimmunized anemic infants) and harm others (e.g., a plethoric twin).

  Placing the newborn on the mother's abdomen before cord pulsations cease has the potential disadvantage that the infant is not secure there and blood drains from the infant to the placenta (usually undesirable).
- *Evaluate and resuscitate if necessary* (Chapter 8) (Fig. 6-15).
- *Clamp and cut the cord when it ceases to pulsate* (or sooner if the infant is premature or in distress, or if isoimmunization is probable). Examine the umbilical cord for the normal *two arteries and one vein.* Apply a *sterile cord clamp,* cord tie of umbilical tape, or rubber band distal to the skin edge at the cord insertion at the umbilicus. Dress the cord stump with dry gauze.

FIGURE 6-15. Resuscitation of the newborn.

- The newborn should be *received into warm clean towels* or blankets, and *avoid chilling. Apply means of identification* (e.g., bracelet).
- At this point, bonding may be initiated with the parents holding the newborn. The mother may begin breastfeeding.

- Next, perform *newborn ocular prophylaxis* (against gonor-rhea and *Chlamydia*). Most commonly, erythromycin or tetracycline ointment is used because they are more protec-tive and provoke less ocular irritation than silver nitrate.
- *Examine the infant and record Apgar scores,* weight, total length, crown-rump length, shoulder circumference, cir-cumference of the head, and cranial diameters. Note facial, peripheral, genital, or other abnormalities (Chapter 8).

IMMEDIATE CARE OF THE MOTHER

- Carefully *inspect the perineum, vagina, and cervix for lac-erations, hematomas, or extension of the episiotomy.* Iden-tify sulcus lacerations, urethral and cervical injury, and other injuries. Lacerations of the birth canal may be described by their extent (expressed as first to fourth degree).

  In *first degree lacerations,* only the mucosa or skin or both are damaged. Bleeding usually is minimal.

  Second degree lacerations include tears of the mucosa or skin or both plus disruption of the superficial fascia and the transverse perineal muscle. (The anal sphincter is spared.) Bleeding often is brisk.

  Third degree lacerations involve the structures indicated in second degree lacerations plus the anal sphincter. Expect moderate blood loss.

  Fourth degree lacerations include the structures included in third degree lacerations and entry into the rectal lumen. Bleeding may be profuse, and fecal soiling is inevitable.
- Control blood loss and repair second to fourth degree lacerations.

MANAGEMENT OF THE THIRD STAGE OF LABOR

AVOID INTERFERENCE IF AT ALL POSSIBLE!

Avoid traction on the cord before placental separation and do not knead the fundus to separate the placenta (Credé maneuver). The former may lead to cord laceration and the latter to hemorrhage, uterine inversion, and shock. Maternal morbidity and mortality rates increase with gross blood loss. A uterus that contracts and remains contracted rarely bleeds excessively.

SEPARATION OF THE PLACENTA

The placenta is attached to the uterine wall only by anchoring villi and thin-walled blood vessels, all of which eventually tear. In some instances, the placental margin separates first. In others, when the central portion of the placenta is initially freed bleeding from the retroplacental sinuses may assist placental separation. Incomplete separation, usually due to ineffectual uterine contractions, may allow the retroplacental blood sinuses to remain open, so that severe blood loss may result.

Normal placental separation is manifested first by a *firmly contracting, rising fundus*. The *uterus becomes smaller and changes in shape from discoid to globular*. The *umbilical cord becomes longer* as the placenta descends. There is a palpable and visible prominence above the symphysis (if the bladder is empty) and a *slight gush of blood from the vagina*. These signs normally appear within about 3–4 min after delivery of the infant. The placenta should present at the internal os after four or five firm uterine contractions, whereupon it is expressed into the vagina for delivery.

These signs often are confused with other conditions: uterine anomaly, a second undelivered infant, feces, a tumor, and lacerations of the birth canal.

RECOVERY OF THE PLACENTA

Spontaneous Uterine Expulsion of Placenta

When the uterus is firmly contracted, the mother who has not been anesthetized may be able to *bear down during a contraction to expel the separated placenta*. Although of historic but little clinical significance, a recording of the placenta presenting with the fetal surface to the introitus (Schultz) or the maternal surface (Duncan) may be made. Spontaneous delivery of the placenta usually is accomplished without difficulty. If it does not occur, however, the following techniques may be used.

Brandt-Andrews Technique (Modified) (Fig. 6-16)

- Immediately after delivery of the infant, *clamp the umbilical cord close to the vulva*. Palpate the uterus gently without massage to determine whether firm contractions are occurring.
- After several *uterine contractions and a change in size and shape* indicate separation of the placenta, *hold the clamp* at the vulva firmly with one hand, place the *fingertips* of the other hand *on the abdomen*, and *press between the fundus*

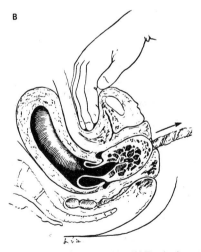

FIGURE 6-16. Brandt-Andrews maneuver. (A) Traction is extended on the cord as the uterus is elevated gently. (B) Pressure is exerted between the symphysis and the uterine fundus, forcing the uterus upward and the placenta outward, as traction on the cord is continued.

(From R.C. Benson, ed. *Current Obstetric & Gynecologic Diagnosis & Treatment,* 4th ed. Lange, 1982.)

and symphysis to elevate the fundus. If the placenta has separated, the cord will extrude into the vagina.
- Further *elevate the fundus, apply gentle traction on the cord,* and *deliver the placenta* from the vagina.

Manual Separation and Extraction of Placenta

Manual separation and extraction of the placenta from the fundus of the uterus is an effective direct technique. This is invasive and, often, effective anesthesia is required. *Manual removal of the placenta should not be undertaken unless it is indicated and the operator is experienced.* Common indications for manual placental removal include: uterine hemorrhage, incomplete separation, prolonged retention, suspected uterine rupture, and retained placental segments.

- *Prepare the perineum* and vulva again with detergent and antiseptic solution.
- Making the hand as narrow as possible, insert gently into the vagina and *palpate for defects in the vagina and cervix.* Slowly probe through the cervix with the fingers, taking care not to lacerate the canal. (Brief moderately deep anesthesia may be required if considerable delay has occurred.)
- *Locate and separate the placenta* if this can be done easily. Do not attempt to force cleavage against unusual resistance (placenta accreta).
- *Palpate the fundus* for defects or tumors.
- Remove the hand while grasping the completely separated placenta, or leave the placenta if it is firmly adherent (placenta accreta).

POSTPARTUM OXYTOCIN

After delivery of the placenta, it is *common practice* (even though not required in the majority of cases) to give *oxytocin.* In the past, 5–10 U IV was frequently given over 5 min to limit blood loss. Currently, it is more common to utilize 20 U of oxytocin in 1000 cc of IV solution and run at 125–250 cc hour.

POSTPARTUM OBSERVATION

The mother should remain *under very close observation for at least 1 h after delivery of the placenta.* Note her *vital signs* and *reactions.* Record the *blood pressure,* the *pulse rate* and regularity, and *the amount of vaginal blood loss* every 15 min, or more often if necessary. Support the uterine fundus. *Massage* it gently and frequently to *maintain firm contraction.* Express clots occasionally and *estimate the total blood loss* after 1 h.

Be alert to complaints of *severe perineal pain suggestive of hematoma* formation. *A rapid pulse* and increasing *hypotension* indicate impending shock, usually due to continued or *excessive blood loss.* Severe *headaches* and *hyperreflexia* may precede *eclampsia. A distended bladder (often visible) will lead to enhanced uterine bleeding.* Catheterize for retention when necessary. *Do not release any patient to room care until her condition is stable.*

POSTPARTUM HEMORRHAGE

Postpartum hemorrhage (PPH) is the rapid or slow loss of >500 mL of blood after delivery. *Early PPH* occurs within 24 h of birth. *Late PPH* may occur 24 h to 4 weeks after birth. Early PPH may be caused by *placental problems* (abruptio placentae, placenta previa, incomplete placental separation), *uterine atony* (anesthesia, marked predelivery uterine distention, abnormal labor, prolonged or excessive oxytocin administration, overdistended urinary bladder), *laceration(s) of the birth canal, rupture of the uterus, blood dyscrasias* (hypofibrogenemia), or *mismanagement of the third stage of labor.* Usually, late postpartum hemorrhage is due to *retained products of conception.* This complication occurs in *5%–10%* of term deliveries. About *2%* of these patients must be *readmitted* to the hospital for transfusion, and *some require surgery.* Further complications of PPH include *shock, anemia, and infection.*

CLINICAL ASSESSMENT

The pulse rate should return to normal within the hour after delivery. Hence, a persistent slight *tachycardia* may indicate a significant uncompensated blood loss. Elimination of the placenta and a contracted uterus will *restore at least 300 mL* of blood to the maternal circulation. This normally causes *a systolic elevation of 10–20 mm Hg* for several hours after delivery. Therefore, *persistent hypotension suggests excessive blood loss,* which may require replacement. Continued, *even moderate postpartum hypertension,* especially with associated headache or hyperreflexia, suggests impending pregnancy-induced hypertension *(PIH).* Magnesium sulfate therapy for the PIH may cause some relaxation of the uterine muscle, but that effect should not deter its indicated usage.

PREVENTION

Properly manage the placenta. Recover the placenta by spontaneous delivery or Brandt-Andrews maneuver. Avoid the Credé maneuver (kneading of the uterus), and never use the fundus as a piston to push out the placenta. Reserve manual extraction for indicated cases.

After placental delivery, give dilute *oxytocin* (5 IU slowly IV). When an atonic uterus is anticipated start dilute oxytocin before delivery of the placenta (once it has been ascertained that there is not a second fetus).

Inspect the birth canal carefully for lacerations.

Explore the uterus in any patient with possible uterine rupture or retained products of conception.

TREATMENT

- Obtain a *CBC, coagulation panel, type and crossmatch.*
- Ensure an *open IV line.*
- Closely *monitor further blood loss and vital signs.*
- Initiate *appropriate blood component replacement.*
- *Manually deliver the partially separated placenta.*
- *Explore the uterus,* and carefully *remove any retained products of conception* (this may require uterine curettage).
- To reverse uterine atony after placental recovery:
    Elevate and maintain the fundus out of the pelvis while performing *gentle uterine massage.*
    Repeat the oxytocin 5 IU slowly IV. If that fails to slow bleeding, consider the addition of prostaglandins or ergonovine (omit the latter if the patient is hypertensive).
- *Repair* the episiotomy and any lacerations promptly.
- Perform *hysterectomy for hemorrhaging placenta accreta.* Alternatively, if availability of the service exists and patient status permits, radiographically guided *embolization of the placental bed* may be attempted.
- *Ligation of uterine arteries or hypogastric arteries* may be lifesaving in certain extreme cases; however, such ligation leads to only a partial, and often transient, decrease in blood pressure and flow.
- *Packing the uterus* to control PPH is now done rarely, except as a temporary measure (e.g., to stop the flow if blood replacement products are not immediately available). Have available many packs of sterilized gauze about 1 yard wide and 5 yards long (packing takes a considerable amount). A Holmes tubular packing instrument may be helpful but is not essential.

PROGNOSIS

The outcome depends on the cause of bleeding, amount of blood lost (in proportion to patient's weight), medical complications, and success of corrective therapy.

AIDS TO NORMAL DELIVERY

THE FATHER

Much has been said of the mother, her needs, and her relationship to the child, but the expectant father (partner, significant other) has been relatively neglected in the process until recently. Preparation for parenthood begins well before courtship and marriage, but the mother's pregnancy is the beginning of the transition leading to fatherhood. Recognition of the father's concerns leads to discussion and solution of many human problems that surround the expectation of a newborn.

Fathers-to-be experience at least five emotional stages (which often overlap): realization or confirmation of pregnancy, awareness of changes in the mother's body and the presence of fetal movements, anticipation of approaching labor, involvement in the delivery process, and new parenthood.

Fears that the father's presence in the delivery room would create a nuisance, add to confusion, or cause infection or legal conflicts have been unjustified. Men who have participated with their spouses in preparation for childbirth have proven helpful, supportive, and reassuring. Moreover, properly conducted delivery room experience is almost always a gratifying one for the father, one that assists him in immediate attachment to the newborn.

The father may act as a coach in addition to the nurse–physician team by assisting with comfort measures. He may be an almost constant companion to the patient to offset the loneliness and anxieties of labor. He can be a messenger, to report problems or call for help, and interpret his wife's needs and wishes to the nurse and doctor. He may serve as an advocate.

In emergencies, when the mother is sedated or in shock, he can give informed consent for treatment that may be life saving. With the father in the delivery room, it is easier for the physician and the parents to welcome a normal newborn or cope with a defective offspring. A well-informed participating father can contribute greatly to the health and well-being of the mother and child, to the benefit of the family relationship and his own self-esteem. All of these factors may prevent or greatly minimize postpartum psychologic problems.

EPISIOTOMY (PERINEOTOMY) AND REPAIR OF EPISIOTOMY AND LACERATIONS

An episiotomy is a pudendal incision, widening the vulvar orifice to permit easier passage of the infant. The advantages of episiotomy are said to be that it prevents perineal lacerations, relieves compression of the fetal head, shortens the second stage of labor (by removing the resistance of the pudendal musculature), and can be repaired more successfully than a jagged tear. It is used in many primiparas and some multiparas. Although currently the utilization of episiotomy is being questioned, the most common indications continue to be: when a tear is imminent, in most operative deliveries, and to facilitate atraumatic delivery of a premature infant.

Types of Episiotomy (Fig. 6-17)

The tissues incised by an episiotomy are (1) skin and subcutaneous tissues, (2) vaginal mucosa, (3) the urogenital septum (mostly fascia, but also the transverse perineal muscles), (4) intercolumnar fascia or superior fascia of the pelvic diaphragm, and (5) the lowermost fibers of the puborectalis portions of the levator ani muscles (if the episiotomy is mediolateral and deep). Currently, only two types of episiotomy are used.

Median Episiotomy

This is the easiest episiotomy to accomplish and repair. It is almost bloodless and is less painful postpartum than other types. Incise the

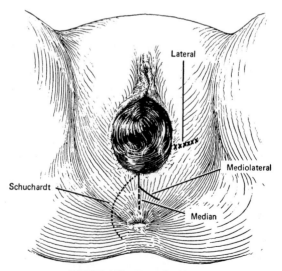

FIGURE 6-17. Types of episiotomy.

median raphe of the perineum almost to the anal sphincter, and extend this separation at least 2–3 cm up to the rectovaginal septum. Occasionally, a third or fourth degree laceration may occur.

Mediolateral Episiotomy

The mediolateral incision is used in operative obstetrics because of its safety. Make the incision downward and outward in the direction of the lateral margin of the anal sphincter and at least one-half the distance into the vagina; however, this incision may bleed excessively and may remain painful even after the puerperium.

Timing of Episiotomy

Episiotomy should be done when the head begins to distend the perineum with a mature fetus, before the head encounters the perineal musculature with an immature fetus, immediately preceding application of forceps, and just before breech extraction.

REPAIR OF EPISIOTOMY AND LACERATIONS (FIGS. 6-18, 6-19)

Episiotomy Repair

Episiotomy repair is actually a fascial repair, not the suture of muscle. *Absorbable suture* (natural or synthetic, usually 00–0000) is preferred. The procedure can employ interrupted or continuous sutures or a combination of both. *Careful reapproximation* of the edges of the divided muscles and surrounding fascia is required. *Avoid mass ligatures and tension on sutures. Do not tie the sutures too tightly,* or pain and necrosis may result. In general, buried sutures cause less discomfort than through-and-through exposed sutures.

Laceration Repair

In repair of fourth degree lacerations, close the rectal submucosal layer with fine interrupted absorbable sutures tied within the lumen of the bowel or a fine continuous suture that everts the mucosal edges. Then approximate the bowel muscularis, with either a running or interrupted fine absorbable sutures, in a manner to invert the previous suture line. Close the rectovaginal septum as in an episiotomy, taking care to reapproximate the internal sphincter ani. This anatomic structure, important to rectal continence, can be appreciated as a thickening of the rectovaginal septum in the lower one third to one half of the vagina. Reapproximate the ends of the external rectal sphincter by interrupted sutures in the sheath of the

1. Continuous suture of mucosa with inverted suture of perineal body

2. Mucosal suture continued in skin and tied with inverted suture

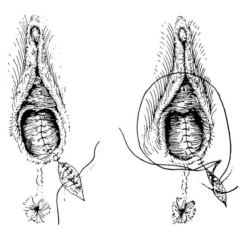

3. Closure of levator ani and perineal musculature

4. Skin closed subcutaneously

FIGURE 6-18. Episiotomy repair.

First-degree tear

Second-degree tear

Third-degree tear

Complete
(fourth-degree) tear

FIGURE 6-19. Perineal tears.

sphincter ani. The perimuscular fascia rather than the friable muscle itself affords a much superior closure. Repair the vaginal mucosal and perineal skin defect in the usual running subcuticular fashion; then, suture lacerations. In all circumstances, absorbable suture is used and care is taken that the sutures approximate, but do not strangulate, the tissue.

OUTLET FORCEPS

Outlet forceps are used to extend the head and to guide the infant beneath the symphysis and over the perineum. Outlet forceps are used only when the vertex is on the perineum (+4 station), with extension beginning. This procedure is indicated (1) *when spontaneous expulsion is inhibited* [e.g., by psychologic circumstances, analgesia, or anesthesia (caudal or spinal anesthesia markedly diminishes the patient's voluntary expulsive efforts)] (2) when *uterine inertia delays or prevents delivery of an infant* whose vertex is distending the perineum, (3) when *fetal compromise* occurs, and (4) to *prevent laceration of the introitus.*

OBSTETRIC ANALGESIA, AMNESIA, AND REGIONAL ANESTHESIA

Pain in childbirth is normally due to traction on the adnexal, uterine, and cervical supports; pressure on the ureters, bladder, urethra, and bowel; *dilatation* of the cervix and lower birth canal; *hypoxia* and the accumulation of catabolites in the myometrium; and *fear, severe tension, and anxiety.* In *dystocia,* or abnormal labor, pain often may be due to cephalopelvic disproportion. Tetanic, prolonged, or dysrhythmic uterine contractions may be painful, and intrapartal infection may cause pain.

The *management of any pain requires individualization.* With proper preparation, however, the patient requires much less medication to spare both herself and her infant. Additionally, the gravida's experience is enhanced, she becomes a team member, and she is able to profit from the birth experience, enhancing her love of the newborn.

The following types of pain relief are in use today: positive conditioning of the patient, hypnotics, analgesics, which decrease the patient's pain threshold; amnesics or hypnotics, which obscure the memory of pain and associated disagreeable experiences; regional anesthesia, which interrupts afferent pain pathways; and general anesthesia, which eliminates central perception of discomfort.

TYPES OF PAIN RELIEF

Positive Conditioning

Positive conditioning of the receptive patient during late pregnancy or early labor may reduce tensions and limit the need for pain relief medication. There are a number of successful techniques for accomplishing this, and they should be encouraged even if both patient and physician recognize that other agents can also be employed. Training and the patient's participation are required and, to be successful, are started antenatally.

Analgesics

The commonly employed analgesics are *narcotic drugs,* for example, 25–75 mg IV or IM (low-dose) Demerol. Injectable narcotics in the usual doses elevate the pain threshold by ≥50% to establish a state of relaxation and lethargy. Most of these drugs have a peak action of <90 min and a duration of effect of at least 1–2 h. *Undesirable side effects are nausea, vomiting, cough suppression, intestinal stasis, and in the early first stage of labor,* diminution in the frequency, intensity, and duration of uterine contractions. Frequently, Phenergan (25 mg) or similar compounds are added because of their antiemetic and potentiating effects. Amnesia is not achieved. *Narcotics adversely affect the infant by depressing all CNS functions, especially those of the respiratory center.* Early preterm status, growth retardation, trauma, or asphyxia enhances the susceptibility of the infant to narcosis.

Amnestics

Hydroxyzine (Vistaril) is an example of an amnestic. It is *useful in the first stage of labor* because of a calming effect tranquilizing action. It may reduce the amount of analgesic drug required. Hydroxyzine has a long half-life. Their use in the first stage of labor in dosages of 5–15 mg every 4 h does not appear to have a deleterious effect on the newborn.

Nerve Blocks

Consider nerve blocks in two categories: *local anesthetics* and the *true regional blocks.* The former is exemplified by paracervical and pudendal blocks and the latter by epidural and spinal anesthetics. It should be recalled that local anesthetics are generally divided into the *ester-linked and the amide-linked.* The ester-linked anesthetics are deactivated locally or in the blood by destruction of the ester linkage. Therefore, they have a shorter action and avoid maternal overdosage. They also have less chance of crossing the placenta in quantities causative of fetal compromise.

Paracervical Anesthesia

A *needle guide* (Fig. 6-20) is useful in directing pudendal and paracervical anesthetic blocks. When using a guide $5\frac{1}{2}$ inches long, a $6\frac{1}{2}$-inch 22-gauge spinal needle will protrude only slightly beyond the guide (desirable).

Paracervical anesthesia (Fig. 6-21) is administered when the *cervix is dilated 4 cm or more*. It relieves pain until the presenting

FIGURE 6-20. Iowa trumpet assembly.

FIGURE 6-21.   Paracervical submucous block.

part reaches the lower vagina, when a pudendal and perineal block or other anesthetic may be required. The needle point is inserted just submucosally (0.1–0.2 cm) into the paracervical tissues at the cervicouterine junction at 4 o'clock and 8 o'clock. Inject no more than 10 mL of 1% procaine on each side.

Exceptional maternal sensitivity to the medication or direct vascular injections (manifest by tachycardia, syncope, seizures) requires 100% oxygen and supportive measures. Paracervical block may cause fetal bradycardia associated with decreased placental blood flow and, perhaps, a reflex mechanism. However, the majority of serious problems are caused by direct fetal injection. In such cases, it is better to allow the fetus to recover in utero than to deliver it in haste.

Pudendal or Perineal Block
(Fig. 6-22). This permits spontaneous, breech, low forceps, or midforceps delivery with little local pain. It is extremely safe and simple, and the patient maintains her ability to cooperate during labor. The infant rarely is depressed, and blood loss is minimal. Disadvantages include discomfort during the injection and a 5-min delay for anesthetic effect.

The two nerves to be blocked on each side of the vagina are the *pudendal and the posterior femoral cutaneous nerves.* The pudendal nerve lies near the inner aspect of the ischial spine and should be blocked there. The posterior femoral cutaneous nerve may be injected beneath the inferior medial border of the ischial tuberosity. The descending branches of the ilioinguinal nerves supply the clitoral region. The perirectal zone is innervated by the hemorrhoidal nerves. The procedure for pudendal and posterior femoral cutaneous block follows:

Develop a wheal of 0.5%–1% procaine (or equivalent) at the base of each labium majus. Perform all injections through this site.

Palpate the ischial spines vaginally or rectally. Slowly guide a 4- or 5-inch, 20- or 21-gauge spinal needle toward each spine while injecting a small amount of procaine ahead of the advancing point. Aspirate, and if the needle is not in a vessel, deposit 5 mL of anesthetic posterior and lateral to the tip of each spine. This blocks the pudendal nerve. Refill the syringe if necessary, leaving the needle in place, and proceed in a similar manner to anesthetize the other areas specified. Keep the needle moving while injecting, and avoid the vaginal mucosa and periosteum.

Withdraw the needle about 3 cm and redirect it toward an ischial tuberosity. Inject 3 mL near the center of each tuberosity to anesthetize the inferior hemorrhoidal and lateral femoral cutaneous nerves.

Withdraw the needle almost entirely and then slowly advance it toward the symphysis pubica almost to the clitoris, keeping it about 2 cm lateral to the labial fold and about 1–2 cm beneath the skin. Inject 5 mL of procaine on each side beneath the symphysis

Needle guide in place on ischial spine

Needle inserted through needle guide

FIGURE 6-22. Use of needle guide (Iowa trumpet) in transvaginal anesthetic block.

to block the ilioinguinal and genitocrural nerves. Expect prompt flaccid relaxation and good anesthesia for 30–60 min.

Although this procedure is optimal, it is far *more common practice* today to merely anesthetize the pudendal nerve using the *transvaginal technique* demonstrated in Figure 6-22. In this technique, the ischial spine is palpated transvaginally and a guide is introduced to facilitate needle placement. The guided needle is placed just inferior and medial to the spine. It is then inserted ~1 cm in the tissue. After aspiration to ascertain that the injection will not be intravascular, the pudendal nerve is blocked by deposition of 5 mL of 0.5%–1% procaine (or equivalent). The procedure is repeated on the contralateral side.

Regional Blocks

Caution: *Special training, skill, and experience are required to administer regional anesthesia.* One must become familiar with the techniques and the pitfalls and be knowledgeable in the selection of procedures. Useful generalizations are noted. Table 6-3 details the indications for regional vs. general anesthesia, and Table 6-4 shows their relative risks.

Anesthetic administration should never be undertaken without having available analeptic drugs, oxygen, endotracheal equipment, and full resuscitation equipment (to treat complications). To prevent complications, it is *crucial to avoid technical errors* (e.g., intravascular injection of anesthetic drugs or accidental intrathecal injection during epidural anesthesia). The prognosis is best for mother and infant (regardless of the type of anesthesia) when obstetric anesthesiologists, obstetricians, and neonatologists work as a team.

TABLE 6-3
INDICATIONS FOR REGIONAL VS.
GENERAL ANESTHESIA

Regional Anesthesia	General Anesthesia
Recent meal	Need for rapid
Respiratory infection or asthma	delivery, severe
Possible airway problems	fetal compromise
	Maternal hemorrhage
	Maternal anxiety,
	hysteria
	Poor uterine
	relaxation
	Blood coagulopathies
	Neuropathies
	(epilepsy excluded)
	Bacteremia, viremia

TABLE 6-4
RISKS OF REGIONAL VS. GENERAL ANESTHESIA

Regional Anesthesia	General Anesthesia
Hypotension	Aspiration of gastric contents
Accidental intravascular or high spinal block	Difficult intubation, e.g., obesity
Postspinal headache	Airway obstruction
Spinal, caudal neuropathy	Prolonged apnea
	Laryngeal pain, edema
	Unfavorable maternal recall

The *major physiologic alterations imposed by gestation must be understood, and necessary alterations in technique must be introduced* (e.g., cardiovascular, respiratory, and gastrointestinal systems and fluid and electrolyte balance). The effective anesthetic dose for epidural or spinal anesthesia is reduced, and maternal uptake and elimination of inhalant anesthetics are increased. In addition, hypoxia is more likely to occur during apnea or airway obstruction. The hazard of hypotension and aspiration of gastric contents is also increased. All of these problems can affect the fetus secondarily. In cases of marked obesity, endotracheal intubation can be difficult. The fetus may be jeopardized directly by undesirable side effects of drugs or indirectly by reduced uteroplacental circulation.

Prevent aortocaval compression by placing the patient in a supported (wedge or pillow) oblique or lateral decubitus position during transport to the delivery room and during delivery. A slight head-down tilt of the bed or table should help also.

Administer *oxygen* by mask to the mother until delivery to improve fetal oxygenation. This is appropriate for both general and regional anesthesia.

Prehydrate the gravida to *avoid hypotension and reduced uteroplacental circulation.* Rapidly infuse approximately 1 liter of Ringer's lactate solution to increase blood volume and ensure osmotic equilibrium before and after the anesthetic block. (Do not use dextrose solution because delayed neonatal hypoglycemia can develop.) Maintain the patient in slight lateral decubitus position.

For *hypotension,* use a drug with *cardiotonic* (as opposed to vasospastic) action (e.g., ephedrine 50 mg IM). Vasopressors with primarily peripheral effects, for example, metaramide (Aramine) and phenylephrine (Neo-Synephrine) increase uterine vascular resistance and can be harmful to the fetus.

Epidural Anesthesia
Epidural anesthesia can be given continuously, that is, during the latter portion of the first and all of the second stage of labor, or terminally, as a single injection just before delivery. The advantages of properly performed epidural anesthesia are that it causes no fetal asphyxia, the mother remains conscious to witness the birth, blood loss is minimal, vaginal and perineal structures remain relaxed, and headache is unlikely. The technique must be exact, however, and inadvertent massive (high) spinal anesthesia occurs occasionally. Undesirable reactions include *rapid absorption syndrome* (hypotension, bradycardia, hallucinations, seizures) and postpartal backache and paresthesia.

The incidence of *persistent occiput posterior positions is increased* because the fetal head is not normally rotated on the relaxed pelvic floor. Forceps rotation and delivery, therefore, is more often necessary.

Spinal Anesthesia
Spinal anesthesia (saddleblock) is widely used to alleviate the pain of delivery. The *advantages* of spinal anesthesia are that *fetal hypoxia rarely occurs, blood loss is minimal,* the *mother remains conscious during delivery,* no inhalation anesthetics or analgesic drugs are required, the technique is not difficult, and good relaxation of the pelvic floor and lower birth canal is achieved. *Spinal headache occurs in about 5% of patients. Operative delivery* is more often required because voluntary expulsive efforts are eliminated. *Hypotension* may result. Respiratory failure may develop if the anesthetic ascends as a result of rapid injection or straining by the patient. The procedure for spinal anesthesia follows:

> With the patient lying on her side or sitting and between contractions, inject 40 mg of procaine (0.8 mL of 5% solution) or comparable drug slowly into the intradaral space (confirmed by flow of CSF) through the third or fourth lumbar interspace. Use a 25-gauge needle to pierce the dura. (This avoids leakage of CSF causative of headache.) Elevate the patient's head on a pillow immediately after the injection. Tilt the table up or down to achieve a level of anesthesia at or near the level of the umbilicus. Anesthesia will be maximal in 10–15 min and will last ≥1 h.
> *Record blood pressure and respirations every 5–10 min.*

Give *oxygen* for respiratory depression. For hypotension, give vasopressors (e.g., ephedrine 25 mg IV).

For cesarean section, tilting the patient about 15–20 degrees to the left by elevating her right hip should avoid vena caval compression by the uterus and possible fetal distress.

GENERAL ANESTHESIA

For occasional deliveries (e.g., instrumented deliveries or cesarean section), general anesthesia may be necessary. This generally is induced by minimal dose short acting barbiturate or equivalent IV, followed by nitrous oxide-oxygen inhalation and succinylcholine by IV drip. Considerable experience is required. For general anesthesia of gravid patients, *endotracheal intubation is essential to prevent aspiration of gastric contents.* Table 6-3 details the indications for general and regional anesthesia, and Table 6-4 shows the relative risks of each. Some useful generalizations for general anesthesia during pregnancy follow.

Prevent hypoxemia by administration of high-flow oxygen for 4–5 min before endotracheal intubation when apnea occurs. *Avoid aspiration of regurgitated gastric contents* by preoperative *administration of liquid antacid, cimetidine, or equivalent,* and insertion of a *cuffed endotracheal tube* after anesthesia induction. Surgery should await adequate lung aeration.

Maintain at least 50% oxygen with anesthetic gas mixtures. Avoid hypoventilation, which results in maternal–fetal hypoxemia and acidosis. Prevent hyperventilation, which causes reduced uteroplacental blood flow and decreased fetal oxygenation. *Maternal oxygen saturation monitoring is recommended.*

DRUGS UNCOMMONLY USED TODAY

Inhalant analgesics (trichlorethylene and nitrous oxide) have been abandoned because of possible overuse and disastrous consequences. Likewise, the use of sedatives has been largely abandoned. They slow mentation, reduce perception of sensory stimuli, and increase suggestion receptivity. In addition, they are poor analgesics, are not amnestics, do not raise the pain threshold appreciably, and they can cause serious fetal depression. Periodic apnea, and even abolition of all movements, may be prolonged barbiturate effects. The amnesics (e.g., scopolamine) have been retired because their effects are unpredictable and they deprive the patient of her ability to participate. Some patients become somnolent or stuporous, whereas others become restless, hallucinating, and delirious. Phenothiazine drugs

(Phenergan) potentiate certain of the desirable (as well as a few of the undesirable) effects of the analgesics, amnesics, and general anesthetics but also have been used less, largely because of their undesirable side effects.

INDUCTION OF LABOR

Induction of labor should be performed only on *specific indications*. There is some risk in any induction, and the *potential benefit must outweigh the risk.*

INDICATIONS

Individual induction of labor, especially in the treatment of abnormal pregnancy (preeclampsia-eclampsia, pyelonephritis), reduces maternal and fetal morbidity and mortality. Recall that delivery is either warranted or it is not. The indication for induction should be so valid that if it fails, delivery is performed by cesarean section. The following indications for induction of labor are valid in no more than 5%–8% of pregnancies.

> *Maternal infections* (e.g., diverticulitis) that fail to resolve and are likely to become more severe unless pregnancy is concluded
> *Partial placental separation* with uterine bleeding
> *Preeclampsia-eclampsia* (delivery is the treatment for this process)
> *Diabetes mellitus with a mature fetus*
> *Renal insufficiency* (from any cause)
> *Premature rupture of the membranes* when delivery is indicated (Chapter 11)
> *Previous precipitate delivery* in a woman who cannot be transported quickly to a hospital
> *Marked polyhydramnios*
> *Placental insufficiency*
> *Isoimmunization* (erythroblastosis)

CONTRAINDICATIONS TO LABOR INDUCTION

Cephalopelvic disproportion
Unfavorable obstetric circumstances, especially floating or deflected vertex or unfavorable presentation (including breech and multiple pregnancy)

Firm, closed, uneffaced posterior cervix (a vaginal examination must be performed before induction so that ripeness of the cervix can be confirmed)

Previous uterine or cervical operations (e.g., cesarean section or multiple myomectomy)

Maternal cardiac disease (functional class III or IV)

Grand multiparity (more than five pregnancies); with oxytocin, the uterus may rupture

Fetal compromise without induction

Placenta previa

DANGERS OF INDUCTION

For the Mother

Emotional crisis (fear and anxiety)

Failure of induction and subsequent attempts to institute labor or to deliver the fetus

Uterine inertia and prolonged labor

Tumultuous labor and tetanic uterine contractions with the possiblity of *rupture of the uterus,* or *cervical lacerations*

Hemorrhagic complications, including abruptio placentae and atonic uterine postpartum hemorrhage

Intrauterine infection from examinations, rupture of membranes, or manipulation

Hypofibrinogenemia or other clotting abnormality

Amniotic fluid embolization

For the Fetus

An *ill-timed induced delivery* exposes the infant to the risks of prematurity

Prolapse of the cord is an early, and infection a late, complication of amniotomy

Violent labor may result in asphyxia, with subsequent damage

Trauma as a result of the labor or delivery or both

DETERMINING APPROPRIATENESS OF INDUCTION (THE BISHOP SCORE)

Bishop devised a scoring system (Table 6-5) to predict the outcome of induction when no contraindications (e.g., placenta previa) exist. *A Bishop score of ≥9 indicates that labor may be induced with only a small chance of failure.* This has been so reliable that it is now applied for many other situations (e.g., premature labor).

TABLE 6-5
BISHOP SCORE*

Cervical Criteria	Score			
	0	1	2	3
Effacement (%)	0–30	40–50	60–70	80
Dilatation (cm)	0	1–2	3–4	5–6
Station of vertex (−3 to +3 scale)	−3	−2	−1, 0	+1, +2
Consistency	Firm	Medium	Soft	
Position	Posterior	Midposition	Anterior	

*From E. H. Bishop. A pelvic scoring for elective induction. *Obstet Gynecol* 1974;24:266.

PREPARATION FOR INDUCTION

The patient must be in a labor and delivery area with full anesthetic, neonatal, nursing, medical, blood banking, laboratory, and emergency facilities. Vital signs must be obtained, and an IV infusion should be started through a large-bore catheter. Fetal monitoring is always required during induction or stimulation of labor.

Prostaglandins (PGE₂, 5 mg in a suppository, gel or strip) applied to the cervix the night before induction ripens the cervix (i.e., increases the Bishop score), thus enhancing the likelihood of initiation of labor.

Enemas and purges for the preparation or induction of labor (by reflex uterine hyperactivity) are harmful and painful and often are unsuccessful. They are contraindicated. Ergot preparations are contraindicated for induction. They cause sustained contractions and must not be used before delivery for any reason.

METHODS OF INDUCTION

SURGICAL METHODS

Amniotomy is the safest (as measured by mortality and morbidity), *easiest, and surest way to induce labor.* Release of amniotic fluid shortens the muscle bundles of the myometrium. The strength and duration of the contractions are thereby increased. Amniotomy is painless and causes few complications.

Rupture of the membranes is accomplished through the partially dilated cervix using a hook or other sharp instrument. Do not displace the infant's head! Keep the patient in bed in Fowler's position after amniotomy so that slow drainage of fluid can occur. Anticipate labor <6 h later if the patient is at term.

Stripping of the membranes (alone) is not recommended, because the result *is unpredictable.* This technique involves inserting a finger between the margin of the partially dilated cervix and the membranes and separating the two by a circular motion. It usually is uncomfortable and can be painful. It probably enhances the natural production of cervical prostaglandins. Unfortunately, untimely membrane rupture, damage leading to bleeding from a low-lying placenta, or mild amnionitis may occur.

MEDICAL METHODS

Parenteral administration of a very dilute solution of oxytocin is a most effective medical means of inducing labor.

The dosage of *oxytocin must be individualized.* The administration of oxytocin is really a biologic assay: the smallest possible effective dose must be determined for each patient and then used to initiate labor. In most cases, it is sufficient to add 0.1 mL of oxytocin (1 U Pitocin or Syntocinon) to 1 liter of intravenous solution. Thus, each milliliter of solution will contain 1 mU of oxytocin.

Begin induction or augmentation at 1 mU/min. Increase oxytocin arithmetically by 2 mU increments (e.g., 1,3,5 . . . mU/min) at 15-min interval.

Doses greater than 15 mU/min are of concern. Those above 40 mU/min cause renal alterations and should not be necessary except in rare circumstances. Administration is controlled by the use of a constant infusion pump.

Constant observation by qualified attendants (preferably a physician) is required.

When contractions of 40–60 mm Hg (internal monitor pressure) or 40–60 sec (on the external monitor) occur at intervals of 1–4 min, the oxytocin dose should not be increased further. If contractions cease or become weak and ineffectual after a satisfactory start, the infusion can be resumed. *The infusion should be slowed or terminated if contractions exceed 60 mm Hg, exceed 60-sec duration, or have an interval of <2 min or if the fetus shows any signs of fetal compromise (Chapter 5).*

It is not uncommon for the first induction attempt to fail; thus repeated (serial) induction must be considered. The criteria for a failed induction include inability to establish a consistent labor pattern (meeting the cited standards) and failure to affect cervical dilatation, effacement, or descent. *Prospective discussion with the gravida and her family concerning the possibility of serial induction is very useful.*

Should labor fail to start in one 6-h interval of induction with intact membranes (e.g., diabetes, preeclampsia) and both mother and fetus remain stable, efforts should cease for 6–18 h. This will allow the mother and myometrium to recover. Prostaglandin E_2 cervical application should be considered. Another 6-h attempt should follow. If this too fails, another 6–18 h rest interval is undertaken (again, if all is stable). At the start of the next 6-h induction, the membranes should be ruptured. If induction should fail, cesarean section is warranted and should be done as soon as it is ascertained that induction is a failure.

Induction with ruptured membranes must proceed more rapidly and should not exceed 24 h from the time of rupture. It is however, still preferable to proceed in approximate 6-h increments.

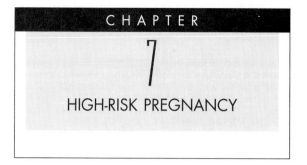

CHAPTER

7

HIGH-RISK PREGNANCY

Although pregnancy can be classified as a normal physiologic condition, it is fraught with considerable risk to both mother and offspring. Fortunately, *most of the risk occurs to a minority of patients.* Thus, it is prudent to *identify those at risk and attempt to prevent the morbidity and mortality.* Some factors contributing to risk are quite obvious, but others are very subtle. Thus, care must be taken in definitions, screening programs, and application of the tools available for diagnosis and treatment. The following is but one of the ways to approach this multifaceted set of circumstances.

DEFINITION, INCIDENCE, AND IMPORTANCE

A high-risk pregnancy is one in which the mother or perinate is or will be in jeopardy (death or complications) *during gestation or in the puerperium/neonatal interval.* Estimates of the incidence of high-risk pregnancy vary widely depending mainly on the criteria used for definition and the accuracy of the data collection. Nevertheless, by most standards, ~20% of established pregnancies in the United States are at some risk and ~5% are at high risk. *About half can be identified antenatally and another quarter during labor* (Table 7-1). For example, *the majority of perinatal deaths are associated with prematurity or congenital anomalies.* If these two conditions are excluded, 60% of fetal and >50% of neonatal deaths are associated with only five obstetric complications: *breech presentation, premature separation of the placenta, preeclampsia-eclampsia, multiple pregnancy, and urinary tract infection.* Certain less common complications (e.g., cord prolapse) also cause an inordinately high proportion or perinatal losses. Of course, a low-risk pregnancy (not endangered by present or foreseeable complications) can become high risk at any time.

The *early identification of risk factors is vital* for both avoidance of serious problems and proper treatment of complications

TABLE 7-1
IDENTIFICATION OF SPECIFIC OBSTETRIC
RISK FACTORS

INITIAL EVALUATION	
Biologic Factors	
High Risk	Some Risk
Maternal age <15 or ≥35 years	Maternal age 15–19 years
Morbid obesity	>20% of standard height for weight
Poor nutrition	<20% of standard height for weight
Maternal malignancy	Short stature (≤60 inches)
Ovarian neoplasms	Uterine leiomyomata
Genetic or familial disorder	Pelvic or spinal deformity
Incompetent cervix	
Cervical malformation	
Uterine malformation	
Congenital anomaly	
Genital tract anomalies	
Obstetric History	
High Risk	Some Risk
Parity of ≥8	Parity of >5
Three or more abortions	Prolonged labor or dystocia
Stillborn or neonatal loss	Infertility
Previous pregnancy with:	Prior ABO incompatibility
Premature labor	Prior fetal malpresentation
Birth weight <2500 g	Previous PIH
Birth weight >4000 g	Genital tract infections
Genetic disorder	Human papillomavirus (HPV)
Congenital anomaly	Herpes
Isoimmunization	Gonorrheal
Eclampsia	*Chamydia*
Birth damaged infant	Group B *Streptococcus*
Special neonatal care	
Medically indicated pregnancy termination	
Molar gestation	

TABLE 7-1
(Continued)

Medical and Surgical History High Risk	Some Risk
Hypertension (moderate to severe)	Mild hypertension
Severe renal disease	Class I heart disease
Class II–IV heart disease	Gestational diabetes
Insulin-regulated diabetes	Recurrent urinary
Endocrine ablation (thyroid)	infections
Abnormal cervical cytology	Positive serology
Sickle cell disease	Sickle cell trait
Pulmonary disease	Epilepsy
Liver disease	Emotional disorders
Recurrent pyelonephritis	Smoking
Collagen vascular disease	Pelvic inflammatory
Malignancy	disease
Gastrointestinal disease	Previous ectopic
Substance abuse	pregnancy
Heavy smoking (>10 day)	Physical abuse

EVALUATION ON EACH PRENATAL VISIT, EARLY PREGNANCY (≤20 WEEKS)

High Risk	Some Risk
Teratic exposure	Antenatal diagnosis
Failure of uterine growth	indicated
Isoimmunization	Unresponsive urinary
Severe anemia	tract infection
(≤9 g Hgb)	Possible ectopic gestation
Multiple gestation	Missed abortion
Fetal anomalies	Severe hyperemesis
Cervical incompetence	gravidarum
Insulin-regulated	Positive serology
diabetes	Sexually transmitted
Fetal anomalies	disease
Nonimmune hydrops	Unresponsive anemia
Renal agenesis	Vaginal bleeding
(Potter's)	Diet-regulated diabetes

(Continued)

TABLE 7-1
(Continued)

EVALUATION ON EACH PRENATAL VISIT, LATER PREGNANCY (>20 WEEKS)	
High Risk	Some Risk
IUGR	Pregnancy ≥41 1/2 weeks
Anemia (≤9 g Hgb)	Preeclampsia
Severe preeclampsia	Breech (for vaginal delivery)
Eclampsia	Placenta previa
Isoimmunization	Premature onset of labor (<36 weeks)
Oligohydramnios	Premature rupture (<38 weeks)
Hydramnios	
Thromboembolic disease	
Abruptio placentae	Chronic or acute pyelonephritis
Abnormal antepartum test (NST, CST, BPP)	Abnormal fetal position
Prolonged membrane rupture	
Fetal infections	

INTRAPARTUM EVALUATION	
High Risk	Some Risk
High-risk factors above	Mild PIH
Severe PIH or eclampsia	Rupture of membranes >12 h
Hydraminos or oligohydramnios	Primary dysfunctional labor
Amnionitis	Secondary arrest of dilatation
Prolonged membrane rupture (>24 h)	Labor >20 h
Uterine rupture	Second stage >2.5 h
Abruptio placentae	Precipitous labor
Placenta previa	Prolonged latent phase
Meconium in amniotic fluid	Uterine tetany
Abnormal presentation	Induction of labor
Multiple gestation	Operative forceps
Fetal weight <1500 g	Vacuum extraction
Fetal weight >4000 g	Nonreassuring FHR patterns
FHR patterns indicating compromise	

TABLE 7-1
(Continued)

| **INTRAPARTUM EVALUATION** | |
High Risk	Some Risk
Breech delivery	General anesthesia
Prolapsed cord	Abnormal maternal vital
Fetal acidosis	signs
Shoulder dystocia	Fetal presentation not
Maternal distress	descending with labor

responsible for increased maternal and perinatal mortality and morbidity. Despite steady improvement, at least three quarters of obstetric deaths (9/100,000 births) and at least one half of newborn deaths (10/1000 births) in the United States are preventable.

PRENATAL CARE: A DIAGNOSTIC AND THERAPEUTIC PROGRAM

Good prenatal care is preventive medicine of a high order. It provides an opportunity to identify the individual's risk status and appropriately individualize care for each patient. Moreover, it has been amply demonstrated that those *gravidas who receive good prenatal care materially improve both their own and their offspring's chance* of successfully negotiating this most hazardous interval of life.

Maternal, fetal, or neonatal hazard often can be foretold by critical assessment of the gravida's history, physical examination, and antenatal course. Dozens of factors during pregnancy, labor, delivery, and the early puerperium suggest added risk; for example, unwanted pregnancy, ignorance, exposure to toxic products, and unwillingness or inability to obtain good early obstetric care relate to high-risk pregnancy. Whatever the problem, prevention, early diagnosis, and proper treatment will greatly reduce the perinatal mortality and morbidity rates. Thus, most clinicians include these factors in their plan for prenatal care (Chapter 5) and actively search for and treat them as the pregnancy progresses.

Additionally, several risk scoring systems to predict jeopardy have been suggested. Although risk scoring systems are not as sensitive or as specific as originally thought, they may provide a useful method to ensure that most of the risk-producing states are screened in each gestation.

HISTORICAL SCREENING

Poverty, ignorance, substance abuse, and unwanted pregnancy are sociologic conditions *associated with high-risk pregnancy.* These may take years to alleviate, and their solutions have little to do with medicine. For example, low socioeconomic and single marital status (in an adolescent) are two important obstetric high-risk factors. Although physicians cannot do much to remedy the underlying problem, proper diet, rest, social support, proper antenatal care, and good patient cooperation can improve the prognosis of such an adolescent to approximate that of most middle-income gravidas. Thus, *our purpose is to deal primarily with factors that can be influenced by medical management* and the currently available diagnostic and therapeutic modalities.

A *uniform perinatal record* is very useful to assist the physician in evaluating high-risk pregnancy. Some commercially available forms may use risk lists, whereas others rate factors according to their importance. Whatever system is used, it must be applied assiduously.

MATERNAL AGE

The lowest rates of maternal and perinatal morbidity and mortality occur at maternal age 20–29 years. Thus, younger and older women are at greater risk.

Adolescent pregnancy has a higher frequency of low birth weight infants, and in those younger than 16 years, there is increased risk of *pregnancy-induced hypertension.* Mothers *age 35 or older are at high risk, and those over 40 years are at extraordinary risk.* The most common problems are *increased chromosomal abnormalities, chronic hypertension, pregnancy-induced hypertension, obesity, uterine leiomyomas, increased incidence of age-related medical problems* (e.g., diabetes), and an *increased risk of being delivered by cesarean section.* The risk of *trisomy* is directly related to age, rising from *0.9% at age 35–36 years to 7.8% at age 43–44* years. Prenatal diagnosis screening questions (Table 7-2) should be asked of each older gravida and the follow-up documented. Starting the screening as early as maternal age 32 has merit. Women with a low level of serum alpha-fetoprotein (AFP), regardless of age, should

TABLE 7-2
PRENATAL DIAGNOSIS SCREENING QUESTIONS

	Circle Appropriate Answer	
1. Will you be age 35 or older when the baby is due?	Yes	No
2. Have you or the baby's father or anyone in either of your families ever had		
a. Down syndrome?	Yes	No
b. Spina bifida or meningomyelocele (open spine)?	Yes	No
c. Hemophilia (blood will not clot)?	Yes	No
d. Muscular dystrophy?	Yes	No
3. Have you or the baby's father had a child born dead or alive with a birth defect not listed in Question 2? If yes, describe:_____	Yes	No
4. Do you or the baby's father have any close relatives who are mentally retarded? If yes, list cause if known:_____	Yes	No
5. Do you or the baby's father or close relative in either of your families have any inherited genetic or chromosomal disease or disorder not listed above?	Yes	No
6. Have you or the spouse of this baby's father in a previous marriage had three or more *spontaneous* pregnancy losses?	Yes	No
7. Do you or the baby's father have any close relatives descended from Jewish people who lived in Eastern	Yes	No

(Continued)

TABLE 7-2
(Continued)

	Circle Appropriate Answer	
Europe (Ashkenazi Jews)? If yes, have either you or the baby's father been screened for Tay-Sachs disease? If yes, indicate results and who screened:_____	Yes	No
8. If patient or spouse is African American: Have you or the baby's father or any close relative been screened for sickle cell trait and found to be positive?	Yes	No

I have discussed with my doctor the above questions which are answered yes and understand that I am at increased risk for:

_____

and that it is usually possible to diagnose an affected fetus by testing amniotic fluid at about 16 weeks of pregnancy or placental tissue at an earlier time in pregnancy and I DO NOT want the test._____

                (Patient Signature)   (Date)

Patient wants amniocentesis and fetal diagnoses for:_____

_____

Patient referred for further testing or counseling concerning: _____

*Modified from *Antenatal Diagnosis,* NIH Publication No. 79-193, April 1979.

be considered for amniocentesis because they have an increased risk of trisomic offspring.

In summary, it is important to ascertain the following. Does the patient, her husband, or their family have heritable disorders (see Table 7-2)? What is the health of first-degree relatives (siblings, parents, and offspring), second-degree relatives (uncles, aunts, nephews, nieces, and grandparents), and third-degree relatives (first cousins)? What are the probable reproductive outcomes? Is there drug exposure (both husband and wife)? What are the parental ages (paternal risk ≥ 55)? What is the ethnic origin (because of enhanced risk of several disease states, e.g., Tay-Sachs disease in Ashkenazi Jews, β-thalassemia in Italians and Greeks, sickle cell anemia in African Americans, and α-thalassemia in Southeast Asians)?

OBSTETRIC HISTORY

The number of previous pregnancies is important. To para 5, there is increased chance of successful pregnancy. However, after 5, the risk from uterine inertia, postpartum hemorrhage, placenta previa, and abruptio placenta begins an almost exponential increase. A history of infertility places a patient at increased risk because of a greater incidence of fetal wastage. There is a correlation between the outcome of previous pregnancies and what may happen to the current pregnancy.

Thus, the following obstetric historical findings signal risk: induced hypertension, baby with known or suspected genetic disorder or congenital anomaly, and birth-damaged infant or infant requiring special neonatal care. Other historical risk factors include operative deliveries (cesarean section, midforceps or breech extraction), prolonged labor or dystocia, severe psychiatric disturbances associated with pregnancy, and closely spaced pregnancies (<3 months).

REPRODUCTIVE TRACT DISORDERS

Abnormalities of the reproductive tract cause at least 25% of recidive reproductive losses. Thus, a *history of incompetent cervix, septate uterus, bicornuate uterus, or uterine leiomyomas may warn of pregnancy risk.* Other reproductive tract aberrations that may place the pregnancy at risk because they can require therapy during pregnancy include *cervical dysplasia and ovarian tumors.* Should intervention be necessary, the safest time to perform surgery is during the second trimester, when both post surgical abortion and preterm labor have the lowest incidence.

EXPOSURE TO FETOTOXIC AGENT

For discussion of the topic, see Chapter 5.

MEDICAL COMPLICATIONS
OF PREGNANCY

Some of the systemic diseases creating risk in pregnancy include: blood disorders (e.g., coagulopathy, sickle cell disease), *cancer, cerebral aneurysms or tumors, chronic hypertension, connective tissue disease* (e.g., systemic lupus erythematosus), *diabetes mellitus, endocrine ablation, epilepsy, gastrointestinal and liver disease, heart disease, pulmonary disease, renal disease* (e.g., glomerulonephritis), and *thyroid disorders* (both hyperthyroidism and hypothyroidism).

FAMILY HISTORY

A detailed family history keyed to *mental retardation* (with particular attention to males—potential fragile X syndrome), *multiple gestation,* and *heritable diseases* is mandatory. Risk assessment is aided by a three-generation pedigree.

PHYSICAL EXAMINATION

STATURE

Women less than 5 feet (150 cm) tall have increased fetopelvic disproportion. Thus, short stature is an indication for careful bony pelvis assessment.

WEIGHT

Ideal weight is necessarily predicated on height and body habitus, and abnormalities of weight must be individualized. *Both underweight and overweight signal risk for the perinate.* Moreover, the maternal prepregnancy weight and gain during pregnancy are related directly to birth weight. The woman who weighs <100 pounds (45 kg) when not pregnant has an increased chance of having an SGA infant. Women who are obese for height have a greater chance of gestational diabetes as well as pregnancy complicated by LGA birth, dysfunctional labor, shoulder dystocia, and birth trauma. Morbidly obese gravidas increase their risk even further.

BLOOD PRESSURE

Hypertension poses risk to pregnancy and requires evaluation (Chapter 13). Although occasional hypotension from orthostasis or from the supine hypotensive syndrome is of concern, it is easily managed symptomatically.

BREASTS

When a mass is found, the usual breast *cancer workup cannot be delayed by the pregnancy.*

HEART

Diastolic murmurs, systolic murmurs ≥grade 3, and arrhythmias always require a medical evaluation.

VASCULAR SYSTEM

Severe varicosities tend to *thrombose* during pregnancy (p. 441).

PELVIC EVALUATION

Pelvic problems relating to risk include genital prolapse, fixation of a retroflexed and retroverted uterus, uterine anomalies, uterine leiomyomata, cervical tumors, cervical laceration, cervical incompetence, genital condylomata acuminata (which may cause neonatal laryngeal papillomas), genital herpes, group B streptococcal infections, abnormalities of the ovaries, abnormalities of the uterine tubes, and abnormalities of the bony pelvis or pelvic capacity.

A *diagnosis and a plan of management for each of the conditions placing the patient at risk may assist in enhancing outcome.*

COURSE OF PREGNANCY

ANTENATAL VISITS

Antenatal visits must be *more frequent for high-risk* than for normal obstetric patients to accurately appraise the pregnancy and identify and correct problems. Antenatal visits also provide an opportunity for education about problems, their solution, and counseling.

The etiologies of many serious problems that develop during pregnancy are reviewed elsewhere. Thus, only the major categories are summarized here.

ABNORMAL VITAL SIGNS

The most frequent aberrations of vital signs signaling risk during pregnancy are abnormal weight or blood pressure. As noted previously, *failure to gain weight during pregnancy often is associated with an SGA perinate,* and *excessive weight gain is associated with an LGA perinate. Fever* can trigger preterm labor and can injure the fetal CNS. *Pregnancy-induced hypertension (PIH)* is most often indicated by a ≥140/90 blood pressure or a ≥30 mm Hg systolic or a ≥15 mm Hg diastolic rise. Other symptoms of PIH include proteinuria and significant edema (Chapter 13).

COMMON LABORATORY ABNORMALITIES

The most common abnormal laboratory values during pregnancy are *urinary* (bacteria, protein, or glucose) or *hematologic.* Significant *bacteriuria* (>100,000 bacteria/mL) places the patient at risk for *pyelonephritis, premature rupture of membranes,* and *premature onset of labor. Diabetes mellitus* (even if only gestational) is related to a number of pregnancy risks (p. 464). Moreover, gestational diabetic mothers require follow-up after delivery because they are at increased risk of developing chemical diabetes. *Hematologic risks,* the most common being *anemia* and *isoimmunization,* are detailed in Chapter 14.

PROBLEMATIC SYMPTOMS OR SIGNS

Symptoms or signs of greatest concern during the course of pregnancy include *vaginal bleeding, uterine growth out of proportion to dates, and the untimely termination of pregnancy.* Uterine bleeding in early or late pregnancy warns of jeopardy to the pregnancy (Chapters 10 and 11). A discrepancy in uterine size for dates requires ultrasonic scanning for explanation. If the *size is less than reasonable for dates,* it is due most frequently to an error in dates, an SGA fetus, a congenital anomaly, or oligohydraminos. If the *uterus is larger than expected for dates,* it most commonly indicates hydramnios, multiple gestation, fetal anomaly, an LGA fetus, or an error in dates. Preterm termination of pregnancy, with or without rupture of membranes, is second only to congenital anomalies as a cause of morbidity and mortality. Postterm pregnancy termination poses risks of uteroplacental insufficiency, meconium-containing amniotic fluid, and complicated labor or trauma during labor and delivery (from excessive size).

SURGERY DURING PREGNANCY

Although not increased by pregnancy, *acute appendicitis is the most common surgical emergency during gestation.* The major pregnancy complications of acute appendicitis (similar to all abdominal surgery) include *premature delivery* and *peritonitis*.

If all *physical trauma* (e.g., assault, motor vehicle accidents, and falls) were categorized as surgical emergencies, trauma would head the list. The patient with significant physical trauma during pregnancy has a marked risk of *abruptio placenta*.

IMMUNIZATIONS DURING PREGNANCY

Current recommendations concerning immunizations during pregnancy are summarized in Table 7-3.

COURSE OF LABOR

Common problems during the course of labor include dystocia, fetal distress, and meconium-stained amniotic fluid.

DYSTOCIA

Dystocia is abnormal or difficult labor. It occurs in <10% of nulliparas and is less common in multiparas. The etiology of dystocia is typically ascribed to one or a combination of the 4 Ps (pelvis, passenger, powers, and placenta).

The most common *pelvic abnormalities associated with dystocia* include *bony size or configuration, birth canal soft tissue aberration* (e.g., congenital anomalies, scarring of the birth canal, conglutination of the external cervix os, or massive condylomata accuminata), and other *reproductive organ neoplasia* (e.g., cervical carcinoma, ovarian cyst, or uterine leiomyoma), including a *distended bladder or bowel.*

ABNORMALITIES OF THE PASSENGER

Abnormalities of the passenger (fetal dystocia) include *excessive fetal size* (>4000 g), *malpositions* (e.g., breech, transverse lie), *congenital anomalies* (e.g., hydrocephalus, sacrococcygeal teratoma), and *multiple gestations* (e.g., malpresentation, locking twins—twin A breech, twin B vertex).

UTERINE DYSTOCIA

Uterine dystocia (i.e., uterine activity that does not elicit the normal progress of labor) is referred to as an *abnormality of the powers.*

TABLE 7-3
RECOMMENDATIONS FOR IMMUNIZATIONS
DURING PREGNANCY

Cholera	Comply only to meet international travel requirements
Hepatitis A	Imunize gravida after exposure
	Newborns of mothers who are incubating or ill should receive 1 dose after birth
Hepatitis B	Newborn should receive hyperimmune globulin soon after delivery, followed by vaccination
Influenza	Immunize gravida following criteria recommended for general population
Measles	Live virus vaccine during pregnancy contraindicated on theoretical grounds
	Pooled immune globulins for postexposure prophylaxis
Mumps	Theoretically contraindicated during pregnancy
Plague	Immunize only if there is substantial infection risk
Poliomyelitis	Not routinely recommended but mandatory in epidemics or when traveling to epidemic areas
Rabies	Same as nonpregnant
Rubella	Contraindicated (although teratogenicity negligible in follow-up of those inadvertently given the vaccine)
Tetanus and diphtheria	Give toxoid if no primary series or no booster in 10 years
	Postexposure prophylaxis in unvaccinated with tetanus immune globulin plus toxoid

TABLE 7-3
(Continued)

Typhoid	Recommended if traveling to endemic area
Varicella	Varicella-zoster immune globulin for exposure
	Indicated for newborns whose mothers developed varicella within 4 days before or 2 days after delivery
Yellow fever	Postpone travel if possible but immunize before travel to high-risk areas

Commonly, uterine dystocia includes *hypertonic, hypotonic, or discoordinate uterine activity,* although *lack of voluntary expulsive effort* during the second stage of labor also may delay delivery.

ABNORMAL PLACENTAL LOCATION

Abnormal placental location (e.g., placenta previa or low-lying posterior implantation) decreases pelvic capacity by lying over the sacral promentory.

PELVIC TYPES

As noted in Chapter 1, the female pelvis is classified into four major types, although various combinations may occur (Fig. 7-1, Table 7-4).

The *gynecoid pelvis* is the most favorable for vaginal delivery and is seen in ~50% of women in the United States. It is characterized by oval inlet (transverse diameter slightly exceeds the anteroposterior diameter), straight sidewalls, nonprominent ischial spines, a wide subpubic arch, and a concave sacrum.

The *android* (male-like) pelvis is found in ~33% of Caucasian and 15% of African American women. The android inlet is wedge-shaped, the pelvic sidewalls are convergent, the ischial spines are prominent, the subpubic arch is narrow, and the sacrum is inclined anteriorly in its lower one third. It is likely to be associated with persistent occiput posterior position and deep transverse arrest dystocia.

TABLE 7-4
PELVIC TYPES[a]

	Gynecoid	Android	Anthropoid	Platypelloid
Inlet	Rounded or slightly heart-shaped Ample anterior and posterior segments	Wedge-shaped or rounded triangle Posterior segment wide, flat; anterior narrow, pointed	Anteroposterior ovoid with length of anterior and posterior segments increased Transverse diameter reduced	Transverse ovoid; increased transverse AP diameter of both segments
Sacrum	Curved, average length	Straight with forward inclination	Normally curved but long and nerrow	Curved, short
Sacrosciatic notch	Medium width	Narrow	Wide, shallow	Slightly narrowed
Side walls (AP view)	Straight, divergent, or convergent	Usually convergent	Straight	Straight or slightly divergent

	Straight, divergent, or convergent	Usually convergent	Often straight	Straight or divergent
Side walls (lateral view: "lateral bore")				
Interspinous diameter	Wide	Shortened	Shortened	Increased
Pubic arch	Curved	Straight	Slightly curved	Curved
Subpubic angle	Wide	Very narrow	Narrow	Wide
Biischial diameter	Wide	Shortened	Often shortened	Wide

[a]After Caldwell and Moloy.

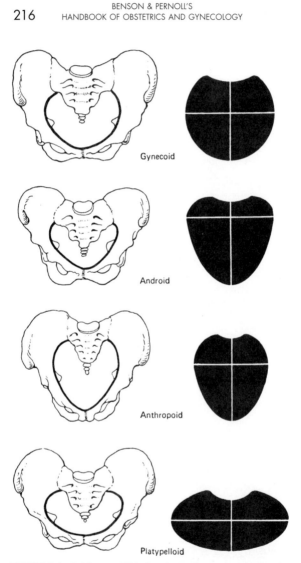

FIGURE 7-1. Pelvic types. White lines in the diagrams at right show the greatest diameters of the pelves at left.

The *anthropoid* pelvis is found in ~20% of Caucasian women and ~85% of African American women. It is marked by an oval inlet (but the anteroposterior diameter exceeds the transverse), the pelvic side walls diverge, and the sacrum is inclined posteriorly. This type pelvis is most likely to be associated with occiput posterior dystocia.

The *platypelloid* pelvis is rare (<3% of all women) and is characterized by a wide transverse diameter of the inlet. Inlet dystocia is common because the fetal head cannot enter the true pelvis. Transverse arrest may occur in the midpelvis because internal rotation is compromised by unfavorable pelvic diameters.

CRITICAL PELVIC MEASUREMENTS

Critical pelvic dimensions (for average-sized fetuses) include a diagonal conjugate ≥12.5 cm, an obstetric conjugate (anteroposterior of the inlet) ≥10 cm, and a transverse of the midpelvis of ≥9.5 cm (Table 7-5).

INLET CONTRACTURE

Inlet contracture can be expected if the anteroposterior is <10 cm or the transverse is <12 cm (or both). This is suggested clinically

TABLE 7-5
MEASUREMENTS IN CLINICAL PELVIMETRY

Measurement	Normal Value	Abnormal Value (Possibly Inadequate)
Biischial diameter (BI)	≥8 cm	<8 cm
Posterior sagittal diameter of outlet (PS)	8–9.5 cm (direct)	<8 cm
Anteroposterior diameter of outlet (AP)	≥11.9 cm	<11.9 cm
Interspinous diameter of midpelvis	≥10.5 cm	<9.5 cm
Diagonal conjugate (DC)	>11.5 cm	<11.5 cm
True conjugate (CV)	>10 cm	<10 cm
Angle of pubic arch	110–120°	<90°

by one or more of the following: a floating vertex presentation at term or in early labor, an inability to perform the Muller-Hillis maneuver (manually pushing the fetal head into the pelvis with gentle fundal pressure), presenting part not well applied to the cervix in labor, an abnormal presentation (e.g., breech, transverse lie), cord prolapse, poor progress in labor, uterine dystocia, excessive molding of the fetal head, or caput succedaneum formation. *Complications* include prolonged labor, prolonged rupture of the membranes, and pathologic retraction ring at the junction of the lower uterine segment and fundus (Bandl's retraction ring, signifying impending uterine rupture). Cesarean section usually is necessary for the true inlet contracture.

MIDPELVIC CONTRACTURE

Midpelvic contracture nearly always occurs as a result of an interspinous diameter of <9.5 cm. This may be suspected if the pelvic sidewalls are convergent and a narrow pelvic arch is present. Other clinical suggestions include prolonged second stage of labor, persistent occiput posterior, deep transverse arrest, uterine dystocia, or excessive molding of the fetal head. As with inlet dystocia, neglected midpelvic dystocia can result in uterine rupture or fistulae due to pressure necrosis. Cesarean section is the treatment of choice because instrumental delivery may lead to fetal or maternal injuries.

OUTLET CONTRACTURE

Isolated outlet dystocia is very rare, but this occurs if the *intertuberous diameter is not >8 cm or the sum of the intertuberous and the posterior sagittal diameter of the outlet is ≤15 cm.*

FETAL ABNORMALITIES CAUSING DYSTOCIA

ABNORMALITIES OF PRESENTATION AND POSITION

Abnormalities of fetal (passenger) *presentation and attitude* (lie) *complicate ~5% of all labors.* The most common of all fetal abnormalities causing dystocia is *breech presentation.* The most common of the *vertex positions* are *occiput posterior* and *occiput transverse* malpositions. Whereas these positions may occur normally, their persistence is abnormal. Occiput posterior is associated with partial deflection of the fetal head and presentation of the larger posterior portion of the head (as opposed to the smaller anterior portion) to the transverse of the midpelvis. The diagnosis is made by vaginal examination (confirmed by palpating the fetal ear). Persistent occiput transverse is associated with pelvic dystocia, platypelloid or android pelves, or uterine dystocia. Deep transverse arrest occurs in the midpelvis and usually is due to an inadequate midpelvic diameter, as in an android pelvis.

Selection of proper treatment that will be the least traumatic to mother and perinate requires clinical acumen.

Sinciput or brow presentations usually are transient fetal presentations with various degrees of deflection of the fetal head, which hopefully convert to face or vertex as labor proceeds. Thus, expectant management is the first recommendation. Of course, fetopelvic disproportion, uterine inertia and arrested progress, prematurity, and grand multiparity may mandate intervention.

Face presentation occurs in ~0.2% of deliveries and is most commonly associated with congenital malformations (e.g., anencephaly), fetopelvic disproportion, prematurity, or grand multiparity. Mentum posterior position, in all but very small prematures, is not safely deliverable vaginally. Delivery of some mentum anterior presentations is possible, but most require cesarean section.

Abnormal fetal lie is most commonly *transverse or oblique* and occurs in ~0.33% of deliveries (*six times more frequent in premature births*). Other causative associations include grand multiparity, pelvic contracture, and abnormal placental implantation. *External cephalic version* during the third trimester is most useful in conversion to a vertex. One of the major risks is a 20 times increase in cord prolapse with rupture of the membranes. A *compound presentation* occurs when the presenting part is accompanied by a prolapsed extremity. Gentle pinching of the digits may cause the fetus to retract the extremity. Should this and spontaneous restitution fail to occur or if dystocia is also a problem, consider cesarean section.

MACROSOMIA

Macrosomia, defined as fetal size >4500 g, occurs in 5%–6% of term deliveries, but is more frequent in pregnancies complicated by diabetes (some 10%–23% of offspring are macrosomic). Macrosomia is associated with increased incidences *of labor induction, prolonged labor, traumatic delivery, and shoulder dystocia.*

Risk factors for macrosomia can be divided into four major categories: *maternal diabetes* (a 2- to 5-fold increase compared to nondiabetic women), *constitutional, postdates pregnancy* (>41 weeks associated with 2- to 4× increase over 38–40 weeks), and *nondiabetic, nonconstitutional.* The constitutional risks (and amount of increased risk) associated with macrosomia include: maternal weight >90 kg (198 lb) at onset of pregnancy (11×), previous macrosomic fetus (10×), maternal birth weight >8 lb (3×), maternal weight gain of >20 kg during pregnancy (2×).

Only recently has the importance of factors other than insulin and hyperglycemia in the creation of fetal somatic overgrowth become apparent. Factors currently being investigated to explain fetal macrosomia in offspring of nondiabetic gravidas without constitutional factors include the following.

Insulin-like Growth Factors. These Include IGF-I, IGF-II, and insulin growth factor binding protein-3 (IGFBP3). IGF-I is statistically higher in the cord blood of large for gestational age (LGA) neonates when compared to average for gestational age (AGA) and appears to be an in utero growth promoter in infants of nondiabetic women. IGF-II expression is associated with fetal somatic overgrowth only when biallelic. Cord blood IGFBP-3 is significantly higher in LGA compared to AGA. Placental lactogen expresses action through regulation of the maternal and fetal beta-cell mass and function. Elevated leptin is observed in asymmetric macrosomic infants of nondiabetic mothers.

Syndromes Associated with Fetal Overgrowth. In the macrosomia associated with the Beckwith-Wiedemann syndrome, biallelic expression of IGF-II may be responsible. However, causation in the majority of syndromes with somatic overgrowth remains unknown. The Sotos and Weaver syndromes are two examples, although they may be different only by locus or allele hetogeneity. These syndromes are characterized by macrosomia, advanced skeletal age, characteristic patterns of facial and radiographic anomalies, and contractures. Sotos syndrome is associated with a higher incidence of cancers. The Simpson-Golabi-Behmel syndrome occurs in males and is associated with macrosomia, a "coarse" face, and a high incidence of cardiac abnormalities. Perlman syndrome is characterized by macrosomia, nephromegaly with renal dysplasia, Wilms' tumor, crytorchidism, multiple facial anomalies, hydramnios, and hypoglycemia. The combination of congenital hypertrichosis, osteochondrodysplasia, and cardiomegaly is emerging as a new genetic syndrome, and includes macrosomia as a portion of the clinical profile. The combination of Sturge-Weber-Krabbe and Kippel-Trenaunay syndromes have been expressed by fetal macrosomia and hydramnios.

Prediction of macrosomia for a given patient is difficult. Historical correlations are less than accurate in predictive value. The physical examination and fundal measurements may be influenced by maternal habitus, imprecise calculations of gestational duration, multiple pregnancy, hydramnios, or uterine tumor. Ultrasonographic measurements of both general obstetric patients and those at risk for macrosomia are no more precise than clinical estimates.

The pregnancy suspected (or known) to be complicated by macrosomia is at risk. Treatment involves both short- and long-term active intervention in several groups. Diabetics and gestational diabetic women will have less macrosomia with rigorously controlled blood sugar levels and carefully timed deliveries (particularly in those with fetus >90th percentile for age, but <4250 g). In glucose intolerant patients with macrosomia (perhaps >4000, but decidedly in >4250 g) an elective cesarean may be considered. Earlier delivery in potential postterm pregnancies may prove useful. Those patients who have previously had a large baby may have the birth weights decreased by elective labor induction, but this may not decrease cesarean rates, shoulder dystocia, or brachial plexus injury. *There is significant recurrence risk for gravidas who have had prior shoulder dystocia (14×, 1% increased to 14%) and traumatic birth (3-fold increase).* Should cesarean not be employed, patients in the latter two categories should be aware of their increased risk with attempting vaginal birth.

Those gravidas with uncomplicated history and prenatal course but with suspected macrosomic fetuses, have an increased incidence of labor abnormalities and cesarean associated with elective inductions. Thus, the wisdom of elective induction for a 4000–4500 g fetus has been questioned. Likewise, the suspicion of macrosomia may not warrant cesarean delivery. Alternatively, with macrosomia, the progress of labor (measured both by contractions and cervical dilation vs. time) should be monitored closely. Labor abnormalities (see p. 223), a lengthened second stage (nullipara >2 h, multipara >1 h), and arrest of descent (<3+) should signal consideration for cesarean.

ABNORMAL LABOR (POWERS)

Consider two components in evaluating labor: *the contractions* per se and *the cumulative effect* of the contractions as determined by the progress of labor.

The evaluation of contractions requires an affirmative answer to the following five questions.

- *Is there fundal dominance?* The relative intensity of contraction normally is greater in the fundus than in the midportion or lower uterine segment. Absence of fundal dominance may indicate lack of a uterine synchrony (as occurs with false labor).

FIGURE 7-2. Normal and dysfunctional uterine contraction types. (After Jeffcoate.) Black, strong contraction; shaded, slight contraction; white, atonic areas.

- *Does the uterus relax between contractions?* Normal resting tone is 12–15 mm Hg. When it is increased without oxytocin stimulation, suspect abruptio placenta.
- *Is the average value of the intensity of contractions >24 mm Hg?* In the active phase of labor, intrauterine pressure often increases to 40–60 mm Hg.
- *Is the frequency of contractions about 3–5 min?* With normal labor, the frequency of contractions progresses from one every 3–5 min to one every 2–3 min during the active phase.
- *Do the contractions last longer than 30 sec?* The duration of effective contractions is abnormal if they exceed 60 sec.

ABNORMAL CONTRACTIONS

Hypotonic Dysfunction

Hypotonic dysfunction is *characterized by contractions with insufficient force (<25 mm Hg) or an irregular or infrequent rhythm or both.* Hypotonic dysfunction is more common in nulligravidas during the active phase of labor but may be associated with excessive sedation, early administration of conduction anesthesia, and uterine overdistention (e.g., multiple gestation, hydramnios). If there is no contraindication (e.g., fetopelvic disproportion, multiple gestation, malpresentation, or allergy), hypotonic dysfunction responds well to oxytocin. Figure 7-2 graphically depicts dysfunctional labor contractions.

Hypertonic Dysfunction

Hypertonic and uncoordinated dysfunction often occur together and may be accompanied by *elevation of uterine resting tone, lack of fundal dominance, and increased uterine pain.* Hypertonic dysfunction generally is associated with overzealous oxytocin use, abruptio placenta, or fetopelvic disproportion. Fetal compromise may be an association. Hypertonic dysfunction may result in precipitate delivery. Treatment is problematic but often includes tocolysis, amyl nitrate, cessation of oxytocin, or cesarean section (if indicated for malpresentation, fetopelvic disproportion, or fetal compromise). The fetus subjected to hypertonic dysfunction is at increased risk of fetal compromise, intracranial hemorrhage, or perinatal injury. Lacerations of the birth canal also may result from rapid delivery.

EVALUATION OF LABOR

Usually, dystocia is heralded by an *abnormal labor pattern.* Figures 6-4 and 6-5 detail one method of assessment and describe the normal course of labor. Decreasing perinatal risk requires the recognition of aberrations of labor and proper intervention.

Abnormal patterns of labor (Fig. 6-6) include a *prolonged latent phase, a protracted active phase (dilatation), protracted descent, a prolonged deceleration phase, the secondary arrest of dilatation, or the arrest of descent.* In contrast, *precipitate labor* may also occur.

ABNORMAL LABOR PATTERNS

The prolonged latent phase begins with the onset of regular contractions and ends at the beginning of the active phase of labor (3–4 cm cervical dilatation). The average latent phase is ~6 h for nulliparas and ~5 h for multiparas, with the upper limit of normal at 20 h for nulliparas and 14 h for multiparas. The usual *causes of a prolonged latent* phase include *excessive analgesics or analgesics administered too early in labor, conduction anesthesia performed before the active phase, an unfavorable cervix* (e.g., a low Bishop score or scarring), *uterine dysfunction* (e.g., weak, irregular, uncoordinated, or ineffective uterine contractions), *and fetopelvic disproportion. False labor* may be the correct diagnosis in 10% of cases in this category. The recommended treatment of prolonged latent stage is the discontinuation of medications or anesthesia, correction of fluid or electrolyte deficiencies, and morphine 8–12 mg (determined on a weight basis) to rest the gravida for 6–12 h. Then, about 5% of patients will require an oxytocin infusion, but nearly all with a prolonged latent phase will proceed to vaginal delivery without fetal complications.

PROTRACTION DISORDERS

The active phase of labor starts at 3–4 cm and ends with complete (10 cm) cervical dilatation. Dilatation is protracted if labor is proceeding at <1.2 cm/h in a nullipara and <1.5 cm/h in a multipara. Descent is protracted if there is <1 cm/h descent in a nullipara and <2 cm/h descent in a multipara. The causes of protraction disorders include *fetopelvic disproportion* (33%), *malpositions* (e.g., occiput posterior), *ineffectual contractions* (e.g., excessive sedation, conduction anesthesia above the T10 dermatome), *and soft tissue dystocia.*

Protraction disorders require an assessment of the quality of labor and the diagnosis (or elimination) of fetopelvic dystocia. The quality of labor usually is investigated using electronic fetal monitoring with an intrauterine catheter to determine pressure changes. In the past, x-ray pelvimetry was used commonly to diagnose fetopelvic disproportion, but today diagnosis is by physical determination of pelvic contours and diameters, often confirmed by ultrasonography.

Cesarean section is indicated for the patient with fetopelvic disproportion. If disproportion can be excluded and if the fetal status remains satisfactory and labor is adequate, avoid oxytocin and inhibitory factors (e.g., analgesia). Ensure support (hydration and close observation) in anticipation of vaginal delivery. If contractions are inadequate but with a satisfactory fetal status, oxytocin stimulation (with close maternal and fetal monitoring) is indicated. Nonetheless, labor may still be prolonged. *Expect about two thirds of these patients to have vaginal delivery.*

ARREST DISORDERS

The deceleration phase starts at nearly 10 cm dilatation and continues to complete dilatation. The deceleration phase is arrested or prolonged if it continues for >3 h in nulliparas or >1 h in multiparas. A secondary arrest of dilatation occurs when there is no progress in dilatation for ≥2 h during the active phase. An arrest of descent occurs with failure to progress for ≥1 h during the active phase of labor. A later failure of descent can occur when there is no descent during the deceleration phase or second stage of labor.

Causes of arrest disorders include fetopelvic disproportion (~50%), fetal malpositions (e.g., occiput posterior, face, or brow), conduction anesthesia labor impairment, and excessive sedation. As with the protraction disorders, each patient must have careful evaluation for fetopelvic disproportion and fetal well-being. If disproportion is present, cesarean section is indicated. In the absence of disproportion or contraindication to its use, oxytocin stimulation is generally effective therapy. This is likely if a post arrest rate of dilatation or descent is greater than or equal to the prearrest rate. Hydration, allowing excessive analgesia or conduction anesthesia to dissipate, and other supportive measures also may be helpful. *Arrest disorders generally carry a poor prognosis for vaginal delivery and have increased perinatal morbidity and mortality.*

PRECIPITATE LABOR

Precipitate labor and delivery may occur as a result of either very rapid dilatation or descent. *Precipitate dilatation is defined as active phase dilatation of ≥5 cm/h in a primipara or ≥10 cm/h in a multipara. Precipitate descent is active phase descent of ≥5 cm/h in a primipara or ≥10 cm/h in a multipara.* Precipitate labor usually results from very forceful contractions (e.g., oxytocin-induced or as a result of abruptio placenta) or low birth canal resistance (e.g., multiparity). Discontinue oxytocin if it is in use. Currently, there is *no effective treatment,* however, and physical attempts to retard delivery are absolutely contraindicated.

Precipitate labor may cause maternal amniotic fluid embolism, uterine rupture, cervical lacerations, or lacerations of the birth canal. There is associated postpartum uterine hypotonicity, with resulting risk of hemorrhage. The *perinate is at extraordinary risk from hypoxia* (impeded uteroplacental exchange because of the contractions) *and perinatal intracranial hemorrhage* (direct or indirect trauma). *Unattended delivery* (direct injury, no resuscitation, chilling) further jeopardizes the newborn.

MECONIUM STAINING OF
AMNIOTIC FLUID

See discussion on page 272.

FETAL COMPROMISE

Fetal compromise is the fetus's critical response to stress, most usually deprivation. It implies that physiologic reserve mechanisms have been exceeded or exhausted and that pathologic changes are occurring or are about to occur that affect vital organ function to the point of temporary or permanent injury or death. The most immediate of fetal needs are (as in the adult) the acquisition of oxygen and the elimination of carbon dioxide. Thus, the metabolic derangements signaling acute fetal distress are hypoxia, hypercarbia, and acidosis.

Usually, asphyxia, or hypoxia, is induced by only three mechanisms: decreased maternal uteroplacental blood flow, decreased maternal oxygenation, and decreased umbilical blood flow. During a moderate asphyxic episode, the fetus can compensate by the diversion of blood flow to the most vital organs, by limiting oxygen consumption over a prolonged interval (e.g., postmaturity), or by shifting to anaerobic metabolism. If the asphyxic stress is severe, prolonged, or becomes more pronounced, these compensatory mechanisms ultimately fail, and fetal distress becomes evident.

Fetal compromise also can be chronic, that is, a longer interval of sublethal fetal deprivation that affects growth and development. This can be associated with a reduction of placental perfusion by placental abnormality or by deficient fetal metabolism. Some degree of either acute or chronic fetal compromise may exist in up to 20% of all patients.

CHRONIC FETAL COMPROMISE

Reduced placental perfusion results from *maternal conditions,* including vascular spasm or inability to adjust to pregnancy (e.g., chronic hypertension, pregnancy-induced hypertension, or diabetes with pelvic vascular calcification), *inadequate systemic circulation* (e.g., severe maternal heart disease, severe anemia), or *insufficient oxygenation of the blood* (e.g., cyanotic heart disease, long-term pulmonary shunting, or residence at high altitude).

Placental causes of chronic fetal compromise include *premature placental aging and diabetes mellitus. Fetal causes* of chronic fetal compromise include the *postmaturity syndrome, multiple gestation, twin-to-twin transfusion, congenital anomalies, maternal–fetal transfusion, and erythroblastosis fetalis.*

Chronic fetal compromise is most *commonly diagnosed by serial ultrasonic examinations or by testing for fetal well-being.* Once diagnosed, chronic fetal compromise or deprivation *requires close follow-up.*

Treatment is supportive but nonspecific. This consists of correcting the underlying condition(s) if possible; maximizing the fetal opportunity to acquire metabolic substrate (oxygen and glucose) by maternal therapy with bed rest, enhanced nutrition, and oxygen; elimination of maternal limitations complicating the underlying condition (e.g., infection); and special surveillance during delivery and in the immediate newborn interval (Chapter 8).

ACUTE FETAL COMPROMISE

Acute fetal compromise usually is caused by compromise of the fetal respiratory lifeline (Table 7-6) and is a true medical emergency. If steps are not taken, the fetus will likely die or be severely compromised. Thus, the health care provider must have a clear and orderly plan of treatment.

Most acute fetal compromise is detected during labor. Often, EFM will reveal decreased placental perfusion with contractions. Most of the criteria for fetal compromise are based on EFM information (p. 239).

The treatment of fetal compromise (rescue) seeks to restore or maintain uteroplacental–fetal blood flow and acid–base balance. The treatment of fetal compromise is straightforward. However, prognosis depends largely on the underlying cause of the fetal compromise and current fetal status.

Change maternal position to relieve pressure on the umbilical cord and improve uterine blood flow, especially from the lateral recumbent position when the uterus impedes blood return via the inferior vena cava.

Correct hypotension. If change of position fails to correct hypotension, shift the uterus off the great vessels by manual pressure, elevate the legs, apply elastic leg bandages, and administer fluids rapidly IV. Cardiotonics (e.g., ephedrine) may be necessary to restore abdominal pressure.

Decrease uterine activity. Discontinue oxytocin if in use. Tocolytics, now being tested, have not yet been approved for general use in acute situations.

Hyperoxygenate. Give 6–7 liters/min of oxygen by mask and guarantee complete maternal oxygenation to enhance maternal–fetal oxygen transfer.

Correct metabolic imbalances. If the mother is acidotic, administer sodium bicarbonate to correct the imbalance. However,

TABLE 7-6
REPRESENTATIVE CAUSES OF ACUTE FETAL COMPROMISE

Maternal	Hypotension (e.g., supine hypotensive syndrome)
	Hypoxia or hypercarbia (e.g., maternal aspiration syndrome)
	Impaired respiration (shock-lung, bronchospasm)
	Pregnancy-induced hypertension
	Shock (hemorrhagic, cardiac, septic)
	Sickle cell crisis
Uterine	Hypertonia or polysystole
	Excessive oxytocin
	Uterine rupture
Placental	Abruptio placentae
	Placenta previa
	Premature placental aging
Cord	Prolapse
	Ruptured vasa previa
	Tight or short cord
	True knot
Fetus	Cardiac failure (hydrops fetalis, tachyarrhythmia, myocarditis)
	Congenital anomaly
	Hemorrhage
	Isoimmunization

the fetus may respond slowly. Maternal hypoglycemia should respond to hypertonic glucose (50 g IV).

Confirm the diagnosis. Fetal scalp blood pH sampling should confirm a presumptive diagnosis of acidosis and hypoxia in life-threatening situations.

Alert necessary personnel of the emergency. Rarely can the obstetrician alone provide the total care necessary for the compromised perinate and mother. Thus, obstetric nursing service, anesthesiology, and the neonatologist or neonatal resuscitation team should be alerted.

Deliver the perinate. If these steps fail, delivery must be effected to save the perinate. The mode of delivery must be individualized based on the status of labor, imminence of vaginal delivery, and maternal factors.

METHODS OF FETAL ASSESSMENT

ULTRASONOGRAPHY

Clinical ultrasound involves high-frequency sound waves produced by applying alternating current to a piezoelectric substance. The transducer is coupled to the patient by a transmitting medium (e.g., mineral oil) and the generated sound waves pass through the soft tissue (ultrasound will not pass through well-mineralized bone) until an interface of different tissue densities is encountered. Part of the sound is then reflected. The transducer broadcasts only a short part of a duty cycle. Most of the time is spent receiving. Thus, the returning sound is collected and subsequently analyzed. One or many transducers may be used, and they can be movable or fixed. A number of such devices are available, and a variety of information may be gathered.

The ability to visualize the fetus probably has contributed more than any other advance in the diagnosis and treatment of the fetus as a patient. Examples of useful ultrasonic scannings include very early identification of normal and abnormal gestation (e.g., blighted ovum, ectopic), measurement of fetal growth, estimation of fetal weight, observation of fetal organs (e.g., the heart) and the determination of fetal well-being, identification of multiple gestation, detailing of fetal anomalies, differential comparison of various fetal parts, demonstration of hydramnios or oligohydramnios, visualization of the cord and measurement of cord blood flows, visualization of the placenta (e.g., maturity, placement, size, blood clot, or tumors), demonstration of placental aberrations (e.g., hydatidiform mole, molar degeneration, or chorioangiomas), visualization of uterine tumors or anomalies, and revelation of cervical abnormalities (e.g., incompetent cervix). Please see p. 113 for a discussion of early (first trimester) ultrasound.

AMNIOCENTESIS

Amniocentesis is the *aspiration of amniotic fluid.* Amniocentesis is useful for antenatal diagnosis, physiologic maturity testing, and the investigation of disorders (e.g., isoimmunization). Amniocentesis is almost always performed transabdominally because of the greater infection risk if performed transvaginally. Occasionally, amniocentesis is used in treatment (e.g., hydramnios).

Perform an ultrasonic scan immediately before amniocentesis and use sonographic needle guidance. The minimal information recorded from the ultrasonic examination should include the number of fetuses, the fetal cardiac activity, the fetal biparietal (and often femur length or abdominal circumference), placental site, and location of the best position for needle placement.

PROCEDURE

Prepare the abdomen with a bactericidal agent and inject a local anesthetic (elective). Use the smallest needle that will adequately remove the sample (usually a 22 gauge) and enter the amniotic cavity for only a short distance. Remove ~15 mL of fluid for diagnostic purposes. Document fetal well-being by ultrasonic scan at the termination of the procedure. Administer Rh-immune globulin to the Rh-negative unsensitized patient receiving amniocentesis.

Amniotic fluid normally is clear to slightly yellow-tinged. It may contain flecks of vernix or lanugo hair in later pregnancy. If bloody, maternal blood probably was aspirated; however, RBC do not interfere with fetal cell growth or other analyses. Examine green to greenish brown fluid under the microscope. If particulate matter (meconium) and not old blood (fetal bleeding) is seen, ~50% fetal mortality is likely. Tobacco brown amniotic fluid usually is associated with fetal death, whereas light brown, dark red, or wine-colored fluid is indicative of intraamniotic hemorrhage (the color depends on the Hgb content). This is associated with pregnancy loss in ~one third of cases. An elevation of AFP in the discolored fluid portends fetal death, spontaneous abortion, or fetal anomaly (e.g., anencephaly).

With experience, transabdominal amniocentesis under ultrasonographic guidance results in <0.5% complications, using a needle ≤20 gauge and only one needle insertion. Complications include maternal bleeding, bruising or hematoma formation, fetal bleeding, possible fetal penetration injury, and infection.

FETAL HEART RATE MONITORING

Observation of the fetal heart rate is the most directly available means of assessing fetal status. Reliable changes in the fetal heart rate are caused by fetal hypoxia and acidosis. Nonetheless, disastrous results have been reported in the presence of a normal fetal heart rate. Thus, to enhance accuracy, the heart rate of the fetus or adult is only one detail that must be evaluated with other available information.

BASAL FETAL HEART RATE

The fetal heart rate (FHR) in early gestation is higher than at term, when it is *120–160 bpm.* Gradual slowing amounts to ~20 bpm and occurs linearly throughout the pregnancy. *The baseline or basal FHR is the average rate prevailing apart from beat-to-beat variability and periodic changes.*

Tachycardia occurs when the *baseline FHR >160 bpm lasting for >10 min.* It is further quantified as *moderate (160–180 bpm) or severe (>180 bpm)* (Table 7-7). *Tachycardia may result from maternal fever, maternal hyperthroidism, fetal infection, fetal dysrhythmia or fetal distress.*

Bradycardia is defined as an *FHR <120 bpm. Moderate bradycardia (100–119 bpm) may be associated with severe fetal distress,*

TABLE 7-7
SUMMARY OF MATURE FETAL HEART
RATE PARAMETERS

Feature	Parameters	Interpretation
Baseline heart rate	120–160 bpm	Normal
Tachycardia		
Moderate	161–180 bpm	Nonreassuring
Marked	>180 bpm	Abnormal
Bradycardia		
Moderate	100–119 bpm	Nonreassuring
Marked	>100 bpm	Abnormal
Short-term variability	5–15 bpm	Reassuring
Long-term variability	Present	Reassuring
Periodic changes		
Accelerations	>15 bpm for >15 sec	Well-being
Decelerations		
Early	10–40 bpm	Head compression
Late	5–60 bpm	Hypoxia/ acidosis
Variable	10–60 bpm	Cord compression
Combinations		Nonreassuring

whereas severe bradycardia (FHR <100 bpm) is likely to be agonal or due to heart block.

There is a beat-to-beat variation of the fetal heart in the mature fetus; that is, *the time interval between heartbeats varies slightly.* The internal EFM normally records small, rapid, rhythmic fluctuations with an *amplitude of 5–15 bpm.* This variation is referred to as beat-to-beat variability, or short-term variability. This is a normal finding in the mature fetus but may not be present in the premature (but normal) fetus, the sleeping fetus, and medicated fetuses (e.g., alphaprodine, atropine, barbiturates, conduction anesthesia, diazepam, general anesthesia, meperidine, morphine, phenothiazines, and magnesium sulfate in large doses). Good FHR short-term variability in the absence of such mitigating factors indicates adequate CNS oxygenation. If normal FHR variability is apparent 5 min before birth, a good Apgar rating is likely, irrespective of earlier periodic changes, assuming no congenital anomalies.

When FHR beat-to-beat variability is significantly decreased and cannot be explained by the above factors, shift the mother to a different position, give her oxygen by mask, and maintain normal blood pressure. With failure of these measures to improve beat-to-beat variability, fetal assessment by scalp sampling or stimulation tests should be undertaken to further test fetal well-being.

There may be a *periodicity to these beat-to-beat alterations* (i.e., the short-term variability appears to have a rhythmic reproducible pattern). This is termed long-term variability. If present, long-term variability is a *sign of well-being but is altered by the same factors affecting short-term variability.*

PERIODIC CHANGES

The periodic changes are deviations from the baseline in response to fetal stimulation, movements, or uterine contractions. Periodic changes may be of two types, accelerations or decelerations.

Accelerations

To be classified as an acceleration, *the FHR must increase >15 bpm, and this must last for >15 sec.* An acceleration usually evokes a rather smooth pattern when viewed on EFM and is *believed to be a solid indication of fetal well-being. Moreover, accelerations may be triggered in the normal mature fetus by body motion, acoustic stimulation, stimulation of the fetal scalp, and other stimuli.*

Decelerations

Decelerations (Fig. 7-3) are *periodic declines in heart rate (from the baseline), usually in response to uterine contractions.* Indeed,

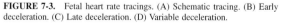

FIGURE 7-3. Fetal heart rate tracings. (A) Schematic tracing. (B) Early deceleration. (C) Late deceleration. (D) Variable deceleration.

(From S.G. Babson et al., *Management of High-Risk Pregnancy and Intensive Care of the Neonate,* 3rd ed. Mosby, 1975.)

FIGURE 7-3. *(Continued)*

on antepartum monitoring, *spontaneous deceleration is a very ominous finding and should be viewed with concern.* Early and late deceleration patterns are uniform, occurring as exact mirror images (on EFM) of the uterine contractions.

With *early decelerations,* the onset of the deceleration occurs with the onset of the contraction, the nadir of the heart rate occurs with the apex of the contraction, and the heart rate increases back to baseline as the contraction ebbs. *Early deceleration is caused by compression of the fetal head and is much more common with ruptured membranes.* It is a benign finding, and *no therapy is required.* If early deceleration patterns are severe, prolonged, persistent, or accompanied by thick meconium staining, however, the problem may be serious. Therapy includes changing of maternal position (lateral recumbent is best) and ruling out umbilical cord compression (sterile vaginal examination). In some cases, with administration of atropine to the mother, the fetus receives enough to block the cause (i.e., vagal stimulation).

Late decelerations appear like early decelerations except with late decelerations, *the pattern occurs later than the contraction;* that is, the onset of FHR deceleration occurs after the contraction onset, the nadir of FHR occurs after the apex of the contraction, and the FHR deceleration continues after the contraction has abated. *Late deceleration is most commonly associated with uteroplacental insufficiency* and is a consequence of hypoxia and metabolic disorders. Thus, this is the *most ominous fetal heart rate pattern.* In less severe cases, the FHR may transiently exceed the baseline after termination of the deceleration. With severely affected fetuses, the FHR takes longer to return to baseline from the deceleration and does not transiently accelerate. In some with severe compromise, however, the fetus will have a baseline tachycardia.

Significant changes during contractions may be subtle, and the FHR may be within the normal range. Thus, *careful interpretation is necessary.* This is particularly true for the postdate fetus because the findings of late decelerations are less obvious than at an earlier stage of gestation. *Treatment involves decreasing uterine activity* (e.g., terminate oxytocin), *correcting maternal hypotension, hyperoxygenating, and expanding maternal blood volume.* Should these steps not be immediately effective, deliver the infant.

Variable decelerations are not uniform and vary widely in configuration. They may *begin at any time in relation to the contraction, and often both onset and cessation are marked by sudden changes in the FHR.* Variable decelerations may be nonrepetitive and are *caused by umbilical cord compression.* Decelerations are classified as *severe if they last >60 sec or lead to an FHR of ≤90 bpm.* If vaginal examination reveals no palpable cord, maternal positional changes do not resolve the pattern, or the decelerations are severe, do fetal scalp blood sampling, if feasible, to determine the degree of fetal compromise. *In the absence of fetal scalp sampling availability, a high presenting part, or other compromising factors, deliver the infant without delay.*

The *most common combined deceleration pattern is that of variable and late decelerations. This is a most ominous pattern* and usually consists of variable onset of the pattern, with a late pattern then developing. Nearly all fetuses with this pattern are severely compromised, and *immediate delivery should be considered* if the simple steps outlined for late decelerations do not cause the pattern to improve.

METHODS OF FETAL MONITORING

The fetal heart rate can be obtained by manual stethoscope, Doppler ultrasound, direct ultrasonic visualization, and direct electrocardiography. Direct ultrasonic visualization is not practical for prolonged observation (e.g., during labor). Availability of equipment, the physician's experience with the various techniques, and the patient's risk state must determine the method for monitoring.

Stethoscopic Monitoring

Stethoscopic monitoring of fetal heart tones to assess fetal well-being currently is adequate for screening low-risk patients. Ascertain the baseline FHR by careful auscultation between contractions and listen for 30 sec after contractions to determine if there are decelerations from the baseline. This should be performed every 30 min during the first stage of labor. In the second stage, auscultation should be accomplished every 15 min and in the delivery room, every 10 min. Stethoscopic monitoring is convincingly inadequate in the high-risk cases.

Electronic Fetal Monitoring

Fetal monitors currently available provide either external or internal sensing of the FHR and the associated contraction sequence while creating a permanent record of the data.

External Fetal Monitoring

Most external fetal monitors use a Doppler ultrasound transducer applied to the mother's abdomen. The transducer detects fetal heart activity and triggers the rate-computing circuitry. A disadvantage of this method is *imprecision in detection of beat-to-beat variability.* What appears to be normal or increased variability may be artifact because of merging of the ultrasound pickup. If the baseline appears smooth when an ultrasound transducer is used, however, the beat-to-beat variability may be decreased. Direct ECG internal monitoring is

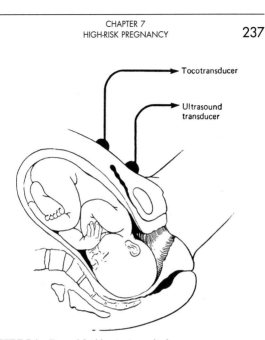

FIGURE 7-4. External fetal heart rate monitoring.
(Redrawn from E.H.G. Hon, *Hospital Practice* 5:91, 1970.)

the only reliable method of achieving recognition of the beat-to-beat variability (Fig. 7-4).

A *tocotransducer* that responds to changes in pressure transmitted from the uterus to the abdominal wall is used to monitor uterine activity externally. Unfortunately, the external monitor does not provide quantitative data regarding the intensity of uterine contractions—only their frequency and duration. Additionally, the input signals often are distorted when the patient moves or if the belt is loosened. Obesity may further reduce the quality of the external FHR recording. Therefore, the abdominal transducer must be readjusted often to ensure good recording. Nonetheless, because external fetal monitoring is noninvasive, it is almost devoid of clinical complications.

Internal Fetal Monitoring
Internal fetal heart monitoring (Fig. 7-5) during labor yields data relatively free of artifacts caused by patient movement. However, internal monitoring cannot usually be used before the cervix is dilated

FIGURE 7-5. Internal fetal heart rate monitoring to develop a beat-to-beat recording that accurately depicts baseline irregularity and the widest ranges of the FHR.

(Redrawn from E.H.G. Hon, *Hospital Practice* 5:91, 1970.)

>1 cm and the membranes are ruptured to permit placement of the scalp electrode. The fetal R wave is used by the rate-computing circuit of the internal fetal monitor.

When an *intrauterine catheter* attached to a pressure transducer can be inserted, an accurate record of intrauterine pressure usually can be obtained. Thus, the *intensity of contractions can be determined, and an abnormal elevation of uterine tone between contractions can be recognized.* This information is useful clinically, especially when oxytocin induction or augmentation of labor is considered or when premature separation of the placenta occurs.

There are *few clinical problems attributable to internal FHR monitoring.* Minor infections can be anticipated in ~1% of cases, but serious fetal scalp infection is rare. Perforation of the uterus or slight placental bleeding with the introduction of the pressure catheter may occur. Amnionitis may develop with prolonged monitoring using an indwelling catheter (>6 h).

It may be difficult to obtain proper pressure readings and ensure subsequent recordings: calibration may not be proper, air bubbles may be present in the line or transducer, pressure leaks or kinks in the catheter system may develop, a valve may be loose, a stopcock may be defective, or a damaged cable or coupling may be the problem. There are few technical problems with the electrode. If the internal electrode is applied to the cervix accidentally, however, the mother's heart rate will be recorded instead of the fetal heart rate.

Retain the entire monitoring strip or representative portions, including abnormal strip recordings, as part of the patient's record.

Most obstetric patients accept fetal monitoring as a part of better perinatal care and insurance against fetal damage or death despite the technology involved.

The *indications for internal fetal monitoring* include advanced maternal age, previous cesarean section, diabetes mellitus, significant cardiac or hypertensive disease, moderate or severe isoimmunization, medical complications of pregnancy, multiple gestation, pregnancy-induced hypertension, moderate or severe anemia, pyelonephritis, uterine bleeding, hydramnios, fetal growth retardation or compromise (abnormal clinical or laboratory tests), premature labor, meconium-stained amniotic fluid, postdatism (≥ 41 weeks), abnormal fetal heart rates or patterns obtained by other methods, augmentation of labor, dysfunctional labor, uterine bleeding, and prolonged first or second stage or labor.

ELECTRONIC MONITORING DIAGNOSIS OF FETAL COMPROMISE

During labor, severe FHR variable decelerations, late decelerations, fetal bradycardia, and decreased FHR variability should be viewed as indicative of fetal compromise. Loss of beat-to-beat variability, together with bradycardia, indicate probable asphyxia. The addition of severe variable or late FHR decelerations is further evidence of asphyxia.

FETAL SCALP BLOOD PH DETERMINATIONS

The fetal blood pH is mediated in the short term by respiratory exchange of O_2 and CO_2 (via the placenta). In the long term, pH depends on the concentrations of lactic and pyruvic acids that accumulate because of anaerobic metabolism. Interruption of placental blood flow (e.g., by cord compression) will produce respiratory acidosis. If the interruption is brief, rapid recovery is likely; however, prolonged hypoxia induces anaerobic metabolism, which leads to metabolic acidosis. Then, recovery takes much longer.

Fetal scalp blood pH determinations can be attempted after the cervix is >3 cm dilated, after the membranes are ruptured and the vertex is engaging or engaged in the pelvis. Proper instrumentation must be available, and laboratory capability must be assured. A sterile drape is applied. The fetal scalp is exposed using a conical endoscope. An antiseptic is applied, then silicone gel is spread over the incision site, and a 2 mm puncture is made. Capillary blood that beads up on the silicone film is collected in several heparinized capillary tubes. The time of collection is recorded, and the specimens are immediately sent to the laboratory for pH determination. Pressure against the puncture site during 1–2 uterine contractions should ensure clotting and prevent fetal bleeding from the incision site. Poor technique or excessive scalp hair may lead to an inadequate blood sample.

Fetal scalp blood sampling should be *considered for persistent late decelerations, for persistent severe variable decelerations, when meconium staining of the amniotic fluid is associated with abnormal FHR patterns, for unexplained fetal tachycardia, or with decreased baseline variability.*

Interpretation of Results

Normal pH	7.25–7.35
Borderline pH	7.20–7.25
Abnormal (low) pH	<7.20

For decisive action, obtain more than one sample report. A *correlation must exist between the FHR monitor pattern and the pH report.* Only a fair agreement between the scalp blood pH and the Apgar score can be expected because of other factors, for example, maternal hyperventilation, drug effect, slow collection, or amniotic fluid contamination. Nonetheless, fetal scalp blood pH monitoring will aid in the confirmation or refutation of otherwise difficult to diagnose cases of fetal distress.

SPECIFIC TESTING FOR FETAL WELL-BEING

EVALUATION OF ABNORMAL ALPHA-FETOPROTEIN (AFP) DETERMINATION

Nearly all AFP is of fetal origin. It is initially produced in the yolk sac, but, by the 13th week, when AFP peaks in both fetal serum and amniotic fluid (AF), it is of hepatic origin. The AFP concentration in the fetal serum is 150 times that in AF. Some of this protein is excreted in fetal urine, however, and AFP eventually passes from the amniotic fluid into the maternal serum (levels ~0.1%–1% of that in the fetal serum).

Over 5% of women screened at 16–18 weeks gestation will have an elevated maternal serum AFP. Normal levels are highly dependent on length of gestation. Thus, exact knowledge of gestational age is critical. The test is used to screen for open neural tube defects. Nonetheless, the *vast majority of elevations will be false positives* caused by inaccurate gestational dating, multiple gestation, fetal demise, a dying fetus, congenital nephrosis (an autosomal recessive trait), bladder neck obstruction, esophageal or duodenal atresia, exomphalos, sacrococcygeal teratoma, pilonidal sinus, Turner syndrome (45,XO), Potter's syndrome (renal agenesis), fetal blood in amniotic fluid, fetomaternal hemorrhage, abdominal pregnancy, some low-birth-weight fetuses, or many noncentral nervous system structural abnormalities. *Therefore, even the false positives may represent serious problems;* hence, an evaluation will be necessary to identify the cause of the elevation. Only 1 in 25 with a single elevated AFP screening study will actually have a neural tube defect. Stated another way, *24 of 25 women with a single elevated AFP value will eventually prove to have a normal fetus.*

The secondary screen generally consists of repeating the maternal AFP determination and performing a detailed ultrasonography (searching for fetal defects and carefully determining the ultrasonic gestational age). This generally will reveal the cause of the initial AFP elevation. However, *if the AFP is ≥2.5 times the mean for the gestational age and ultrasonography does not yield a specific diagnosis, further studies will be necessary.*

Perform amniocentesis for *amniotic fluid AFP, AF acetylcholinesterase, and possibly for a karyotype. AF acetylcholinesterase levels* (if available) *are significantly elevated in open neural tube defects, and it is more specific than AFP.*

False negative tests are uncommon, but *low maternal serum AFP* levels require investigation because they may be associated with genetic abnormalities, especially *trisomies.*

ANTENATAL GENETIC DIAGNOSIS

Eliciting genetic information is discussed earlier in this chapter. A complete evaluation of those potentially affected with genetic disorders is beyond the purpose of this text. Nonetheless, we summarize the conditions amenable to prenatal diagnosis and the techniques available for obtaining tissue for analysis.

CONDITIONS AMENABLE
TO ANTENATAL DIAGNOSIS

About 90% of antenatal diagnostic tests are done to diagnose or rule out chromosomal disorders. The most common indication for study is advanced maternal age ($\geq$35 years, although $\geq$32 seems more logical). It is known that with aging, women have a greater chance of having a chromosomally abnormal baby. Although mothers $\geq$35 have ~6% of all pregnancies, they account for >25% of all neonates with Down syndrome.

Other indications for antenatal diagnosis include a previous offspring with a chromosomal defect, three or more spontaneous abortions, patient or husband with chromosome anomaly (e.g., a parent who is a known translocation carrier), possible X-linked disease (e.g., hemophilia—usually only able to tell gender of offspring), risk of an inborn error of metabolism (e.g., Tay-Sachs), and risk of a neural tube defect. Many other disorders will soon be detectable. Thus, when a specific case is encountered, the practitioner should consult a center that performs antenatal genetic diagnosis to ascertain testing available for the specific condition, the techniques usually applied, and at what stage of gestation the testing is best accomplished.

REQUIREMENTS TO PROVIDE
ANTENATAL DIAGNOSIS

Antenatal diagnosis is complex and requires experienced personnel: an obstetrician experienced in the techniques, a medical genetics group with biochemical and cytogenetic expertise, a genetic counseling service, and professional referral services.

ANTENATAL DIAGNOSIS
TECHNIQUES

The tissue for analysis may be acquired by several routes.

Amniocentesis is ideally performed at 14–16 weeks, when there is approximately 200 mL of amniotic fluid and many viable cells in the fluid. Although diagnosis of many genetic diseases can be made using chorionic villus sampling, others will require amniocentesis (e.g., anomalies associated with marked elevation of AFP).

Chorionic villi sampling (CVS) offers a newer, earlier approach to the prenatal diagnosis of many genetic disorders. Between 8 and 12 weeks, the fetus is enclosed by the amniotic sac with a space between the thin inner amniotic membrane and the thicker outer chorionic membrane. On the external surface of the chorion are delicate, fernlike villous projections, the chorion frondosum. During the late first trimester, these villi are evenly distributed. Later, some of the villi develop into a dense, shaggy concentration that finally attaches to the uterine wall to form the placenta.

To accomplish CVS, insert a thin, soft plaster catheter transcervically into the chorion frondosum under high-resolution linear array ultrasonography, and gently suction portions of the villi for study. The timing is important because, much earlier or later, the risk of complications increases. The recovered 5–8 g of tissue is useful for preliminary direct evaluation, but many chromosomal, DNA, or enzyme studies require fetal cell culture.

The advantages of CVS are that it is feasible at 8–12 weeks gestation, same-day determination of fetal gender and chromosome number is possible, and it avoids membrane puncture. The main disadvantages are that some chromosome morphology is less precise on direct tissue preparation, great care must be taken in preparation or an artificially high incidence of mosaicism may result (i.e., the syncytiotrophoblast must be removed), spontaneous abortion may be more frequent than with amniocentesis, an enhanced number of limb-reduction defects may occur, and serious infections may result.

Direct Fetal Blood Sampling. Some disease states are so problematic and the diagnosis is so important that cordocentesis may be required to sample fetal blood directly. This complicated procedure, although quite safe in experienced hands, is best performed in a limited number of centers.

TESTS OF PHYSIOLOGIC MATURITY

The physiologic maturity of the fetus can be determined by the amniotic fluid lecithin/sphingomyelin ratio (LS ratio), phosphotidylglycerol (Pg) determinations, and other tests for pulmonary surfactant. Creatinine content, bilirubin concentration, and fluid osmolality tests have largely been abandoned.

The **rapid surfactant test (RST, bubble test)** is a simple, rapid, and reliable technique for predicting fetal lung maturity. Amniotic fluid is centrifuged at 2000 rpm for 15 min, and the supernatant is then drawn off. Two dilutions of supernatant and 95% ethanol are made (1:1 and 1:2). The tubes are capped and shaken vigorously for 30 sec and observed for the appearance of bubbles at the surface. The predicted fetal pulmonary maturity has been correlated with the LS ratio as shown in Table 7-8.

The presence of **phosphatidylglycerol** is determined in the phosphatidylglycerol test. Phosphatidylglycerol (Pg) constitutes

TABLE 7-8
CORRELATION OF RAPID SURFACTANT TEST (RST)
WITH LECITHIN/SPHINGOMYELIN (LS) RATIO

Predicted Fetal Pulmonary Maturity	LS Ratio	RST
Mature	>2	Complete ring of bubbles persists 15 min at 1:1 and 1:2 dilutions
Intermediate	1.5–2	Complete ring of bubbles persists 15 min at 1:1 dilution only
Immature	<1.5	No complete ring of bubbles at either dilution

about 10% of surfactant phospholipids, and its presence appears to improve the functioning of lung surfactant. Unfortunately, double thin-layer chromatography is required for the Pg determination.

NONSTRESS TESTING

The nonstress test is an appraisal of fetal well-being based on the observation that the normal fetus will have characteristic periodic accelerations in the FHR patterns, and the unhealthy fetus will not. Average baseline variability and acceleration of the FHR in response to fetal movement indicate that the fetus is not in jeopardy and has a good reserve. This is assessed by external fetal monitoring without stimuli (stress) to the fetus.

If the fetal CNS is depressed because of hypoxia, acidosis, or drugs, the baseline variability may be reduced and FHR acceleration with fetal movement absent. These patterns may be noted also during fetal sleep. If sleep is likely, the fetus should be stimulated by abdominal palpation.

Major indications for nonstress testing are a history of stillbirth or serious anomaly, drug abuse, possible asphyxia or other circulatory problem (e.g., meconium-stained amniotic fluid before labor, hemoglobinopathy, Rh isoimmunization), suspected intrauterine growth retardation, medical complications of pregnancy (e.g., diabetes mellitus of classes B–H, chronic renal disease, systemic lupus erythematosus), hypertensive disorders complicating pregnancy, and prolonged pregnancy.

The first nonstress test is rarely required before the 28th week of pregnancy. The maternal history or status generally indicates the time for the initial test (e.g., about the 32nd week in mildly diabetic women).

PROCEDURE

Place the patient in bed in the semi-Fowler position at ~30 degrees elevation. Record maternal blood pressure on the FHR record every 10 min. Continue the test for 20 min.

If the test is reactive (see below), end the test and repeat in 7 days. If nonreactive, continue the test for 20 min more. If the test remains nonreactive, proceed to manual stimulation, acoustic stimulation, administration of food or glucose to the mother or, in the very high-risk patient, to the contraction stress test.

INTERPRETATION

The test is reactive if there are ≥2 accelerations of FHR that reach >15 bpm above the baseline and are at least ≥15 sec in duration in a 20 min interval. A nonreactive test does not meet the criteria for the reactive test. If there is no fetal movement, the test is unsatisfactory.

CONTRACTION STRESS TEST

The contraction stress test (CST) is a useful method for *determining fetal well-being.* It is a stress test based on the fact that *uterine contractions decrease uteroplacental blood flow.* This transient decrease may be enough to evoke a significant response in the compromised fetus.

Before the onset of labor, mothers with obstetric problems associated with *uteroplacental compromise* (e.g., small-for-dates fetus) *are candidates for the CST fetal evaluation. Contraindications include* placenta previa and women at high risk for premature labor (e.g., those with incompetent cervix, multiple pregnancy, or ruptured membranes with a premature offspring).

Although prognostication may be difficult, the incidence of perinatal mortality and morbidity is much higher in high-risk patients with a positive CST than in those with a negative CST.

There are *two methods* of evoking contractions: the nipple (or breast) stimulation and the oxytocin contraction test.

NIPPLE STIMULATION TEST

Nipple stimulation, which releases oxytocin in late pregnancy, is used to accomplish the uterine contraction test. Nipple stimulation is effective in about 90% of cases, is noninvasive, and overdosage is unlikely.

The test is conducted like the oxytocin challenge test with the same end points. There is no standardized nipple stimulation procedure as yet. However, an effective plan requires the gravida to roll one nipple between her fingers for 1 min. (Longer stimulation may evoke exaggerated uterine activity.) After 3 min, if moderate uterine contractions have not ensued, she may manipulate both nipples for 5–10 min. If this is not effective, proceed to an oxytocin challenge test.

THE OXYTOCIN CHALLENGE TEST (OCT)

The gravida is placed in the semi-Fowler position and slightly on one side. An external FHR monitor (usually Doppler ultrasound) and a uterine activity (toco) monitor are placed on the mother's abdomen. FHR and uterine activity are observed for 10–30 min (baseline). Oxytocin is then administered by controlled IV infusion pump at 0.5 mU/min. Oxytocin dosage is increased slowly until at least *three contractions develop in a 10 min period.* Slow (every 20 min) step up may be required, but *hyperstimulation*—contractions at intervals of 2 min or less or contractions over 90 sec in duration—*must be avoided,* or fetal distress and emergency cesarean section may be necessary. The CST requires 60–90 min to perform. Interpretation depends on strict adherence to the protocol to avoid false positive CSTs.

A positive CST is one in which persistent late deceleration occurs (i.e., a drop in FHR with onset at or beyond the peak of uterine contraction). The minimal degree of deceleration in FHR (bpm) has not been acceptably defined. Some specialists have agreed on 5, and others regard any perceptible deceleration as significant. Nonetheless, decelerations must occur and persist with most contractions.

When the *CST is positive, about 10% of fetuses will die within 1 week if undelivered.* When the state of the cervix is favorable, a closely monitored labor may be chosen. Before vaginal delivery of any high-risk patient is attempted, place an internal electrode and monitor the patient by direct means during labor.

In most cases, a convincingly positive CST is an indication for prompt cesarean section because 50%–75% of these patients who are allowed to go into labor have late decelerations.

A suspicious or equivocal CST hyperstimulation or an unsatisfactory test cannot be interpreted and must be repeated in 24 h.

A negative CST is temporarily reassuring, but the outcome of any high-risk pregnancy must be guarded. Intrauterine death is unlikely to occur within 7 days with a negative CST. The *CST should be repeated in 1 week or less.* If labor, unfavorable symptomatology, or serious laboratory indices develop, the need for cesarean section must be assessed.

DAILY FETAL MOVEMENT COUNTING

Frequent movements of the fetus (as perceived by the mother) have been a reassuring sign for centuries. Investigators have reported a marked decrease in fetal movements during fetal distress or just before fetal death. Comparisons of daily fetal movement counts (DFMC) with movement recorded electronically for a 12 h period have revealed that almost *90% of all fetal movements can be identified by the mother.* Thus, this simple, cost-effective test can be used as a first screening in complicated pregnancies, as a routine test in normal gestation, or as a supplement to other testing.

Normally, the number of fetal movements decreases late in pregnancy. In uteroplacental insufficiency (fetal distress), however, the frequency of fetal movement decreases markedly, to cease at fetal death. Although the test has not yet been standardized, fewer than 10 fetal movements in a 12 h period probably mandates additional evaluation.

BIOPHYSICAL PROFILE

In high-risk patients, high-resolution dynamic ultrasonography may be used to obtain a fetal biophysical profile (*BPP*). This is derived from assessment of the following variables: *fetal movement, tone, breathing, nonstress test, and approximate amniotic fluid volume.* Chronic asphyxia, a common cause of perinatal death with associated diminished fetal movements and oligohydramnios, results in depressed fetal CNS activity. During ultrasound examination (10–30 min), fetal movements are observed and are assigned a score of 2 when normal and 1 when abnormal. When the results of this screening test are markedly abnormal, a 50- to 100-fold increase in perinatal mortality is likely.

Ideally, this type of testing should be begun in high-risk patients at about 30 weeks gestation and repeated at weekly intervals.

OTHER TESTS OF FETAL WELL-BEING

Estriol determinations have been largely abandoned for fetal assessment.

APPRAISAL OF FETAL HEALTH IN LABOR

- Consider pertinent details in the history, the general physical and obstetric examination, pelvimetry, and fetal heart tones (monitored externally or internally).
- Evaluate the character and progress of labor (e.g., Friedman's curve) and the passage of blood or meconium-stained amniotic fluid.
- Identify fetal distress (i.e., abnormal FHR patterns either direct or indirect), with special concern for bradycardia or late severe variable deceleration, and acidosis in samples of fetal scalp blood.

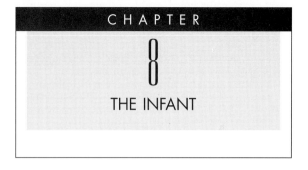

NEWBORN

The neonatal, or newborn, period is defined (e.g., for mortality data) as the first 28 days of life. Thus, it is the first portion of infancy, which extends from birth through the first year of life. There is a greater mortality during the tumultuous neonatal period than in all ensuing life until the eighth decade.

Obviously, the infant's status at birth is affected by its status in utero, especially during stressful labor and delivery. The condition at the moment of birth varies from an active, crying, normal newborn, to one who is totally unresponsive and likely to die without immediate resuscitation. Thus, providers of obstetric and newborn care must be prepared (with trained personnel, proper equipment, and necessary medications) to render comprehensive emergency support and care for the newborn.

IMMEDIATE EVALUATION AND CARE AT DELIVERY

APGAR SCORE

A *rapid evaluation* is mandatory during the first few seconds after birth as the cord is being clamped. *Muscle tone and activity* can be assessed even before delivery of the body is complete. Most infants are *slightly blue in color at birth, but they rapidly turn pink* with effective respiration except for the distal extremities (acrocyanosis). Palpating the cord pulsations or auscultating the chest for 15 sec affords a *contemporary heart rate.*

These parameters are combined into a screening assessment of the newborn's immediate adjustment, the Apgar score, recorded at *1 and 5 min after birth.* This scoring system provides points between *0 and 2 for each of five categories,* including *color, tone, respiratory effort, reflex activity, and heart rate* (Table 8-1). The best possible Apgar score is 10; the lowest score is 0.

Interpretation of the score often guides immediate therapy: ≥ 7 *is considered normal, 4–6 is compromised, and 0–3 is a medical emergency.* The scores should be recorded every 5 min until a score of 7 or above is reached. Thus, an Apgar score recorded as 1, 3, 5, 8 would be interpreted as 1 at 1 min, 3 at 5 min, 5 at 10 min, and 8 at 15 min.

The Apgar scores are not a good measure of asphyxia or of long-term outcome. Moreover, certain groups of neonates will not score well, including the *premature* (when the neonate lacks sufficient neuromuscular development), the *narcotized fetus,* and the *traumatized fetus.* A variety of problems apply to the fetus, including maternal general anesthesia sufficient to anesthetize the fetus. The narcotized newborn may have no tone, no respiratory effort, no reflex activity, and blue color. Nevertheless, he or she may have a good heartbeat for an Apgar score of 2, with a normal cord pH and no asphyxia. Of course, asphyxia will rapidly ensue if respiratory support is not provided until recovery is sufficient for spontaneous respiration.

ARTERIAL CORD pH

The arterial cord pH is another indicator of status at birth. Normally, arterial cord pH is ≥ 7.21. A pH < 7.00 indicates significant acidosis, although an isolated sample cannot determine if the fetal condition is improving or deteriorating. Nonetheless, an arterial cord blood gas is useful in the high-risk patient, cases of unexpectedly low Apgar score, premature infants, the narcotized newborn, the traumatized newborn, and uncertain or unexplained situations.

DRYING, WARMING, POSITIONING, SUCTIONING, IDENTIFICATION, AND PROPHYLAXIS

The wet newborn rapidly chills due to evaporative heat loss. *Rapid gentle drying* with warm towels or blankets under a radiant warmer or a warming surface *minimizes cold stress.* Cold stress can result in hypothermia, hypoglycemia, and respiratory distress. While drying, continue to evaluate responsiveness. If the infant is not breathing (apneic), tactile stimulation may be sufficient to initiate respiratory effort. Because the infant may be draining fluid from the lungs or gastric contents (vomiting), the *head should be keep flat*

TABLE 8-1
APGAR SCORE OF NEWBORN INFANT

		Score	
	0	1	2
A Appearance (color)	Blue or pale	Body pink, extremities blue	Completely pink
P Pulse (heart rate)	Absent	<100	>100
G Grimace (reflex irritability in response to stimulation of sole of foot)	No response	Grimace	Cry
A Activity (muscle tone)	Limp	Some flexion of extremities	Active motion
R Respiration (respiratory effort)	Absent	Slow, irregular	Good, crying

251

or somewhat lower than the feet, and oropharyngeal suction should be applied (gently) as necessary to prevent aspiration. Routinely aspirating gastric contents by orogastric or nasogastric tube is contraindicated because of the potential vagal induction of bradycardia when passing the tube. The fluid is also a source of glucose immediately after birth.

When the newborn has stabilized, place *identity bands* and administer *prophylactic ophthalmic treatment* against gonorrhea and *Chlamydia* using 1% silver nitrate, erythromycin (0.5%), or tetracycline (1%) ointment. The last two are preferred therapy against *Chlamydia.* The newborn should be kept warm while bonding with the parent(s).

INITIAL PHYSICAL AND LABORATORY OBSERVATIONS

Next, record the *vital signs* (temperature, respiratory rate, and heart rate), *weigh,* and *measure* (head circumference and length). Do a gestational assessment using either a complete Dubowitz evaluation of neurological and physical characteristics or a modified Dubowitz (Ballard) examination (Table 8-2).

Evaluate the *appropriateness of growth for gestation* in every newborn by plotting weight, length, and head circumference against norms for gestational age. Morbidity varies significantly within a single weight group depending on maturity. Infants below the 10th percentile in weight for gestation are classified small for gestational age (SGA). SGA is associated with many causative factors, including intrauterine infection, genetic abnormalities, maternal drug ingestion, maternal small stature, multiple gestation, placental insufficiency, and maternal hypertension.

Infants weighing above the 10th percentile for gestation are large for gestational age (LGA). LGA is associated with infants of diabetic mothers, maternal obesity, hydrops fetalis, postdatism, multiparity, advanced maternal age, large maternal stature, and congenital disorders (e.g., Beckwith-Weidemann syndrome).

A *physical examination* should be performed by the nursing staff as well as the baby's physician. Administer vitamin K to prevent hemorrhagic disease of the newborn because vitamin K stores are low at birth and vitamin K in breast milk is minimal. *Blood glucose screening for hypoglycemia* is recommended, and some centers will also obtain a hematocrit level at the same time to determine anemia or polycythemia. If the blood glucose level is low (<45 mg/mL) on the initial screening test, obtain a true blood glucose level and initiate therapy. If the *hematocrit* is abnormal, undertake appropriate studies.

TABLE 8-2
NEWBORN MATURE RATING AND CLASSIFICATION: ESTIMATION OF GESTATIONAL AGE BY MATURITY RATING

Neuromuscular Maturity

NEURO-MUSCULAR MATURITY SIGN	SCORE							RECORD SCORE HERE
	−1	0	1	2	3	4	5	
POSTURE								
SQUARE WINDOW (Wrist)	>90°	90°	60°	45°	30°	0°		
ARM RECOIL		180°	140°-180°	110°-140°	90°-110°	<90°		
POPLITEAL ANGLE	180°	160°	140°	120°	100°	90°	<90°	
SCARF SIGN								
HEEL TO EAR								

TOTAL NEUROMUSCULAR MATURITY SCORE

Physical Maturity

PHYSICAL MATURITY SIGN	SCORE							RECORD SCORE HERE
	−1	0	1	2	3	4	5	
SKIN	sticky friable transparent	gelatinous red translucent	smooth pink visible veins	superficial peeling &/or rash, few veins	cracking pale areas rare veins	parchment deep cracking no vessels	leathery cracked wrinkled	
LANUGO	none	sparse	abundant	thinning	bald areas	mostly bald		
PLANTAR SURFACE	heel-toe 40-50 mm:-1 <40 mm:-2	>50 mm no crease	faint red marks	anterior transverse crease only	creases ant. 2/3	creases over entire sole		
BREAST	imperceptible	barely perceptible	flat areola no bud	stippled areola 1-2 mm bud	raised areola 3-4 mm bud	full areola 5-10 mm bud		
EYE/EAR	lids fused loosely:-1 tightly:-2	lids open pinna flat stays folded	sl. curved pinna; soft; slow recoil	well-curved pinna; soft but ready recoil	formed & firm instant recoil	thick cartilage ear stiff		
GENITALS (Male)	scrotum flat, smooth	scrotum empty faint rugae	testes in upper canal rare rugae	testes descending few rugae	testes down good rugae	testes pendulous deep rugae		
GENITALS (Female)	clitoris prominent & labia flat	prominent clitoris & small labia minora	prominent clitoris & enlarging minora	majora & minora equally prominent	majora large minora small	majora cover clitoris & minora		

TOTAL PHYSICAL MATURITY SCORE

(Continued)

TABLE 8-2
(Continued)

Birth Date _____ Hour _____ am / pm

Apgar _____ 1 min _____ 5 min

SCORE

Neuromuscular _____

Physical _____

Total _____

MATURITY RATING

Score	Weeks
-10	20
-5	22
0	24
5	26
10	28
15	30
20	32
25	34
30	36
35	38
40	40
45	42
50	44

GESTATIONAL AGE (weeks)

By dates _____

By ultrasound _____

By exam _____

Scoring system modified from J.L. Ballard et al., New Ballard Score, expanded to include extremely premature infants. J Pediatr 1991; 417–423. Reprinted by permission.

Vital signs should be continued even if stable and monitored every 1 h during the transition, then every 4–8 h thereafter. A *bath* using mild soap and water is usually given during this period to wash off blood and meconium.

NEWBORN EXAMINATION

Many physical and neurological findings are recorded as part of the gestational assessment examination. These are summarized in Table 8-2.

GENERAL APPEARANCE

Note the infant's activity, proportions, obvious defects, cry, and respiratory effort.

SKIN

Look for skin tags, moles, discolorations, and other defects of skin. The skin will vary in thickness depending on the length of gestation, ranging from very thin and red in the preterm infant to pale and leathery in the postterm infant. Vernix (a whitish fatty coating most evident from 36 to 39 weeks) may be present (before a bath). Perfusion can be assessed by capillary refill (normally <3 sec) after blanching the skin of the extremity or chest by finger pressure. Bruising is not uncommon. Localized petechiae are not unusual (especially on the head and back), but generalized petechiae warrant further investigation. Jaundice at birth is abnormal. Meconium staining may be present, especially around the nails or umbilical cord, but should not be confused with jaundice. Acrocyanosis (blueness of the hands and feet) is normal because of the high hemoglobin levels present. Plethora (ruddy color) may be noted with crying if the baby is polycythemic.

HEAD

Note the shape of the head (round, elongated, asymmetric), separation or fusion of sutures, presence and size of the anterior and posterior fontanelles, and edema of the scalp (caput succedaneum), which was the presenting part.

EYES

Check pupil size and shape and look for conjunctival hemorrhage.

EARS

Note auricular size, shape, and placement and determine the presence of an open auditory canal.

NOSE

Ascertain that both nares are patent by gently occluding one nostril at a time, and observe for air flow while holding the mouth closed. Note abnormalities in size, shape, septum, philtrum, and nasal bridge.

MOUTH AND PHARYNX

A cleft lip will be obvious if present. Inspect the gums for cysts or neonatal teeth. Check the palate for clefts. A submucous cleft of the palate may not be seen but can be palpated with a finger in the mouth. Note the presence of the uvula and whether it is bifid. A frenulum below the tip of the tongue is not uncommon. Look for symmetric movement of the lips with crying.

NECK

Assess the neck length and check for webbing, cysts, masses, or torticollis.

CHEST

Note intercostal or subcostal retractions. Check the spacing of the nipples. Asymmetry of the chest may indicate pneumothorax.

LUNGS

Auscultate to evaluate the presence of rales or rhonchi. Are breath sounds equal? Diaphragmatic hernia and pneumothorax must be excluded.

HEART

Record rate and rhythm as well as presence, timing, and location of murmurs (fully one third of all newborns will have a murmur detected in this transition period). Muffled heart tones suggest pneumomediastinum. Displaced heart tones suggest dextrocardia, pneumothorax, or diaphragmatic hernia. Palpate brachial and femoral pulses for presence and strength. Absent or diminished femoral pulses suggest coarctation of the aorta.

ABDOMEN

Observe movement with each breath, protuberance, or scaphoid appearance. Palpate for masses or enlargement of the liver, spleen, kidneys, or bladder. Check the umbilical cord for evidence of herniation or infection and the number of vessels, normally three. Anomalies in an infant with a two-vessel cord are increased.

GENITALIA

The male penis should be evaluated for length, torsion, chordee, hypospadias, or epispadias. The scrotum should contain two testicles of similar size. Asymmetry may indicate a unilateral hydrocele. Bilateral hydrocele is not uncommon, especially with breech position. If the testis is not felt in the scrotum, feel along the inguinal canal for incomplete descent before diagnosing cryptorchidism.

In the female, the relative size of the labia majora and minora should be noted, and vaginal patency should be assessed. Vaginal tags are not unusual. Whitish discharge may often be found. Look for introital cysts.

ANUS

Check for anal location, patency, and tone.

HIPS

Gently assess for range of motion and signs of dislocation.

CLAVICLES

Palpate the clavicles to ascertain presence, crepitus (fracture), and symmetry.

EXTREMITIES

Count the numbers of fingers and toes. Exclude syndactyly (webbing of fingers or toes). Assess the shape, symmetry, and length of each extremity or digit and check range of motion.

SPINE

Observe for curvature and evidence of spina bifida or masses.

CENTRAL NERVOUS SYSTEM (CNS)

Evaluate tone and general activity levels. Is the cry normal? Do all extremities move equally? Birth injury to the brachial plexus may be present in an upper extremity that does not move or has limited movement. Test the Moro reflex. Assess the tonic neck reflex and Babinski reflex. The normal infant makes a stepping motion if the foot is placed on a hard surface. Check the grasp reflex. Test cranial nerve II by observing the newborn fix and follow a bright object 10–12 inches in front of the face for about a 60-degree arc. Suck and swallow tests cranial nerves V, VII, X, XI, and XII. The ocular movement with the doll's eyes maneuver (rotating the infant upright at arm's length in both directions) will evaluate cranial nerves III, IV, VI, and VIII (vestibular only). Testing the auditory portion of VIII requires observation of the infant's response to sound (awakens if asleep, quiets if awake).

CORD CARE

The cord may be painted once with triple dye to speed drying and minimize bacterial infection. To help keep the cord dry, apply isopropyl alcohol several times a day until the cord separates (<2 weeks). Erythema or purulence should be evaluated for the possibility of omphalitis.

FEEDING

The initial feeding may occur shortly after delivery. Sterile water or glucose/water has no advantage over milk with regard to chemical pneumonitis if aspiration occurs. Formula feeding should be offered at least every 3–4 h, but breastfeeding may be more frequent because relatively small amounts of colostrum and breast milk are produced for the first 24–48 h.

VOIDING AND DEFECATION

The newborn will void within the first 24 h unless an abnormality is present. The first voiding frequently occurs in the delivery room.

Hence, accurate recording then and later should be used to avoid undue concern. *The normal newborn will pass meconium in the first 48 h of life (~10%–15% before birth).* Meconium is the accumulation of bile salts, swallowed lanugo, shed intestinal cells, and intestinal secretions. It is sticky and dark green to black in appearance. With the initiation of feeding, the stool undergoes a transition phase that is partly meconium and partly food residue. Eventually, the stool becomes yellow to green and seedy in appearance. Stool passage may be as infrequent as every other day to as frequent as a small stool with each feeding.

CIRCUMCISION

Circumcision (surgical removal of the penile foreskin) usually is performed by either the pediatrician or the obstetrician. Although circumcision has been practiced for many centuries (for religious reasons), *there is controversy as to the medical value of routine circumcision.* Circumcision should not be performed on infants with bleeding disorders or when penile anomalies are present (e.g., hypospadias) because the foreskin may be needed for reconstructive surgery. Recent reports have suggested that the incidence of urinary tract infection in uncircumcised males is higher than in the circumcised population. The major risks of circumcision are bleeding, infection, and scar formation. The advantages and disadvantages must be discussed with the parents to obtain informed consent for the procedure. Because of the pain involved, local anesthesia should be administered.

SCREENING FOR METABOLIC DISORDERS

All states have screening programs for certain metabolic disorders causing mental retardation that are preventable by diet or medication if begun early enough in life. The most common of these disorders are phenylketonuria and hypothyroidism. However, galactosemia, Tay-Sachs disease, and others are screened with increasing frequency. Testing for sickle cell disease or trait in the African American population should be routine.

DISCHARGE

On the day of discharge, the *physical examination should be repeated* because some findings not evident on the day of birth (e.g., heart murmurs, cephalhematoma, jaundice) may have appeared.

Routine baby care should be discussed and arrangements made for follow-up care. Follow-up in 24–48 h is especially important with early discharge (often <24 h after delivery). Hypoplastic left heart may only manifest itself after closure of the ductus arteriosus and is rapidly fatal without therapy. Signs of sepsis may not appear before discharge. Thus, *parents must be made aware of the need to seek assistance at the earliest sign of trouble. Parents should be informed of positioning the infant on the back to sleep.* Indeed, sudden infant death syndrome (SIDS) has decreased markedly since positioning on the back to sleep has been promoted. *The proper use of an infant car seat must be impressed on the family* because a babe in arms is at high risk in a moving vehicle.

RESUSCITATION

Anticipation is the key to the best possible outcome. A low-risk pregnancy can suddenly change into high risk (e.g., predelivery cord prolapse or postdelivery diaphragmatic hernia). Resuscitative equipment and personnel trained in resuscitation should be present. Ideally there should be three people, one to manage the airway, another to assess the cardiac function, and another to provide necessary drugs and equipment and record the time and the procedures performed. Rapid drying and a radiant heat source are essential to minimize hypothermia during resuscitation. *Newborn resuscitation follows the same ABCs applied to resuscitation of the adult.*

AIRWAY

A patent airway is essential. Because the newborn frequently has mucus or meconium in the oropharynx, use suction devices to aspirate mucus or meconium from the oropharynx. Bulb suction can clear the oropharynx, but a suction catheter or endotracheal tube connected to suction will be required to clear the trachea. Because of the risk of AIDS, avoid mouth-to-mouth and mouth-to-endotracheal tube suction unless there is no other option available (e.g., home delivery). *Provide a source of oxygen (Fio_2 1.0) once the airway is clear if the infant is cyanotic.* When spontaneous breathing is well established with good color, maintain oxygen therapy until the infant is stable. The risk of oxygen toxicity in a term infant after a brief period is negligible. It is better to give too much rather than too little oxygen initially because the infant may be acidotic and at high risk for persistent pulmonary hypertension. A preterm infant often requires an oxygen saturation monitor. This is easily applied to an extremity, with adjustment of the oxygen level to maintain saturation between 90% and 95%.

BREATHING

Mask and Bag

If the infant is not breathing spontaneously but has an Apgar score of ≥4, *gentle stimulation with drying and warmth may initiate respirations.* Without response, begin assisted ventilation by bag and mask using 100% oxygen (Fio_2 1.0). A self-inflating bag should have a reservoir or rebreathing device, or only about 40% oxygen (Fio_2 ~0.40) will be available to the infant. Check the Fio_2 setting if the gas source is attached to a blender and adjust to 1.0.

The mask should be the proper size for the baby (preterm and term sizes are available). Adjust the mask so that it is snug to avoid air leaks. Be careful not to inadvertently press the top of the mask against the eyes. The newborn tongue is relatively large, *so lift the mandible toward the mask by fingers at the angle of the jaw rather than pressing the mask down on the face.*

A few breaths may be necessary to inflate the lungs and initiate spontaneous respiration. Watch the infant closely, and auscultate the chest to ensure adequate air exchange whether respiration is spontaneous or assisted. Continue bag and mask resuscitation at ~40–60 breaths/min. If the infant is not receiving adequate ventilation via bag and mask, use endotracheal intubation.

Endotracheal Tube

If the apnea persists or if respiration is insufficient with bag and mask resuscitation, perform endotracheal intubation. Multiple attempts at intubation by the unskilled can do more harm than good (e.g., perforation of the hypopharynx, trachea or esophagus, prolonged hypoxemia as attempts are made, or intubation of the esophagus). *This is a skill that any provider delivering babies must have acquired.*

The endotracheal tube size should be determined by the infant's size and weight. A 3.5-mm internal diameter tube is appropriate for most term infants except the large for gestational age, which may require a 4.0. A 2.5-mm tube is the smallest that should be used and should be able to accommodate infants up to 1250 g. Between 1250 and 2500 g, a 3.0-mm tube should be adequate. If a tube is too small, the work of breathing will be increased and air can leak around it (cuffed endotracheal tubes are never to be used in newborns). If the endotracheal tube is too large and is forced into the trachea, damage and stenosis can follow.

Do not insert the endotracheal tube too far into the airway. To prevent this, estimate the depth of insertion based on the infant's weight. Use only endotracheal tubes with markings in centimeters. The tip of the tube to the lip edge should be remembered as the rule of 1-2-3-4 and 7-8-9-10. For a 1 kg infant, the tip to lip distance should be 7 cm. For 2 kg, the tip to lip distance should be 8 cm. For 3 kg, it should be 9 cm, and for 4 kg, 10 cm. For weights in between, estimate the distance (e.g., 7.5 cm for 1500 g).

Always auscultate for equal air exchange and air leaks after insertion before taping the tube in place. Another method of endotracheal tube location can be applied by feeling in the suprasternal notch as the tube is inserted. Stop advancement of the tube just after the tip passes the examining finger. *X-ray confirmation of tube location will be necessary later if the endotracheal tube remains in place.*

Frequently, the infant will become vigorous, with good respiratory effort, after several minutes of assisted ventilation, and the endotracheal tube can be removed. Observe for recurrence of respiratory distress or cyanosis. *Insert an orogastric or nasogastric tube to allow decompression of the stomach from insufflated gas.*

CARDIAC

Assessment of heart rate should be performed by both auscultation of the chest and palpation of brachial pulse. Feeling the cord for pulsations immediately after birth may be helpful in determining heart rate. *Bradycardia (<100 bpm) usually responds rapidly to the administration of oxygen and assisted ventilation.* If heart rate persists at ≤60 bpm or remains 60–80 without increasing despite respiratory support, chest compressions should be initiated.

The sternum should be depressed using finger pressure over the middle of the sternum (not the lower one third) 1–1.5 cm. The overlapping thumbs can be used with the hands encircling the chest or the index and third fingers pressing simultaneously at a rate of three compressions and one ventilation in a 2-sec period. Assisted ventilation should be continued with periodic auscultation to ensure adequate air exchange and heart rate.

If the infant does not respond, administer 1:10,000 concentration of epinephrine 0.1–0.3 mL/kg into the endotracheal tube or intravenously. This can be repeated every 3–5 minutes if required. If the heart rate increases to over 100, discontinue the epinephrine. If hypovolemia or acute blood loss is suspected (signs of pallor, weak pulses, low blood pressure) give a *volume expander* (e.g., normal saline, 5% albumin, or Ringer's lactate) 10 mL/kg intravenously over 5–10 minutes.

For *prolonged* arrest that does not respond to other therapy, use *sodium bicarbonate in a 4.2% solution (0.5 mEq/mL) in a dose of 2 mEq/kg intravenously over at least 2 minutes (no faster than 1 mEq/kg/min)*. Effective ventilation must precede and accompany the administration of sodium bicarbonate. Because sodium bicarbonate is caustic if extravasated, administration into a large peripheral vein, the umbilical artery, or an umbilical venous catheter preferably positioned above the diaphragm (to avoid hepatic necrosis) is recommended.

While intravascular access is being attempted, *epinephrine* can be absorbed via the trachea using the *endotracheal tube* in a dose of 0.1 mL/kg of a 1:10,000 solution. Because epinephrine is less effective in an acidotic environment, repeat the dose intravascularly after the bicarbonate has been administered if bradycardia persists.

Once an adequate heart rate has been established, discontinue cardiac massage and observe for adequate pulses and assess blood pressure. For isolated *respiratory depression due to narcotics* given to the mother, *administer naloxone hydrochloride* (Narcan) in a dosage of 0.1 mg/kg via endotracheal, IV, IM, or subcutaneous routes. Narcan should not be given to the newborn of a narcotic addicted mother because it can precipitate seizures in the infant.

PROBLEMS ASSOCIATED WITH PREMATURITY

RESPIRATORY DISTRESS SYNDROME (RDS)

Respiratory distress syndrome (also called hyaline membrane disease) *is the most common cause of mortality and morbidity in the nonanomalous preterm infant.* The *incidence is directly related to gestational age*—the more preterm the infant, the greater the risk (as high as 60% at 30 weeks, 20% at 34 weeks). Term infants can develop RDS, but this is uncommon, except perhaps in infants of diabetic mothers (IDM), where the overall incidence of RDS is two to three times higher than in infants of nondiabetic mothers.

The pathophysiology of RDS is a vicious cycle of *decreased alveolar surfactant leading to increased alveolar surface tension, resulting in generalized atelectasis.* This atelectasis causes both hypoventilation and uneven ventilation–perfusion, which in turn cause CO_2 retention and hypoxemia. These in turn cause acidosis and subsequent capillary endothelial damage. Capillary damage results in leakage of plasma proteins and fibrin, which produces a diffusion gradient, further increasing CO_2 retention, hypoxemia, and acidosis, which in turn reduce surfactant synthesis, storage, and release. If this cycle cannot be broken, the patient dies. If hypoxemia and acidosis can be brought under control, the alveolar cells have the opportunity to recover sufficiently to produce and release surfactant, thereby reducing atelectasis and allowing better ventilation and perfusion.

RDS is exacerbated by predelivery or postdelivery asphyxia, acidosis, or hypothermia. Assess pulmonary maturity antenatally by determining the lecithin–sphingomyelin (LS) ratio of amniotic fluid or the presence or absence of phosphatidyl glycerol (Pg). *The incidence of RDS is decreased in infants experiencing certain types of stress* (e.g., IUGR, prolonged rupture of the membranes, maternal hypertension). RDS (both amount and severity) can also be decreased by administration of glucocorticoid to the mother at least 24–48 h before delivery at 28–34 weeks gestation when preterm delivery is anticipated. *RDS is now being prevented or treated postdelivery by synthetic or bovine surfactant administered into the trachea.*

RDS may be present at birth or within the first 4–6 h of life. Consider other causes if respiratory distress begins thereafter. The infant will have any combination of tachypnea (RR >60), retractions (substernal, intercostal), nasal flaring, grunting respirations, or cyanosis. The chest x-ray shows intermediate expansion of the chest with a reticulogranular (ground glass) appearance and air bronchograms. The blood gases show progressive acidosis (predominantly respiratory) with hypoxemia and hypercarbia.

Assisted ventilation frequently is necessary to assure adequate oxygenation and gas exchange. Reduce the Pa_{CO_2} to a normal or near normal range to correct acidosis, maintain a neutral thermal environment, and provide appropriate IV glucose to maintain adequate blood sugar levels and to provide some caloric intake. Avoid fluid overload, which can contribute to significant PDA.

PULMONARY AIR LEAK

Microscopic tears in the airway and alveolar lining allow air to pass along the vascular sheath, into the interstitium or the pleural space. *The location of the free air determines its designation as pneumothorax, pneumomediastinum, pulmonary interstitial emphysema, pneumopericardium, or pneumoperitoneum.* The estimated incidence is ~1% of all live births. Air leak is not limited to preterm infants. Not all infants with pulmonary air leak will be symptomatic.

Air leak is more common in meconium aspiration syndrome than in RDS.

Suspect air leak in any newborn with respiratory distress, especially after resuscitation, and in infants on ventilators with deterioration or with muffled heart tones.

The *diagnosis of air leak is made by chest x-ray*, and both anteroposterior (AP) and lateral views are necessary initially to determine location and size. Thereafter, an AP view will be sufficient in most cases for follow-up.

Transillumination of the chest also can be used to diagnose pulmonary air leak, but it requires a dark room. The area of free air shows greater transmission of light around the light source than does the unaffected side. Treatment ranges from simple observation to hyperoxygenation to needle thoracentesiss and chest tube insertion, depending on the baby's condition.

PATENT DUCTUS ARTERIOSUS (PDA)

The ductus arteriosus (between the aorta and pulmonary artery) is necessarily patent in utero to allow circulatory bypass of the lungs, but the ductus closes rapidly after the first breath in a vasoconstrictive response to increased Pao_2. This response is mediated by prostaglandin. *Final closure can take 1–8 days in the term infant, but in the preterm, this process can take weeks.* As many as 75% of preterm infants <1000 g have a clinically evident PDA.

PDA can cause a range of problems from an asymptomatic intermittent murmur at the left upper sternal border to florid congestive heart failure. Echocardiography can make the diagnosis and evaluate the degree and direction of shunting.

INTRACRANIAL HEMORRHAGE

Four relatively common types of intracranial hemorrhage are recognized: *subarachnoid, subependymal germinal matrix/intraventricular (SEH/IVH), subdural, and cerebellar.*

Fetal intracranial hemorrhage occurs, but most significant hemorrhages occur after birth in the preterm infant, although term infants are not immune.

SUBARACHNOID HEMORRHAGE

Subarachnoid hemorrhage is the *most common hemorrhage in term newborns* (presumably either due to trauma involving molding of the head for delivery or related to asphyxia). Most do not result in significant bleeding, and the infant is asymptomatic. A lumbar puncture can reveal RBCs. Cranial ultrasonography or CT scan will eliminate or elucidate other origins of the bleeding.

SUBEPENDYMAL GERMINAL MATRIX/ INTRAVENTRICULAR (SEH/IVH)

Because the germinal matrix (a highly vascularized area adjacent to the ventricular area of the brain) is present until ~35 weeks gestation, intraventricular and periventricular hemorrhages are common (10%–20% at 1000–1500 g and 50%–60% <1 kg) in preterm infants. Ultrasonography or CT scan should provide the diagnosis.

Because the germinal matrix is most prominent at the head of the caudate nucleus at the level of the foramen of Monro, this is the site of most hemorrhages. Bleeding limited to the subependymal area of the germinal matrix is termed subependymal hemorrhage (SEH). When the bleeding ruptures through the germinal matrix and into the ventricular system, it is called intraventricular hemorrhage (IVH). IVH is mild when there is no ventricular dilation. It becomes moderate when the ventricle(s) dilate and severe when the hemorrhage extends into the parenchyma of the brain. The latter two gradations are associated with increased incidence of morbidity and mortality. *Many affected infants will develop posthemorrhagic hydrocephalus within 2–3 weeks of the original hemorrhage.* Some cases of hydrocephalus will resolve spontaneously, whereas others will require drainage procedure(s). Developmental delay or neurologic deficits or both will be present in as many as two thirds of the infants with moderate to severe IVH.

SUBDURAL HEMORRHAGE

Subdural hemorrhage occurs with trauma when there is excessive molding of the head and sudden tearing of the superficial veins over the cerebral cortex or the venous sinuses of the posterior fossa during delivery of the head. The usual circumstances are *precipitous labor and delivery in a primigravida, high or midforceps delivery, or an LGA baby. If hemorrhage occurs in the cerebellar fossa, death occurs rapidly* due to compression of brainstem. When the hemorrhage occurs over the cerebral hemispheres, the early symptomatology can be anemia, unexplained jaundice, seizures, or other signs of increasing intracranial pressure (bulging fontanel, altered states of consciousness). Later signs (4–6 weeks) can include increasing head circumference, failure to thrive, or vomiting. CT scan is better than ultrasonography in defining the exact location, quantity of blood, and extent of hemorrhage.

CEREBELLAR HEMORRHAGE

Cerebellar hemorrhage *most commonly occurs in the preterm infant concomitant with asphyxia or trauma.* Such hemorrhage frequently results in a progressive downhill course to death. Symptoms in those with nonlethal hemorrhage are apnea, high-pitched cry, hypotonia, vomiting, absent Moro reflex, and rapidly increasing head circumference. Although cerebellar hemorrhage can be diagnosed by cranial ultrasonography, CT scan may give better delineation.

SUBGALEAL HEMORRHAGE

Subgaleal hemorrhage, or *bleeding in the potential space between the periosteum of the skull and the scalp,* can occur with any form of delivery, but is highest with instrumented and vacuum assisted deliveries. Acute blood loss into this space can cause severe anemia, shock, and death.

RETINOPATHY OF PREMATURITY (ROP)

Formerly known as retrolental fibroplasia, ROP *is a disorder of the immature retinal vascular system.* The retinal vessels are incompletely developed until about 34–36 weeks gestation, with the temporal area the last site to mature. *The more preterm the infant, the greater the risk of developing ROP.*

Vasoconstriction of the retinal arteries occurs in response to increased arterial oxygen tension (Pao_2), similar to the vasoconstriction of the ductus arteriosus after birth in response to the sudden increase in Pao_2. This vasoconstriction may be a protective response and cause no harm to fully developed retinas, but localized hypoperfusion and hypoxemia in the incompletely vascularized retina may stimulate proliferation of new vessel formation (neovascularization) in an attempt to supply the underperfused areas. The subsequent hemorrhage(s) into the vitreous and retina causes fibrous proliferation, scar retraction, and in the worst case, retinal detachment and blindness.

Relative hyperoxemia can occur in infants breathing room air. Thus ROP has been reported in preterm infants who have never received supplemental oxygen. Likewise Fio_2 1.0 is not necessarily harmful to the retina if normoxemia is maintained. Because of fluctuating Pao_2 despite constant Fio_2 delivery, *continuous monitoring of blood oxygen is a necessity in small preterm infants.*

APNEA

Apnea in the newborn is *cessation of respiration for 15–20 sec, frequently accompanied by cyanosis or bradycardia.* Respiratory irregularity is common in preterm infants due to immaturity. Practically all preterm infants <34 weeks will have apnea at some point. Before deciding that apnea is secondary to immaturity of the neonatal respiratory control centers, other causes must be investigated and treated if present. These include drugs, both maternal (e.g., magnesium, narcotics) and neonatal (e.g., narcotics, Prostin), infections (e.g., sepsis, meningitis, NEC), metabolic disturbances (e.g., hypoglycemia, hyponatremia, or hypocalcemia), CNS abnormalities (e.g., seizures, intracranial hemorrhage), temperature abnormalities (e.g., hypothermia or hyperthermia), gastroesophageal reflux, decreased oxygenation (e.g., hypoxemia, anemia, or left to right shunt from PDA). *Apnea may be obstructive* (chest wall moves with respiratory effort but no nasal air flow occurs), *central* (CNS) in origin, or *mixed* (a combination of the two).

Treatment of apnea of prematurity consists of multiple modalities ranging from stimulation for infrequent episodes, changing position (may be helpful in obstructive apnea), methylxanthines (theophylline, caffeine) for recurrent apnea, to nasal CPAP or assisted ventilation for intractable apnea.

BONDING/SEPARATION ANXIETY

Parents are frequently and legitimately concerned about bonding with their sick or preterm infant. With more liberal visiting and handling policies of current neonatal intensive care units (NICUs), visiting is more often a problem when the mother and baby are in different locations (hospital, city, or state) or have transportation problems. This is one advantage of maternal transport for delivery rather than neonatal transport after birth.

Nursing personnel can be a tremendous asset in helping parents cope with the stresses associated with prematurity. Recording the *frequency and length of parental visits (or lack thereof) and parental response* (e.g., talking to the baby, making eye contact) is the first step in recognizing a problem and finding resources to solve it. Weekly letters and Polaroid pictures sent to the parents can help. *Parent support groups* can also relieve some anxiety. *NICU social workers* are available in most centers and can be invaluable in helping parents deal with financial worries, etc. Because the typical weight at discharge has decreased to the 4 to $4\frac{1}{2}$ pound range, more and more NICUs are providing facilities for the *parents to room in with the baby* for 1 or 2 nights before discharge to allow a better transition from hospital to home. This assists in assuring parental competence and confidence in handling the preterm infant, giving medication, and home monitor usage.

INFECTION

Because the immune system is incompletely developed in the newborn, *infection is one of the more common causes of morbidity and mortality.* Mortality is higher in the preterm than in the term infant. Sepsis and pneumonitis predominate in the first few days of life. Meningitis and urinary tract infection become more frequent after the first week.

Many infants are born prematurely because of chorioamnionitis and are infected before or at birth. *Determining the offending organism in the neonate can be difficult for several reasons:* only a small blood sample is available for culture (1 mL or less); the organism may be bacterial (aerobic or anaerobic), fungal, or viral; and skin contaminants are relatively common because of difficulty in obtaining free-flowing blood.

Laboratory findings associated with neonatal infection include leukocytosis (WBC >30,000), leukopenia (WBC <5000), increased immature neutrophils (left shift, immature: total neutrophils >0.2), thrombocytopenia (platelets <100,000), metabolic acidosis, and increased WBC in CSF (>30). *Chest radiographs* may show pneumonitis, and *Gram's stain of the tracheal aspirate* may reveal organisms. *Culture and Gram's stain of the gastric contents* immediately after birth can indicate the presence of amnionitis but not necessarily neonatal infection. Since group B beta-hemolytic streptococcus is the most common neonatal bacterium causing infection, *latex agglutination testing* of blood, urine, and CSF may be helpful, especially if cultures are negative.

Treatment consists of broad-spectrum antibiotics until the offending organism can be isolated and antibiotic sensitivity can be determined.

PROBLEMS ASSOCIATED WITH THE TERM INFANT

TRANSIENT TACHYPNEA OF THE NEWBORN (TTN)

TTN may result from delayed clearing of pulmonary fluid. It is not an aspiration syndrome. Pulmonary fluid is produced by the lungs and has a different protein and electrolyte content from amniotic fluid. TTN occurs more frequently after cesarean delivery without labor, presumably because the onset of labor terminates production of pulmonary fluid, and fluid is more effectively squeezed out of the lungs when the chest is compressed passing through the birth canal. The respirations typically are 80–120 per min, usually without grunting. The tachypnea is present shortly after birth. Cyanosis will be present if the spontaneous hyperventilation is inadequate to maintain oxygenation. Blood gases in room air usually show normal pH and $Paco_2$ (CO_2 diffuses 20 times faster than O_2), with low to normal Pao_2. The chest x-ray shows good chest expansion with some haziness and, frequently, fluid in the interlobar fissures (seen best between RUL and RML).

TTN is usually self-limiting and generally resolves in <36 h. *Maintain adequate oxygenation,* usually by oxyhood, until the fluid can resorb spontaneously. Assisted ventilation is rarely necessary, and mortality is unusual.

HYPERBILIRUBINEMIA

Jaundice (icterus, yellow skin) is *present in ~50% of all newborns.* Unconjugated hyperbilirubinemia (level >1.0–1.5 mg/mL) is present in almost all. It is important to distinguish between physiologic and pathologic hyperbilirubinemia to provide appropriate therapy.

Bilirubin is produced primarily as the breakdown product of heme from RBCs. Free bilirubin rapidly binds with albumin and is transported to the liver, where it is conjugated with glucuronic acid to form a water-soluble product for excretion in bile. Once in the intestine, the bilirubin becomes unconjugated and may be reabsorbed via the portal system, converted to urobilinogen, and excreted via the kidneys or excreted in stool.

The *two forms of bilirubin* that are of clinical significance in the newborn are the *unconjugated fraction* (indirect reaction, fat-soluble, commonly elevated) and the *conjugated fraction* (direct reaction, water-soluble, less commonly elevated). Physiologic elevation of unconjugated bilirubin is a combination of increased production (e.g., naturally shorter life span of fetal RBCs, bruising) and decreased excretion (e.g., increased enteric resorption of bilirubin, decreased activity of hepatic glucuronyl transferase).

Physiologic hyperbilirubinemia can be as high as *12 mg/mL* in term infants (mean peak at 3 days) and *14 mg/mL* in preterm infants, with a later mean peak (5 days). Note that a physiologic level does not exclude the risk of harmful effects (especially in the premature infant). *Elevated conjugated bilirubin* (level >1.5–2 mg/mL) *is never physiologic.* Causes include primary hepatitis (e.g., viral, bacterial, protozoal, or idiopathic), toxic hepatitis (e.g., drugs, necrosis, sepsis, or parenteral alimentation), metabolic disorders (e.g., galactosemia, alpha$_1$-antitrypsin deficiency, cystic fibrosis, or Gaucher's disease), and ductal disturbances (e.g., biliary atresia, choledochal cyst).

Pathologic causes of unconjugated hyperbilirubinemia secondary to increased production include *isoimmunization* (Rh, ABO, and other blood group incompatibilities), RBC *biochemical defects* (e.g., G6PD deficiency, pyruvate kinase deficiency), *infection* (bacterial, viral, or fungal), and *blood sequestration* (e.g., cephalhematoma, IVH, bruising, or abdominal hemorrhage). Pathologic causes of *decreased excretion* include *conjugation defects* (e.g., Crigler-Najjar, type II glucuronyl transferase deficiency, or breast milk jaundice) and *increased reabsorption* (e.g., intestinal obstruction, gastrointestinal hemorrhage). Unconjugated hyperbilirubinemia of *undetermined etiology* may be seen in infants of diabetic mothers and hypothyroidism.

Bilirubin encephalopathy results from cytotoxic effects of unconjugated bilirubin on neurons (especially basal ganglia, hippocampal cortex, and subthalamic nuclei). Severe disease progresses from lethargy and hypotonia to rigidity, opisthotonos, high-pitched cry, fever, and seizures, which may end in death. The survivors may have residual choreoathetoid cerebral palsy, hearing deficits, paralysis of downward gaze, and occasionally, mental retardation. Infants having sequelae of subclinical disease are categorized as having minimal brain dysfunction. Conditions that increase the risk of bilirubin encephalopathy are prematurity, hypoxia, sepsis, acidosis, hypoglycemia, rapid hemolysis, drugs that compete for bilirubin binding sites (e.g., sulfonamides), and low albumin states.

Appropriate initial *laboratory studies* include *both total and direct bilirubin levels, CBC with platelet count, blood type,* and *Coombs' test.* Further studies are indicated depending on results and clinical findings.

Treatment is intended to decrease the unconjugated bilirubin level before damage can occur and to eliminate the cause if possible. The recommended maximum tolerance of total bilirubin levels ranges from 10 to 20 mg/dL depending on birth weight, gestational age, associated risk factors, and etiology of hyperbilirubinemia. There is some suggestion that breast milk jaundice is better tolerated, and higher levels may not be harmful.

Double volume exchange transfusion is the most rapid and effective method to decrease bilirubin levels (usually ~50%) but carries the risk inherent in simple blood transfusion as well as hypoglycemia, sepsis, acidosis, platelet washout, arrhythmia, and death. The most frequent treatment is phototherapy, which uses wavelengths in the blue spectrum to photoisomerize bilirubin to allow excretion without conjugation. The eyes must be shielded, and increased water loss from the skin and gastrointestinal tract (diarrhea is a common side effect) necessitates adequate fluid intake. Phototherapy is not helpful and may be contraindicated in significant direct hyperbilirubinemia. Phenobarbital stimulates protein synthesis and hepatic enzyme production and can decrease both direct and indirect bilirubin levels over a period of 24–48 h and may be helpful especially when phototherapy is contraindicated.

PROBLEMS ASSOCIATED WITH THE POSTTERM INFANT

MECONIUM ASPIRATION SYNDROME WITH PERSISTENT PULMONARY HYPERTENSION

Postterm infants have the highest incidence of meconium passage in utero. They also are at greater risk of asphyxia during labor and delivery as a result of progressive uteroplacental insufficiency.

PATHOPHYSIOLOGY

When asphyxia occurs, the postterm fetus may gasp and swallow meconium (often very thick from the large volume passed and lower amniotic fluid available for mixture), filling both the airway and stomach. With the first breath after birth, the meconium is inhaled further into the small airways and subsequent breaths (spontaneous or with resuscitative efforts) may cause pulmonary air leak (from the ballvalve effect of the meconium obstructing the airway on exhalation), further compromising ventilation, perfusion, and oxygenation. The meconium causes a chemical pneumonitis. *The resultant respiratory distress can persist for 7–10 days.*

Because these infants are frequently acidotic and hypoxemic, vasodilation of the pulmonary arteries is inhibited, resulting in *persistent pulmonary hypertension of the newborn (PPHN),* formerly called persistent fetal circulation (PFC). PPHN is responsible for a vicious cycle in which the lungs receive insufficient cardiac output to properly oxygenate the systemic circuit. High pulmonary artery pressure causes right to left shunting of blood across the patent foramen ovale or PDA where pressures are lower. Continued hypoxemia or acidosis results in further vasoconstriction of the pulmonary circuit and even less pulmonary blood flow. PPHN may also be associated with RDS, hypoglycemia, sepsis, or hyperviscosity or can be idiopathic in origin.

Chest x-ray may reveal coarse infiltrates more on the right than left due to the takeoff position of the left mainstem bronchus. Pulmonary air leak should be evaluated and treated if present.

TREATMENT

The best treatment of meconium aspiration is prevention. Suctioning the nasopharynx and oropharynx (trachea in skilled hands) before delivery of the body can be extremely helpful. Tracheal suctioning need not be performed in every meconium-stained baby but should be performed in cases of thick (pea soup) meconium, depression, or respiratory distress at birth. A 14 F suction catheter has the same external diameter as a 3.5 mm endotracheal tube and is large enough to remove most particulate meconium.

Meconium regurgitated into the oropharynx from a stomach overdistended by bag and mask ventilation often is aspirated. Thus, this is one instance where emptying the gastric contents can be beneficial.

Antibiotic therapy is indicated in the patient with residual respiratory distress or infiltrate on chest x-ray for two reasons. Sepsis may have been the precipitating factor in meconium passage in utero; and meconium is a good culture medium.

PERINATAL ASPHYXIA

Although asphyxia can occur without regard to gestational age, the *incidence is higher in preterm and postterm infants than in term infants.* Factors associated with increased risk for asphyxia include:

- Sudden disruption of fetoplacental exchange (e.g., cord prolapse, placental abruption, bleeding placenta previa, or nuchal cord)

- Chronic decreased fetoplacental exchange (e.g., postmaturity, IUGR)
- Decreased maternal/placental blood flow (e.g., hypotension, hypertension, or uterine tetany)
- Decreased maternal oxygenation (e.g., cardiopulmonary disease, hypoventilation, or hypoxia)
- Delayed or improper resuscitation

Physical damage varies with gestational age. The periventricular area and subependymal germinal matrix are more susceptible in the preterm infant. In the term newborn, the typically affected areas are the cortical and CNS subcortical gray matter. Damage to the latter results in hypoxic ischemic encephalopathy (HIE). The most severe degree of asphyxia results in brain necrosis (if survival is more than 24 h postinsult) and death. During the asphyxial episode, all organs of the body are exposed (some more than others due to the redistribution of blood flow to the vital organs). Renal failure or cardiac failure, or both, postasphyxia indicate significant insult and, of themselves, can cause further CNS damage, impede recovery, or cause death.

Signs of CNS dysfunction include an altered state of consciousness, poor sucking, poor feeding, respiratory pattern abnormalities (including apnea), seizure activity, abnormal pupillary response, decreased oculovestibular response, and a tight or bulging fontanel. When it occurs, *seizure activity usually begins 12–24 h after birth, but it can occur as early as 2–6 h.* When status epilepticus or serial seizures persist for over 24 h, the risk of death or sequelae is highest, but not without exception. Seizures should be treated promptly, and efforts should be made to maintain adequate glucose levels and oxygenation because apnea frequently accompanies seizure activity. The two signs most predictive of long-term sequelae are duration of seizure activity and altered states of consciousness.

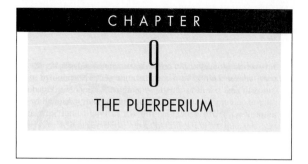

The puerperium, arbitrarily designated as *the 6 weeks following childbirth,* is the period of adjustment after pregnancy, when lactation usually occurs and the mother's body returns to the nonpregnant state.

PHYSIOLOGIC EVENTS OF THE PUERPERIUM

CARDIOVASCULAR AND BLOOD

Cardiac output peaks immediately after delivery, at which time it is 80% above the prelabor value in most normal patients. This is accompanied by elevated *venous pressure and increased stroke volume.* Rapid changes toward normal nonpregnant values occur thereafter, particularly during the first week, with a gradual decline during the next 3–4 weeks to prepregnancy values.

The HCT *rises ~5% above the predelivery value* in patients having an uncomplicated vaginal delivery. This occurs, despite the average blood loss of ~500 mL, as a result of renal elimination of both intravascular and extravascular fluids that have accumulated during pregnancy. Indeed, *blood volume decreases by ~20% by the 5th postpartum day.* Following cesarean delivery, there is an ~5% drop in hematocrit by the 5th day postpartum as a result of the average blood loss of 1000 mL. The average puerperal fluid loss is ~4 kg (9 pounds). Gradual weight loss follows.

Most women with normal blood values during pregnancy and an average blood loss at delivery show *a relative polycythemia* during the 2nd week postpartum. Iron supplementation is not necessary for normal nonlactating postpartum women if the HCT or hemoglobin concentration 5 days after delivery is about the same as the normal predelivery value.

The normal slightly *hypercoagulable state found during pregnancy is further enhanced during the puerperium,* thus predisposing to *thrombosis.* By 3–5 days after delivery, platelet adhesiveness will have increased considerably, with lesser increases in platelet count and factor V and VIII values. Despite fibrinolytic activity also increasing, *thromboembolism is 3–5 times higher in the puerperium than during pregnancy.* The hypercoagulable state peaks at 6–14 days after delivery, and returns to normal by the 4th postpartum week.

The increased concentrations of cholesterol and triglycerides which characterize the second and third trimesters of pregnancy gradually decline to their prepregnancy levels during the puerperium. *Lactation is associated with a more rapid decline of both cholesterol and triglycerides.*

LUNGS, RENAL, REPRODUCTIVE TRACT, AND SKELETON

Postpartum lung volume and capacity changes are at nonpregnant levels by 6 weeks. The hypotonic and slightly elongated and *dilated ureters and renal pelvis revert to normal* by the third month. Nearly 50% of patients have mild proteinuria during the first week, but renal function returns to prepregnant levels during the early puerperium.

The uterus involutes most rapidly after delivery and is complete by the 6th week postpartum. This is chiefly a result of contraction and decrease in the size of individual myometrial cells (Fig. 9-1). Following a term gestation, however, the uterus remains slightly larger than before pregnancy because of some added connective tissue and a persistent slightly augmented vasculature. Endometrial regeneration is complete by the 3rd week postpartum, except for the placental site, which requires 5–6 weeks. Microscopic evidence of placental implantation (primarily fibrous tissue) remains permanently.

Lochia rubra, the bloody discharge that follows delivery, normally becomes more serous and lighter in color (lochia serosa) after 2–3 days. In another week, the lochia becomes mucoid and yellowish due to the inclusion of leukocytes and disintegrating decidual elements. Discharge usually ceases 22–34 d after delivery; however, ~10% of women will have lochia lasting >40 d.

The *cervix gradually closes* during the puerperium. The external os is converted to a transverse slit ~2 weeks after delivery. The distended vagina gradually *returns to its prepartum state by the third week after vaginal delivery.* The rugae remain flattened and the torn hymen heals irregularly.

The *voluntary muscles of the pelvic floor gradually regain their tone,* although trauma during vaginal delivery may weaken the musculature

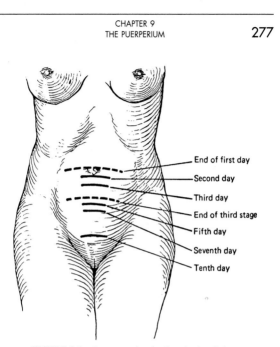

FIGURE 9-1. Postpartum levels of uterine involution.

and predispose to genital hernias. Additionally, the first vaginal delivery poses the greatest risk of mechanical anal sphincter injury, and women with transient fecal incontinence or occult anal-sphincter injury after their first vagina delivery are at increased risk of fecal incontinence after a second vaginal delivery. Overdistention of the abdominal wall during pregnancy can cause rectus diastasis (separation).

Lactation is associated with temporary decreases in bone mineral. Although residual effects persist after cessation of lactation, these seem more related to the losses of pregnancy and less related to the duration of lactation.

RETURN OF OVULATION AND MENSTRUATION

Hormone changes immediately after delivery are abrupt. *Estrogen, progesterone, and hCG levels fall to the nonpregnant range within 1 week.* The *prolactin level increases* considerably during the first week, especially in patients who are nursing, and remains high during lactation. A state of relative estrogen deficiency occurs during the puerperium, especially in women who nurse their babies. This may lead to a menopausal appearing vagina and dyspareunia. Vaginal cytologic studies will reveal near-atrophic smears.

Nursing mothers rarely menstruate in <6 weeks postpartum. However, ~50% will ovulate on or before that time. After abortion, ≤15th week, the average time required for return of ovulation is 2–3 weeks, and menstruation should occur within 4–5 weeks. If pregnancy was >15 weeks duration, ovulation should occur within 4–6 weeks, and menses should resume within 6–7 weeks. The time of the *first ovulatory cycle after delivery is variable.* In nonlactating women, ovulation may occur as early as the 25th–35th day postpartum. *Menstruation resumes in about 40% of nonlactating women by the 6th week.* By 12 weeks after delivery, 70%–80% of nonlactating women will have begun to menstruate again.

CARE DURING THE FIRST WEEK OF THE PUERPERIUM

LENGTH OF HOSPITALIZATION AND VITAL SIGNS

Most patients can return home safely 1–2 days after vaginal delivery. To effectively screen for puerperal problems (especially sepsis), however, the *temperature, pulse, and respiration rate should be ascertained every 4 h for 2–3 days.* Give $Rh_o(D)$ immune globulin (300 μg IM within 72 h of delivery) to unsensitized Rh-negative women who deliver Rh-positive offspring.

EXERCISE AND EARLY AMBULATION

Early ambulation is encouraged. It provides a sense of well-being, hastens involution of the uterus, and may reduce the incidence of thrombosis. Nonetheless, the patient should avoid lifting, straining, or pushing. Rest periods are essential.

DIET

Regular diet may be resumed as soon as the patient desires and is free from the effects of analgesics, amnesics, or anesthetics. High-protein foods, fruits, and vegetables are recommended. A high fluid intake is advised, especially for nursing mothers. Even lactating women probably require no more than 2600–2800 kcal/day, and caloric excess has the usual consequences.

BLADDER CARE

Avoid overdistention of the bladder, which is normally hypotonic immediately after delivery. *Postpartum polyuria* for several days after delivery causes the bladder to fill in a relatively short time, and *frequent voiding is necessary.* The gravida may be unaware of the distending bladder, and thus timed voiding (every 1–2 h) may be necessary. If overdistention occurs, decompression by catheter can be required. If catheterization yields >1000 mL or is required ≥3 times/day during the first several days after delivery, a retention catheter for 12–24 h may assist in regaining bladder tone.

BOWEL FUNCTION

Normally, bowel function continues without serious problems. A mild ileus may follow anesthetics or some analgesics. This can generally be reversed by a mild laxative (e.g., milk of magnesia). A rectal suppository, such as bisacodyl (Dulcolax), or a small tap-water enema may be required.

ANALGESICS AND SEDATIVES

Acetaminophen (325–550 mg every 4 h) is usually sufficient for pain, but in more severe cases, codeine 30–60 mg every 4 h may be added. If the latter is insufficient for pain relief, seek a more serious problem (e.g., hematoma) as the cause of the pain.

Hospital procedures, noise, and strange surroundings are not conducive to sleep. *Mild sedatives at bedtime may be necessary* to ensure a good night's rest. The medication selected should allow the gravida to awaken easily and be alert to care for the baby without a later hangover effect.

CARE OF EPISIOTOMY AND LACERATIONS

Gently cleanse the perineum with soap or detergent and water at least once or twice each day and after defecation. Keep the pudendum clean and dry. However, sitz baths bid or tid may be very beneficial, especially if hemorrhoidal discomfort is a problem. Healing should occur rapidly. Dry heat applied to the perineum with an infrared lamp for 20–30 min tid often relieves discomfort and promotes healing. Greasy ointments or salves to the perineum cause skin maceration and can foster infection.

Inspect the episiotomy or repaired lacerations daily. Perform vaginal or rectal examination if a hematoma or infection seems likely. Drain the sutured area if suppuration develops.

BATHS

As soon as the patient is able, she may take a shower, sitz bath, or tub bath. Water does not ascend into the vagina with the patient sitting in a bathtub.

CARE DURING CONVALESCENCE

Hygiene, diet, and other care are essentially the same as noted. Discuss with the gravida the normally decreasing amounts of *sanguineous vaginal discharge,* which lasts about 3 weeks. Mention the possibility of a "small period" during the 4–5 weeks after delivery. This should allay later concerns. The seriousness of *infection* should be stressed and its signs (local heat, pain, redness, fever) reiterated. Instruct the patient as to what to do should any of these signs develop. A *brassiere,* worn constantly, especially if she is nursing, may assist with breast discomfort. A girdle is rarely necessary. Vaginal douches should be used only on specific indication. *Coitus should not be resumed until an episiotomy or lacerations have healed* (generally 4 weeks). The postpartum dialogue is an opportunity for the patient to voice her *desire for future reproduction* and for the physician to assist (if necessary) with contraception.

Activity and responsibility should increase gradually. During the first 3–4 weeks postpartum, a limited regimen is recommended (light duty), but *full activity should be anticipated by about 6 weeks postpartum.*

Active exercise involving the pubococcygeus muscles *(Kegel exercises)* may enhance resolution of pelvic floor relaxation and urinary stress incontinence even if significant anatomic defects (e.g., cystocele) are present. Repeated contraction of the pubococcygeus muscle (as with attempts to stop voiding or a bowel movement in progress) for 5–10 min 3–4 times daily may restore muscle tone and function.

POSTPARTUM EXAMINATIONS

FIRST POSTPARTUM EXAMINATION

Examine the patient about *4–6 weeks after delivery.* By this time, *healing of the perineum should be complete, the lochia should have ceased, the cervix should be closed, and the uterus should have nearly returned to its prepartum size.* Hopefully, the examination will occur before intercourse so that any minor abnormalities can be corrected and, again, the type of contraception can be discussed. General inquiry and examination should estimate the time for return to full activity and employment. Specifically the first postpartum examination should include the following.

Weight. Ideally, the patient will have returned to her *approximate prepregnancy weight.* The abdominal muscle tone will be improving, but this is largely exercise dependent.

Breasts. *Note abnormalities* of the nipples, lactation, the adequacy of support, and the presence of redness, tenderness, or masses.

Uterine Bleeding. *Heavy or persistent uterine bleeding* requires definitive investigation and treatment. A course of an oxytocic (e.g., ergonovine) may be beneficial. However, dilatation and curettage may be required.

Vaginal Discharge. *Leukorrhea* ceases in about two thirds of the patients by 4–5 weeks. Infections require diagnosis and specific treatment.

Pelvic. *Do a complete pelvic examination:* speculum, bimanual, and rectovaginal evaluation. The postpartum examination should afford the best opportunity for bimanual examination of the intraabdominal organs because some abdominal relaxation will have persisted. Examine the vagina, rectovaginal septum, sphincter ani, and perineum. Check episiotomy and/or repaired lacerations. Perineovaginal support should be ascertained.

Uterine subinvolution can be the result of infection, retroposition, or retained products of conception. Treatment must be directed toward correction of the specific problem. If uterine prolapse (descensus) is present, its degree should be noted and related to symptoms. If prolapse is marked and persists for 4 months, consider surgical correction.

Repeat specific **laboratory tests** that were abnormal during pregnancy. *Treat problems identified (e.g., anemia).*

Contraception. *Discuss family planning.* Prescribe the contraceptive method most suitable and acceptable to the couple.

FURTHER EXAMINATIONS

If further therapy is necessary other visits should be scheduled. A gynecologic examination and cervical cytologic study should be performed ~6 months after delivery. At that time, menstrual or other problems should be evaluated.

LACTATION

Lactation begins about 48–72 h after delivery, with sudden engorgement of the breasts. However, the infant can begin nursing almost immediately after birth because colostrum will be available.

PHYSIOLOGY AND PATHOPHYSIOLOGY OF LACTATION

Estrogen and progesterone, present in large amounts during pregnancy, *stimulate the ductal and alveolar systems of the breast,* respectively. This causes proliferation and differentiation of the mammary glands and the production of clear, thin, serumlike colostrum as early as the third month of pregnancy. Colostrum continues to be secreted to term. Nonetheless, the high level of estrogen during pregnancy inhibits the binding of prolactin (hPL) in breast tissue, so milk is not produced. *After delivery, estrogen, progesterone, and hCS levels fall sharply, and hPL stimulates the mammary alveoli to produce milk.* Interestingly, the hPL level needed to maintain lactation is lower than that achieved during pregnancy. Optimal levels of insulin and thyroid and adrenal hormones play a secondary roles in lactation.

Suckling is not required for the initiation of lactation; however, nursing is necessary for continued milk production (suckling stimulates periodic hPL secretion). Suckling also stimulates release of oxytocin from the posterior pituitary via a breast-to-pituitary neural reflex. In addition to its effect on uterine smooth muscle, oxytocin contracts the periacinar muscle fibers of the breast, causing ejection of milk into the major collecting sinuses that converge on the nipple. This is called the *milk ejection or milk letdown reflex.* Tension and fatigue inhibit the letdown reflex, but the infant's cry and nursing stimulate it.

The infant does not nurse by developing intermittent negative pressure but by a rhythmic grasping of the areola. Thus, milk is worked into the mouth. Very little force is required in nursing because the breast reservoirs can be emptied and refilled independent of suction. Nursing mothers develop a sensation of drawing and tightening—a draught or concentration—within the breast at the beginning of suckling after the initial breast engorgement disappears. Mothers are thus conscious of the milk ejection reflex, which may even cause milk to spurt or run out. The milk letdown phenomenon is inhibited by drugs, pain, breast engorgement, or adverse psychic conditioning, such as embarrassment.

For several days after initial milk production (breast filling), the milk ejection reflex may be deficient. Then, the breasts become so distended that the nipples appear retracted, the areolas are unyielding to the nursling's efforts, and the infant obtains little or no milk. Manual expression of milk or the administration of oxytocin (or both) will usually start the flow and relieve the engorgement, whereupon nursing may be more successful.

The mother should nurse her infant at both breasts at each feeding because *overfilling of the breasts is the main cause of decreased milk production.* Nursing at only one breast at a feeding leaves the other breast full, and the distention of the full breast inhibits the letdown reflex. This causes a reduction in milk output in both breasts. Thus, alternating breasts from one feeding to the next may increase engorgement distress and reduce milk output. It is also advisable to move the infant from one breast to the other every 5–10 min to minimize nipple maceration.

ADVANTAGES AND DISADVANTAGES OF BREASTFEEDING

FOR THE MOTHER

Breastfeeding is convenient, costs nothing, is emotionally satisfying for most women, and speeds uterine involution. Suckling promotes favorable maternal–infant interaction. Moreover, mothers who breastfeed may derive some protection against breast cancer.

The disadvantages are that regular nursing may restrict activities and nipple tenderness or mastitis can develop.

FOR THE INFANT

Breast milk is digestible, readily available, at the proper temperature, and free from bacterial contamination. The composition is ideal. As a result, breastfed infants have fewer digestive or allergy problems. The child receives passive antibodies, infant–maternal bonding is enhanced, and the child is less likely to become obese (compared to formula-fed babies). There are no known disadvantages to the breastfeeding of an infant if the mother is healthy and willing and the supply of milk is adequate.

CONTRAINDICATIONS TO BREASTFEEDING

Absolute contraindications to breastfeeding are *epidemic mastitis, HIV infection, breast cancer, active pulmonary tuberculosis, and maternal intake of antithyroid medications, radioactive iodine, cancer chemotherapeutic agents, or certain other toxic drugs.* Indeed, when prescribing medications for the nursing mother, it is essential to *consider their potential impact on the infant.* Breastfeeding may be impossible for weak, ill, or very premature infants, or those with cleft palate, choanal atresia, or phenylketonuria (PKU). However, expressed breast milk may be saved and given at a later date, except in the case of PKU.

DRUGS IN BREAST MILK

Innumerable drugs can be detected in a parturient's blood and milk. Numerous drugs harmful to the nursing infant pass into breast milk, including chloramphenicol, metronidazole, nitrofurantoin, sulfonamides, and antithyroid drugs. Again, prior to administering or prescribing mediations to a nursing mother, the provider must consider their potential impact on the infant.

TEACHING BREASTFEEDING

Success or failure of breastfeeding is related to the amount of factual information and emotional support available to the mother. Although this may be useful at the time of delivery, it may be much more effective if included as part of the prenatal educational program. Organizations, such as the La Leche League, the Nursing Mothers of Australia, and the Plunkett Society in New Zealand, have been very effective in promoting breastfeeding. Demonstrations of infant care and formula preparation are also generally a part of nursing service programs. Several important points bear emphasis.

- The patient should wash the nipples daily with unscented mild soap and water, using a washcloth (beginning in the last trimester). After drying, she may apply hydrated lanolin. Perfumed soaps and skin or hand creams should not be used because they may contain irritants. The application of alcohol is inadvisable because it dries and hardens the skin.
- Inverted or short nipples should be drawn gently outward each day to increase their length temporarily.
- The nipples should be protected with plastic film or nipple shields.
- A well-fitted brassiere (worn even at night) supports the breasts, improves circulation, and avoids trauma.
- Expressing colostrum gently several times each day during the last 4–6 weeks of pregnancy stimulates the flow of the fluid.
- Beginning on the first postpartum day, if not contraindicated, the normal newborn should nurse at each breast on demand or approximately every 3–4 h for 3 min total nursing time per breast per feeding. Increase the time by 1 min each day, not exceeding 7 min per breast per feeding. The average infant obtains 60%–90% of the milk in 4 min of nursing. Suckling for longer than 7 min often causes maceration and cracking of the nipples (with subsequent risk of mastitis).
- A glass of cool water 5 min before nursing or another method of psychological preparation (especially fluids) strengthens the reflex of milk ejection. Ample fluids are especially important, but beer, wine, and spirits will not increase milk production more than water.
- Avoid engorgement and trapping of milk by gentle expression of excess milk before nursing or by use of oxytocin, 10 units in 0.25 mL of normal saline as a nasal spray, just before infant feeding.

MILK PRODUCTION

Normally, *the mother's yield of breast milk is directly proportionate to the infant's demand,* assuming that free secretion of milk has been established and feedings are given every 3–4 h. With nursing, the average milk production on the 2nd postpartum day is about 120 mL, on the 3rd postpartum day at least 180 mL, and by the 4th day about 240 mL. A rule of thumb for calculation of milk production for a given day during the first week after delivery is to *multiply the number of the postpartum day by 60.* This gives the approximate milliliters of milk/24 h. Sustained milk production

should be achieved by most mothers after 10–14 days. A yield of
120–180 mL of milk per feeding is common by the end of the 2nd
week.

*Oral contraceptives and estrogens adversely affect the amount
of milk produced,* but few other commonly used drugs have this
capability.

NIPPLE FISSURES

Fissured nipples have painful cracks that can lead to mastitis. Apply dry heat and nonmedicated, nonperfumed hydrous lanolin for
benefit. Prefeeding manual expression of milk will reduce breast
engorgement and make nursing easier. A nipple shield can also be
used. Finally, the nursing infant should alternate from breast to
breast after no more than 5 min to promote healing.

SUPPRESSION OF LACTATION

If the patient does not choose to nurse her infant, *estrogen or androgen administration (or a combination of both) decreases hPL,
or mechanical inhibition of lactation (breast binding) may be effective.* All are most *effective only if started immediately after delivery,* and all have a *high failure rate.* Moreover, concerns about
the undesirable side effects of estrogen particularly (e.g., thromboembolism) have led to decreasing use of sex steroids.

A dopamine-agonist, bromocriptine (Parlodel) 2.5 mg orally for
14 days, inhibits prolactin secretion and will suppress lactation. Prolonged treatment with this drug may be necessary, however, and
side effects are sufficiently worrisome as to make this therapy currently uncommon.

MECHANICAL SUPPRESSION

The patient should not nurse and should not express milk or pump
her breasts. A tight compression uplift binder for 72 h and a snug
brassiere thereafter are necessary. Ice packs and analgesics (e.g.,
acetaminophen or aspirin and codeine) may be used if necessary
Fluid restriction and laxatives are not helpful in suppression of
lactation.

At first, the breast will become distended, firm, and tender. After 48–72 h, lactation usually ceases and pain subsides. Involution
will be complete in about 1 month.

PUERPERAL PATHOLOGY

Puerperal pathology is so highly weighted to infectious disease that even the definition of postpartum morbidity remains a definition implying infection (i.e., a temperature of $>101.8°F$ on two consecutive occasions 6 h apart more than 24 h after delivery). The *three major problems are urinary tract infection, puerperal mastitis, and puerperal sepsis.* Nevertheless, other noninfectious problems can complicate the puerperium.

PUERPERAL MASTITIS

Puerperal mastitis is breast infection during the 6 weeks following childbirth. Generally, it is unilateral. The usual cause is *Staphylococcus aureus.* About 0.5%–1.0% of parturients are affected, and most of these are primiparas. There are two types of puerperal mastitis.

- The *sporadic form is an acute cellulitis* involving interlobular connective and adipose tissues. A nipple fissure is the usual avenue of infection. Localized pain, tenderness, segmental erythema, and fever result. The milk is not infected.
- *Epidemic mastitis is a fulminating infection* of the breast glandular system, with symptoms and signs similar to but more acute than those of sporadic mastitis. A nursery *Staphylococcus* carrier is most often incriminated, where an infant acquires the infection, which is then spread into its mother's ductal system after the regurgitation of a small amount of infected milk.

Diagnostically, it is crucial to culture the milk and to culture the neonate. Perform serial CBCs, blood cultures, and other laboratory tests as indicated.

Treat both types of acute mastitis with antibiotics capable of destruction of penicillinase-resistant pathogens (e.g., oxacillin, cephalothin, or equivalent). In the sporadic form, continued suckling is advisable because nursing prevents engorgement and decreases the likelihood of abscess formation. Often, a nipple shield will decrease maternal discomfort. In the epidemic form, the infant harbors the pathogenic organism. Hence, antibiotic therapy, prompt weaning, suppression of lactation, cold packs, and a snug breast binder are recommended.

Usually, if proper antibiotic therapy is initiated before the onset of suppuration, the signs and symptoms of infection should begin to resolve within 24 h. Puerperal mastitis that has not subsided in 2–3 days has most likely progressed to an abscess. Then, surgical drainage of all infected loculations is necessary to resolve the abscess.

Prevention is obviously more effective in the sporadic type and involves good hygiene (i.e., cleansing the nipples with plain soap and water, avoiding topical alcohol, and prevention of nipple fissures). Helpful methods to prevent the latter are (1) to place a finger in the corner of the infant's mouth to break its sucking force at the end of feeding and (2) to not allow lengthy feeding at one breast or maceration may occur.

Therapy for the infant is not usually necessary, even in the epidemic form.

PUERPERAL SEPSIS

Any infection of the genital tract occurring as a complication of abortion, labor, or delivery is termed puerperal sepsis (see also Septic Shock, p. 342). Streptococci, staphylococci, clostridia, coliform bacteria, or Bacteroides are the pathogens most often identified. Cellulitis resulting from vaginal or cervical lacerations may be the initial site of infection, as may the endometrium, particularly in the zone of placental attachment (the equivalent of a large surface wound). Debility (anemia, undernutrition), serious systemic disorders, prolonged rupture of the membranes, protracted labor, and traumatic delivery predispose to puerperal infection.

The *incidence of puerperal sepsis in U.S. hospitals is <3%* in low-risk, vaginally delivered patients. The incidence rises (nearly exponentially) with increasing obstetric risk and operative delivery. Puerperal sepsis is exceeded only by hemorrhage and preeclampsia-eclampsia as a major cause of maternal death in this country.

CLINICAL FINDINGS

Many genital tract infections are mild and cause few or slight symptoms. Others are fulminating and may be fatal within a short time.

Symptoms and Signs
Malaise, headache, anorexia, and remittent slight elevations in temperature and a rise in pulse rate generally begin 3–4 days after delivery. Vague discomfort in the perineum or lower abdomen and nausea and vomiting may follow. Often, the lochia becomes foul or

profuse. *High fever (childbed fever), rapid pulse, ileus, localization of pain, and tenderness in the pelvis may be observed during the next 1–2 days. Bacteremic shock may develop.*

Physical Examination

At the first suspicion of puerperal infection, conduct a careful aseptic pelvic examination. The repair of any laceration or episiotomy must be *scrutinized for signs of sepsis.* A sterile ring forceps should be used to open the cervix to *guarantee free flow of lochia.* Perform a careful bimanual examination (including rectovaginal) to identify potential sites of infection. *Culture the cervical canal,* and obtain a *urine culture* for predominant organisms and their sensitivity to major antibiotics. If improvement does not follow after 48–72 h of intensive multiple antibiotic therapy, *careful reexamination for an abscess* should be conducted.

Laboratory Findings

Polymorphonuclear leukocytosis and an increased sedimentation rate indicate infection. Identification of pathogens from cervical and uterine lochia by culture and sensitivity tests will require 24–48 h, but stained smears should be obtained immediately for a preliminary diagnosis.

Ultrasonography and X-Ray Findings

X-ray studies are not helpful except to exclude gastrointestinal, urinary, or pulmonary problems. Ultrasonography may be useful for the localization of an abscess or to diagnose or rule out retained products of conception or pelvic thrombophlebitis.

COMPLICATIONS AND SEQUELAE

Genital tract infections commonly progress from endometritis to endomyometritis to pelvic cellulitis and peritonitis or septic pelvic thrombophlebitis. Abscess formation, septicemia, pulmonary embolism, septic shock, and death may result.

DIFFERENTIAL DIAGNOSIS

Febrile complications of the puerperium unrelated to genital tract infection include *mastitis, urinary and respiratory infection, and enteritis,* in that order of frequency.

PREVENTION

Avoidance of puerperal sepsis requires strict aseptic technique during pelvic examination and delivery. Minimize obstetric trauma because injured tissues are susceptible to infection.

TREATMENT

Emergency Measures
Treat septic shock (see p. 350).

General Measures
- Place the patient in the semi-Fowler position.
- Order a clear liquid diet for at least several days if ileus is not present.
- Administer IV fluids to maintain proper electrolyte and fluid balance. Dilute oxytocin in the infusion should maintain a contracted uterus.
- Administer analgesics, sedative-hypnotic drugs, or laxatives as required.

Specific Measures
- Initial high dose antibiotic therapy with both aerobic and anaerobic coverage is key to successful therapy. Knowledge of the usual organisms causing such infections in the physician's community may be useful in altering the otherwise emperic therapy. When the results of culture and sensitivity studies are reported, continue therapy with the antibiotics of choice in large and repeated doses.
- For the serious infection, it is often necessary to admit the patient to an intensive care unit and to perform hemodynamic monitoring.
- For treatment of disseminated intravascular coagulation, see p. 348.

Surgical Measures
- Surgical drainage of abscesses usually is necessary, and the pelvic approach is preferred.
- Percutaneous insertion of an inferior vena caval umbrella may be necessary in cases of septic pulmonary thromboembolism.
- Hysterectomy is indicated for serious uterine infections unresponsive to antibiotics (e.g., a postabortal uterine abscess or an infected hydatidiform mole). In such cases, it may be possible to spare the ovaries using continued high-dose antibiotics. However, the outcome may still be uncertain.

- Ligation of the ovarian veins may be life saving in repeated septic pulmonary embolization from septic pelvic thrombophlebitis.

PROGNOSIS

The maternal mortality due to puerperal sepsis in the United States is about 0.2%, but it is vastly greater in some developing countries. Puerperal infections have the potential to cause abscesses in the remaining pelvic organs (e.g., ovaries), impair subsequent fertility, and require subsequent surgery.

PUERPERAL INVERSION OF UTERUS

An inverted uterus is one partially or completely turned inside-out. Inversion of the uterus can be partial (herniation of the fundus into the uterine cavity) or complete (extrusion of the corpus through the cervix into or beyond the vagina). Either type can be spontaneous or induced and acute or chronic. Acute spontaneous puerperal inversion is due to straining by the patient soon after delivery. *Acute induced puerperal inversion* may be due to:

- Traction of the cord before placental separation
- Severe kneading of the fundus to induce placental separation or expulsion
- Improperly executed manual separation or extraction of an adherent placenta

Chronic induced puerperal inversion is due to the same causes as the acute variety that are unrecognized after delivery. The incidence of uterine inversion is about *1:15,000 deliveries* (lowest where obstetric care is of the highest quality).

CLINICAL FINDINGS

- Acute complete inversion causes *sudden agonizing pain and an explosive sensation of fullness* extending downward into the vagina. *Hemorrhage and profound shock* occur in >50% of patients. If inversion is partial, pain and bleeding will be less severe.
- In complete inversion, *a large bleeding mass* will be obvious outside the introitus, often with the placenta still attached.
- In partial inversion, bimanual examination will reveal a *cup-shaped depression at the fundus* with a mass palpable above or bulging through the cervix.

- Chronic partial uterine inversion is characterized by *persistent, otherwise unexplained bleeding and discomfort.* Bimanual examination or an instrument passed through the partially closed cervix may reveal the abnormality.

DIFFERENTIAL DIAGNOSIS

A *large submucous leiomyoma* at the external cervical os can cause the same signs as inversion, but the fundus will be large and rounded without a craterlike depression.

COMPLICATIONS

Shock, hemorrhage, or death may ensue in acute complete inversion, especially when mismanaged. Anemia, infection, or embolization may develop in partial or chronic cases.

PREVENTION

Avoid traction on the cord until definite separation of the placenta has occurred. Do not knead the fundus. Supervise the patient until the uterus is rounded and firmly contracted.

TREATMENT

- *Control shock* with IV fluids, plasma, whole blood, and oxytocin before attempting definitive treatment. *Caution: do not give ergotrate, or cervical contraction may block fundal replacement.*
- *Attempt to replace the uterus by abdominovaginal means. If the placenta is still attached, leave it attached* (this limits additional bleeding). Deep brief general anesthesia may be required. Cervical constriction can be relaxed by whiffs of amyl nitrite vapor or epinephrine 0.3–0.6 mL of a 1:1000 solution IM. Countertraction on the cervix while directing the inverted portion of the uterus upward facilitates replacement.

  Another method of correcting acute or subacute puerperal uterine inversion is as follows. Under general anesthesia, lift the uterus out of the pelvis by grasping the inverted fundus with the vaginal gloved hand, then apply steady pressure toward the umbilicus. Retain the fist within the uterus until the corpus is well contracted (prostaglandins or ergot may be desirable) to prevent recurrence of inversion. Packs are not effective and maintain distention.

- *If correction cannot be accomplished quickly by manipulation, surgical replacement may be mandatory.* This must be accomplished by abdominal laparotomy. Visualization generally reveals that the ovaries are close together in the midline, and the uterus is not visible. The ovarian ligaments, tubes, and round ligaments disappear into a tightly closed hole. A linear incision in the posterior wall of the cervix at the level of the uterocervical junction (usually between the uterosacral ligaments) relaxes the stricture, and with gentle manipulation from above and below, the uterine fundus is replaced. The incision can then be repaired in at least two layers with an absorbable synthetic suture. Oxytocics are administered after the fundus is delivered.

PROGNOSIS

Manual replacement is effective in >85% of cases. Prophylactic administration of antibiotics may be warranted because there is a high rate of infection after uterine inversion. *Recurrence* of inversion or in a subsequent pregnancy may occur.

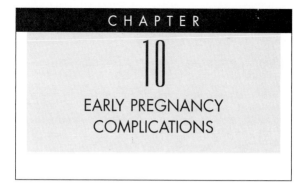

CHAPTER 10

EARLY PREGNANCY COMPLICATIONS

SPONTANEOUS ABORTION

Spontaneous abortion (miscarriage) is the termination of pregnancy before completion of the 20th gestational week. The term applies to both live and stillborn fetuses weighing ≤500 g. However, a fetus need not be identified if other products of conception are present (e.g., placenta or membranes). Familiarity with the local legal definition is mandatory because there is considerable state to state variation.

Loss of pregnancy is very common. Recent estimates are that only 62.5% of pregnancies result in live births, 21.9% end in legal abortions, 13.8% have spontaneous abortions, 1.3% are ectopic gestations, and 0.5% end in fetal deaths. Other estimates place spontaneous abortion at 15%–40%. *The earlier in gestation, the more likely is spontaneous abortion.* About 75% occur before 16 weeks, and approximately 60% occur before 12 weeks. A major difficulty in detailing exact numbers is the variability of methods for pregnancy diagnosis. For example, a serum beta-subunit hCG determination will detect very early pregnancies (and thus more losses) than the available standard urine pregnancy tests. At least 80% of all pregnancies terminate spontaneously before the woman or physician is aware of the pregnancy (*subclinical or undiagnosed spontaneous abortion*). Table 10-1 estimates the losses with in vitro fertilization (which would be included in the subclinical category).

Mortality is rare (0.7 per 100,000) with spontaneous abortion, but risk factors include: women age >35 years, races other than white, and abortion in the second trimester. Direct causes of deaths include: infection (~59%), hemorrhage (18%), embolism (13%), complications from anesthesia (5%), and other (5%). Disseminated intravascular coagulation complicates many of the cases proceeding to death.

295

TABLE 10-1
IN VITRO FERTILIZATION LOSSES

- 16% of fertilized ova do not divide
- 15% of fertilized ova are lost before implantation (first gestational week)
- 27% are lost during implantation (second gestational week)
- 10.5% are lost following the first missed menses
- Total loss is 68.5%

ABORTION DEFINITIONS

Many different variables apply to abortion, and a number of definitions are required. It is assumed that all definitions refer to spontaneous abortion, if not otherwise specified.

Early abortion occurs <12th gestational week.

Late abortion occurs between 12 and 20 weeks gestation.

Threatened abortion refers to intrauterine bleeding <20th week of completed gestation, with or without uterine contraction, without cervical dilatation, and without expulsion of the products of conception (POC). Moreover, ultrasound must reveal the fetus to show signs of life (e.g., heartbeat or motion). In threatened abortion, the previable gestation is in jeopardy, but the pregnancy continues.

Inevitable abortion is intrauterine bleeding before the 20th completed gestational week, with continued cervical dilatation but without expulsion of the POC. In inevitable abortion, momentary evacuation of part or all of the conceptus is likely. Abortion is considered inevitable with two or more of the following:

- Moderate effacement of the cervix
- Cervical dilatation >3 cm
- Rupture of the membranes
- Bleeding for >7 days
- Persistence of cramps despite narcotic analgesics
- Signs of termination of pregnancy (e.g., absent mastalgia)

Incomplete abortion is the expulsion of some but not all of the POC <20th completed gestational week.

Complete abortion is expulsion of all the POC <20th completed gestational week. When the entire conceptus has been expelled, pain ceases, but slight spotting persists for a few days.

Missed abortion is death of the embryo or fetus <20th completed gestational week, but the POC are retained in utero for ≥8 weeks. Symptoms of pregnancy disappear, and there may be a brownish vaginal discharge but no free bleeding. Pain and tenderness are absent, the cervix is semifirm and closed or only slightly patulous, the uterus becomes smaller and irregularly softened, and the adnexa are normal. Fetal death at 18–26 weeks followed by missed labor and retention for >6 weeks may be associated with maternal fibrinogen depletion (*dead fetus syndrome*). Consider administration of cryoprecipitate to prevent hemorrhage from hypofibrinogenemia before evacuation of the uterus (Fig. 10-1).

FIGURE 10-1. Top. Complete abortion. At right, product of complete abortion. Bottom. Incomplete abortion. At right, product of incomplete abortion.

Infected abortion is that associated with infection of the internal genitalia.

Septic abortion is infected abortion with dissemination of bacteria via the maternal circulation.

Habitual abortion is the spontaneous, consecutive loss of 3 or more nonviable pregnancies.

Induced abortion is the purposeful interruption of pregnancy by medical or surgical techniques.

ETIOLOGY OF SPONTANEOUS ABORTION

EARLY ABORTION

Abnormal products of conception are the overwhelming cause of spontaneous abortion. At least 10% of human conceptuses have chromosomal abnormalities, and most of these are aborted. Indeed, 50%–64% of first trimester spontaneous abortions have an abnormal karyotype (vs. ~7% in elective induced abortion). The most common karyotypic abnormalities are autosomal trisomy (52%–62%), triploidy (16%), monosomies (11%–15%), and tetraploidy (4%). The single most common karyotypic anomaly is trisomy 16 (19%).

The aneuploidies most commonly associated with spontaneous abortion occur in the following chromosomes: XY, 13, 14, 15, 16, 18, 21, and 22. *Major interruptions of embryogenesis* (e.g., failure of the fetus to develop or neural tube defects) account for some of the rest. These are largely *multifactorial* in etiology (an admixture of genetic and environmental). Additional factors include *infections* (e.g., cytomegalovirus), *autoimmune disorders* (e.g., lupus), *endocrine abnormalities* (e.g., failure of the corpus luteum), and *genital tract abnormalities* (e.g., subseptate uterus). The cause of a significant number of early abortions remains unknown.

LATE ABORTION

Worldwide, the major causes of abortion during the second trimester are infections (e.g., syphilis, malaria), *circumvallate placenta, maternal metabolic imbalances* (e.g., diabetes mellitus, severe hypothyroidism), *maternal physiologic impairment* (e.g., cardiac disorders, hypertension), *maternal dietary insufficiency* (e.g., bulimia, avitaminosis B or C), *isoimmunizations, exposure to fetotoxic factors* (e.g., lead poisoning, substance abuse), *trauma* (e.g., direct or indirect abdominal injury), *and uterine or cervical defects* (e.g., cervical incompetency). A wide variety of other etiologies may induce abortion, including severe electric shock, although there is no convincing evidence that abortion may be induced by psychic stimuli (e.g., severe fright, grief, anger, or anxiety).

DIAGNOSIS OF ABORTION

CLINICAL

Obtain a complete history and perform a general physical (including pelvic) examination on every patient to determine if special laboratory or other studies are necessary to detect diseases or deficiency states.

Classically, the *symptoms of abortion are uterine cramping (with or without suprapubic pain) and vaginal bleeding in the presence of previable pregnancy.* The integration of the physical examination with these symptoms allows a tentative diagnosis.

LABORATORY STUDIES

In many cases, a serum pregnancy test is useful. Minimal laboratory studies should include culture and sensitivity of cervical mucus or blood (to identify pathogens in infection) and a complete blood count. In some cases, determination of progesterone levels may be useful to detect corpus luteum failure. When hemorrhage is present, blood typing and crossmatching as well as a coagulation panel are necessary.

Genetic analysis of aborted material may determine chromosomal abnormality as the etiology. This often provides invaluable information for counseling.

DIAGNOSIS OF FETAL DEATH

The immunoassay (IA) and radioimmunoassay (RIA) pregnancy tests identify hormones produced by the trophoblast. A steep rise of hCG is the hallmark of normal pregnancies in the peri-implantation interval. *Abnormal pregnancies may have a deficiency in hCG levels* as well as the rate of increase. Finally, in some abnormal pregnancies, hCG has a lower biologic activity.

However, even with death of the embryo or early fetus, groups of trophoblastic cells may remain attached and temporarily viable. Therefore, these pregnancy tests can remain positive for a time. In any event, when a negative RIA test is reported, the pregnancy is over, although gestational debris may be retained.

With a clinical diagnosis of inevitable abortion, ultrasonography is less useful than it is in threatened abortion, when ultrasonography may distinguish a living from a nonliving gestation. Using real-time ultrasonography, the *absence of gross motion and especially heartbeat is indicative of fetal death.* In some cases, *absence of a fetus or fetal disorganization* also can be detected. Rarely, *gas in the great vessels* will be observed.

If cardiac motion is present, as is normally noted <8 gestational weeks (mean sac diameter 2.5 cm), the prognosis is more favorable.

DIFFERENTIAL DIAGNOSIS

Ectopic gestation is differentiated from spontaneous abortion by the additional symptoms and signs of *unilateral pelvic pain or tender adnexal mass. Membranous dysmenorrhea* may closely mimic spontaneous abortion, but decidua and villi are absent in the endometrial cast and pregnancy tests (even RIA) are negative. *Hyperestrogenism* can lead to marked proliferative endometrium with symptoms of cramping and bleeding. *Hydatidiform mole* usually ends in abortion (<5 months) but is marked by a very high hCG titer and fetal absence. *Pedunculated leiomyoma* or *cervical neoplasia* may also be confused with spontaneous abortion.

COMPLICATIONS

Hemorrhage and *infection* are major causes of maternal mortality or morbidity. Although very rare, about three fourths of cases of *choriocarcinoma* follow abortion. Infertility may result from inflammatory tubal occlusion after infected abortion. Rh sensitization may be avoided by administration of Rh immune globulin (see p. 321).

The immediate period of pregnancy loss is often accompanied by *grief, dysphoria, and anxiety.* Longer term grief is characterized by *perceived stress and high levels of depressive symptoms* (including self-blame). The latter phase lasts for at least a year. Those at risk of developing more intense or longer lasting distress include: those highly desirous of pregnancy, those waiting a long time to conceive, those with no living children, those who had elective abortions or prior losses, those with few warning signs of loss, late pregnancy losses, and younger women with multiple miscarriages. Little social support, marital and/or family problems, and a history of coping poorly further increase the emotional sequelae of spontaneous abortion. In addition to depression, the more severe distress may be characterized by anxiety disorders, guilt, and concerns about future reproduction.

Following spontaneous abortion, *a high percentage of patients indicate anger and dissatisfaction with medical care,* primarily relating to physician insensitivity and lack of opportunity to discuss personal significance of the loss. These responses may be *mitigated by: a more caring demeanor at the time; a follow-up appointment soon after the loss; answering why the abortion occurred, and whether it may happen again; and allowing adequate focus on the patient's feelings.*

PREVENTION

Some abortions can be prevented by *treatment of maternal deficiencies or disorders* before or during pregnancy (e.g., diabetes mellitus, hypertension). Closure of an incompetent cervix may prevent certain abortion.

FIGURE 10-2. Cerclage of the cervix (Shirodkar) with incompetent os in pregnant patient.

The usual technique for correction of cervical incompetency, *cervical cerclage,* involves placement of a suture or a nonabsorbable Mersilene or comparable strand, ribbon, or band beneath the mucosa and pericervical fascia at the cervicouterine junction. It may be done during the pregnant state for correction of cervical incompetence (Fig. 10-2) or accomplished between pregnancies. The physician must then decide whether to release the ligature during labor for vaginal delivery or to perform cesarean section near term.

TREATMENT

Rapid assessment of the patient's hemodynamic status should be performed (e.g., blood pressure, pulse rate). A rare critical case will require hemodynamic monitoring. In all except those with minimal bleeding (e.g., a stable complete abortion or an early threatened abortion), establishing an intravenous line is necessary. Administer *antishock therapy,* including fluid and blood replacement when indicated.

COMPLETE ABORTION

In nearly two-thirds of all patients *observation* (at least 1 h) for further bleeding may be sufficient. Criteria for these expectantly managed patients include: *being afebrile, stable blood pressure, normal heart rate, minimal bleeding, minimal pain, and a hemogram not indicative of infection or anemia. Transvaginal sonography* may assist in determining that minimal products of conception are present.

Less than 20% of women have hemorrhages. If the products of conception are available, they should be studied for completeness and may be submitted for genetic analysis or other pathologic assessment. In questionable cases, ultrasonic uterine scanning may detail remaining products of conception. After observation, the patient suffering complete abortion may return home with instructions to note signs of *infection* (fever, chills, or pain), which occurs in 0.8%–3.1%, observe for *vaginal hemorrhage,* and *refrain from intercourse or douching* until *reexamined in about 2 weeks* to determine lack of cervical closure or other abnormalities.

THREATENED ABORTION

Place the patient at *bedrest* after immediate danger from hemorrhage and infection has passed. Clinical judgment dictates whether bedrest may be accomplished at home (generally only in a nontroubling situation) or in the hospital. *Coitus and douches are contraindicated.*

Ultrasonic scanning is useful to determine fetal well-being. Obviously, a major determinant of prognosis is the recognition of fetal life and normality of fetal structures. Abortions without signs of fetal life should be managed as inevitable or incomplete abortions after appropriate discussion with the patient and family.

Progesterone therapy has theoretical value in <5% of abortions (those due to documented deficiency). In such cases, one may administer progesterone parenterally or by vaginal suppository. However, *progesterone treatment remains controversial.* The main points of contention include proper case selection, questionable efficacy, the potential to continue the retention of an abnormal pregnancy (i.e., missed abortion), and possible teratogenesis. *Other therapy* (e.g., tocolytics) *is even more questionable.*

In case of questionable fetal viability, the *prognosis is best when bleeding and cramping quickly subside, with evidence of cervical closure. The longer the symptoms persist, the more ominous the situation.*

The prognosis for the patient is good if all products of conception are evacuated or removed and if hydatidiform mole and choriocarcinoma can be ruled out.

Correction of maternal disorders may make future successful pregnancies possible. If an aborted fetus is found to have an abnormal karyotype, however, it may be desirable for the parents to obtain a genetic workup. In such cases, genetic investigation involving chorionic villus sampling or amniocentesis may be prudent during the next pregnancy. In certain severe transmissible genetic disorders, a determination of the exact defect in one or both parents will assist them and the practitioner to select artificial insemination (AID), in vitro fertilization of donor egg or in vitro fertilization with donor egg and donor sperm, adoption, or sterilization.

INEVITABLE AND INCOMPLETE ABORTION

Once the patient's hemodynamic status has been assessed and treatment started, *retained tissue must be removed* or bleeding will continue. *Oxytocics* (e.g., oxytocin 10 IU/500 mL of 5% dextrose in Ringer's lactate solution IV at ~125 mL/h) should contract the uterus, limit blood loss, aid in the expulsion of clots or tissue, and decrease the possibility of uterine perforation during dilatation and curettage. Ergonovine should be given only after the diagnosis of complete abortion is certain.

In some cases, *tissue at the external os may simply be removed with sponge forceps.* In others, it will be necessary to perform a *suction D & C.* Although it is rarely required, a sharp curettage may be lightly performed after the suction D & C to ascertain completeness. A heavy or extensive sharp curettage is potentially hazardous because it may lead to uterine synechia.

The removal of products of conception usually may be performed safely under *paracervical block* in an outpatient facility. However, a limiting factor is the ability to adequately observe the patient after the procedure. In cases of heavy bleeding or if the abortion has occurred in the second trimester, hospitalization is usually necessary.

The majority of *patients receiving outpatient care may be released after observation (1–6 h) confirms the return of physiologic function and absence of early complications.* Discharge instructions for the uncomplicated case are as noted for complete abortion.

The *major complication of D & C is uterine perforation.* If this is suspected, the patient must be observed in the hospital for signs of intraperitoneal bleeding, rupture of the bowel or bladder, or peritonitis. Exploratory laparotomy and broad-spectrum antibiotic therapy may be necessary.

OTHER ABORTION PROBLEMS

MISSED ABORTION

Ultrasonic scanning is usually definitive in the diagnosis of fetal death. It also assists in the differential diagnosis of a normal pregnancy with *inaccurate dates, pelvic tumor, or the loss of a multiple gestation.*

Current *treatment of missed abortion is induction of labor* using prostaglandin E_2 suppositories, enhanced if necessary with dilute IV oxytocin.

The major risk of missed abortion is the possibility of hypofibrinogenemia. Thus, if the products of conception are contained longer than 4 weeks after fetal death, close monitoring of the serum fibrinogen is mandatory.

INFECTED OR SEPTIC ABORTION

With infected abortion, *expect pelvic and abdominal pain and fever* (100–105°F). On physical examination, there is often *suprapubic tenderness and signs of peritonitis.* The pelvic examination will likely, but may not necessarily, reveal a *malodorous cervical discharge, pain on motion of the cervix, or uterine tenderness.* Hypothermia may precede endotoxic shock, and jaundice may be due to hemolysis. Oliguria or renal failure is a serious complication.

The necessary laboratory information includes a *complete blood count, urinalysis, culture of cervix or uterus or both, serum electrolytes, and a coagulation profile. Chest and abdominal x-ray* films are necessary to diagnose or rule out septic emboli, gas beneath the diaphragm (uterine perforation), foreign body in the uterus (possible criminal abortion), and gas in the pelvic tissues from gas-forming organisms.

Treatment consists of *hospitalization, high-dose IV antibiotic therapy* (individualized to the suspected organisms), *fluid and electrolyte support, and careful monitoring of vital signs and urinary output.* These patients must be considered serious, even potentially critical. *Hemodynamic monitoring* may be necessary in the more severe cases (for determination of cardiac output, blood volume, and blood gases).

The uterus must be emptied, and this should be accomplished by D & C as soon as the patient is stable. All products of conception must be removed, even though a thorough curettage of infected uterus greatly enhances the risk of uterine synechia (Asherman's syndrome). Abdominal hysterectomy may be necessary when *Clostridia* or *Bacteroides* are the causative organisms, when there is necrosis of the uterus, with complete uterine perforations (e.g., bowel injury), or when the patient responds poorly to septic shock treatment.

Pelvic thrombophlebitis and septic emboli may be grave sequelae of septic abortion. Consider additional, more specific antibiotic and also anticoagulant therapy. Pelvic vein ligation or percutaneous umbrella occlusion of the vena cava may be necessary for septic embolization.

HABITUAL (RECURRENT) ABORTION

Based on very conservative data (a 15%–40% chance of loss of any given pregnancy), three consecutive losses are required to approach statistical significance (<1%). The risk of first trimester abortion after one loss is 24%, after two losses 26%, and after three losses, 32%. Thus, data from a series of cases with only two consecutive losses may not be valid.

The most likely causes of habitual abortion are genetic abnormality, reproductive tract anatomic abnormalities, hormonal (endocrinologic) abnormalities, infections, abnormal immunologic factors, or systemic disease (environmental). However, the *cause remains unknown at least in one third* of all habitual abortions. Currently, investigations are most active in the autoimmune factors (e.g., anti-cardiolipin, antithyroid, antinuclear, and antiphospholipid antibodies) and alloimmune factors (e.g., natural killer cells, cytotoxic T cells), and embryotoxic factors.

Thus, the *incidence of habitual abortion varies* with parental genetic abnormalities (e.g., balanced translocation carrier parent, hyperploidy), maternal systemic diseases (e.g., hypertension, diabetes mellitus, SLE), maternal hormonal abnormalities (e.g., hypothyroidism), maternal genital tract abnormalities, and parental sharing of similar HLA-A and HLA-B (and possibly abortion, stillbirth, or infant with malformations).

Possible *etiologies for genetic errors* include parental chromosome translocation, recombination defects, other genetic factors (e.g., homozygous dominant inheritance), environmental agents (i.e., radiation, chemicals, medications), or delayed fertilization. In an abortion with an abnormal karyotype, there is an ~80% chance of the next abortus having an abnormal karyotype (vs. ~50%–60% if the first has a normal karyotype).

Even after three spontaneous abortions, the probability of a fourth is <1 in 3. However, even this chance justifies investigation to determine a demonstrable cause. In addition to routine history and physical examination, the following are useful.

- Prepare a three-generation pedigree for both partners and complete a thorough reproductive history (including pathologic and karyotypic information from previous abortions).
- Obtain a karyotypic study of both parents. Structural chromosome rearrangements in couples with recurrent fetal wastage is as high as 5.34%. Two thirds of the chromosomal rearrangements are autosomal balanced translocations, with the others including: Robertsonian translocations, inversions, and sex-chromosomal abnormalities.
- Perform a hysterosalpingogram, hysteroscopy, or laparoscopy to rule out anatomic abnormalities of the reproductive tract.
- Order laboratory studies for T_3, T_4, TSH, glucose abnormality screening (1 or 2 h postprandial), SMA, and antinuclear antibodies or antibodies to double-stranded DNA.
- Arrange for immunologic screening for both parents. Currently, controversy exists over appropriate testing. An immunologic consultation may be useful.
- Biopsy the endometrium during the luteal phase, or obtain serum progesterone to assess the corpus luteum, or do both.
- Perform infectious screening of cervical or endometrial tissue by culture for *Listeria monocytogenes, Chlamydia,*

Mycoplasma, U. urealyticum, Neisseria gonorrhoeae, cytomegalovirus, and herpes simplex and serum titers for
Treponema pallidum, Brucella abortus, and *Toxoplasma
gondii.*

Therapy must be guided by the diagnostic workup.

- *Genetic error.* Consider artificial insemination by donor or
  in vitro fertilization with donor ova or sperm.
- *Anatomic abnormalities of the reproductive tract.* Employ
  hysteroscopic removal of polyps or uterine septum, uterine
  operations (e.g., Jones, Tompkins, Strassman procedure, myomectomy), cervical cerclage (abdominal or vaginal), or cervical reconstruction.
- *Hormonal abnormalities.* When deficient, administer thyroid,
  progesterone, or clomiphene citrate. Additionally, it may be
  necessary to treat hyperprolactinemia and hyperandrogenism.
- *Infection.* Give appropriate antibiotics.
- *Immunologic factors.* The use of purified paternal lymphocytes is currently questioned and increasingly, intravenous
  immunoglobulin is suggested as a potential treatment for immunologic associations of recurrent pregnancy loss. Other
  therapies include heparin, aspirin, and both heparin and aspirin. Prednisone (alone and in conjunction with aspirin)
  may be necessary to treat the underlying condition, but has
  largely been replaced by heparin and aspirin therapy for recurrent fetal wastage.
- *Treat systemic disorders* appropriately using disease-specific
  therapy. Recently, the therapy of hypercoagulable states with
  aspirin, heparin, or both, has been suggested.
- *Encourage the creation of an environment most conducive
  to pregnancy.* This involves: stopping fetotoxins (e.g., alcohol, tobacco, cocaine), decreasing stress, and utilization of
  folic acid prior to the onset of pregnancy (see p. 139).
- *Even when the interval of most likely abortion is successfully navigated, fetal risk continues* (e.g., IUGR is increased
  2-fold, gestational hypertension is increased 2-fold, preterm
  delivery is increased 3-fold, and cesarean section is twice as
  common).

ECTOPIC PREGNANCY

*A fertilized ovum implanted outside the uterine cavity is an ectopic
pregnancy.* Ectopic pregnancy usually results from conditions that

delay or prevent the transit of a fertilized ovum through the fallopian tube. Over 50% are associated with tubal inflammatory changes (previous or chronic salpingitis). Other important etiologic factors include zygote abnormalities, transmigration of the ovum, postmidcycle ovulation–fertilization, or exogenous hormones.

The *incidence of ectopic pregnancy has risen dramatically* during the past two decades in the United States to at least >1:100 pregnancies (from ~1:500), and in some reports as high as 2% of all pregnancies. The increase, most notable among nonwhite women, is attributable to tubal infection, endometriosis, and an enhanced chance of ectopic gestation after failed laparoscopic tubal ligation. Unknown factors also are likely.

Morbidity and mortality are directly related to tubal rupture. There are some associations with risk of rupture, including: never having used contraception, a history of tubal damage together with infertility, induction of ovulation, and a high level of hCG when ectopic pregnancy is suspected. Unfortunately *tubal rupture cannot be safely predicted* by any known risk factor, serum hCG level, or sonographic finding and *occurs in approximately 20%* of patients in developed countries. Only early diagnosis and treatment will prevent the sequelae of tubal rupture. Ectopic pregnancy is a major cause of maternal mortality mainly because of uncontrolled hemorrhage and shock (0.1%–0.2% in the United States, but the rate is higher in developing countries). Fetal mortality in ectopic pregnancy is nearly universal.

CLASSIFICATIONS

Ectopic pregnancy is classified according to the site of implantation (the following is in decreasing order of occurrence).

Tubal (98–99%) ectopic pregnancies are further subdivided into the anatomic section involved: ampullary (55%), isthmic (25%), fimbrial (17%), interstitial (angular, cornual) (2%), and bilateral (very rare) (Fig. 10-3).

Ovarian pregnancy (0.5%) may follow fertilization of an unextruded ovum.

Abdominal (~1/15,000 pregnancies) pregnancy may be primary, with the initial implantation of the zygote outside the tube (e.g., on the liver), or secondary to expulsion or rupture of a tubal pregnancy.

Cervical implantation (rare) is suggested by a greatly enlarged cervix (often as large as the nonpregnant uterus, known as the "hourglass sign"). This is an enlarged, highly vascularized, bleeding cervix, with tight internal os and a gaping external os.

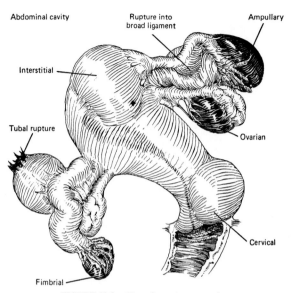

FIGURE 10-3. Sites of ectopic pregnancies.

Uterine ectopic gestations (rare) may occur with implantation in the cornua, a uterine diverticulum, uterine sacculation, rudimentary horn, or the muscular wall (intramural).

Combined intrauterine pregnancy (*heterotopic*). This occurs in 1/17,000–30,000 pregnancies. Other rare possibilities include intraligamentous. Pregnancy even follows hysterectomy.

PATHOLOGIC PHYSIOLOGY

Whereas the usual early signs of pregnancy are noted in the cervix, the uterus becomes minimally enlarged and slightly softened with an ectopic gestation. The endometrium contains decidua (but no trophoblast) and has a characteristic microscopic appearance termed the *"Arias-Stella reaction."*

In ectopic gestation, the corpus luteum of pregnancy functions as long as the trophoblast remains viable. Amenorrhea results from trophoblast production of hCG and corpus luteum secretion of progesterone. *Slight endometrial bleeding generally* occurs, presumably with abnormal hormonal patterns, *following a variable interval of amenorrhea.* Endometrial separation and bleeding occur when the trophoblast is withdrawn (e.g., with rupture). Only in uncommon interstitial pregnancy does blood from the tube drain via the uterus into the vagina.

Lower abdominal, pelvic, or low back pain may be secondary to tubal distention or rupture. Isthmic pregnancy usually ruptures in about 6 weeks, and hemorrhage due to ampullary pregnancy occurs at 8–12 weeks. *Cornual pregnancies are most commonly carried to the second trimester before rupture.* Intraabdominal pregnancy may terminate anytime with bleeding. A pelvic mass is caused by enlargement of the conceptus, hematoma formation, bowel distortion by adhesions, or infection. If the fetus dies without extensive bleeding, it may become infected, mummified, calcified (lithopedian), or an adipocere (fatty replacement).

DIAGNOSIS, HISTORY, AND PHYSICAL EXAMINATION

Before the advent of high-resolution ultrasound, <2% of ectopic pregnancies were unruptured when discovered. Now, however, almost 50% are diagnosed at this stage. Abdominal pain is reported by 97% of ectopic pregnancy patients and 99% report some abdominal or pelvic pain. In ~80% this is associated with abnormal vaginal bleeding. Secondary amenorrhea of <2 weeks duration is reported by 68% of patients. Characteristically, pain associated with ectopic gestation is described as moderate to severe, lateral, or sharp. Other historical items of significance include infertility (15%), with tubal factor being the most important, and previous ectopic gestation (11%). Emerging associations include difficult embryo transfer (particularly in association with a history of tubal damage or prior ectopic gestation) and possibly myomectomy. Physical findings with ectopic pregnancy frequently include abdominal tenderness (~90%), a tender pelvic mass (54%–70%), but the *most consistent sign is adnexal tenderness (96%).* Unilateral tenderness on turning the patient (positive Adler sign) is inconsistent but important if present.

Sharp unilateral lower abdominal or pelvic pain or both (and possible backache) after brief amenorrhea and irregular bleeding are also the usual complaints with an acute (rupturing or recently ruptured) ectopic gestation. Collapse and shock (from bleeding), which may be precipitated by a vaginal examination, occur in at least 10%.

With *chronic ectopic gestation (now unusual)* pelvic discomfort is variable. Expect an adnexal or cul-de-sac mass. This eventually may become crepitant. A bluish discoloration in or about the umbilicus (Cullen's sign of hematoperitoneum) may appear in neglected cases. By this time, the pregnancy usually is over, but pain persists and infection may intervene.

In addition to the above symptoms and signs, ruptured ectopic pregnancies usually demonstrate *hemodynamic instability* and/or peritoneal signs (accompanying the blood loss with a ruptured ectopic gestation). As in other circumstances, these internally hemorrhaging patients present a surgical emergency, requiring resuscitation (fluid, colloid, blood products, and oxygen) and surgical intervention. Although sonography may be helpful, it should not delay definitive therapy. Surgical intervention, usually accomplished by either laparoscopy or laparotomy, may be accompanied by a D & C.

Culdocentesis (transvaginal passage of a needle into the cul-de-sac) has largely been replaced by transabdominal or transvaginal ultrasound for the diagnosis of hematoperitoneum. Sonography compared to culdocentesis is more sensitive (100% vs. 66%), more specific (100% vs. 80%), and has a better negative predictive value (100% vs. 25%—nondiagnostic culdocentesis) in the diagnosis of hemoperitoneum. When sonography is unavailable, however, culdocentesis may be useful for the determination of free blood in the abdominal cavity. Grasp the posterior lip of the cervix with an Allis clamp or tenaculum and cleanse the vagina (e.g., with povidone—iodine). Infiltrate local anesthetic into the vaginal wall between the uterosacral ligaments. Pass an 18-gauge spinal needle (attached to a 10 mL syringe) 1–4 mm into the cul-de-sac while exerting gentle countertraction on the cervix.

Blood recovered by culdocentesis is evidence of hematoperitoneum if the blood does not clot (having already clotted and partially liquefied in 95% of ruptured ectopic gestations), red blood cells (RBC) rouleaux are absent, and the RBCs are crenated.

Laparoscopy usually is diagnostic in early and unruptured ectopic pregnancy. However, if culdocentesis reveals free intraperitoneal blood and the patient is a surgical emergency, laparoscopy will unduly delay therapy. Proceed to laparotomy.

LABORATORY FINDINGS

In hemodynamically stable, nonemergent patients, the next step in diagnosis is a quantitative hCG and sonography. The two tests are frequently done concurrently, unless there is significant doubt concerning pregnancy (then the hCG is performed first). When patients have a beta-hCG <1000 mIU/mL, a single serum progesterone may be useful in determination of normal and abnormal pregnancies, including ectopic gestation. A single progesterone <5.0 ng/mL in patients with beta-hCG <1000 has a sensitivity of 94% (95% CI 86%–98%) and specificity of 100% (95% CI 78%–100%) in detection of all abnormal pregnancies. Thus, while nonspecific, it may provide useful overall information.

Another alternative in the stable and nonemergent patient is serial quantitative hCGs. The serum hCG increases less rapidly in most ectopic pregnancies than in normal pregnancies (when it should double every 2–4 days). Sonography is also useful in these questionable patients, because ~90% of patients with ectopics will have suggestive sonographic findings (i.e., fluid in the cul-de-sac, complex adnexal mass, or cystic mass). In those patients with beta hCG <1000 and indeterminate pelvic ultrasound, the serial change in hCG values may be most useful. Those at highest risk are those with hCG increases of <66% over 48 hours with an empty uterus.

Although transabdominal ultrasound is also usually used, the sensitivity of transvaginal sonography in detection of ectopic gestation is 87% (specificity 94%, positive predictive value 92.5%, and negative predictive value 90%). Diagnostic accuracy may be improved further in the very difficult cases by the still investigational laparoscopy-assisted intrapelvic sonography using a high-frequency, real-time miniature transducer for assessment of the fallopian tube. The highest diagnostic accuracy is obtained by correlating clinical findings, sonography, and beta-hCG values.

DIFFERENTIAL DIAGNOSIS

Conditions clinically similar to ectopic pregnancy include *appendicitis, salpingitis, ruptured corpus luteum cyst, ruptured ovarian follicle, abortion, ovarian torsion, and urinary tract infection* (Table 10-2, pp. 313–315).

TREATMENT

Increasingly the treatment of tubal pregnancy is being divided into two categories. At the time of presentation, *20%–25% of ectopic gestations will have tubal rupture and/or active bleeding.* These patients have immediate threat to life, present a spectrum of surgical emergencies, and are operated immediately on diagnosis. Delay is justified only to correct shock. The second category of ectopic gestation patients are generally diagnosed at an earlier gestation, have

TABLE 10-2

DIFFERENTIAL DIAGNOSIS OF ECTOPIC PREGNANCY

	Ectopic Pregnancy	Appendicitis	Salpingitis	Ruptured Corpus Luteum Cyst	Uterine Abortion
Pain	Unilateral cramps and tenderness before rupture	Epigastric, periumbilical, then right lower quadrant pain; tenderness localizing at McBurney's point; rebound tenderness	Usually in both lower quadrants, with or without rebound	Unilateral, becoming general with progressive bleeding	Midline cramps
Nausea and vomiting	Occasionally before, frequently after rupture	Usual, precedes shift of pain to right lower quadrant	Infrequent	Rare	Almost never

(*Continued*)

TABLE 10-2
(*Continued*)

	Ectopic Pregnancy	Appendicitis	Salpingitis	Ruptured Corpus Luteum Cyst	Uterine Abortion
Menstruation	Some aberration: missed period, spotting	Unrelated to menses	Hypermenorrhea, menorrhagia, or both symptoms start near end of menses	Period delayed, then bleeding, often with pain	Amenorrhea, then spotting, then brisk bleeding
Temperature and pulse	37.2–37.8°C (99–100°F); pulse variable: normal before, rapid after rupture	37.2–37.8°C (99–100°F); pulse rapid: 99–100	37.2–40°C (99–104°F); pulse elevated in proportion to fever	Not over 37.2°C (99°F); pulse normal unless blood loss marked, then rapid	To 37.2°C (99°F) if spontaneous; to 40°C (104°F) if infected
Pelvic examination	Unilateral tenderness,	No masses	Bilateral tenderness on	Tenderness over affected	Cervix slightly patulous;

314

	especially on movement of cervix; crepitant mass on one side or in cul-de-sac		movement of cervix; masses only when pyosalpinx or hydrosalpinx is present	ovary; no masses	uterus slightly enlarged, irregularly softened; tender with infection
Laboratory findings	White cell count to 15,000/µl; red cell count strikingly low if blood loss large; sedimentation rate slightly elevated	White cell count 10,000–18,000/µl (rarely normal); red cell count normal; sedimentation rate slightly elevated	White cell count 15,000–30,000/µl; red cell count normal; sedimentation rate markedly elevated	White cell count normal to 10,000/µl; red cell count normal; sedimentation rate normal	White cell count 15,000/µl if spontaneous; to 30,000/µl if induced (infection); red cell count normal; sedimentation rate slightly to moderately elevated

an *unruptured ectopic pregnancy, do not have active bleeding, and are hemodynamically stable.*

EMERGENCY TREATMENT

- Hospitalize the patient.
- Insert a large-bore IV into a large vein.
- Obtain hemogram, clotting panel, and blood for type and crossmatch.
- Administer antishock measures as indicated: IV crystalloids, blood component transfusion, keep the patient comfortably warm, give oxygen, and apply MAST compression trousers or moderately snug tourniquets around the upper legs.

SURGICAL TREATMENT (EITHER LAPAROSCOPY OR LAPAROTOMY)

- Choice of procedure (laparotomy or laparoscopy) depends on surgical judgment. Currently, laparoscopy with antimesenteric linear salpingostomy (preferably by laser) is being increasingly used.
- Control hemorrhage (blood and clots need not be completely removed; they will be absorbed and limit anemia, or the filtered citrated blood may be used for autotransfusion).
- Remove the products of conception (secondary implantation may occur with incomplete removal).
- Preserve normal or minimally damaged tubes or other organs. If the pregnancy is early or if tubal missed abortion has occurred, perform salpingostomy to enucleate the pregnancy and preserve the tube. Ligate bleeding points. Suture closure is not necessary.
- Indications for organ removal include:
  Uncontrollable hemorrhage.
  Severely damaged tube (requires cornual excision—not resection—to prevent repeat ectopic pregnancy and endosalpingosis of the stump).
  Hysterectomy may be required in ruptured interstitial or cervical pregnancy.
  Oophorectomy is necessary in ovarian pregnancy but is not recommended in cases where tubal removal is required.

Laparoscopy has been used as the standard by which other therapy is measured. However, surgical treatment is very dependent on the experience and expertise of the surgeon, the equipment and the facilities available, as well as the patient's status. As surgeons, equipment, and facilities have advanced, laparoscopy has far exceeded the original guidelines: a hemodynamically stable patient, an hCG <6000, a history suggestive of minimal pelvic adhesions, and the pregnancy confined within the tube (by ultrasound). A note of caution is that this is also accompanied by a higher rate of complications and several reports suggest that in more complex cases, laparotomy results in fewer complications. The highest rate of complications (nearly 25%) is in complex cases undergoing after conservative laparoscopic surgery.

Overall, comparing laparoscopy to medical therapy, the mean hospital stay is longer, but follow up is significantly shorter, return to normal hCG is shorter (13 vs. 29 d), and laparoscopy requires fewer clinical examinations, sonograms, and hCGs. A few laparoscopically treated patients will have retained trophoblastic tissue and require medical therapy to achieve normal hCG levels.

MEDICAL TREATMENT

Medical therapy is increasingly utilized for treatment of unruptured ectopic gestations with minimal bleeding. Medical therapy is most safe and efficacious in ectopic gestations with the following: beta-hCG <5000 IU/mL, hematosalpinx <3 cm, peritoneal fluid <300 cc, and the patient is capable of complying with the necessary follow-up. *Methotrexate is the current choice of medical agents* and is either administered systemically or instilled into the gestation's amniotic sac by ultrasonic (or less commonly by laparoscopic) guidance. The potential advantages of the intraamniotic injection include: a greater local antitrophoblastic effect, a shorter treatment interval, reduced dosage, and fewer side effects. A number of dosage regimens are under investigation (e.g., systemic 50 gm/m² IM, 0.5 mg/kg IM, 1 mg/kg IM, 15 mg IV, and gestational sac 10–12.5 mg, 100 mg). With each administration of methotrexate, folic acid 0.1 mg/kg po (Citrovorum Factor) is usually given.

This rapidly emerging treatment plan has a number of issues to be resolved, for example: Are these criteria too conservative? Are best results obtained by systemic or intra-amniotic injection? What is the most effective yet safest dosage and administration regimen (an important consideration given the toxicity of methotrexate)? Does dosage and technique need altered for further advanced cases (e.g., fetal cardiac activity, initial hCG >3500, gestational mass >3.5 cm)? Are other therapeutic adjuncts useful?

The preliminary results are encouraging with each of the several protocols. The rate of resolution of the ectopic gestation with intraamniotic injection has been reported to be *71% after a single dose and 84% after another injection.* Side effects (usually minor) were experienced by ~25%, and ~10% will suffer ruptured ectopic.

The rate of resolution with systemic methotrexate (1–3 doses) is 90%–92% overall, but recent information indicates that resolution is related to the length of gestation, with earlier gestations having a higher rate of resolution. For example, when the hCG is <3500 IU/mL, there is a higher success rate (nears 100%) with a single injection and less patients require hospitalization. Overall, ~$\frac{3}{4}$ of patients are treated as out-patients and time to resolution of hCG (<10 IU/mL) is 27 d.

Follow-up consists of serial clinical exams, beta-hCG assays, liver tests and blood cell counts. The follow-up interval is longer than that necessary with laparoscopy.

Side effects are noted in at least one third of medically treated patients, the most common and problematic being abdominal pain. Such patients may require surgical intervention if hemodynamically unstable, but some stable patients may be monitored closely despite rebound or free peritoneal fluid. Other potential side effects include negative impact on: physical functioning, role functioning, social functioning, health perceptions, and energy. Indeed, the potential side effects plus depression are all reported with a higher incidence in medically vs. surgically treated patients.

Medical management has been suggested for two specific and very dangerous ectopic pregnancies, the interstitial and the cervical. These complex circumstances often involve pregnancy much further advanced than those tubal pregnancies recommended for medical treatment.

A useful adjunct to medical therapy, particularly in further advanced ectopic gestations, may be the antiprogesterone mifepristone. In preliminary studies, unruptured ectopic pregnancy resolves quicker in women given the combination of methotrexate (50 mg/m^2) and mifepristone (600 mg) po compared to women given only methotrexate.

SUPPORTIVE TREATMENT

- Give broad-spectrum antibiotics for infection.
- Prescribe oral or IM iron therapy or both to replenish iron stores.

PROGNOSIS

Ectopic pregnancy is a life-threatening disorder in >10% of cases, and >1% of these patients die of internal hemorrhage and shock or of later complications. Survival of the fetus in extrauterine pregnancy is exceptional.

Ectopic pregnancy (and probably its antecedents) severely limit future reproductive potential, with only is similar to one third of affected women ever subsequently having a live-born infant. Fertility following ectopic gestation appears more dependent on the normalcy of the contralateral fallopian tube than the treatment modality. Women who have experienced two ectopic gestations are at such risk that some recommend that they are candidates for assisted reproduction. Currently, there are limited comparisons between laparoscopy and medical therapy concerning future reproduction, but preliminary data indicate potentially higher overall intrauterine pregnancy and fewer repeat ectopic gestations with medical therapy. Ectopic pregnancy recurs in about 15% of cases.

In combined extrauterine and intrauterine pregnancy, one or the other usually is diagnosed—rarely both. Generally, the extrauterine pregnancy succumbs, and 60% of the intrauterine pregnancies go on to viability.

COMPLICATIONS

Without surgical intervention, a ruptured ectopic pregnancy can cause life-threatening hemorrhage. Infection often follows neglected ruptured ectopic pregnancy. Sterility or other reproductive failure may occur after or as a result of ectopic pregnancy (in 30%–50% of patients who have had surgical removal of a tube for an ectopic gestation). Obstruction and fistulas may develop after hematoperitoneum, peritonitis, or lithopedian formation. Rh immune globulin administration prevents Rh isoimmunization (see p. 321).

PREVENTION

Other than properly treating salpingitis, preventive measures for ectopic gestation remain unclear.

ISOIMMUNIZATION

Isoimmunization is the development of antibodies against the antigens of a genetically dissimilar individual. Antigens may be transferred by exposure to blood products or by mingling of fetal blood with the maternal blood. The latter occurs throughout pregnancy but usually reaches levels sufficient to provoke a response in late gestation or during delivery. Once the mother is immunized, even minute amounts of subsequent antigen act as a stimulus, causing a rise in maternal antibody production.

When the mother becomes sensitized, a variety of antigens are produced. The gamma globulin antibodies (IgG) can cross the placenta and destroy fetal RBCs. If the fetal hematopoietic system is not able to compensate for the *RBC destruction, hemolytic anemia* occurs. The increased destruction of RBC results in heme as well as increased levels of unconjugated bilirubin. Both heme and unconjugated bilirubin are neurotoxic. In utero these are efficiently transferred across the placenta. When the cord is severed, however, the immature liver cannot conjugate bilirubin efficiently (due to low levels of glucuronyltransferase), and hyperbilirubinemia develops. Jaundice ensues, and as bilirubin and heme accumulate in the plasma, bilirubin may cross the blood–brain barrier to be deposited in the nuclear zones of the midbrain and brainstem, causing kernicterus.

The Rh antigen (Rh factor) is the most common cause of maternal isoimmunization. Individuals who carry the Rh factor are described as Rh positive; those who lack the factor are termed Rh negative. Rh isoimmunization occurs only in the Rh-negative individual. If an Rh-negative woman is carrying an Rh-positive fetus, the stage is set for fetal isoimmune hemolytic disease.

Other blood groups causing isoimmunization with an IgG response and, thus, the potential for fetal hemolytic disease include (in descending order of occurrence) Kell, Duffy, Kidd, MNS, Diego, and P factors. Although Lutheran and Xg groups may cause fetal hemolysis, it is usually less severe.

RH ISOIMMUNIZATION

Severe isoimmune hemolytic disease has the potential to occur in ~1/200 pregnancies in the United States. The vast majority of these are due to Rh isoimmunization. *The incidence of Rh negativity differs markedly among races:* Basques (30%–35%), other Caucasians (10%–12%), African Americans (8%), Native American (1%). The risk of isoimmunization for an Rh-positive ABO-compatible infant with an Rh-negative mother is ~16%. Of these, ~2% will occur antepartum, 7% within 6 months of delivery, and 7% early in the subsequent pregnancy. ABO incompatibility affords some protection from isoimmunization, but not enough for reliance. It is imperative that every pregnant woman be screened for her Rh status because with the administration of immune globulin (RhIgG), kernicterus can be virtually eliminated.

DIAGNOSIS

- Screen all pregnant women (including those who have aborted or have ectopic pregnancy) for ABO type, Rh, and other pertinent antibodies (e.g., Hemantigen screen).
- If the woman is Rh-negative and unsensitized
    Test the husband for ABO and Rh.
    Repeat the antibody screen at 28 and 35 weeks.
    Administer prophylactic RhIgG.
- If the mother is sensitized
    Serial dilutions of the indirect Coombs' test are a guide to the maternal response but do not correlate well with the fetal status. Any dilution of $\geq 1:8$ must be investigated by amniotic fluid analysis. Positive tests of lesser dilutions warrant a repeat study in ~ 2 weeks.
    Spectrophotometric analysis of the amniotic fluid will determine the relative degree of fetal jeopardy (Fig. 10-4). This should start at 16–18 weeks.
    Serial fetal ultrasonography (start at 14–16 weeks) is used to determine normal growth as well as presence of ascites or hydramnios.
- Investigate for fetomaternal hemorrhage
    Determine significant blood loss by newborn hematocrit or hemoglobin determination or both.
    Ascertain the presence of fetal hemoglobin in the maternal circulation (e.g., Kleihauer-Betke, hemoglobin electrophoresis).

PREVENTION

All of the *following information pertains to Rh-negative pregnancies because immune globulins are not available for the other blood group isoimmune hemolytic disorders.*

- **Abortion.** Approximately 2% of spontaneous abortions and 4%–5% of induced abortions will undergo isoimmunization. Spontaneous early first trimester abortions may be treated adequately with 50 μg RhIgG, However, later abortions and induced abortions require the usual dose (300 μg).
- **Amniocentesis.** There is an 11% chance of sensitization if the needle enters the placenta. Administer 300 μg of RhIgG after amniocentesis in the unsensitized patient.
- **Routine prophylaxis.** In the unsensitized, Rh-negative woman with a negative antibody screen, 300 μg of RhIgG should be administered at 28 weeks. This confers relative protection for ~ 12 weeks and substantially reduces the chance

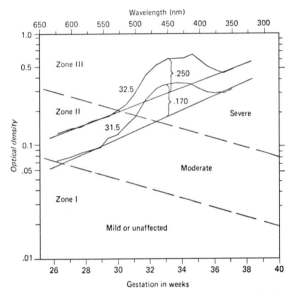

FIGURE 10-4. Transabdominal amniocentesis: spectrophotometric analysis of amniotic fluid surrounding an erythroblastotic fetus. Amniocentesis was performed at $31\frac{1}{2}$ and $32\frac{1}{2}$ weeks. The spectral absorption curve was obtained by plotting the optical densities at various wavelengths on 2-cycle semilogarithmic graph paper. A tangential line joining the lowest portions of this curve approximates the values for unstained amniotic fluid and is the baseline for calculations. The difference between the involved and uninvolved curves is measured at 450 nm (the wavelength at which maximum absorption by bilirubin or bilirubin-like products occurs) and plotted at the appropriate number of weeks of gestation (dotted line). The case illustrated shows rapid progression from moderate to severe disease. Under such conditions, fetal death often is imminent. Immediate delivery usually is necessary if the gestational age will permit. Otherwise, intrauterine fetal transfusion may be considered.

(From S.G. Babson and R.C. Benson, *Clinical Perinatology*. Mosby, 1971.)

of becoming sensitized before delivery. The 28-week prophylaxis does not alter the delivery plan. If the pregnancy goes beyond 40 weeks, however, it may be prudent to administer antepartum prophylactic RhIgG again.

- **Antepartum hemorrhage.** Patients with placenta previa or abruptio placenta who do not deliver immediately should receive 300 μg of RhIgG. If the pregnancy is carried 12 weeks from the time of the first administration, another prophylactic dose is recommended.

- **Abdominal trauma.** Auto accidents, physical assault involving the abdomen, or external version may result in the release of fetal RBC into the maternal circulation. Hence, to prevent isoimmunization, 300 μg of RhIgG is recommended after the incident.

- **Fetal death.** In cases of fetal death, there is often loss of fetal RBCs into the maternal circulation and occasionally, fetomaternal exsanguination. Thus, investigation for fetal hemorrhage and dose-specific RhIgG (minimally 300 μg) are both necessary.

- **Delivery.** If the infant of an Rh-negative woman is Rh-positive or Du-positive, administer 300 μg of RhIgG within 72 h.

- **Fetomaternal hemorrhage.** Fetomaternal hemorrhage may result with multiple gestation, manual removal of the placenta, cesarean section with placental incision, precipitous delivery, tetanic labor, abruptio placenta, and placenta previa. When the approximate amount of fetal blood has been ascertained, the amount of RhIgG to be administered is based on 25 μg/ml of fetal blood.

TREATMENT AND PROGNOSIS

Mildly affected fetus (Liley zone 1). Continue ultrasonic monitoring every 2 weeks, repeat amniocentesis in 2–3 weeks, and plan for delivery at term or with fetal pulmonary maturity. Testing for fetal well-being may be desirable. In summary, intervention is usually not necessary, and only minimal neonatal treatment leads to a good prognosis.

Moderately affected fetus (lower Liley zone 2). Continue ultrasonic monitoring and add weekly biophysical profile testing. Repeat amniocentesis every 1–2 weeks. Deliver before term as soon as pulmonary maturity is compatible with survival. If delivery is necessary before pulmonary maturity, administer betamethasone within 48 h before delivery. In summary, careful monitoring is necessary to determine that the fetus is not worsening. If the fetus remains in lower zone 2, usually only early delivery and neonatal therapy are necessary for a satisfactory prognosis.

Severely affected fetus (upper Liley zone 2 and zone 3). Intervention generally is necessary for the fetus to reach a gestational age when delivery and extrauterine risks are less than risks of in utero therapy. Weekly or more frequent ultrasonic scans and tests of fetal well-being are necessary. Amniocentesis is done approximately weekly to determine fetal status and pulmonary maturity. Intrauterine transfusion, using O-negative, low-titer, glycerolized RBC may be required to save the immature, severely anemic fetus. Although this procedure is beyond the scope of this text, it may be accomplished safely by ultrasonically guided intravascular transfusion. Once started, repeated in utero transfusion is necessary because fetal hematopoiesis decreases or ceases. In summary, with this poor prognostic situation, direct intervention is usually necessary to save the perinate's life.

ABO HEMOLYTIC DISEASE

Potential maternal–infant ABO incompatibility occurs in 20%–25% of pregnancies but *causes a recognizable neonatal problem in only 10% of those at risk.* Moreover, the problem nearly always affects A (especially A1) or B infants of group O mothers, and 40%–50% of cases occur in the firstborn (vs. 1%–2% of Rh problems). The maternal antibodies are variable, and the neonatal direct Coombs' test may be either positive or negative. Although ABO isoimmunization produces an IgG response, for unknown reasons, it generally causes a much milder hemolytic disease. Serious fetal anemia is rare, and such sequelae as stillbirth or hydrops almost never occur.

Characteristically, during the first day after birth, the neonate with ABO hemolytic disease shows the onset of indirect hyperbilirubinemia. The neonate may have hepatosplenomegaly. Usually, management requires only bilirubin surveillance and phototherapy (~10% of cases), although occasionally (~1%), exchange transfusion is necessary. *Serious sequelae are rare.*

THIRD TRIMESTER HEMORRHAGE

DEFINITION AND ETIOLOGY

The only bleeding that normally occurs during late pregnancy is a very small amount (<15 mL), with loss of the mucous plug prior to delivery. All other bleeding is abnormal and merits investigation. A useful list of the causes of third trimester bleeding is contained in Table 11-1.

The health care provider *must distinguish between obstetric and nonobstetric bleeding* (the two major classifications). Nonobstetric causes are much less common in pregnancy and generally are less hazardous. Of the *obstetric causes, various forms of placental bleeding account for the vast majority.* The most frequent are *placenta previa or premature separation of a normally implanted placenta. Rupture of the uterus,* rare without previous uterine surgery, occurs in up to 1% of patients previously delivered by cesarean section. Uterine rupture may cause vaginal bleeding, but most of the loss will be concealed. *Nonplacental bleeding,* rare during pregnancy, may be due to *blood dyscrasia or lower genital tract disorders* (e.g., cervical or vaginal infections, neoplasms, or varices). Generally, the bleeding is slight, even with carcinoma of the cervix.

INCIDENCE AND IMPORTANCE

Second trimester vaginal bleeding of obstetric origin is more common in multiparous women and those with a history of prior preterm delivery. *Second trimester bleeding is ominous,* being associated with an increased risk of *preterm delivery* (relative risk 1.9), *fetal*

TABLE 11-1
ETIOLOGIC CLASSIFICATION OF THIRD
TRIMESTER BLEEDING

| | Causes | |
Risk	Obstetric	Nonobstetric
High	Placenta previa	Coagulopathies
	Abruptio placentae	Cervicouterine
	Uterine rupture	neoplasms
	Vasa previa	Lower genital
	with fetal	malignancies
	bleeding	
Moderate	Circumvallate	Vaginal varices
	placenta	
	Marginal sinus	Vaginal lacerations
	rupture	
Low	Cervical mucous	Cervicitis, eversion,
	extrusion	erosion, polyps
	(bloody show)	

death (relative risk 5.4), and *perinatal death* (5-fold increase). If sonography reveals an intrauterine clot, membrane separation, or placenta previa, there is further risk and in these patients, perinatal mortality exceeds 250 per 1000. The etiologies of *second trimester bleeding include: circumvallate placenta, early abruptio placenta, and placenta previa.* Currently, expectant management is the most common treatment option for pregnancies complicated by second trimester bleeding.

Significant vaginal bleeding occurs in 5%–10% of third trimester pregnancies and must be carefully evaluated because *obstetric hemorrhage is the largest cause of maternal morbidity and mortality.* Two of the major causes of late pregnancy hemorrhage (placenta previa and placenta abruption) are associated with cigarette smoking.

Additionally, it is a significant factor in perinatal morbidity and mortality. Most patients have <500 mL bleeding, but *serious hemorrhage >500 mL will occur in 2%–3% of pregnancies.* Overall, multiparas are more commonly affected.

DIAGNOSIS OF THE CAUSE OF BLEEDING

INITIAL EXAMINATION

There are *three principles* of investigation of third trimester hemorrhage.

- Because of the extreme hazard of uncontrollable bleeding with placenta previa, *vaginal or rectal examination must be avoided until that diagnosis can be excluded.*
- All third trimester vaginal bleeding must be investigated in a hospital with the *capability of dealing with maternal hemorrhage and perinatal compromise.*
- *Immediate assessment of blood loss and hemodynamic status guides the earliest stage of therapy.* Recall that the signs and symptoms of hypovolemic shock include pallor with clammy skin, orthostatic hypotension, syncope, thirst, dyspnea, restlessness, agitation, anxiety, confusion, declining blood pressure, tachycardia, and oliguria.

CRITICAL HEMORRHAGE (HEMODYNAMICALLY UNSTABLE PATIENTS)

Antishock therapy must be immediately instituted in all hemodynamically unstable patients. The following is one method of initiating that therapy. The patient is placed in the *Trendelenburg position.* Care is taken that this is not so steep that respiration is compromised. An *adequate airway* is guaranteed by a plastic oral airway, or endotracheal tube. A *large-bore* ($\geq$18 gauge) *IV* is inserted for *crystalloid replacement* (saline or lactated Ringer's solution). Blood is obtained from another vein for *CBC, platelets, fibrinogen, PT and PTT, fibrin split products, type and crossmatch for 4–6 units of whole blood or packed red blood cells.* In severe cases, it may also be necessary to obtain *fresh frozen plasma, platelet packs, electrolytes, and blood gases. The necessity of hemodynamic monitoring is considered.* The *use of vasoactive drugs is weighed.* They are desirable for their pharmacologic effects (e.g., increasing myocardial contractility) or if volume expansion is ineffective. One effective agent is dopamine, 200 mg in 500 mL saline at 2–5 mg/kg/min increasing to 20–50 mg/kg/min.

Once the acute measures are taken, an *indwelling Foley catheter* may be inserted to measure urinary output and obtain details of the acute episode.

Use the *clot fragility observation test* if serial determinations of fibrinogen levels are not immediately available. This is performed by drawing venous blood (2–3 mL) into a clean test tube q 1h. If clot formation fails to occur within 5–10 min or if dissolution of a formed clot follows gentle shaking, a clotting deficiency due primarily to lack of fibrinogen and platelets is likely.

Examination of the abdomen is gently conducted and the fundus measured or the uterine apex marked. The *fetal heart rate* is frequently recorded and *electronic fetal monitoring* initiated. *Uterine tone, fetal presentation, and possible engagement of the presenting part* (engagement largely excludes total placenta previa) *are all observed.* Next, it is decided whether the patient must be taken to *surgery immediately or* if blood transfusions and *stabilization* must be accomplished first.

The patient is readied for surgery (prepare abdomen, obtain informed consent, notify the operating room, anesthesia department, and neonatal–pediatrics). *Frequent vital signs and FHR* (every 2–15 min depending on status) are continued until definitive therapy is accomplished. *Delivery and control of hemorrhage* are accomplished as soon as practical. In postpartum hemorrhage, it is evaluated whether selective arterial embolization, prophylactic uterine, or hypogastric artery ligation will be of assistance. In all cases of hemorrhage, erythropoietin use after the acute episode is considered.

LESS THAN CRITICAL HEMORRHAGE (HEMODYNAMICALLY STABLE PATIENTS)

The patient is placed at *bedrest* and the history of the acute episode obtained. Also, the *obstetric history* is obtained and the patient's *vital signs* ascertained. A *gentle abdominal examination* is conducted and the fundus measured or the uterine apex marked. *Fetal heart rate* is ascertained and *electronic fetal monitoring initiated.* If electronic fetal monitoring is not available, the FHR is frequently recorded. *Uterine tone, uterine irritability, fetal presentation, and the likely station of the presenting part are determined.* A large-bore (≥18 gauge) *IV is started to initiate crystalloid maintenance* replacement (saline or lactated Ringer's solution). Venous blood is obtained for *CBC, platelets, fibrinogen, PT and PTT, fibrin split products, type and crossmatch for 2–4 units of whole blood or packed red blood cells* from another vein. A gentle vaginal examination is considered. Vaginal examination is indicated before ultrasonic examination only if delivery may be imminent, the presenting part is unquestionably engaged, or the patient is in active labor.

If vaginal delivery is not imminent, an *ultrasound examination assists in determination of placental location* (possible placenta previa) *and status* (perhaps abruptio placenta). Additionally, the ultrasound examination should *include assessment of fetal well being, estimation of gestational age,* and *amount and localization of amniotic fluid.* In cases of borderline maturity when a few days delay (if possible) may mean the avoidance of respiratory distress, amniocentesis and subsequent fetal maturity determination may be useful.

At this time, sufficient information has usually been obtained to assist in determining which of the three general management options is most desirable based on the maternal status, fetal status, and probable cause of the bleeding.

- *Immediate delivery is indicated when there is fetal or maternal compromise, or persistent heavy bleeding.*
- *Continued labor is warranted with a mature fetus, active labor (>4 cm), ruptured membranes, bleeding at a controllable rate, or if there are additional complications* making vaginal delivery desirable.
- *Expectant management is possible in almost 90% of cases* because third trimester bleeding will usually subside within 24 h.

By *saving all pads,* a reasonably accurate estimate of blood loss can be made. Generally, the patient is *observed for 24 h.* If bleeding materially decreases or ceases, and she is not near term, she may be transferred for less intensive observation. If placenta previa can be excluded, a gentle cervical visualization and pelvic examination may be performed to assist in ascertaining the cause of bleeding.

ABRUPTIO PLACENTAE (PREMATURE SEPARATION OF THE PLACENTA, ABLATIO PLACENTAE, AND ACCIDENTAL HEMORRHAGE)

DEFINITIONS AND INCIDENCE

Abruptio placenta is defined as *placental separation from a normal implantation site before delivery of the fetus.* It occurs in 1:86 to 1:206 advanced pregnancies, depending on the diagnostic criteria employed, and *is responsible for ~30% of all late antepartal bleeding.* About *50% of abruptions occur before labor, but 10%–15% are*

TABLE 11-2
GRADES OF ABRUPTIO PLACENTAE

Clinical Finding	Grade		
	1	2	3
Vaginal bleeding	Slight	Mild to moderate	Moderate to severe, (but may be concealed)
Uterus	Irritable,	Irritable tetanic	Tetanic, painful
Maternal pulse	Normal	Increased	Elevated
Maternal blood pressure	Normal	Maintained, but postural hypotension	Hypotension to shock
Fetal status	Normal	Fetal compromise (FHR criteria)	Fetal death
Fibrinogen level	Normal	Reduced (150–250 mg%)	<150 mg% and thrombocytopenia or factor depletion
% of total (approximate)	15	20–40	>45

not diagnosed before the second stage of labor. Abruptio placenta may be classified into three groups by clinical and laboratory findings (Table 11-2).

ETIOLOGY AND IMPORTANCE

The exact *cause* of placental separation *is usually unknown,* although there are a number of common associations. A previous placental separation carries a *recurrence rate of 10%–17%;* following two previous separations, the incidence is >20%. The *hypertensive states of pregnancy impose a 2.5%–17.9% incidence* of abruptio placenta. However, of those cases severe enough to *cause fetal demise,* ~50% are associated with hypertensive states of pregnancy (with one half associated with chronic hypertension and one half associated with pregnancy-induced hypertension). Other frequent predispositions to placental separation include *high parity, smoking, uterine over distention* (e.g., multiple pregnancy, hydramnios), *vascular disease* (e.g., diabetes mellitus, collagen disorders), *microangiopathic hemolytic anemia, Factor V Leiden mutation, cocaine usage, and uterine anomalies or tumors.* There are *direct precipitating causes* (in only 1%–5%) of *abruptio placenta, including circumvallate placenta, direct uterine trauma* (e.g., external version, automobile and other accidents), *sudden reduction of amniotic fluid, or short cord.*

DIAGNOSIS

The *symptoms and signs are variable and are largely predicated on the extent of the problem* (Table 11-2). However, the usual symptoms of abruptio placenta are *dark red vaginal bleeding (80%), uterine irritability (two thirds), and lower abdominal or back pain (two thirds).* The erroneous diagnosis of premature labor will be assigned to about 20%. *Fetal compromise* (determined by electronic-fetal heart rate criteria) *is present in >50% of cases.*

Because of the protective factors in healthy gravidas, there may be a considerable acute blood loss before anemia develops. Thus, with abruptio placenta, the amount of blood loss is all too frequently out of proportion to the degree of anemia. A peripheral blood smear may reveal *schistocytes* (suggesting disseminated intravascular coagulation, DIC). *Reduced platelet counts* and *fibrinogen depletion* are common in more severe cases. With DIC, elevated levels of fibrin split products will be present. Thrombomodulin, a marker of endothelial cell damage, has been localized to the placental syncytiotrophoblast. It is a highly sensitive and specific marker for acute placental separation. To date, it has not been of value in detection of those where abruption is imminent.

PATHOLOGY AND PATHOPHYSIOLOGY

Various pathophysiologic mechanisms have been suggested as being operative in abruptio placenta, including *local vascular injury* leading to decidua basalis vessel disruption, an *abrupt rise in uterine venous pressure* leading to intervillous space engorgement and separation, *mechanical factors* (e.g., short cord, trauma, sudden loss of amniotic fluid), and possible *extrinsic initiation of the coagulation cascade* (e.g., trauma with the release of tissue thromboplastin).

Hemorrhage may occur into the decidua basalis or directly retroplacental, from rupture of a spiral artery. In either case, bleeding occurs, a clot forms, and the placental surface cannot provide exchange between mother and placenta. The clot compresses the adjacent placenta, and nonclotted blood courses from the site. In either concealed or external (apparent) bleeding (Fig. 11-1), blood may rupture

FIGURE 11-1. Types of premature separation of the placenta.

(Redrawn from Beck and Rosenthal, *Obstetrical Practice*, 7th ed. Williams & Wilkins, 1957.)

through the membranes or placenta. The latter has grave significance, for it may lead to maternal–fetal hemorrhage, fetomaternal hemorrhage, maternal bleeding into the amniotic fluid, or amniotic fluid embolus. Occasionally, extensive intramyometrial hemorrhage leads to a purplish, ecchymotic, and indurated uterus (uteroplacental apoplexy, Couvelaire uterus) and loss of contractility.

With *severe placental separation there may be DIC.* Clinically, the *hemorrhagic diathesis consists of widespread petechiae, active bleeding, hypovolemic shock, and failure of the clotting mechanisms.* Although not directly observable, *fibrin is being deposited in small capillaries,* resulting in dire complications, for example: renal cortical and tubular necrosis, acute cor pulmonale, and anterior pituitary necrosis (Sheehan's syndrome).

DIFFERENTIAL DIAGNOSIS

- *Nonplacental causes of bleeding.* These usually are nonpainful. Rupture of the uterus may cause vaginal bleeding but, if extensive, is associated with pain, shock, and death of the fetus.
- *Placental causes of bleeding.* Placenta previa is associated with painless hemorrhage and is commonly diagnosed by sonography.
- *Undetermined causes of bleeding.* In at least 20% of cases, the cause of antepartum bleeding cannot be determined. If serious problems can be ruled out, however, undiagnosed bleeding rarely is critical.

TREATMENT

EMERGENCY MEASURES

If deficient, the clotting mechanism must be restored before any attempt is made to deliver the infant. Administer cryoprecipitate, fresh frozen plasma, or fresh blood. Institute antishock therapy. Monitor the fetus continuously. Rupture the membranes, if possible, irrespective of the probable mode of delivery.

SPECIFIC MEASURES

Grade 1. *When the patient is not in labor, watchful expectancy* is indicated, because bleeding ceases spontaneously in many cases. *When labor begins, prepare for vaginal delivery* in the absence of further complications.

Grade 2. *Anticipate vaginal delivery if labor is expected within about 6 h,* especially if the fetus is dead. *Cesarean section should be performed if there is persistent evidence of fetal compromise,* and the infant is likely to survive.

Grade 3. *The patient is always in shock, the fetus has died, the uterus is tetanic, and a coagulation defect may be present.* After correction of the coagulopathy, deliver the patient vaginally if this can be done within about 6 h. Vaginal delivery is probably best for the multiparous patient. *Otherwise, do a cesarean section.*

SURGICAL MEASURES

Cesarean section is indicated when *labor is expected to be of long duration (over 6 h), when hemorrhage does not respond to amniotomy and cautious administration of dilute oxytocin, and when early (not prolonged) fetal compromise is present and the fetus is likely to survive.* Hysterectomy rarely is indicated. Even a Couvelaire uterus will contract, and bleeding will almost always cease when the coagulation defect is corrected.

PROGNOSIS

Worldwide maternal mortality rates are currently between 0.5% and 5%. Most women die of *hemorrhage* (immediate or delayed) or cardiac or renal failure. Early diagnosis and definitive therapy should reduce maternal mortality rates to 0.3%–1%.

Fetal mortality rates range from 50% to 80%. About 30% of patients with premature separation of the placenta are delivered at term. Almost 20% of those with abruptio placenta have no fetal heartbeat on admission to the hospital, and in another 20%, fetal compromise is soon noted. When maternal transfusion is urgently required, the fetal mortality rate will probably be at least 50%. Birth is preterm in 40%–50% of cases of premature separation of the placenta. Infants die of hypoxia, prematurity, or delivery trauma.

PLACENTA PREVIA

Placenta previa occurs when the placenta develops implants low, within the zone of dilatation–effacement of the lower uterine segment. Thus, the placenta precedes the fetus and can block vaginal delivery. *Placenta previa complicates 1:200–1:250 pregnancies* that continue beyond the 28th week. There is a *strong association between previous lower uterine segment cesarean section and subse-*

quent risk of placenta previa. Moreover, the risk increases with the number of previous cesarean sections: one cesarean increases the risk 2.2-fold, two cesareans increase the risk 4.1-fold, and three cesareans increase the risk 22.4-fold. Other *maternal associations of placenta previa include: cigarette smoking, higher gravidity, higher parity, and higher numbers of abortions.*

The types of placenta previa are *complete,* in which the placenta totally covers the internal os (Fig. 11-2); *partial,* where a portion of the internal os is overlaid by the placenta (Fig. 11-3); and *low-lying,* in which the placenta is just above the os but situated where it may deflect or obstruct the presenting part (e.g., over the sacral promontory) (Figs. 11-4 and 11-5).

Painless vaginal bleeding is the presenting complaint in placenta previa. *Breech or an abnormal presentation is common* because the

FIGURE 11-2.   Complete placenta previa.

FIGURE 11-3. Partial placenta previa.

fore-lying placenta alters the usual intrauterine space available. Even a small vertex may not engage.

DIAGNOSIS

No laboratory tests will aid in the diagnosis of placenta previa. Blood studies however, (e.g., Hgb, Hct), should be obtained periodically because of blood loss and the threat of anemia. Approximately *15% of patients require transfusion,* but the vast majority (>80%) of these are postpartum; thus, the *patient should be typed and the determination made that blood is available.* The cross matching and keeping specific blood available for the gravida is necessary in only selected circumstances. X-ray and radioisotope studies to determine the site of the placenta have been abandoned in favor of safer, more accurate *sonography.*

FIGURE 11-4. Normal placenta.

SONOGRAPHY

Sonography is the modality of choice for the diagnosis of placenta previa. False negative reports of placenta previa with sonography in early pregnancy are uncommon. However, there are enough false positives to warrant confirmatory sonography at 26–30 weeks if placenta previa is suspected in mid-pregnancy. Late in pregnancy, it may be difficult to diagnose placenta previa because the presenting part may preclude optimal visualization of the placenta and its relation to the internal cervical os. This can usually be overcome, unless engagement has occurred, by placing the patient in the Trendelenburg position and applying gentle upward traction on the presenting part. Confirmatory sonography may be obtained translabially or in some circumstances, by a gentle low transvaginal approach.

FIGURE 11-5. Low implantation.

If sonography or another means of diagnosis of placenta previa is unavailable, vaginal examination may be required. In this case, arrange a double setup examination, that is, have the operating room readied for cesarean section because even slight penetration or separation of the placenta may cause hemorrhage.

DIFFERENTIAL DIAGNOSIS

Rule out local causes of painless vaginal bleeding, for example, cervical cancer or polyp, by visualization of the cervix, biopsy, or similar means. Caution: Do not do a pelvic examination before sonography has *excluded placenta previa.* Exsanguinating hemorrhage may be induced by vaginal examination of the patient with placenta previa. Even after sonography, penetration of the cervix may be harmful and of no value.

Slight marginal separation of the placenta, impossible to diagnose by sonography or clinically, must be considered, but bleeding probably will cease after bedrest. Because blood loss may be fetal as well as maternal, all gravidas with placenta previa should have a test for fetal blood in the discharge [e.g., APT (potassium hydroxide), Kleihauer-Betke test, identification of nucleated RBC].

COMPLICATIONS

MATERNAL

Hemorrhage and shock may follow ill-conceived examination in lieu of sonography. Slight premature separation of the portion of the placenta over the os probably occurs in most cases. Localized placentitis may develop here also. Uterine sepsis before delivery is rare, but postpartum endometritis often complicates placenta previa.

FETAL

Preterm delivery occurs in 46%–60% of infants of mothers with placenta previa and is the prime cause of neonatal complications. Other major fetal and neonatal complications of placenta previa are *major congenital anomalies* (odds ratio 2.48), *respiratory distress syndrome* (odds ratio 4.94), and *anemia* (odds ratio 2.65). In addition to early or chronic blood loss, acute fetal bleeding may occur during cesarean section when an anterior placenta previa is torn. Entry below or above the placenta, as indicated by sonography, should minimize the risk. However, the fetal blood loss is directly proportional to the time lapse between laceration of a cotyledon(s) and clamping of the cord. For reasons yet to be determined, there is a strong association between placenta previa and male gender at birth.

TREATMENT

Usually, *brief hospitalization and expectant management* are essential because most gravidas are preterm and bedrest alone will be accompanied by cessation of bleeding within 24 h. The patient or her fetus *almost never die during the first occurrence of bleeding* (assuming no pelvic examination). *Monitor the fetus carefully.* Asymptomatic patients with placenta previa diagnosed by 32 weeks, with a Hgb >11 gm/dL may be offered *autologous blood donation*. Recently, *tocolysis* (in very well-controlled investigational circumstances) has been reported to be safe and to prolong pregnancy in selected cases of symptomatic placenta previa. *Cervical cerclage* (to decrease bleeding associated with cervical dilatation and effacement) has been reported to be of value and not to be of value in the recent literature. Subsequent bleeding episodes may require continued hospitalization.

However, selected patients may receive outpatient management. *Both inpatient and outpatient management have the goal of delaying delivery.* Delivery should be delayed, if possible, to ensure increased fetal maturity. If sonography was performed before the 30th week, it should be repeated by the 32nd week to determine the placental site, fetal age, and growth.

With *rupture of the membranes, labor, or if heavy bleeding* occurs, *expeditious delivery by the safest means* will be necessary. This is necessary regardless of fetal status. Most primigravidas with placenta previa should be delivered by cesarean section. Some multiparas with partial or low-lying placenta previa can be delivered safely from below unless hemorrhage is marked. *Electronic fetal monitoring* should be employed in all labors involving placenta previa.

PROGNOSIS

Clinical outcomes of placenta previa are variable and cannot be predicted from antenatal events. However, several generalizations may be useful. *Over 70% of patients with placenta previa will have at least one episode of bleeding.* There is no difference in the grade of previa between those bleeding and those who do not bleed. There are no known antecedents to predict who will experience bleeding; however, *bleeding results in both earlier diagnosis (usually >4 weeks) and delivery (usually >1 week).* Emergency cesarean is more common (by a factor of almost 2) in women with bleeding.

FOR THE MOTHER

With proper management, the maternal prognosis in placenta previa is good. With sonography and expectant therapy, the *maternal mortality in the United States has dropped from >1% to <0.2%.*

FOR THE INFANT

The perinatal mortality rate associated with placenta previa in many hospitals in the United States before expectant treatment was approximately 15%, or more than 10 times that of normal term pregnancy. This has dropped, and the rate probably can be reduced to *<10% with current management.*

PLACENTA ACCRETA

When the *placenta directly adheres to, penetrates into, or entirely traverses the myometrium,* it is termed placenta accreta. This condition occurs when trophoblasts come into direct contact with the myometrium. This implies either overly invasive trophoblastic tissue or an *absence of the usual layer of decidua and Nitabuch's layer separating placenta from myometrium.* Placenta accreta may be subclassified according to the depth of trophoblastic penetration as well as the amount of placenta involved in the abnormal process. *Placenta accreta vera (~80% of cases)* is when the villi adhere to the superficial myometrium. *Placenta increta (~15% of cases)* is the term for villus penetration into the myometrium. With *placenta percreta* the villi penetrate the full thickness of the myometrium. Focal, partial, or total adherence refers to whether a single cotyledon, several cotyledons, or the entire placenta is involved.

The incidence (all classifications) of placenta accreta is *1/2000–7000 deliveries.* Unfortunately, placenta accreta, like placenta previa, is *increasing in direct proportion to the increase in cesarean section.* Indeed, prior cesarean section patients with antepartally diagnosed placenta previa should be considered at high risk for placenta accreta. Other clinical associations include *grand multiparity, previous uterine curettage, and previously treated Asherman's syndrome* (the latter leads to an 8% incidence). Additionally, *recurrence of placenta accreta is common.*

Placenta accreta *rarely causes antepartum complications,* although if the placenta invades adjacent organs (e.g., bladder), there is the potential for hemorrhage as a presenting sign. Placenta accreta of any extent increases the incidence of *postpartum hemorrhage and the potential for hemorrhagic shock.* The diagnosis is suggested by delayed *spontaneous separation of the placenta, retained portions of placenta, and difficulty in establishing a cleavage plane* during manual removal of the placenta. Persistent efforts to manually remove a placenta accreta are futile and increase blood loss.

Treatment should begin with fluid and blood replacement, for *90% of patients with placenta accreta lose >3,000 mL.* Evaluation of puerperal hemorrhage should be performed as outlined previously. Usually, placenta accreta of any extent, particularly if associated with placenta previa, requires hysterectomy. Invasion of adjacent organs may necessitate resection of the areas involved if there is active bleeding. *Conservative treatment* of placenta accreta (including involvement of other organs) is gaining favor for the hemodynamically stable patient. The placenta is left in situ and will later slough. The resolution process may be enhanced by utilization of methotrexate or selective arterial embolization.

PUERPERAL SEPSIS.

Any infection in the genital tract that occurs as a complication of abortion, labor, or delivery is termed puerperal sepsis (see also Shock, p. 345). Streptococci, staphylococci, *Clostridia,* coliform bacteria, and *Bacteroides* are the pathogens most often identified. Although the *group A streptococcus (beta-hemolytic)* may cause a variety of infections, it has recently been identified in *severe invasive infections, circulatory insufficiency, and multiple organ failure.* With the latter two circumstances, this is termed the streptococcal toxic shock-like syndrome. This is likely a variant of the systemic inflammatory response syndrome and multiple organ dysfunction syndromes (American College of Chest Physicians/Society of Critical Care Medicine, 1992).

Cellulitis resulting from vaginal or cervical lacerations may be the site of infection. *Incisions* may be the focus of infection (cesarean or episiotomy), as the *endometrium* (particularly when endometritis occurs in the zone of placental attachment—the equivalent of a large surface wound). *Debility* (anemia, undernutrition), *serious systemic disorders, premature or prolonged rupture of the membranes, protracted labor, and traumatic examinations or delivery predispose to puerperal infection.* A few cases of fulminant group A streptococcal infections have occurred in late pregnancy (prior to delivery), preceeded only by an episode of upper respiratory infection. This is followed by septicemia, acute myometritis, shock, and multiorgan failure. The maternal and fetal prognosis is very poor.

The incidence of puerperal sepsis in hospitals in the United States is at least 5%. Puerperal sepsis is exceeded only by hemorrhage and preeclampsia–eclampsia as a cause of maternal death in this country.

CLINICAL FINDINGS

Many genital tract infections are so mild as to cause few or slight symptoms. Others are violent, fulminating, and fatal within a short time.

SYMPTOMS AND SIGNS

Malaise, headache, anorexia, and remittent slight elevations in temperature and pulse generally begin 3–4 days after delivery. Vague discomfort in the perineum or lower abdomen and nausea and vomiting may follow. High fever (childbed fever), rapid pulse, ileus, and localization of pain and tenderness in the pelvis may be observed during the next 1–2 days. The lochia may become foul and profuse. Bacteremic shock may occur.

If improvement does not follow after 48–72 h of antibiotic therapy, reexamine the patient; an abscess may be forming. If the infection is related to septic endomyometritis and postpartum ovarian vein thrombosis and does not respond to appropriate antibiotics and intravenous heparin, surgical intervention (total abdominal hysterectomy, bilateral salpingo-oopherectomy, and ovarian vein removal) may be necessary. In cases of the streptococcal toxic shock-like syndrome, additional features may include sore throat, diarrhea, muscle aches (all limbs), edema, and macular and vesicular erythrodemia (especially of the trunk).

LABORATORY FINDINGS

Polymorphonuclear leukocytosis and an increased sedimentation rate indicate infection. Identification of pathogens from cervical and uterine lochia by culture and sensitivity tests will require 36–48 h. In fulminant infections, there may be *disseminated intravascular coagulation as well as increased C-reactive protein, creatine kinase, creatinine, and urea.*

IMAGING

X-ray studies are not helpful except to exclude gastrointestinal, urinary, or pulmonary problems.

COMPLICATIONS AND SEQUELAE

Genital tract infections commonly progress to *peritonitis, pelvic cellulitis, pelvic thrombophlebitis* (including ovarian vein thrombosis), *abscess formation, septicemia, pulmonary embolism, septic shock, and death.*

DIFFERENTIAL DIAGNOSIS

Febrile complications of the puerperium unrelated to genital tract infection include *mastitis, urinary infection, respiratory infection, and enteritis,* in that order of frequency.

PREVENTION

Avoidance of puerperal sepsis requires aseptic technique during manual examination and delivery. Obstetric trauma should be minimized because traumatized tissues are susceptible to infection.

TREATMENT

EMERGENCY MEASURES

Patients with puerperal sepsis are *treated for septic shock* (see p. 350).

GENERAL MEASURES

Placing the patient in the *semi-Fowler position* allows any free pus in the peritoneal cavity to collect in the pelvis. *IV fluids* are administered to maintain electrolyte and fluid balance. If the patient is able to maintain oral intake, it is commonly initially limited to clear liquids. Analgesics, sedative-hypnotic drugs, oxytocics, or laxatives are administered, as required.

SPECIFIC MEASURES

Initially, *antibiotics are administered in large doses.* One starting antibiotic regimen is ampicillin (2 g IV every 6 h), gentamicin (2 mg/kg IV loading dose), and clindamycin (900 mg IV every 8 h). The maintenance dose of gentamicin is 1.5 mg/kg every 8 h, but peak and trough levels should be monitored. When the results of culture and sensitivity studies are known, therapy is continued with the antibiotic of choice in large and repeated doses. In cases of group A streptococcus, penicillin G and tobramycin have been recommended. For treatment of disseminated intravascular coagulation (DIC), see p. 348.

SURGICAL MEASURES

Hysterectomy is indicated for serious puerperal infections (e.g., intractable myometritis, a postabortal uterine abscess, infected hydatidiform mole, or myoma). *Clipping or ligation of the vena cava and ovarian veins may be life saving in case of repeated* (often septic) *pulmonary embolization.* Pelvic drainage may be necessary. Abscesses may require surgical drainage.

PROGNOSIS

The *maternal mortality rate* due to puerperal sepsis in the United States is *about 0.2%,* but in some areas of the world, the mortality rate is vastly greater. The morbidity of severe sepsis is related to the *multiple organ dysfunction syndrome* manifest by disseminated intravascular coagulopathy, respiratory insufficiency, hypotension, cardiac insufficiency, and renal insufficiency. Later sequelae may include encephalopathy, cardiomyopathy, pulmonary hypertension, and peripheral neuropathy. The *acute renal failure is usually due to acute cortical necrosis (>80%),* but in some, there is tubular necrosis.

SHOCK

Shock is a syndrome characterized by prostration and hypotension due to diminished circulating blood volume to the point of failure of perfusion of the vital organs.

CLASSIFICATION

The shock syndromes encountered in obstetrics and gynecology may be classified clinically as follows:

- *Hypovolemic shock* follows hemorrhage, trauma, and dehydration. It is characterized by an absolute or relative decrease in blood volume.
- *Septic shock* most frequently occurs following bacteremia due to gram-negative organisms and their endotoxins.
- *Toxic shock* (see p. 581) is often caused by an exotoxin produced by some coagulase-positive strains of *Staphylococcus aureus.* It is seen most often in menstruating women who use tampons and is characterized by headache, vomiting, diarrhea, fever, rash, and hypotension.
- *Vascular obstructive shock* may occur as a result of blockage of major blood vessels by amniotic fluid, air, or blood clots. Supine hypotension in obstetric patients may be a contributing factor.
- *Neurogenic shock,* as seen in simple fainting, spinal anesthesia, and central nervous system injury, is usually associated with peripheral vasodilation.
- *Anaphylactic shock* produces marked vasodilatation with relative hypovolemia. This may be due to allergy to medications, sera, or other sensitizing agents.

- *Drug shock* may follow excessive administration of hypnotic drugs, anesthetics, vasodilators, vasoconstrictors, and other drugs.
- *Cardiogenic shock* may result from acute diminution of cardiac output and usually is associated with varying degrees of vasoconstriction (e.g., myocardial infarction, heart failure, paroxysmal tachycardia, myocardial depressant drugs).
- *Metabolic shock* occurs mainly in hypoadrenocorticism. Fluid, electrolyte, and other chemical abnormalities in diabetic acidosis and in acute pulmonary hepatic or renal insufficiency may impair cardiovascular mechanisms and lead to metabolic shock.

CLINICAL FINDINGS

IMPENDING SHOCK

A variable period of *intense sympathetic activity* generally precedes hypotension. Weakness, pallor, cool, moist skin, orthostatic hypotension and tachycardia develop. (Caution: Do not confuse with simple fainting.) Fever and shaking chills precede collapse in septic shock. Marked orthopnea, arrhythmia, and severe chest pain are warning signs or cardiogenic shock.

ESTABLISHED SHOCK

Hypotension (systolic pressure <100 mm Hg) is superimposed on the early signs of impending shock, and *tachycardia* (>100) usually develops. *Thirst, air hunger, severe prostration, and dulling of the sensorium are advanced signs. Coma, cardiac arrest, and death are imminent at this point.*

SEPTIC SHOCK

Chills, high fever, tachycardia, anorexia, and occasional nausea and vomiting are often preceded by a history of infected abortion, traumatic delivery, or recurrent pyelonephritis. Between *3 and 9 h after the first shaking chill, a precipitous drop in body temperature to subnormal levels often heralds shock.* (Also see p. 350.)

TREATMENT

Shock is an *acute emergency that takes precedence* over all other problems except acute hemorrhage, cardiac arrest, and respiratory failure. To act effective, the *primary cause* of shock must be determined promptly. A brief history (if available) and the gross physical findings often permit the differentiation of hemorrhagic, cardiogenic, septic, and allergic shock. Except in neurogenic shock due to fainting—a self-limiting condition treated by placing the patient in the recumbent position and administering stimulant—proceeding with antishock measures may be lifesaving. Additional therapy may be required for specific problems.

GENERAL MEASURES

Place the Patient in the Recumbent Position
The Trendelenburg position is best avoided because it may interfere with breathing. In some cases, military antishock trousers (MAST suit), if available, may be useful.

**Establish an Adequate Airway and Ensure
Pulmonary Ventilation**
Oxygen by nasal catheter, mask, or endotracheal tube is administered as required, especially when *dyspnea or cyanosis* is present.

Keep the Patient Comfortably Warm
This is best accomplished with blankets because external heat will cause peripheral vasodilatation.

Control Pain and Relieve Apprehension
Shock patients often have very little discomfort. A sedative, such as pentobarbital sodium, 100 mg IV, may be given. (Caution: Narcotics are contraindicated for patients in coma, those with head injuries or respiratory depression, and pregnant women who are likely to deliver within 1–2 h.) *Care must be taken to avoid overdosage of all drugs. Shock materially alters pharmacokinetics, generally resulting in less clearance, higher levels, and longer therapeutic effect.*

FLUID REPLACEMENT

If superficial veins have collapsed, puncture a large vein (e.g., femoral vein) for temporary infusion before cutdown or perform percutaneous canalization of a major vessel, such as the jugular vein, for infusion and another for monitoring. The latter procedure also provides a direct route for therapy to the heart in cases of extreme blood loss, septic shock, or serious electrolyte imbalance.

Restore Adequate Blood Volume Immediately!

Whole Blood

The most effective replacement fluid for blood loss is usually whole blood, especially if the hematocrit is <35%. Whole blood must be correctly grouped and crossmatched for possible transfusion. Treatment in cases of shock may require 4–5 liters of whole blood delivered under pressure in 30 min to restore CVP to 10–13 cm H_2O. Use large needles and multiple infusions if transfusion is needed urgently.

Plasma

Plasma, serum albumin, and Plasmanate (a reconstituted blood product) are particularly valuable for the treatment of plasma loss. *Posttransfusion hepatitis* may occur in patients receiving pooled plasma; the risk is *about 10%*.

Plasma Expanders

Dextran 40 (Rheomacrodex) is a low-molecular-weight dextran that is superior to other dextrans in reducing the viscosity of the blood and maintaining the microcirculation. Administer 1–1.5 g/kg in 10% solution in normal saline IV at a rate of 20–40 mL/min, but do not give more than required to sustain the blood pressure at 85–90 mm Hg. (Caution: Patients with cardiac or renal disease may develop pulmonary edema.) Because dextrans interfere with blood typing, blood samples should be obtained before dextran is administered. Dextrans can impair blood coagulation mechanisms and may cause infrequent but serious anaphylactoid reactions.

Saline and Dextrose Solutions

Lactated Ringer's solution, is the crystalloid of choice, normal saline solution or 5% dextrose may be used as initial therapy or to provide water and electrolytes. The amount necessary to correct acidosis is determined by the blood pH (normal 7.35–7.45) or serum or plasma P_{CO_2} (normal 24–29 mEq/L). Serial determinations of these values should guide correction.

Adjustment of Acid–Base Balance

Restore serum sodium, calcium, chloride, etc. to normal values, using periodic blood chemistry determinations as a guide.

Pure Component Therapy

Some now recommend that hemorrhagic shock be treated by *pure component therapy*. This includes: adequate volume resuscitation with *crystalloids and colloids* and the utilization of *plasma-poor red cells.* With this therapy, plasma content is minimal; thus, deficits of plasma and *coagulation factors develop earlier than with whole blood and packed red blood cells.* Characteristically, *hypofibrinogenemia develops first followed by other coagulation factor deficits* and later by *thrombocytopenia.* The plasma and coagulation factors are treated primarily with *fresh frozen plasma* whereas *platelet replacement is guided by repeated platelet counts.*

VASOACTIVE DRUGS

Vasopressors have *almost no place in resuscitation* if the patient is *in shock.* The *exception is cardiogenic shock,* where a brief use of pressor drugs may increase myocardial contractility and thus improve cardiac function.

The vasoactive drugs should not be considered primary therapy in shock. Volume replacement, correction of hypoxia and fluid and electolyte imbalance, and a search for treatable causes should come first. Unless volume replacement is adequate, the administration of vasodilators may result in prompt failure of the circulation due to a fall in blood pressure and circulatory collapse. Vasodilators are never indicated until the vascular volume has been restored to normal and the CVP is in the high normal range. At that point, use of drugs that dilate the peripheral vasculature may decrease vascular resistance and, thus, decrease the work of the heart and improve cardiac output and tissue perfusion.

The drug of choice for *cardiac resuscitation has been isoproterenol (Isuprel).* This drug has two modes of action. It stimulates myocardial contractility and simultaneously lowers peripheral resistance. Give 1–2 mg in 500 mL of lactated Ringer's solution IV at a rate that produces optimal circulatory benefit. Because of its inotropic effect, an increased incidence of cardiac arrhythmias precludes its use if the heart rate exceeds 120/min.

CORTICOSTEROIDS

Corticosteroids *may be beneficial in shock* because they support the patient in a serious stress state, aid in the transfer of fluids from intracellular to extracellular compartments, and, in septic shock, block intense sympathomimetic effects of endotoxin and restore vascular tone. They also have a beneficial antiallergic effect.

TREATMENT OF SPECIFIC
TYPES OF SHOCK

CARDIOGENIC SHOCK

The treatment of cardiogenic shock includes: *Conversion of arrhythmias, the use of digitalis to correct myocardial insufficiency, the relief of cardiac tamponade, and, potentially, the administration of adrenergic drugs.*

ANAPHYLACTIC SHOCK

Epinephrine, 1:1000 solution, 0.1–0.4 mL in 10 mL of normal saline solution slowly IV is usually the first medication. Diphenhydramine hydrochloride or tripelennamine hydrochloride, 10–20 mg may be administered IV, if the response to epinephrine is not prompt and sustained. Hydrocortisone sodium succinate (Solu-Cortef), 100–250 mg IV over a period of 30 sec, may be used as an adjunct to epinephrine and diphenhydramine. The dosage depends on the severity of the condition. The drug may be repeated at increasing intervals (1,3,6,10 h, and so on) as indicated by the clinical condition. Aminophylline, 0.25–0.5 g in 10–20 mL of normal saline is administered slowly IV for severe bronchial spasm. The duration of action is 1–3 h, after which the drug may be repeated.

HYPOVOLEMIC SHOCK

The usual steps in treating hypovolemic shock include; volume replacement, correction of hypoxia, treatment of fluid and electrolyte balance, and seeking treatable causes. Treatment is monitored as discussed on pages 347–348.

SEPTIC SHOCK

Septic shock associated with pregnancy is most often caused by septic abortion, postpartum infections, pyelonephritis, peritonitis, ruptured viscus, and septic thrombophlebitis. During pregnancy, treat septic shock with antibiotics and volume infusion.

In most types of shock, initial volume infusion is accomplished with 2 liters of lactated Ringer's solution. If the systolic blood pressure remains <80 mm Hg, a pulmonary artery catheter should be inserted and volume expansion continued until the pulmonary capillary wedge pressure (PCWP) is ≥14–16 mm Hg. Should the blood pressure fail to respond to volume expansion and if the left ventricular function curve is depressed, begin inotropic therapy with dopamine and digoxin. If there is no improvement in left ventricular function curve, add dobutamine or isoproterenol or both. If the blood pressure fails to respond to this treatment (systolic ≤ 80 mm Hg) and the systemic vascular resistance index is ≤ 1500 dynes/sec/cm^{-5}/M^2, phenylephrine may be initiated. If this fails, norepinephrine may be used. Electrolyte imbalances must be corrected, and administration of *oxygen may be useful.* If the site of infection is not known, studies are initiated to determine the source.

EVALUATION OF ANTISHOCK THERAPY

Patients are usually *observed continuously for clinical and laboratory signs of responses to therapy.* Characteristically, tachycardia subsides, and the skin becomes warm and dry as blood pressure rises above 100 mm Hg. Blood pressure, pulse rate, and respiratory rate are usually determined every 15 min. Fluid intake and output charts, noting time and amount of replacement fluid given and measuring urine output every 30 min are routinely maintained. Acute renal failure often is a sequela to deep, unresponsive, or prolonged shock. The PCWP response, especially to initial rapid infusion or transfusion, is useful as a guide both to diagnosis and to subsequent treatment. *The goal is to rapidly achieve and maintain a normal PCWP with avoidance of both underreplacement or overreplacement of fluids.* The heart is minimally evaluated by periodic auscultation of the chest for arrhythmia, rales, muffled tones (cardiac tamponade), or murmurs. An ECG and appropriate medical consultation are obtained in severe cases.

PROGNOSIS

This decade has witnessed *significant advances in management of all forms of shock.* Examples of practical steps taken include the establishment of massive transfusion protocols, more precise component therapy, and detailing endpoints to transfusion. Generalizations are of limited usefulness, but *approximately one half of all trauma and hemorrhagic shock patients survive.* Among those surviving >24 h, more than a third will develop life-threatening infections and one quarter will develop multiple organ failure. Current research into the pathophysiologic mechanisms, including immunological alterations, should provide insights that will enhance therapeutic approaches. Further two types of artificial oxygen carriers are being experimentally and clinically investigated.

COMPLICATIONS OF LABOR

PRETERM OR PREMATURE LABOR

About 7% (6.9%–10.0%) of infants born in the United States *are preterm* (i.e., <37 weeks gestational age). These may or may not be small-for-dates. Preterm labor may be associated with many disorders or diseases (Table 11-3).

Premature delivery is one of the most urgent problems in medicine. The *death rate of the low-birthweight neonate is about*

TABLE 11-3
CONDITIONS ASSOCIATED WITH PREMATURE LABOR

Primary risk factors
  Multiple gestation (associated with 17% of preterm
    births)
  Chorioamnionitis
  Previous preterm births
  Uterine or cervical anomalies
  Placenta previa
  Abruptio placentae
  Intrauterine growth retardation
  Premature rupture of the membranes
  Hydramnios
  Genetic anomalies
  Congenital malformations
  Genital infections (e.g., Bacterial vaginosis, gonorrhea,
    chylamydia)

Secondary risk factors
  Adolescent pregnancy (younger maternal age)
  Previous pregnancy
  Multiple induced abortions
  Cervical or uterine laceration
  Onset of pregnancy within four months of prior
    delivery

Current or previous pregnancy
  Chronic hypertension
  Severe pregnancy-induced hypertension

TABLE 11-3
(*Continued*)

Current pregnancy
  Malnutrition
  Severe anemia
  Inadequate weight gain during pregnancy (particularly
    when coupled with low prepregnancy body mass)
  Pulmonary or systemic hypertension
  Renal disease
  Heart disease
  Substance abuse
    Heavy cigarette smoking (may contribute to 11% of
      preterm births)
    Alcohol abuse
    Drug abuse
  Peritoneal irritation
    Adnexal torsion or leaking cysts
    Perforated peptic ulcer
    Appendicitis
    Intraabdominal procedures
  Trauma or burns
  Infections (for example)
    Pyelonephritis
    Acute systemic infections
    Fetotoxic infections
  Severe violence or abuse
  Gravida having been preterm at birth

40 times that of full-sized infants born at term. Moreover, the association of *cerebral palsy* with preterm delivery may be as high as *10 times and mental deficiency 5 times that of the term neonate.* Visual and hearing deficits, emotional disturbances, and social maladjustments of prematures far exceed those of mature infants.

Continuation of fetal development, in the absence of contraindications, may be imperative. For example, pulmonary maturation of a fetus of 24–25 weeks gestational age is so incomplete that the infant has a high chance of dying of respiratory distress syndrome or complications of prematurity. If the otherwise normal fetus is carried to 33 weeks in utero, however, it is most likely to survive.

CLINICAL DEFINITION OF PREMATURE LABOR

The clinical definition of premature labor involves four criteria.

- A gestation of >20 weeks but <37 weeks
- Regular, painful uterine contractions occurring at least twice every 10 min for at least 30 min
- Demonstrated cervical effacement or dilatation (those at 80% effacement and >1 cm dilatation are at particular risk for both preterm labor and rupture of the membranes)
- Intact membranes (ruptured membranes highly associated with delivery in <1 week)

Other symptoms may include *vaginal bleeding, increased vaginal discharge, and vaginal pressure.* Necessary assessments include *ascertaining that the maternal health will tolerate therapy, that the membranes have not ruptured, that the fetus is truly premature, that fetal compromise is not occurring, and that there is not an abnormal fetal presentation* (as so frequently occurs with the premature infant).

The laboratory studies include blood for *CBC with differential, C-reactive protein, serum electrolytes, and glucose, urine for analysis and culture and sensitivity, and ultrasonography for fetal size, position, anatomy, and placental location.* Amniocentesis may be necessary in borderline cases to determine fetal maturity (LS, Pg, or RST) or to check for fetal infection (bacteria on microscopic analysis). Checking for infection is particularly important, because *7%–26% of premature labors have intrauterine infection.*

The following protocol is extremely helpful in management of these patients.

MANAGEMENT

Observation

- *Observation* is conducted for 30–60 min with electronic fetal monitoring.
- *Confirmation* that the gestational age <37 weeks may require sonography.
- *Examination and tests are performed to rule out any contraindication to sedation-hydration therapy* (Table 11-4). This is very important for suppression of labor is indicated in only ~25% of cases, whereas the remaining 75% have either contraindications or do not require tocolysis.

TABLE 11-4
RELATIVE CONTRAINDICATIONS TO LABOR SUPPRESSION

Mature fetus
Probable lethal fetal defects
Fetal death
Fetal compromise (including that occurring with tocolysis)
Chorioamnionitis
Ruptured membranes
Bulging membranes
Cervical dilation of >4 cm and effacement >80%
Polyhydramnios
Erythroblastosis fetalis
Severe intrauterine growth retardation
Severe pregnancy-induced hypertension
Maternal pulmonary or cardiac disease (e.g., pulmonary edema, adult respiratory distress syndrome, cardiac failure)
Maternal hemorrhage (e.g., placenta previa, abruptio placentae, DIC)

First Decisions
Decisions regarding the next step in management are based on criteria in Table 11-5.

Sedation and Hydration
Morphine sulfate 8–12 mg IM (provided there are no allergies, delivery is not imminent, and Narcan is available), may be used for sedation. *Hydration is achieved by giving 500 mL 5% dextrose in 0.5 normal saline* (or lactated Ringer's solution 5% dextrose) IV over 30 min. Observation of the patient is continued for 1 h, with continuous fetal monitoring.

Second Decisions
At the end of 1 h, decisions are made into which of three therapy categories the patient is placed.

- *Cervical effacement and dilatation are progressing.* Proceed to first-line tocolytics. Generally, this is only a small percentage of patients.

TABLE 11-5
DIAGNOSIS AND MANAGEMENT OF PRETERM
LABOR BASED ON OBSERVATION OF UTERINE
CONTRACTIONS AND CERVICAL CHANGE

Uterine Contractions	Cervical Effacement and Dilatation	Diagnosis	Management
No	No	No labor	None
Yes	No	Premature labor	Hydration and sedation
No	Yes	Incompetent cervix	Bed rest, cerclage
Yes	Yes	Premature labor	Tocolytic protocol

- *There is no cervical change, but uterine contractions continue.* This group should also be placed on first-line tocolytics. This group is usually less than half of the patients, and even if suppression is currently successful, they still have a risk of subsequent labor and delivery.
- *Uterine contractions cease and there is no cervical change.* Observation should continue for 6–12 h. More than half of patients will be in this group, and here, too, there is a continued risk of labor and delivery, but the majority of these patients may be monitored by an outpatient regimen.

Tocolytics

Before initiating tocolytic drugs *several evaluations are useful.* This includes, serial measurement of blood pressure and pulse rate, a baseline ECG, establishing a record of fluid intake and output, and continuous FHR monitoring.

Magnesium sulfate, the safest tocolytic, may be given in a 4–6 g bolus IV over 10 min, followed by an IV infusion of 2 g/h for 6–8 h. Additional fluids should be given by mouth. Monitor vital signs and ECG closely (q30–60 min), and closely watch the deep tendon reflexes and urinary output. Diminution or absence of either indicates the possibility of overdosage. With this program, other serious adverse effects of magnesium administration, (e.g., hypotension, sinoatrial or atrioventricular block, or cardiac arrest) are exceptional. However, each time blood is drawn for a magnesium level (q6h), a calcium level also should be determined to ascertain that acute hypocalcemia has not occurred. The fetus should be minimally affected by this regimen. *Calcium is the antidote for magnesium overdosage and should be administered IV (10 ml of a 10% calcium solution) if magnesium overdosage occurs.*

Ritodrine is a more effective tocolytic than magnesium sulfate and is FDA approved for tocolysis. Prepare ritodrine by dissolving 150 mg in 5% dextrose water. This IV solution will yield 0.3 mg/mL. Begin with 0.1 mg/min, gradually increasing by 0.05 mg/min every 10 min until satisfactory uterine inhibition has been achieved. The maximum IV dosage, established mainly by tachycardia, is about 400 mg/min. Ritodrine IV should be continued at effective dosage for at least 2 h after cessation of contractions. Then, it should be slowly reduced over 1–2 h. The maintenance dose of ritodrine is 20–30 mg orally bid, for weeks if necessary.

Adverse reactions, all dose-related, include hyperglycemia, hypoinsulinemia, and hyperkalemia. Pulmonary edema may occur if ritodrine is given IV in saline solution, especially with excessive drug dosage or prolonged treatment, or when over-hydration occurs or in the presence of infection. Unpleasant cardiovascular, gastrointestinal, or neurologic side affects must be expected, but these usually are mild. Fetal tachycardia may occur with any beta-adrenergic drug therapy. With proper selection of patients, correct dosage, and cautiously maintained tocolysis, however, there should be no harm to the infant. *The use of oral or subcutaneous terbutaline has not been cleared for tocolysis by the FDA, but has been widely used in clinical practice.*

PREVENTION

Predicting preterm labor has been attempted using risk scoring systems, home uterine activity monitoring, cervical assessment, and biochemical methods. Risk scoring systems have not proven effective. Consensus regarding usefulness of home uterine activity monitoring is lacking. Transvaginal ultrasound cervical assessment, although promising, requires additional study. A variety of biochemical methods are currently aimed at detection of those at particular risk for preterm labor so that special care may be administered and preterm delivery prevented. Foremost among these tests is fetal fibronectin (determined from cervicovaginal smear). Indeed, a positive *fetal fibronectin* in the late second and early third trimester appear an important risk factor for preterm labor in asymptomatic women with either singleton or multiple gestations. Additionally, there is recent interest in estriol (salivary) as a means of detecting those at risk. Given the heterogeneous, interactive, pathogenesis of preterm labor, it is likely that multiple biochemical markers will be necessary to detect the process with reasonable sensitivity and specificity.

USE OF CORTICOSTEROIDS

Overall, >80% of women in preterm labor and >50% of those presenting with >4 cm cervical dilation will deliver >48 h after presentation. Thus, *there is ample opportunity for the majority of women in preterm labor with intact membranes to receive a complete course of corticosteroid therapy.*

Antenatal administration of corticosteroids has proven of benefit to the preterm neonate. Specifically, accelerated lung maturation occurs with physiologic stress levels of corticosteroids. Clinically, between 24–34 weeks gestation antenatal corticosteroids reduce the risk of: respiratory distress syndrome (RDS), intraventricular hemorrhage (IVH), and mortality. Importantly, this increased survival is not accompanied by an increase in medical morbidity, and has resulted in reduced medical costs of care for these risk neonates.

The mechanism(s) of other beneficial effects are currently less well understood. These effects include: fewer patent ductus arterioses requiring treatment, a lower rate of necrotizing enterocolitis, fewer low Apgar scores in newborns <1000 g, less need for blood pressure support in extremely premature infants, and protection against the development of retinopathy of prematurity (ROP) as well as against severe forms of ROP. Finally, in pregnancies with umbilical-artery absent end-diastolic flow, betamethasone treatment is associated with decreased placental vascular resistance. Although the beneficial or harmful fetal effect of the latter currently remains unknown, this may prove a valuable tool in these very compromised fetuses.

Current clinical applications generally follow the recommendation of an NIH Consensus Statement (Effect of corticosteroids for fetal maturation on perinatal outcomes. *NIH Consensus Statement.* 1994, Feb 28–Mar 2:12(2)1–24) paraphrased as follows:

- *All fetuses between 24–34 weeks' gestation at risk of preterm delivery should be considered candidates for antenatal treatment with corticosteroids* unless there is evidence that corticosteroids will have an adverse effect on the mother or delivery is imminent.
- *Treatment consists of betamethasone, two doses of 12 mg IM 24 h apart.* An alternative is dexamethasone, four 6 mg doses IM 12 h apart.

- *Optimal benefit begins 24 hours after initiation of therapy* and lasts 7 d. Because treatment for <24 h is still associated with some beneficial effects, corticosteroids should be given unless immediate delivery is anticipated.
- *Neonatal benefits occur from 24 h to 7 d* after initiation of therapy.
- *With preterm premature rupture of the membranes* (PPROM), *corticosteroid therapy is appropriate in fetuses of <30–32 weeks in absence of chorioamnionitis.*

Despite the last statement, one of the most controversial areas is the utilization of corticosteroids with PPROM. This utilization has been said to be based on extrapolation, but the benefit of a small decrease in severe IVH outweighs the potential harm of a large increase in the rate of neonatal sepsis. Additionally, although corticosteroid use in PPROM has been the subject of numerous publications since the NIH Consensus statement, definitive information has not been forthcoming. However, several important observations bear on the specific issue of corticosteroid use in PPROM.

Betamethasone does not alter CRP level or impede leukocyte response to infection; thus, standard tests to determine intrauterine infection may be employed.

Ampicillin-sulbactam *prophylaxis in combination with corticosteroids in PPROM significantly lowers the total frequency of neonatal mortality, sepsis, and RDS.* Additionally, antibiotic prophylaxis and antenatal corticosteroids extends pregnancy (as measured by increased birth weight) compared to steroids alone. Corticosteroids with preterm rupture of membranes is of no apparent benefit to neonates weighing <1000 g.

Multiple courses of corticosteroid with PPROM are associated with an increased risk of early-onset neonatal sepsis. Corticosteroids are not recommended at >34 weeks gestation unless there is evidence of pulmonary immaturity. Insufficient data exists to fully indicate the benefit of antenatal corticosteroids in pregnancies complicated by: hypertension, diabetes, multiple gestation, IUGR hydrops. Nevertheless, the NIH Consensus Statement indicates that "it is reasonable" to utilize antenatal corticosteroids in pregnancies with these complications prior to 34 weeks if delivery is anticipated.

It would be remiss to not mention several areas that are currently subject to investigation. Even optimal corticosteroid therapy failed to alter RDS in multiple gestation. Thus, dosage for multiple gestations remains to be determined. The clinical trials of thyrotropin releasing hormone (TRH) have been disappointing. TRH should not be utilized outside a clinical trial setting. There is conflicting data concerning the potential synergistic beneficial effects of corticosteroids and tocolytics. There is, however, no data to suggest harmful results from utilization of both modalities.

The optimal number of courses of antenatal corticosteroids (CS) for lung maturation remains unclear. Although it is clear that the effect of antenatal corticosteroids lasts for only 7 days, there is controversy about whether it is useful to repeat another course of corticosteroids after that time. Some investigators indicate that there are no harmful effects, but recently, a worrisome series of reports have indicated several potentially deleterious outcomes. In one series, repeated doses of corticosteroids did not improve outcome and were associated with increased mortality, decreased fetal growth, and prolonged adrenal suppression. In another series, increased rates of transient hypertrophic cardiomyopathy was reported in newborns that had received repeated antenatal doses of corticosteroids. Finally, a third report indicated that repeated antenatal corticosteroids were associated with adverse effects on size at birth without apparent benefit.

PROLONGED PREGNANCY (POSTDATES)

There is no accurate end point of pregnancy; however, prolonged pregnancy is defined as one that has continued for ≥294 days, or 14 days beyond the EDC, as calculated from the LMP or other means (280 + 14 = 294 days, or 42 weeks.) About 5% of all pregnancies go beyond 294 days. Prolonged pregnancy *may be recidive* (a woman who has had one postdate pregnancy has 2 times the likelihood of another). It occurs in *fetal anencephaly* (due to adrenal hypoplasia and altered hormonal production) and *placental sulfatase deficiency and is more prevalent in certain families.* The cause, however, is not determined in the vast majority.

Among postdate fetuses, *30%–40% are dysmature* and are at increased perinatal risk. They may be underweight, with reduced subcutaneous fat, appear wrinkled with peeling skin, and are often meconium stained. *Oligohydramnios* frequently is an associated finding. These neonates may have or have had fetal compromise. However, the *majority of postterm infants appear to be normal or are macrosomic.* Therefore, in the absence of presumed placental insufficiency (causing the fetal alterations noted), fetuses continue to grow slightly even after the EDC. Thus, *ascertaining which fetuses are jeopardized and which are not is essential.* Recent studies suggest that *the risk after 41 weeks gestation is little different from that at 42 weeks.* Therefore, delivery should be considered or careful monitoring initiated.

EVALUATION OF THE POSTTERM PREGNANCY

Accurately Date the Pregnancy

The EDC may not yet have been reached! Of course, accurate dating should have been performed prospectively (during the course of pregnancy), but that so often is not the case. Thus, if three of the following four clinical criteria are met, the patient should not be considered postdate.

- Less than 36 weeks have elapsed since a positive pregnancy test.
- Less than 32 weeks have elapsed since Doppler recording of the fetal heart (FHTs).
- Less than 24 weeks have elapsed since observed fetal movements.
- Less than 22 weeks have elapsed since FHTs were noted by auscultation.

Two satisfactory ultrasonographic fetal biparietal (or other) measurements, at least 1 month apart, can establish gestational age by ±1 week. Therefore, a precise determination is more likely. The earlier in gestation the ultrasonic examinations are accomplished, however, the more accurate dating will be. The EDC cannot be established accurately or confirmed when the fetal biparietal diameter is >9.5 cm by a single ultrasonography.

Fetal surveillance is essential to assess fetal well-being. Once the due date is past, until the 41st week, it may be wise to implement all or part of the surveillance noted below (e.g., weekly instead of biweekly determinations). Clinical parameters include full maternal evaluation.

- Biweekly recording of fundal height and abdominal girth (decreasing uterine contents signals oligohydramnios).
- Maternal fetal motion counting (Chapter 5).
- Visualization of the membranes (if possible) through the cervix to determine if meconium has been passed. Meconium is a nonspecific reaction to stress and should not be taken as a sign of fetal compromise, but as a warning signal that the fetus may be near the limits of placental reserve.
- *Biweekly biophysical profile testing* or, minimally, *biweekly NSTs* will assist in determining fetal well being.
- Additionally, at least *one definitive (level III) sonography,* specifically examining fetal size parameters, fetal organ systems, presentation, and the placenta (including grading) may be of assistance.
- *Contraction stress testing* may be utilized if any parameter is questionable.

Amniocentesis is rarely indicated but may be useful in the patient who has totally unknown dates and appears without any prospective monitoring. Analysis of the amniotic fluid does not assist in determining the gestational age but can definitively describe fetal pulmonary maturity, even when a sample is contaminated by blood or meconium.

TREATMENT

The *safest time for delivery to occur is 39–41 weeks.* After the 41st week, there is steadily rising mortality (e.g., stillborn, uteroplacental insufficiency) and potential morbidity. The mortality is 5%–7% in infants delivered at or after 42 weeks. By the 42nd week, the risk is equal to that at <35th week. The exact time for delivery must be individualized (e.g., parity, fetal size). The ideal time for delivery is when the minimal risk of induction is surpassed by the ever increasing risks of postdate gestation. However, it seems unquestionable that delivery by or during the 42nd week is indicated. An increased rate of labor induction at >41 weeks of gestation may contribute to decreasing stillbirths.

When Definite Prolonged Pregnancy is Confirmed (≥42 weeks)
A thoughtful review all the available information facilitates decisions as well as discussions with the gravida and her family. The postdate status should be reconfirmed. Sweeping (or *stripping*) *of the membranes* is accomplished by inserting a gloved finger through the cervix and circumferentially sweeping the finger between the membranes and the cervix. This has been demonstrated to reduce the interval to the spontaneous onset of labor. However, there is no evidence that it assists in reducing maternal or neonatal morbidity or mortality. *If feasible, labor may be induced.* About 70% of postterm gravidas have an unripe cervix (low Bishop score) and seem to lack preparation for labor. In these patients, induction of labor often is unsuccessful. In those who have a low Bishop score, consider attempting to enhance the score by preinduction administration of cervical prostaglandin E_2.

Monitor the Fetus Continuously During Induction
Dysmature fetuses withstand labor poorly, particularly when oxytocin stimulation is used. They are prone to fetal compromise and may die of intrapartum asphyxia. Given the risk of these patients, it is useful to use *continuous electronic fetal monitoring,* observe for *meconium on rupture of membranes,* and should fetal compro-

mise occur, maternal complications intervene, or serial induction of labor fail, undertake *cesarean section* immediately.

RUPTURE OF THE UTERUS

Uterine rupture, complete or partial, occurs in about 1:1500 (0.05%–0.086%) deliveries (Figs. 11-6 and 11-7). *Complete* rupture extends through the myometrium and the serosal peritoneum, whereas *partial* is anything less, including scar dehiscence. The rupture most commonly *(~90%) occurs in the lower uterine segment.* Rupture can be *spontaneous or traumatic.* Complete rupture can occur in late pregnancy or during labor in patients who have had classic cesarean section or extensive uterine surgery. *Prior uterine surgery is a major correlation* to subsequent uterine rupture with scarred uteri rupturing with a ratio of at least 3:1 to unscarred. Examples of uterine surgery that may increase subsequent rupture include myomectomy, instrumental perforation during induced or incomplete abortion, and resection of a uterine septum. Even *prior low transverse cervical cesarean increases the incidence to 0.038%–0.8%.* Traumatic rupture is most commonly associated with motor vehicle accidents and probably contributes 20%–25% of uterine ruptures. *Other causes associated with complete rupture* (multiple associations per case results in percentages not equaling 100) are obstructed labor (20%), oxytocin overstimulation of labor (as high as 40%), prostaglandin use (30%), grand multiparity (20%), and operative delivery (as high as 30%) (e.g., vacuum or forceps delivery, version-extraction). *Incomplete or occult rupture* during labor may follow partial dehiscence of a low-cervical cesarean section scar or uterine trauma during late pregnancy, (e.g., lap-type seatbelt injury). Instrumental perforation of the uterus during induced or incomplete abortion also occurs. Although uncommon, *corneal (isthmic) pregnancies appear to be increased by in vitro fertilization-embryo transfer and may cause spontaneous, and usually second trimester, uterine rupture. Intervention is usually prompted by fetal heart rate decelerations (70%) and/or severe hemorrhage (30%). Retroperitoneal bleeding may accompany concealed rupture, with late signs and symptoms.*

The *classic symptomatology of rupture of the uterus is bleeding during labor, suprapubic pain and tenderness, cessation of uterine contractions, disappearance of fetal heart tones, recession of the presenting part, or vaginal bleeding.* Hematoperitoneum and hypovolemic shock soon follow. Persistent, uncontrollable uterine bleeding during the third stage of labor in the absence of cervical or other laceration also suggests ruptured uterus.

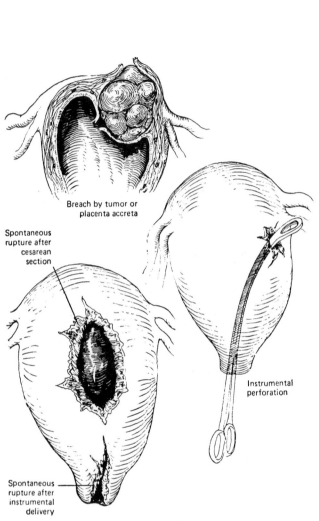

Breach by tumor or
placenta accreta

Spontaneous
rupture after
cesarean
section

Instrumental
perforation

Spontaneous
rupture after
instrumental
delivery

FIGURE 11-6. Types of uterine rupture.

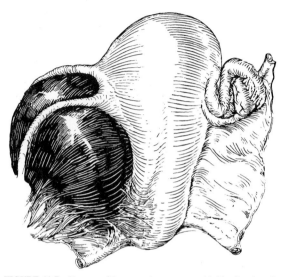

FIGURE 11-7. Rupture of lower uterine segment with bleeding into the broad ligament.

Recent data suggest that *acute abdominal pain is a feature of 60% of cases, maternal tachycardia occurs in ~50%, bloody amniotic fluid in 20%, and severe hypotension in 20%–33%.* Retroperitoneal bleeding may accompany concealed rupture, with late signs and symptoms.

DIAGNOSIS

Sonographic measurement of the lower uterine segment at 36–38 weeks gestation may assist in detection of those with defective lower uterine scars. The defect is thinner than surrounding tissue. In one series, the suggested value of 3.5 mm, in relation to subsequent rupture or dehiscence, provides sensitivity of 88%, specificity of 73.2%, positive predictive value of 11.8%, and negative predictive value of 99.3%.

An index of suspicion is necessary to make the diagnosis, for the *symptoms are by no means diagnostic.* There is no one common feature in fetal heart rate patterns or uterine activity hearlding uterine rupture. However, variable and/or late decelerations may occur before the onset of a fetal bradycardia in some cases. If the cervix will admit the examining hand after delivery, uterine exploration usually makes the diagnosis. Ultrasonography or x-ray films frequently reveal an abnormal fetal position or extension of fetal extremities in complete uterine rupture.

COMPLICATIONS

Complications of ruptured uterus are *hemorrhage, shock, infection, bladder or ureteral injury, hematomas, thrombophlebitis, disseminated intravascular coagulation, pituitary hypofunction,* (e.g., failure to lactate), *or death.* If the patient survives, infertility or sterility may result. The incidence of *fetal loss is high; and those that are saved have a higher rate of compromise.*

PREVENTION

Supervise oxytocin induction and stimulation of labor. Avoid difficult vaginal delivery. Perform low-cervical, not classic, cesarean sections. Consider ultrasonic measurement of the lower uterine segment in patients who are undertaking vaginal birth following cesarean.

TREATMENT

Surgical repair of the uterus is possible in the majority of cases. This is particularly true in case occurring in a prior scar. Generally, those occurring in an unscarred uterus are more catastrophic. Ligation of the uterine or internal iliac arteries may check otherwise uncontrollable hemorrhage. Packing of the uterus may temporarily control bleeding. Hysterectomy may be necessary in some cases, and circumstances may dictate subtotal hysterectomy, is the preferred treatment for uterine rupture, but careful repair may be warranted when future childbearing is important.

PROGNOSIS

Rupture of the uterus imposes a *significantly increased risk of maternal mortality and morbidity* (5%–40%) directly related to the severity, placement, and immediacy of care. Perinatal mortality and morbidity is also increased at least 50%, again directly related to the immediacy of care. Cases of successfully repaired uterine rupture are usually delivered by cesarean in subsequent pregnancies.

MULTIPLE PREGNANCY

DEFINITIONS, ASSOCIATION, INCIDENCES AND IMPORTANCE

Multiple pregnancy involves more than one embryo (fetus) in any one gestation. Two independent mechanisms may lead to multiple gestation: *segmentation of a single fertile ovum* (identical, monovular, or monozygotic) or *fertilization of separate ova by different spermatozoa (fraternal or dizygotic)* multiple pregnancy.

In the development of twins (the most frequent higher-order gestation), *monozygotism is constant (~2.3–4/1000 deliveries),* whereas *dizygotism has certain predispositions.* Dizygotic twinning is inherited as a *recessive autosomal trait via the female descendants.* The father's being a twin has little influence on the rate of twinning in his offspring. *Race* is of special importance: blacks have the greatest incidence of dizygotic twins (about 50/1000 births in Western Nigeria), whites are intermediate, and Asians have the fewest (~1–2/1000 births in Japan). *Other factors* influencing dizygotism include greater maternal height or weight, increasing maternal age (peaks at 35–45 years), and white mothers of blood group O or A. In developed countries, two of the major causes of multiple gestation are *cessation of oral contraception* and *artificial ovulation induction.* The latter is of particular concern for higher-order multiple gestations (triplets and above) are increasingly common (1.2- to 2-fold increase in developed countries) as a result of assisted reproductive technologies (ART). Although these pregnancies are not at significantly increased risk from the ART, they are at exceptional *risk for immature or premature delivery and other morbidity and mortality* associated with higher-order multiple gestations.

In the heterogeneous population of the United States, slightly >30% of twins are monozygotic, and nearly 70% are dizygotic (Fig. 12-1). In such a population, a useful estimate of the natural frequency of multiple gestation is that *twinning occurs ~12 per 1000 births (1:88). Each increase in birth number may then be estimated*

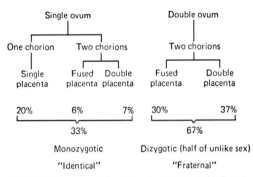

FIGURE 12-1. Placental variations in twinning. (After Potter.)

by raising the ratio 1:88 to the exponential of the birth number minus 1. For example, triplets occur $1:88^{(3-1\ =\ 2)} = 1:7744$; quadruplets occur $1:88^3 = 1:681,472$.

In multiple births, males predominate (but more die early). About 75% of twins are of the same gender. Both are males in ~45% of cases, and both are females in ~30%.

Maternal morbidity and mortality are much higher in multiple than in singleton pregnancy. There is increased frequency and severity of *anemia;* increased occurrence of *urinary tract infection;* more *preeclampsia-eclampsia, hydramnios, and uterine inertia* (overdistention); and a *greater chance of hemorrhage* (before, during, and after delivery).

The perinatal mortality rate of twins is 4–6 times higher—and for triplets much higher again—than for singletons because of prematurity and associated difficulties. Indeed, as the number of fetuses rises, their average size and length of gestation decrease. Twins are delivered, on average, at ~36 weeks, triplets at ~32 weeks, and quadruplets at <30 weeks. Moreover, *intrauterine growth retardation* (IUGR) is more common in all multiple gestations (as opposed to singletons). *Congenital abnormalities* of all organ systems are as high as 18% among twins (considering both monozygotic and dizygotic). Other perinatal risks of multiple gestations include *abnormal presentation and position, hydramnios, hypoxia because of cord prolapse* (~4%, 5 times more common in multiple pregnancy), *placenta previa,* and *premature separation of the placenta* after the first twin or operative manipulation. *Collision, impaction, and interlocking of twins* are additional critical but uncommon complications (Figs. 12-2, 12-3, and 12-4). Because of maternal and perinatal risk, many authorities

FIGURE 12-2. Locked twins.

recommend that no less than qualified obstetricians care for twins and that maternal–fetal consultation be utilized. Additionally, triplet and higher birth order risk is such that maternal–fetal specialists should be involved in, or provide their care.

FIGURE 12-3. Both twins presenting by the vertex.

FIGURE 12-4. One vertex and one breech presentation.

Monozygotic multiple fetuses are far more likely to be jeopardized than dizygotic twins. For example, monozygotic twins have 3 times the incidence of serious congenital abnormalities compared to double-ovum twins. Conjoined twins and enhanced early loss of one or both fetuses (probably two thirds of all implanted multiple gestations) result in a single birth. Moreover, a parasitic fetus without a heart (fetus acardiacus, complicating ~1%) is also a potential problem of monozygous twinning. Other unique monozygotic complications include placental vascular shunts resulting in the twin-to-twin transfusion syndrome (to some degree complicates 5–35%), in which the smaller but cardiomegalic twin pumps its arterial blood into the lower pressure venous system of the larger, plethoric, and macrosomic twin. Cord abnormalities, more common in monozygous twins, include two-vessel cords and velamentous cord insertion (7% incidence). Cord entanglement in a single monoamniotic sac may occur, and this leads to a ~50% loss. Monozygotic twins are smaller and are more likely to die in utero than dizygotic twins. This may be because a single (monochorionic) placenta is less efficient than a fused dichorionic placenta.

The time of segmentation is crucial to the outcome of monozygotic fetuses. Division before the morula and differentiation of the

Double-ovum twin

Amnion and chorion
on both sides

1 2 3 4 5

Two amnions,
no decidua

Single-ovum twin

Monoamniotic
single-ovum twin

FIGURE 12-5. Amniotic membranes of twins.

trophoblast (day 5) lead to separate or fused placentas with two chorions and two amnions. Division after trophoblastic differentiation but before amnion formation (5–10 days) is the pattern of two thirds of all monozygotic twins. This results in a single placenta, a common chorion, and two amnions. Division after amnion differentiation (10–14 days) leads to a single placenta with one chorion and one amnion. Division >14 days results in incomplete twinning. Division just before that (8–14 days) may lead to conjoined (Siamese) twinning.

Monozygotic multiple gestations share the same genetic features (e.g., blood group, histocompatibility, and basic karyotypes). Therefore, skin grafting and organ transplantation are possible and become the ultimate test of monozygotic vs. dizygotic twinning. Monozygotic twins are termed identical, but they often have considerable phenotypic variation. Dizygotic (fraternal) twins may be of the same or different genders and bear only the resemblance of brothers or sisters. They may or may not have sufficiently similar genetic features to serve as organ donors for each other.

Examination of the placenta and membranes assists in zygosity determination. At delivery, careful inspection and dissection of the placenta(s) and membranes, particularly the membraneous T-septum or dividing membrane between the twins, may reveal microscopic evidence of the probable type of twinning. Monozygotic twins have a thin septum made up of two amniotic membranes only (no chorion and no decidua). Indeed, ~1% of monozygotic twins are monoamniotic. By contrast, dizygotic twins have a thick septum composed of two chorions, two amnions, and intervening decidua (Fig. 12-5). In some circumstances, it is necessary to resort to definitive genetic testing to determine monozygosity or dizygosity. The early diagnosis of twins is mandatory, and assessment of the placenta is the key.

CLINICAL FINDINGS

The clinical suggestions of multiple pregnancy include the following:

- A uterus larger than expected for the duration of pregnancy (>4 cm than anticipated);
- Excessive maternal weight gain not explained by eating or edema;
- Hydramnios;
- Iron deficiency anemia;
- Maternal reports of increased fetal activity;
- Eclampsia-preeclampsia;
- Uterus containing ≥3 large parts or multiple small parts;

- and simultaneous auscultation or recording of two fetal hearts varying >8 beats per min and asynchronous to the maternal heart.

LABORATORY FINDINGS

Commonly encountered *laboratory findings in multiple pregnancy include:* abnormal elevation of maternal hCG and/or alpha-fetoprotein, moderate reduction in Hct (also Hgb and RBC count, i.e., iron deficiency anemia), blood volume increased over normal pregnancy values, and an increased incidence of glucose intolerance. Cervicovaginal secretion of fetal fibronectin (Ffn) is a sensitive predictor of preterm delivery in twins, but has low specificity. Thus, Ffn is best used in conjunction with other criteria (e.g., sonographic evaluation of cervical length). Currently, there is little Ffn data for higher-order multiples.

SONOGRAPHY

Sonography is vital in modern management of multiple gestations. Areas of utility include: assisting in *zygosity determination,* detecting and assessing *fetal anomalies,* determination of *growth,* assessing *amniotic fluid,* determining *well being,* management of *antenatal testing,* and caring for *uncommon complications.* Therefore, a standardized approach to sonographic evaluations is useful.

EARLY SONOGRAPHY

Sonography (no later than the early second trimester) assists in determination of chorionicity. Multiple pregnancy may be demonstrated by vaginal ultrasonography before 6 weeks, and multiple pregnancy should be routinely detected by other scanning methods at <8 weeks. A pitfall of multiple gestation sonography, particularly those done at <6 weeks, is both undercounting and overcounting fetuses.

Sonographic visualization of the chorion(s) can be assessed as early as 6–7 weeks (after LMP), with dichorionic being visualized earlier. Although reliable imaging of the amnion is not usually possible before the 9–10th week. This determination is important because of the disproportionate outcomes related to chorionicity and amnionicity. Differential findings include: placental masses, septal thickness, "twin peak" sign, as well as fetal gender.

At 16–20 weeks, a detailed sonographic anatomic survey screens for congenital anomalies and provides a baseline for further testing.

Serial sonographic examinations may vary by chorionicity. Sonography for dichorionic pregnancies are often started later (26 weeks v. 23 weeks) and subsequently, performed less frequently (4 weeks v. 3 weeks) than monochorionic twins, although optimal schedules have not been articulated. Serial examinations are useful in determination of growth patterns, assessing amount of amniotic fluid, determining fetal position, ascertaining placental maturation, and a host of other useful information.

Serial sonographic assessment of cervical length as well as screening for cervical funneling is a useful adjunct in management of multiple gestations. Premature cervical shortening and cervical funneling both indicate the potential for premature labor and delivery.

Prior to or at the onset of labor, sonography is useful in planning management (see the discussion that follows).

DIFFERENTIAL DIAGNOSIS

Single large pregnancy, hydramnios, hydatidiform mole, abdominal or pelvic tumors complicating singleton pregnancy, and complicated multiple gestation (e.g., triplets) must all be considered in the diagnosis of multiple gestation.

TREATMENT

PREVENTION OF MULTIPLE PREGNANCY

Currently there are *few possibilities* for preventing multiple gestation, but those known follow. Use of a barrier type of contraception for the first cycle off oral contraceptives may prevent fertilization of multiple ova. Administering clomiphere initially, if ovulation is to be induced results in fewer multiple gestations. However, dizygous twins still occur in 5%–10% of clomiphene-stimulated cycles. Avoiding the use of human menopausal gonadotropin therapy unless the proper dosage can be established and daily sonography is available for ovulation monitoring assists in lowering multiple gestation. Selective reduction of fetuses (i.e., selective elimination) is a new and controversial technique of elimination of one or more fetuses. This technique employs ultrasonic-guided methods for reducing the number of fetuses, with the rationale that intact survival of a few is better than nonintact survival of many. Initial reports support this approach in selected cases.

AVOIDING MATERNAL COMPLICATIONS IN MULTIPLE PREGNANCY

A thoughtful approach is necessary for the mother with multiple gestations. This plan begins with *early diagnosis* of multiple pregnancy. This goal may be achieved by obtaining sonography (ideally on all and certainly on questionable pregnancies) no later than 12–16 weeks. A *high-protein, high-vitamin diet;* with no limitation of weight gain assists in prevention of fetal intrauterine growth retardation. Dietary supplements demonstrated to be useful in multiple gestations include: *a prenatal vitamin per day, folic acid of 1.0 mg per fetus per day, supplemental iron preparations as indicated* by hemogram and *calcium to a total intake of 1500 mg/day* beneficially influences birth weight.

Because of the number of potential problems, it is common to *examine the patient with multiple pregnancy more often* than most during pregnancy (individualized, but in most cases at least twice as often). *Physical activity is usually limited* to ensure adequate uterine blood flow (e.g., cancel regular exercise programs). Frequent rest periods are initiated after the 24th week (e.g., 1 week of bedrest at 26 weeks and again at 32–33 weeks). *Ultrasound examinations* and *blood counts are obtained more frequently.* Ultrasound examinations for growth progress may be useful monthly from diagnosis until the 32nd week, when both ultrasonography and BPP on each fetus may be useful on a weekly basis. Cervical length sonography may be performed as often as every other week in the latter half of pregnancy.

Given the risk, *consideration is given to deliver all patients with multiple pregnancy in a tertiary medical facility if possible.* Psychoprophylaxis is often stressed, and the patient introduced to a support group. Additionally, patients find literature concerning multiple gestation and preterm birth prevention education helpful. At the time of delivery, *increased blood loss may be anticipated* (hemorrhage is 5 times increased over singletons). Thus, seeking donors acceptable to the patient in advance may be worthwhile. In cases where one fetus delivers untenably early (e.g., 22 weeks), some now recommend *delaying delivery of the remaining fetuses* (especially if membranes are intact) in an attempt to decrease morbidity and mortality in the remaining fetuses. Although the delayed delivery of remaining fetuses improves prognosis, there is no consensus regarding technique or enough cases to demonstrate true statistical relevance. In sum, care of the mother with a multiple pregnancy requires enhanced sensitivity to, as well as frequent assessment of, maternal symptoms and cervical status.

PREVENTION OF FETAL COMPLICATIONS OF MULTIPLE GESTATION

Details concerning identifying congenital anomalies are noted previously (see "Imaging"), as are techniques to maximize fetal growth (see "Maternal Care"). Preventing early preterm delivery is an objective best realized through *maximizing maternal antenatal care* (as above). The utilization of fetal fibronectin screening may be useful in detection of preterm labor. Utilization of home uterine activity monitoring, salivary estriols, and other modalities may be considered. Cervical cerclage may delay preterm birth in selected cases. Indeed, some now recommend this in triplet and higher-order gestations. Further study is necessary, however, prior to recommending this approach.

Tocolytic drugs to prevent early birth may be effective (Chapter 11); however, these agents must be used with great care in multiple gestation because of *possible maternal pulmonary edema*. Appropriate fetal therapy is initiated if early delivery is anticipated (Chapter 11).

ASCERTAIN FETAL PROBLEMS

It is important to *ascertain fetal problems early*. Certainly, some of these may be determined by repeated sonography to screen for fetal defects, IUGR, fetus-to-fetus transfusion syndrome, and fetal well-being. Antenatal diagnosis is used as indicated. The twin-to-twin transfusion syndrome is usually manifest in monozygous twins by discordant fetal growth (a difference of >20%) and one fetus having polyhydramnios while the other has oligohydramnios. Individual testing for pulmonary maturity studies is utilized (if necessary). If selective reduction is an option, the patient may be referred to an appropriate center.

LABOR

During labor, *special vigilance is warranted*. Labor is conducted with full preparations for cesarean section, should the need arise. This includes: starting IV lactated Ringer's solution with a large-bore needle, obtaining a complete blood count, and blood type and crossmatch for a minimum of 2 units packed red blood cells or whole blood. Maternal and fetal oxygenation is enhanced by mask or nasal prong oxygen therapy (7 liters/min). Sonography assists in ascertaining the fetal presentations. In practice, this nearly always

TABLE 12-1
DELIVERY SITUATIONS ACCORDING TO
PRESENTATION OF TWINS

Situation	Twin A	Twin B	%
A	Vertex	Vertex	>40
B	Vertex	Nonvertex	~40
C	Nonvertex	Other (any)	~20

involves one of the three situations outlined in Table 12-1. In most obstetric units, only twins are considered for vaginal delivery. All those of higher birth orders, with the exception of certain centers familiar with vaginal birth of high-order multiples, should be delivered by cesarean section.

All fetuses should be separately electronically monitored. In the United States, if fetal monitoring of this type is not primarily available, consideration should be given to referring the gravida to a medical center. Psychoprophylaxis or local anesthesia is used in so far as possible to limit maternal analgesia and anesthesia. It is particularly important to keep the mother off her back! The degree of aortocaval compression with subsequent hypotension may be profound.

DELIVERY

Cesarean section is recommended for monoamniotic twins because of the ~10% delivery loss from cord entanglement. Other standard *indications for cesarean include: any birth number exceeding twins* (e.g., triplets), *twins <2500 g, or if the first twin is nonvertex (situation C).* It is recommended that all twin gestations be delivered in an operating room with full preparation (including maternal abdominal preparation), equipment, and personnel in attendance for cesarean section. The first twin may be delivered vaginally if it presents by the vertex (situation A and situation B). A significantly shorter first stage of labor (compared to singletons) may be anticipated. A generous episiotomy reduces fetal cranial compression. With delivery of the first fetus, clamp the cord promptly. Should there be twin-to-twin vascular communication, a second monozygotic twin can exsanguinate through the first cord.

A *vaginal examination immediately after the first delivery* is performed to identify a possible forelying or prolapsed cord and establish the position of the second fetus. If B has continued as a vertex (situation A), a second vaginal delivery may be performed. If the second fetus is anything but vertex (situation B), there are three alternatives.

- Bringing the head into the inlet by external guidance (version); if successful, allows labor to proceed for another vertex vaginal delivery.
- Perform cesarean section immediately if external version is unsuccessful or if the fetus is not a candidate for a vaginal breech delivery.
- Complete a vaginal breech delivery if the external version is unsuccessful and the fetus is a candidate for a vaginal breech delivery.

Rupture of the second sac (if present) is accomplished *as late as possible to avoid prolapse of the cord.* Continuous electronic fetal monitoring of the second twin is employed. Should fetal compromise supervene (e.g., persistent cord compression or premature separation of the placenta) and the second twin cannot be delivered easily or immediately, an immediate cesarean section is recommended.

The *three major preventable causes of morbidity* in twins are *immaturity, trauma, and manipulative delivery* (with associated asphyxia), and preventing their occurrence is a primary goal. To assist with care of the newborns, a neonatologist or pediatrician should be in attendance.

POSTPARTUM

Oxytocin 5–10 units IV slowly but promptly after delivery of the second twin assists in making sure the atonic uterus properly resumes tone. An IV infusion of dilute oxytocin may be used if uterine atony becomes a problem. Elevating the uterus out of the pelvis and massaging it gently (Chapter 11) also is useful in treating uterine atony.

CLASSIFICATION

The hypertensive disorders of pregnancy have been variously classified without consensus being achieved as to a lasting classification. A practical classification may be achieved by modification of the system proposed by the American Committee on Maternal Welfare (1985).

I. Pregnancy Induced Hypertension (Preeclampsia-eclampsia, toxemia, EPH, and gestosis)

- Gestational hypertension[*]
- Preeclampsia
  1. Mild[*]
  2. Severe[*]
- HELLP Syndrome[*]
- Eclampsia[*]

II. Chronic hypertension

- Primary (essential, idiopathic)
- Secondary (to some known cause)
  1. Renal: e.g., parenchymal (glomerulonephritis, chronic pyelonephritis, interstitial nephritis, and polycystic kidney disease), renovascular nephritis
  2. Adrenal: cortical-Cushing's disease, hyperaldosteronism, medullary-pheochromocytoma
  3. Other: coarctation of the aorta, thyrotoxicosis, etc.

III. Chronic hypertension with superimposed preeclampsia
IV. Transient (atypical, undiagnosed) hypertension (a nebulous group of patients who develop hypertension in labor or immediately postpartum)

[*]Modifications

PREGNANCY-INDUCED HYPERTENSION

DEFINITIONS, INCIDENCE, ETIOLOGY, AND IMPORTANCE

Preeclampsia-eclampsia, a multisystem disorder of unknown etiology peculiar to pregnant women, remains a major contributor to maternal and perinatal morbidity and mortality both in developing as well as industrialized nations. Currently, it is *not possible to predict who will acquire the processes.* There are *no strategies for prevention.* This group of conditions are *progressive, but with variable presentations and rates of progression.* Moreover, after clinical symptoms have occurred, there are only symptomatic therapeutic options. *One or another of the hypertensive disorders will complicate approximately 10% of pregnancies.*

The mildest form of the process is **gestational hypertension,** which consists of *systolic blood pressure >140 with a rise of >30 mmHg and/or diastolic blood pressure of >90 mmHg with a rise of >15 mmHg.* Only 15%–25% of women having gestational hypertension will develop preeclampsia. This progression is more likely with earlier presentation or if the woman has had a prior spontaneous abortion. Women with gestational hypertension >36 weeks have ~10% risk of developing preeclampsia.

Preeclampsia is characterized by *hypertension (as previously defined), plus generalized edema, and/or proteinuria occurring after the 20th week of pregnancy* (usually in the last trimester or early puerperium). Any two of the three signs are diagnostic. The only exception to the 20th week for onset is when pregnancy-induced hypertension (PIH) is associated with trophoblastic disease. Preeclampsia is divided into *mild and severe,* based on blood pressure and laboratory abnormalities (see below).

Although up to 40% of patients with preeclampsia will have some hemostatic abnormalities, for reasons yet unknown, some preeclamptic patients will develop the **HELLP syndrome.** This includes the signs of preeclampsia (as above) plus hemolysis (H), elevated liver enzymes (EL), and low platelets (LP, see below). These gravidas deserve even more special consideration because of the potential for *poor perinatal and maternal prognosis* without early diagnosis and proper therapy, including expeditious delivery.

Eclampsia, the most fulminating degree of PIH, is characterized by *convulsions or coma, in addition to the other signs and* *symptoms of preeclampsia.* Uncontrolled preeclampsia may progress to eclampsia, with resultant permanent disability or death.

Chronic hypertension (CH) alone or with **superimposed preeclampsia** (SIPE) must be differentiated from PIH. *The risks of chronic hypertension in pregnancy (abruptio placenta, fetal growth restriction and prematurity) are worsened by the superimposition of preeclampsia.* Additionally, the maternal and perinatal risk increase in relation to the severity of the preexisting chronic hypertension.

About 8% (recent reports range from 5%–10%) of all pregnant women in the United States develop preeclampsia; however, there is great geographic variation in incidence. Approximately 5% of these cases progress to eclampsia, and about 5% of women with eclampsia die of the disease or its complications. At least *95% of cases of PIH occur after the 32nd week,* and about 75% of these patients are primigravidas. The incidence is at least doubled with multiple pregnancy, hydatidiform mole, and polyhydramnios. Primigravidas of all ages are affected. PIH is more prevalent among blacks and Native Americans than whites.

Other factors predisposing to PIH include age <20 and >35, vascular or renal disease, diabetes mellitus, gestational diabetes mellitus, obesity, chronic hypertension, pheochromocytoma, systemic lupus erythematosus, nonimmune fetal hydrops, malnutrition, and low socioeconomic status.

Interestingly, if a multigravida remarries, her chance of having PIH with her next pregnancy is similar to what it would be as a nullipara. Pregnancies achieved through assisted reproductive technology with a male donor to whom the gravida has not previously been exposed have the same risk as a primigravida, even if they are a multipara. In preliminary data, donated gametes further increase the risk of preeclampsia (to >18%). All of these conditions contribute to maternal and perinatal morbidity and mortality; however, given the spectrum of the processes, the amount and type of risk is variable. This information is summarized as follows.

Although many associations have been detailed (see previous discussion), the cause of preeclampsia-eclampsia remains unknown and speculation has been so rife that this disorder has been called a disease of theories. Currently there are four popular hypotheses:

- *Placental ischemia.* Increased trophoblast deportation, as a consequence of ischemia, may inflict endothelial cell dysfunction. Certainly evidence for endothelial involvement in this condition abounds.
- Preeclampsia is the *manifestation of a toxic reaction.* At least two areas are being investigated: *Very low density lipoprotein toxicity prevention.* In pregnancy, nonesterified fatty

acids are mobilized to compensate for increased energy demands. Albumin, which has a specific antitoxic activity, also transports the nonesterified fatty acids from adipose tissues to the liver. Low albumin concentrations may allow an expression of very low density lipoprotein toxicity. *Impaired antioxidant activity and the reduction of antioxidant levels,* which increase the level of lipid peroxidation products, may cause peroxidative damage of vascular endothelium.

- *Immune maladaptation.* The immune interaction between mother and invading cytotrophoblast may be aberrant, leading to shallower endovascular cytotrophoblastic cell invasion of spiral arteries. This dysfunction may lead to increased decidual release of cytokines, proteolytic enzymes, and free radial species. Preeclampsia is associated with widespread apoptosis of placental cytotrophoblasts with the uterine wall.

- *Genetic imprinting.* Genetic imprinting for pregnancy induced hypertension could be based on a single recessive gene or a dominant gene with incomplete penetrance (depending on fetal genotype). Preeclampsia during the pregnancy of a mother is a risk factor for development of preeclampsia during the pregnancy of her daughters.

PATHOLOGIC PHYSIOLOGY

VASOSPASM

Arteriolar spasm, consistently observed in the retinas, kidneys, brain, and splanchnic region, promotes hypertension. Furthermore, the normal refractoriness to angiotensin II (A-II) is lost weeks before the onset of preeclampsia. In contrast, normal pregnant women lose their refractoriness to A-II after receiving prostaglandin synthetase inhibitors (e.g., aspirin, which implicates prostaglandin as a mediator of vascular reactivity to A-II during pregnancy). Moreover, A-II refractoriness can be restored to preeclamptic individuals by drugs that increase levels of cyclic AMP (cAMP) (e.g., theophylline). An imbalance between prostacyclin (PGI_2), a vasodilator and inhibitor of platelet aggregation, and thromboxane (TXA_2), a vasoconstrictor and platelet aggregator in preeclampsia, also occurs because PGI_2 production is decreased months before the clinical onset of preeclampsia. Mild preeclampsia is associated with lower systemic daytime production of prostacycline, elevated plasma norepinephrine levels, and blunting of the normal diurnal variations of brain natriuretic peptide, atrial natriuretic peptide, norepinephrine, and aldosterone.

SODIUM AND WATER RETENTION

Sodium retention is an adjunct of growth and is normal during pregnancy, but sodium retention, particularly *intracellular, is exaggerated in PIH*. Nonetheless, sodium retention does not cause this disorder. However, an alteration at the cellular membrane level may inhibit the usual exchange of sodium. Reduced serum levels of albumin and globulin resulting from proteinuria account for the diminished oncotic pressure of the blood despite hemoconcentration. Increased excretion of corticosteroids (including aldosterone) and vasopressin in certain patients suggests increased tissue concentrations of these substances. This results in enhanced sodium and water retention.

PROTEINURIA

Degenerative changes in the glomeruli permit loss of protein via the urine. The albumin–globulin ratio in the urine of patients with preeclampsia-eclampsia is approximately 3:1 (vs. 6:7 in patients with glomerulonephritis). In this case, renal tubular disease contributes only slightly to the leakage of protein.

HEMATOLOGIC ALTERATIONS

The Hgb and Hct are elevated due to hemoconcentration. Preeclampsia is a hypercoagulative status that may be explained by a derangement of the platelet L-arginine-nitric oxide pathway. Severe preeclampsia-eclampsia shares similarities with the disorders of coagulation because disseminated intravascular coagulation (DIC) of varying degrees so frequently occurs. The magnitude of the coagulation defect does not always correlate with the severity of preeclampsia-eclampsia. The alterations may include thrombocytopenia, decreased coagulation factors (especially reduced fibrinogen), and the presence of fibrin split products. Microfibrin emboli may occur in the lungs, liver, or kidneys. Occasionally, hemolysis (e.g., microangiopathic hemolytic anemia, deformed red blood cells), elevated liver enzymes, and thrombocytopenia occur in patients with preeclampsia-eclampsia. This combination is termed the HELLP syndrome.

BLOOD CHEMISTRY ABNORMALITIES

Uric acid levels are generally >6 mg/dL. Serum creatinine is most often normal but may be elevated in severe cases. Some serum albumin and globulin are lost via the urine, but blood proteins must also be lost or destroyed in other ways, since proteinuria alone is not sufficient to explain the abnormally low protein levels in severe cases. Acidosis occurs after convulsions. Elevated levels of hepatic enzymes indicate hepatic dysfunction. Placental clearance of dehydroepiandrosterone sulfate (DHEAS), as a measure of placental perfusion, decreases before the onset of preeclampsia.

In summary, PIH is marked by vasospasm. Whereas normal pregnancy is marked by sodium and water retention, together with increased blood volume, in preeclampsia, there is enhanced sodium and water retention with a contracted plasma volume. Swan-Ganz catheter studies in preeclampsia reveal normal wedge pressures and normal or elevated cardiac output.

PATHOLOGY

KIDNEY

In severe preeclampsia and eclampsia, the only typical lesion is *glomerular capillary endotheliosis* (i.e., swelling of the glomerular capillary endothelium, narrowing of the capillary lumen, and subendothelial fibrinoid deposition). These abnormalities are totally reversible and disappear by 6 weeks postpartum. In patients with the clinical diagnosis of preeclampsia, renal biopsy reveals glomerular capillary endotheliosis in ~70% of primigravidas <25 years, and ~25% have unsuspected renal disease. Other electron microscopic abnormalities include massive subendothelial and mesangial deposits of lipids and fibrillar fibrins, monocyte invasion in the mesangium, and rupture and duplication of the glomerular capillary wall.

CARDIOPULMONARY

Pulmonary edema may occur with severe preeclampsia or eclampsia from cardiogenic or noncardiogenic causes. It is most common postpartum and also may be related to fluid overload and decreased plasma colloid oncotic pressure. Preeclampsia is usually characterized as a hyperdynamic state, with increased cardiac output, normal wedge pressure, and normal or slightly elevated systemic vascular resistance. *Aspiration of gastric contents* may occur as a complication of eclamptic seizures. Death may result from particulate matter obstructing airways or from chemical pneumonitis, leading to the *adult respiratory distress syndrome.*

GASTROINTESTINAL

In the liver, chronic passive congestion and subcapsular hemorrhages may develop.

FETUS

As a result of the poor intervillous blood flow, *intrauterine growth retardation* may be marked. Fetal death may follow hypoxia or acidosis. This is further compounded by both severe hypertension and maternal multiple organ involvement, which may necessitate early delivery.

PLACENTA

Grossly, no specific placental lesions are typical of preeclampsia-eclampsia, although the placenta is often *smaller than normal,* and *intervillous fibrin deposits (red infarcts) are common.* Increased and more severe endarteritis and periarteritis, a thinned and broken syncytium, and calcium and intervillous fibrin deposition may appear (grossly, microscopically, and sonographically) as premature aging. There are two very serious microscopic placental alterations in patients with preeclampsia: *the spiral arteries in the myometrium fail to lose their musculoelastic structure,* and *acute atherosis develops in the myometrial segment of the spiral arteries.* This leads to increased vascular resistance and a compromise of the vessel lumen. Thus, the fetus receives less intervillous blood flow.

SYMPTOMS AND SIGNS

Except for an abnormal blood pressure, patients with gestational hypertension are *usually asymptomatic.* Preeclampsia-eclampsia is characterized by *hypertension, generalized edema, and proteinuria* in the absence of vascular or renal disease. The manifestations develop from the *20th week of pregnancy through the 6th week after delivery.*

HYPERTENSION

Hypertension is the key sign in the diagnosis of PIH. Gestational hypertension is a rise in systolic blood pressure of ≥ 30 mm Hg, a rise in diastolic pressure of ≥ 15 mm Hg, or a blood pressure of $\geq 140/90$. Some (Canadian Hypertension Society Consensus Conference) consider only the diastolic blood pressure. *Except for very high diastolic readings (>110), it is recommended that all diastolic readings be confirmed after 4 hours.* Hypertension also exists with a mean arterial pressure rise of 20 mm Hg. The levels described must occur at least twice, 6 h or more apart, and be based on previously recorded blood pressures. Occasional patients with hypertension during pregnancy must remain unclassified until studies can be evaluated after the puerperium.

EDEMA

Edema is the *least precise sign of PIH* because dependent edema is normal in pregnancy and up to *40% of patients with PIH do not have edema.* However, the following criteria may facilitate the diagnosis.

- Generalized accumulation of fluid in tissues (i.e., >2+ pitting edema after 1 h bedrest).
- A weight gain of ≥2 pounds/wk because of the influence of pregnancy.
- Nondependent edema of the hands and face present on arising in the morning.

PROTEINURIA

Gestational proteinuria is often the last sign to develop and is defined as ≥0.3 g/liter in a 24-h specimen or >1 g/liter (1+ to 2+ by dipstick methods) with urinalysis on random midstream or catheter specimens. Up to 30% of patients with eclampsia will not have proteinuria, but when present, proteinuria signals increased fetal risk (more SGA infants and enhanced perinatal mortality). If only the noted criteria for preeclampsia are present, it is classified as mild preeclampsia. The criteria for severe preeclampsia follow.

- Blood pressure >160 systolic or >110 diastolic (at bedrest, on two occasions at least 6 h apart)
- Proteinuria >5 g/24 h (3+ to 4+ on dipstick)
- Oliguria (≤500 mL/24 h)
- Cerebral or visual disturbances
- Epigastric pain
- Pulmonary edema or cyanosis

OTHER

Severe, persistent, generalized headache, vertigo, malaise, and nervous irritability are prominent symptoms in cases of severe preeclampsia. *Scintillating scotomas* and partial or complete blindness are due to edema of the retina, retinal hemorrhage, or retinal detachment. *Epigastric pain, nausea, and liver tenderness* are the result of congestion or thrombosis of the periportal system and sub-capsular hepatic hemorrhages.

There are *no consistent symptoms of the HELLP syndrome.* This nonspecificity is problematic for early diagnosis. Similarly, eclampsia may occur with little or no warning.

COMPLICATIONS

Maternal complications are related directly to progression from gestational hypertension to preeclampsia, the HELLP syndrome or eclampsia. The fetal complications are related to acute and chronic uteroplacental insufficiency (e.g., asymmetric or symmetric SGA fetus, stillbirth, or intrapartum fetal compromise) and early delivery (complications of prematurity).

LABORATORY STUDIES

All patients with PIH may need the following studies (additional studies or repetition may also be necessary): *Hct, or Hgb, WBC; urinalysis, urine culture and sensitivity; serum protein and albumin/globulin ratio; and serum uric acid and creatinine.* Also, depending on the gestational age and seriousness of the situation, it may be useful to determine *fetal physiologic maturity* by amniocentesis and appropriate tests. A *24-h urine collection is* collected for *total protein, creatinine clearance, and vanillylmandelic acid* (if BP varies greatly). *Baseline coagulation studies* usually include a *platelet count, total fibrinogen, prothrombin, partial thromboplastin time, and split fibrin products (if DIC is suspected).* A *liver function profile* is usually added to rule out HEELP syndrome. This includes *bilirubin and liver enzymes (lactate dehydrogenase, aspartate aminotransferase, alanine amniotransferase).*

Recently, some have recommended that the laboratory evaluation of patients suspected of preeclampsia may be abbreviated in certain circumstances. Specifically, if there is no evidence of bleeding or of a condition that could produce coagulopathy and if the platelet count and lactate dehydrogenase level are both normal, a PT, a PTT, or fibrinogen test is not necessary.

IMAGING

Sonography is useful in detailing the *fetal size and position* and in *estimation of well-being.* Additionally, Doppler evaluation of the *uterine artery velocimetry* may be useful in predicting adverse pregnancy outcomes from compromised fetuses.

MANAGEMENT

The *objectives* of treatment of all hypertensive states complicating pregnancy are to *prevent or control convulsions, ensure survival of the mother without (or with minimal) morbidity, and deliver a surviving infant without serious sequelae.*

GENERAL MEASURES

If the patient is *stable* and not severely preeclamptic or eclamptic, general diet without sodium restriction may be appropriate, as is unrestricted fluid intake (but with recorded intake and output). The *lateral recumbent position* increases renal blood flow, which assists in resolving edema. Therefore, the patient is encouraged to assume right or left lateral recumbency as much as possible. High-risk obstetric care and treatment of complications is required to optimize outcomes. The keys to treatment are *bedrest and delivery at a time of fetal maturity.*

Those who have *gestational hypertension* may be followed under *close supervision as outpatients.* Such supervision usually involves *bedrest* (lateral recumbent position as much as possible), *blood pressure evaluation (while awake) every 4 h, a daily urine dipstick evaluation for proteinuria, a minimum of twice weekly physician visits, weekly nonstress testing* (or other evaluation of fetal well-being), and *maternal fetal motion counting.*

Careful patient education is necessary concerning *signs that would require immediate hospitalization: proteinuria, increasing blood pressure, severe headache, and epigastric pain.*

In some circumstances, for gestational hypertension and in all preeclamptic women, *maternal hospitalization may help prevent premature delivery* and thus be less expensive (compared to premature neonatal care). An example of hospital care includes *bedrest* (again, in the lateral recumbent position), *daily weights, blood pressures every 4 h (because the highest pressures of the day occur at 3–5 AM, it is worthwhile to screen these occasionally); daily urine dipstick for proteinuria, and 24-h urine once or twice weekly (for creatinine clearance and total protein).* On admission and weekly thereafter, the following laboratory studies may be employed: *hemogram, liver function studies, uric acid and creatinine, electrolytes, serum albumin, and a coagulation profile.*

Sonography for gestational age is usually obtained on admission and every 2 weeks thereafter. *Weekly testing for fetal well-being* may be performed by serial BPPs, or NSTs. Should an abnormality arise, a CST may be necessary. *Glucose tolerance testing* is indicated after 20 weeks gestation if the patient has hyperglycemia or multiple pregnancy. A *vanillylmandelic acid study* is effective in ruling out pheochromocytoma if wide blood pressure fluctuations occur.

Criteria to allow nonhospital care for the patient commonly include an *environment where bedrest is possible, BP reduction to ≤120/80, proteinuria ≤150 mg/24 h and normal renal function, and no evidence of CNS irritability. Any relapse or complications require readmission to the hospital.* If possible, delivery is delayed until physiologic maturity (>36 weeks amniocentesis and testing) occurs. If early delivery is required, induction is attemped. When the cervix is not favorable (Bishop score <6–7), a prostaglandin ripening agent may be useful. If induction is not a good option, if labor is delayed, or if fetal compromise develops, cesarean section may be a better option.

INDICATIONS FOR DELIVERY

While there are few absolutes, given the large number of variables in fetal states, fetal maturity, intercurrent diseases, maternal status, and so forth, some of the criteria commonly employed for delivery follow.

Hypertension is the issue that mandates delivery in the vast majority of patients. Blood pressure elevations forcing this delivery are consistently >100 diastolic for 24 h, and a single BP diastolic >110 despite bedrest. *Laboratory abnormalities* signaling sufficient risk to warrant delivery consideration include: proteinuria >1 g/24 h, increasing serum creatinine, abnormal liver function studies, and thrombocytopenia. *Maternal complications* signaling the consideration for delivery comprise the HELLP syndrome, eclampsia, severe preeclampsia (including signs such as epigastric pain and cerebral symptoms), pulmonary edema, cardiac decompensation, coagulopathies, and renal failure. *Fetal abnormalities* indicative of risk sufficient to warrant delivery include: fetal compromise by electronic monitoring criteria; abnormal NST, CST, or BPP; and an SGA fetus with growth failure on sonography.

SEVERE PREECLAMPSIA

Severe preeclamptics and their offspring are best cared for in tertiary centers. The goals of management are prevention of convulsions, control of maternal blood pressure, and delivery.

For gestations of <27 weeks, conservative management (delaying delivery) may be warranted, but maternal complications (abruptio placenta, eclampsia, coagulopathy, renal failure, hypertensive encephalopathy, and hepatic rupture) are directly related to the length of time delivery is delayed. In some pregnancies distant from term, however, attempting to lengthen gestation is the most rationale choice to avoid the morbidity and mortality of early preterm delivery. Patient and family participation is necessary.

Severe preeclampsia is a *high-risk situation* that may end in maternal complications or poor perinatal outcomes despite maximal medical efforts. For those ≥28 weeks with a tertiary care nursery available, delivery after short-term maternal stabilization is the treatment of choice. Laboratory assessment should be similar to the mild preeclamptic, but it may be necessary in extreme cases to add electrocardiography and hemodynamic monitoring. Determination of fetal pulmonary maturity is necessary to properly time delivery. This may be repeated at weekly intervals to accomplish delivery as soon as survival is likely. Corticosteroid therapy for gestations of 26–34 weeks is indicated to enhance fetal lung maturity.

The *severe preeclamptic may be started on magnesium sulfate to help in preventing seizures* (see dosage under "Eclampsia"). Magnesium sulfate prevents seizures by direct central nervous system action; however, magnesium sulfate decreases acetylcholine release at the neuromuscular junction and causes paralysis at a serum level of ~15 mg/dL. Magnesium sulfate potentiates both depolarizing and nondepolarizing muscle relaxants. In patients requiring hypertensive control, hydralazine and labetalol have traditionally been the safest agents. *Blood pressures of 170/110 are an emergency and treatment with hydralazine, labetalol, or nifedipine should be initiated immediately.* Although the benefits and risks of antihypertensive treatment should be considered in all cases of hypertension in pregnancy, it is particularly important to treat those with *sustained systolic BP > 160 mm Hg or sustained diastolic BP > 100.* With lesser hypertensions, the decision to utilize antihypertensive therapy may be much more individualized. In *milder cases (e.g., gestational hypertension), methyldopa is the treatment of choice.* Labetalol, pindolol, oxprenolol, and nifedipine are second-line drugs.

Those patients with *nausea, vomiting, and epigastric pain are at particular risk.* Additionally, these patients may have *laboratory findings that indicate a greater maternal risk:* lactate dehydrogenase level >1400 IU/L, aspartate aminotransferase >150 IU/L, alanine aminotransferase >100 IU/L, uric acid level >7.8 mg/dL, serum creatinine >1.0 mg/dL, and 4+ urinary protein by dipstick. These factors are independent of the rising maternal risk associate with the decreased platelet count found in full expression of the HELLP syndrome. Prompt delivery must be considered for the indications noted previously.

PREVENTION

Since there are no known specific causes of preeclampsia-eclampsia, prevention can be achieved only in a general way by providing the highest-quality prenatal care. The *diet* during pregnancy should be high in protein and contain adequate vitamins and minerals. The patient should be permitted to *gain about 12 kg* (25 pounds) more than her ideal nonpregnant weight. A *moderate salt intake* is reasonable. *Diuretics should not be used.* Alert diagnosis and effective management of prodromal symptoms prevent clinical preeclampsia in the third trimester. Low dose aspirin has been extensively studied and has not prevented the onset of pregnancy induced hypertension. Another compound under investigation is *prenatal calcium* supplements of 600 mg to 1.5 g/day. Those receiving calcium have reduced vascular sensitivity to angiotensin II and, preliminarily, a reduction in the rate of preeclampsia.

HELLP SYNDROME

There are no specific symptoms of the HELLP syndrome. The signs, which are all abnormal laboratory values, should be screened for in all preeclamptic patients. *The platelet count is the most reliable indicator of the HELLP syndrome.* The earlier in the course of the HELLP syndrome that the diagnosis is made, the better it is for both maternal and perinatal prognosis.

Usually treatment is directed to: *seizure prophylaxis, blood pressure control, correction of the several hematological defects (transfusion of blood products), and expeditious delivery.* However, recent reports indicate that *nonmineralocorticosteroid therapy* (high dose dexamethasone, betamethasone 12 mg twice 12 h apart) may assist in amelioration of the hematological abnormalities to the point that pregnancy may be prolonged in those distant from a time for delivery of reasonable perinatal safety. Patients with refractory HELLP syndrome may benefit from *plasmapheresis.* The *maternal morbidity and mortality* rates associated with HELLP syndrome approaches *25%.*

ECLAMPSIA

DEFINITION, INCIDENCE, ASSOCIATIONS

A patient with signs of preeclampsia who has at least one convulsion or episode of coma between the 20th week of pregnancy and the end of the 6th week after delivery must be presumed to have eclampsia if other causes can be excluded. Eclampsia occurs in *0.2%–0.5% of all deliveries.* The occurrence is influenced by the same factors noted for preeclampsia. Eclampsia is classified according to the *time of occurrence of the first convulsion* with respect to the time of delivery. *Prepartum eclampsia* (~75% of total) denotes convulsions before delivery. About *50% of postpartum eclamptic convulsions occur within 48 h of delivery.* In most series, eclampsia will be associated with >20% of total maternal mortality. Those women dying with eclampsia tend to be relatively older, multiparous, have underlying chronic hypertension, an early onset of preeclampsia-eclampsia, and have multisystemic manifestations (primarily hematological, hepatic and neurological).

SYMPTOMS AND SIGNS

Patients *usually have no aura and may have one to several seizures with a variable interval of unconsciousness.* The seizures are of the *tonic-clonic* type and are marked by *apnea.* Hyperventilation (to compensate for the respiratory and lactic acidosis) is common after the seizure. *Fever is a poor prognostic sign. Tongue biting* is common, and other complications include *aspiration, head trauma, broken bones, and retinal detachment.*

LABORATORY AND IMAGING FINDINGS

A *chest x-ray to rule out aspiration* is necessary for the patient who has had a seizure. If the patient has not been evaluated previously, the studies noted above (see p. 387) should be obtained. Eclampsia is associated with proteinuria of 3+ to 4+, hemoconcentration, a greatly reduced blood CO_2 combining power, and increased serum uric acid, blood nonprotein nitrogen, and blood urea nitrogen levels. An ophthalmoscopic examination may reveal papilledema, retinal edema as manifest by increased sheen, retinal detachment, vascular spasm, arteriovenous nicking, and hemorrhages. Repeated examination is helpful in determining improvement or failure of treatment in preeclampsia-eclampsia. Deep tendon reflexes are exaggerated and there may be pathological reflexes.

DIFFERENTIAL DIAGNOSIS

Although convulsions may be due to hypertensive encephalopathy, epilepsy, thromboembolism, drug intoxication or withdrawal, trauma, hypoglycemia, hypocalcemia (of parathyroid or renal origin), hemolytic crisis of sickle cell anemia, or the tetany of alkalosis, during pregnancy, eclampsia is the first consideration. *A brief coma usually follows the convulsions of eclampsia, but coma may also occur without convulsions.* Other causes of coma (in descending order of probability) are epilepsy, syncope, alcohol or other drug intoxication, acidosis or hypoglycemia (diabetes), stroke, and azotemia.

MANAGEMENT

EMERGENCY MANAGEMENT

Immediate management aims to *assure maternal well-being.* The first step is to obtain an *unobstructed airway and to prevent maternal oral injuries.* This may be accomplished by insertion of an oral airway or padded tongue depressors. Both of these methods minimize tongue biting or tooth fracture, which may occur with seizures. *Suctioning of the oropharynx* may be initiated as soon as it can be ascertained that the patient will not bite the suction catheter. Administration of *oxygen by nasal prongs or mask* will increase oxygen saturation during this precarious interval. The next step in immediate *management is to control seizures.* This is generally achieved by *administration of magnesium sulfate* in a 4–6 g IV loading dose followed by IV infusion of 1.5–2 g/h, attempting to reach a therapeutic level of 4.8–8.4 mg/dL. When magnesium sulfate is being administered, a *urinary catheter* is usually desirable to ascertain that adequate urinary output is occurring. Magnesium sulfate is largely excreted by the kidneys, and the *drug may reach dangerous levels if urinary output is impaired.* If seizures recur >20 min after the loading dose and therapeutic levels are confirmed, consider diazepam 5–10 mg IV or up to 250 mg amobarbital (be aware of their effect on the fetus and neonate). Additionally, it is often necessary to *control hypertension* (usually initiated for sustained systolic BP >160 mm Hg or sustained diastolic >100 and with a goal to bring the diastolic to 90–100). Labetalol may be given every 10 min: 20 mg first dose, 40 mg second dose, 80 mg subsequent doses (to a maximum 300 mg or until blood pressure is controlled). The second-line drug is hydralazine, although diazoxide, sodium nitroprusside, trimethaphan, and nitroglycerin also have been used acutely to lower blood pressure. Each of the drugs has side effects that must be weighed carefully to individualize therapy. It may be necessary to gently restrain the patient to prevent bony or soft tissue injury.

GENERAL MEASURES

Hospitalization is mandatory. The patient is placed in a *darkened, quiet place at absolute bedrest, with bedrails in place for protection* during convulsions. *Continuous intensive nursing* is required and every effort is made to reduce stimuli, including absolute minimization of visitors. The patient is also not disturbed for unnecessary procedures (e.g., tub baths, leave the blood pressure cuff on her arm). The patient is maintained on her sides to prevent inferior vena cava syndrome or aspiration of vomitus. A padded tongue blade is kept at hand to be placed between the patient's teeth during convulsions. As well, a bulb syringe and catheter or suction apparatus is maintained at the bed side to *aspirate mucus or vomitus* from the mouth, glottis, or trachea, and an *oxygen* mask or tent (masks and nasal catheters produce excessive stimulation).

Typed and crossmatched whole blood (or blood products) are kept available for immediate administration because patients with eclampsia often develop premature separation of the placenta with the associated-hemorrhage. Their hemodynamics are such that they are also susceptible to shock.

LABORATORY TESTS

A retention catheter is necessary to *accurately measure urinary output* (50–100 mL/h is desirable). *Quantitative protein content* of each 24-h urine specimen is obtained until the 4–5 postpartum day. Also, *creatinine clearance tests* are obtained as a measure of renal function. Elevated levels of *hepatic enzymes* may presage liver failure. *Coagulation studies may suggest DIC.*

PHYSICAL EXAMINATION

The *blood pressure is obtained at least hourly* during the acute phase and *every 2–4 h thereafter.* Similarly, *fetal heart tones are monitored continuously* or, at the minimum, every time the mother's blood pressure is obtained. An *ophthalmoscopic examination* may be useful on a daily basis. Additionally, examination of the face, extremities, and especially the sacrum (which becomes dependent when the patient is in bed) is helpful in *detection of edema.* A patient undergoing stabilization for delivery should *remain NPO. Fluid intake and output for each 24-h period is measured and recorded.* If the urine output exceeds 700 mL/day, the output plus insensible fluid loss (approximately 500 mL/day) is usually replaced with salt-free fluids (including parenteral fluids). This may include

200–300 mL of 20% dextrose in water 2–3 times daily during the acute phase to protect the liver, to replace fluids, and to aid in nutrition. Do not give 50% glucose, since it scleroses the veins. The use of sodium-containing fluids (e.g., physiologic saline, Ringer's solution) must be monitored carefully.

Delivery is mandatory once the gravida has been stabilized and is accomplished by the safest, most expeditious method, individualized to each patient. *Cesarean section* is preferred for primigravidas, but *induction by rupture of the membranes and vaginal delivery* may be appropriate for some multiparas. Note if *meconium* is present in amniotic fluid. Indications for cesarean section have been liberalized, but cesarean section may be lethal for a patient with continuing convulsions or coma. Seizures and insensibility should be absent for a period of ~4 h before cesarean section is performed on a maternal indication.

For cesarean section, *general anesthesia or well-controlled epidural or caudal anesthesia* is generally employed. Spinal anesthesia is less commonly used because it may cause sudden, severe hypotension. If an anesthetist is not available, procaine, 0.5% or 1% (or its equivalent), can be used for local infiltration of the abdominal wall. For vaginal delivery, pudendal block or local anesthesia is preferred, but increasingly, epidural anesthesia is proving useful.

Postpartum magnesium sulfate is continued for at least 24–48 h. Phenobarbital (120 mg/day) may be used in patients with persistent hypertension and no spontaneous postpartum diuresis. If the diastolic blood pressure is consistently >100, the administration of a diuretic and methyldopa or other antihypertensives may be considered.

COMPLICATIONS

EARLY

Convulsions increase the maternal mortality rate 10-fold and the fetal mortality rate 40-fold. The causes of maternal death due to eclampsia are (in descending order of frequency) *circulatory collapse* (cardiac arrest, pulmonary edema, and shock), *cerebral hemorrhage, and renal failure.* The *fetus usually dies of hypoxia, acidosis, or placental abruption.* Blindness or paralysis (due to retinal detachment or intracranial hemorrhage) may persist in patients who survive eclampsia.

About 30% of patients who develop premature separation of the placenta have one of the hypertensive disorders. Approximately half of such patients will be found to have hypertensive disease and about one quarter will have preeclampsia-eclampsia.

Postpartum hemorrhage is common in patients with hypertensive syndromes during pregnancy. *Toxic delirium* in patients with eclampsia, either before or after delivery, poses serious medical and nursing problems. *Injuries* incurred during convulsions include lacerations of lips or tongue and fractures of the vertebrae. *Aspiration pneumonia* may also occur. *Renal or hepatic failure and DIC* are rare maternal complications.

Preterm delivery with all attendant neonatal morbidity and mortality is a marked risk with preeclampsia-eclampsia.

LATE

Fifteen to thirty-three percent of patients with severe preeclampsia or eclampsia (without known preexisting hypertensive or renal disease) *suffer a recurrence of preeclampsia-eclampsia* with subsequent pregnancies. If, however, their problem was not preeclampsia but undiagnosed chronic hypertensive cardiovascular disease, the rate of recurrence is nearly 100%. *Permanent hypertension, the result of vascular damage, may occur as a result of severe preeclampsia-eclampsia in 30%–50%.*

PROGNOSIS

FOR THE MOTHER

Maternal morbidity (defined by severe hypertension or multisystem involvement) and potential mortality is enhanced even with gestational hypertension. *Approximately 16% of nulligravidas with gestational hypertension but no proteinuria eventually develop severe hypertension or multisystem involvement.* With gestational hypertension and even one plus proteinuria, severe maternal complications eventually occurs in ~42% of all nulligravidas (of total, severe hypertension 80%, multisystem disease 20%). The *outlook for patients with preeclampsia is materially worse, with nearly two thirds of nulligravidas developing severe hypertension (33%) or multisystem disease (67%).* Death from preeclampsia is <0.1%. If eclamptic seizures develop, 5%–7% of these patients will die. The *causes of death include intracranial hemorrhage, shock, renal failure, premature separation of the placenta, and aspiration pneumonia.* Moreover, chronic hypertension may be a sequel of eclampsia. Although platelet counts are significantly increased postpartum after normotensive pregnancy, there is a further 2- to 3-fold rise in preeclamptic patients. Peak values occur 6–14 d after delivery. Most authorities recommend a *complete evaluation 6 weeks to 6 months postpartum* for the women who have had eclampsia or severe preeclampsia.

FOR THE INFANT

Preterm birth and small for gestational age infants occur more frequently (Odds Ratio, OR 1.7) in gestational hypertension compared to normotensive nulligravidas. Preeclampsia further increases both preterm birth and small for gestational age infants (OR 14.6). Perinatal mortality may be as high as 20%. With early diagnosis, antenatal therapy, and intensive neonatal care, however, this loss can be reduced to <10%.

CHRONIC HYPERTENSION

DEFINITION AND INCIDENCE

It is often *difficult to distinguish chronic hypertension from preeclampsia,* especially when the patient registers late in pregnancy (Table 13-1). Chronic hypertension may be present before conception or <20 weeks gestation, or hypertension may persist for >6 weeks postpartum. *Superimposed preeclampsia on chronic hypertension is defined by ≥30 systolic or ≥15 diastolic increase from previous levels* with either nondependent edema or proteinuria. The correct diagnosis can be made by renal biopsy, but this carries a considerable risk during pregnancy. Moreover, the exact diagnosis may be academic, for (as noted previously) ~25% of patients with preeclampsia have underlying renal disease and ~20% of patients with the clinical diagnosis of chronic hypertension and superimposed preeclampsia have renal disease. *Chronic hypertension occurs in 0.5%–4% of pregnancies (averaging 1.5%).* Approximately 80% of chronic hypertension is idiopathic, and 20% is due to renal disease. *Common associations* include >30 years of age, obesity, multiparous, diabetes mellitus, nonwhite, and family history of hypertension. There is a *>50% chance of maternal or perinatal morbidity* occurring in women who enter pregnancy with severe chronic hypertension in association with other renocardiovascular complication.

Chronic hypertension complicating pregnancy carries significant *perinatal risk: abruptio placenta, fetal growth restriction, and prematurity.* These complications are encountered more frequently in cases of severe hypertension, preexisting cardiovascular diseases, preexisting renal diseases, as well as target organ damage from

TABLE 13-1
DIFFERENTIAL DIAGNOSIS OF CHRONIC HYPERTENSIVE CARDIOVASCULAR DISEASE AND PREECLAMPSIA

Features	Hypertensive Disease	Preeclampsia
Onset of hypertension	Before pregnancy; during first 20 weeks of pregnancy	After 20th week of pregnancy (exception: trophoblastic tumors)
Duration of hypertension	Permanent; hypertension persists beyond 3 months postpartum	Hypertension usually absent at 6 weeks postpartum; always by 3 months postpartum
Family history	Often positive	Usually negative; may be positive
Past history	Recurrent toxemia	Psychosexual problems common
Age	Usually older	Generally teenage, early 20s
Parity	Usually multigravida	Usually primigravida
Habitus	May be thin or brachymorphic	Usually eumorphic
Retinal findings	Often arteriovenous nicking, tortuous arterioles, cotton wool exudates, hemorrhages	Vascular spasm, retinal edema; rarely, protein extravasations
Proteinuria	Often none	Usually present (see definition); absent at 6 weeks postpartum

From RR de Alvarez. In R.C. Benson, ed., *Current Obstetric & Gynecologic Diagnosis & Treatment,* 4th ed. Lange, 1982.

hypertension. The use of *antihypertensive therapy* during pregnancy in all of preceding high-risk chronic hypertensive patients has been demonstrated to *improve both maternal and perinatal outcomes.* However, in lower risk chronic hypertensive states, the data for antihypertensive therapy to improve maternal or perinatal outcomes is less convincing.

DIAGNOSIS

SIGNS

The designation of chronic hypertension in pregnancy is based on *documented hypertension before conception or hypertension <20 weeks gestation or >6 weeks postpartum.*

LABORATORY EVALUATION

Hypertensive patients should be evaluated as soon as feasible in pregnancy. The following *baseline laboratory studies* (in addition to the customary prenatal laboratory tests and those for preeclampsia) are recommended. SMA-6 or SMA-12, serum uric acid (>5.5 mg/dL identifies women with increased likelihood of superimposed preeclampsia), urine culture and sensitivity, 24-h urine collection for creatinine clearance (decreased in 5%–10% of patients, who will also have elevated serum creatinine and proteinuria) and total protein, *chest x-ray films* (rule out cardiomegaly because those with increased heart size are at greater risk of superimposed preeclampsia, pulmonary edema, and arrhythmias), and *electrocardiogram* (expect left ventricular hypertrophy in 5%–10% of patients).

MANAGEMENT

Obstetric patients with chronic hypertensive cardiovascular or renal disease should be managed similarly to those with preeclampsia. Many of the former will have superimposed preeclampsia, and it may not be possible to decide what the basic problem actually was until at least 3–4 months after delivery, when appropriate tests and studies should be ordered.

If the *diastolic BP exceeds 100 mm Hg, antihypertensive drug therapy is initiated* to prevent maternal stroke or cardiac failure. The aim should be *maintenance of BP at 80–90 mm Hg.* Whether or not uterine blood flow is autoregulated is still undecided. If it is, antihypertensive therapy is not likely to decrease blood flow. On the other hand, if uterine blood vessels are always fully dilated and the flow is not autoregulated, lowering of the maternal BP should decrease uterine blood flow—possibly harmful to the fetus. Hence, *antihypertensive drugs must be used cautiously* because they carry an uncertain risk–benefit ratio.

Methyldopa, a popular antihypertensive drug, has been used extensively during pregnancy and is considered by some to be the first agent of choice. However, the drug is responsible for contraction of the blood volume in chronic hypertension-preeclampsia after recent diuretic therapy. Therefore, it may not be the drug of choice in many preeclamptic patients. Another effective therapy is *Labetalol.* Beta-blockers may cause hypoglycemia and respiratory depression. Moreover, these drugs blockade the tachycardiac response of neonates of mothers on beta-blocker therapy. Alternative drugs probably are safer and are at least as effective in late pregnancy.

FETAL ASSESSMENT

Fetal activity determinations and nonstress and stress tests are important assessment parameters because they may indirectly indicate reduced uterine blood flow and placental function, which may become critical factors in preeclampsia-eclampsia. *Fetal maturity* (LS ratio or rapid surfactant test) should be determined and the fetal status monitored closely to properly plan delivery.

CHRONIC HYPERTENSION WITH SUPERIMPOSED PREECLAMPSIA

Patients with chronic hypertension with superimposed preeclampsia (about *one third of all chronic hypertensives in pregnancy*) on hospitalization may seem to stabilize but then deteriorate rapidly. One of the complications is *premature separation of the placenta,* noted in >10% of patients with chronic hypertension (>10 times the incidence in normal pregnancy). Other problems include *thrombocytopenia, oliguria, and retinal detachment.* Even if chronic hypertensive patients have apparently normal renal function, the incidence of superimposed preeclampsia is 15%–30%. If there is renal insufficiency, almost all these patients will develop preeclampsia-eclampsia. *Intrauterine growth retardation* is a major fetal hazard if preeclampsia is superimposed on chronic hypertension. Prematurity is often another problem because preterm delivery may occur spontaneously or by necessity.

The seriousness of the preeclampsia-eclampsia is directly related to the severity of the underlying cardiovascular disorder. The perinatal mortality rate is much higher than that in normal pregnancies or in preeclampsia-eclampsia not associated with chronic hypertensive cardiovascular disease.

NONVERTEX PRESENTATIONS, SHOULDER DYSTOCIA, AND CORD ACCIDENTS

BREECH PRESENTATION

DEFINITIONS, ASSOCIATIONS, INCIDENCES, AND IMPORTANCE

Breech is a longitudinal presentation in which the cephalic pole occupies the fundus and the caudal (podalic) pole lies in the lower segment of the uterine cavity or within the birth canal. Overall breech presentation occurs in *3%–4% of singleton pregnancies* commencing labor, but has a much *higher incidence in multiple gestations* (e.g., ~25% of first twins and ~50% of second twins are breech). The incidence rises further in higher order multiple pregnancies. Other associations with breech presentation include: *earlier gestations* (35% at <28 weeks, 25% at 28–32 weeks, 20% at 32–34 weeks, 8% at 34–35 weeks, 2%–3% at >36 weeks), a *prior breech* (over 4-fold increase after one and up to 30-fold after three), *placental placement* (i.e., placenta previa), *oligohydramnios, fetal congenital anomalies* (e.g., hydrocephalus), *pelvic tumors impinging on the uterus or birth canal* (e.g., leiomyomata), and *uterine anomalies* (e.g., bicornuate, septate uterus).

As presentations are thought to be a matter of fetal–uterine accommodation, breech presentation may be caused by any aberration of this adaptive process or of the fetal attitude. Thus, breech presentation is not a disease or an abnormality. However, breech presentation may be an important sign of *congenital fetal compromise*. For example, breech presentation is increased with *chromosomal anomalies* (e.g., trisomies 18 and 21), *neuromuscular abnormalities* (e.g., familial dysautonomia), and *skeletal malformations* (e.g., spina bifida, meningomyelocele). The incidence of *major congenital anomalies* (e.g., anaencephaly, hydrocephaly) in breech presentations is more than double (~6%) that found in vertex. Additionally, *delivery of the breech fetus imposes perinatal risks* of birth anoxia and birth trauma as well as maternal risks of traumatic delivery, or cesarean section.

There are three types of breech presentation (Fig. 14-1): *frank* (legs flexed at the hip and extended at the knee), *complete* (legs flexed at the hip and flexed at the knee), and *footling* (legs extended at the hip and extended at the knee). The amount of both hip and knee extension in footling breech is variable and may involve one

FIGURE 14-1. The three types of breech presentation.

(single footling) or both *(double footling)* feet as the presenting part. The *incidence of frank breech increases as size increases* (40% <2500 g, 65% over 2500 g), whereas complete breech represents ~10% at all sizes and *footling breech decreases in relation to size* (50% <2500 g, 25% >2500 g). In breech presentations (all three types), the *fetal reference point to describe position and station is the sacrum.* Knowledge of the type of breech presentation is essential to management.

DIAGNOSIS

Physical examination is generally the first clue to breech presentations. Leopold's maneuvers discover the softer and less well-defined breech above the pelvic inlet and the firm, well-defined head in the uterine fundus. The fetal heart (heard best over the back) is found higher on the maternal abdomen. Vaginal examination (with cervical dilatation) reveals the softer and irregular breech presentation, a foot, or feet as opposed to the usually encountered firm, smooth, rounded cephalic presentation with readily identified sutures. The *diagnosis is usually confirmed by sonography.*

Sonography is also useful to determine multiple gestation, the type of breech, attitude, size (and gestational age), location of the placenta, and amniotic fluid volume. Given the incidence of congenital anomalies (>6%) associated with breech presentation, *an anatomic survey is also helpful.* If the sonography has been accomplished at some time prior to labor, it is useful to repeat the ultrasound at the onset or early in labor to *confirm fetal presentation, head position,* and to *estimate fetal size.* Radiography is rarely necessary.

MANAGEMENT

PRENATAL

Confirmation, Follow-up, and Counseling

Given current utilization of sonography during pregnancy, breech presentations are usually detected in the second trimester. However, some breech presentations remain undetected prior to the onset of labor. A recent report from a large managed care program indicated that *~21% of term breeches were not detected before the onset of labor and an additional 15% not detected until after 38 weeks of gestation.* On those that are detected earlier, follow up sonography (often ~32 weeks and ~36 weeks) is useful to ascertain if the usual course of spontaneous version to vertex occurs, to determine fetal size and attitude, and to screen for fetal defects. *Breech patients are considered at risk and their care plans are customarily individualized and more rigorous than vertex, low-risk patients.*

When breech presentation persists, *parental involvement is encouraged.* This usually involves dissemination of information, counseling concerning the presentation, detailing available management options, and discussion of the parent's concerns and questions. The goal of this counseling is to *formulate a plan for delivery that meets the parents' desires, can be executed by the health care provider(s), and affords maximal safety for both mother and child.*

Patients with breech presentations are warned to come to the hospital as soon as labor begins or spontaneous rupture of membranes occurs. The latter is particularly important because of the increased incidence of cord prolapse. As noted previously, admission sonography is necessary.

External Cephalic Version

External cephalic version (ECV) is the term describing *maneuvers performed through the maternal abdominal wall attempting to convert the presentation from breech to vertex* (Fig. 14-2). Antenatally, ECV is limited to singleton gestations and is usually performed *after the 36th week,* but prior to the onset of labor. Although ECV has been performed as early as the 28th week of gestation, early attempts are currently less favored because of a high recurrence to breech and to avoid preterm delivery if complications occur.

ECV is more successful in: *multigravidas, pregnancies with sufficient amniotic fluid, and in unengaged complete and footling breech presentations. ECV is contraindicated by: prior uterine surgery* (myomectomy, cesarean section or metroplasty), *suspected or documented congenital malformations, indications of fetal compromise* (e.g., intrauterine growth retardation, abnormal biophysical testing), *placenta previa, anterior placentation* (i.e., placenta between the fetus and the abdominal wall), *abruptio placenta, premature rupture of the membranes, marked oligohydramnios, and engagement of the presenting part.* Relative contraindications include those conditions limiting the use of tocolytic agents (maternal cardiac disease, diabetes mellitus, or thyroid disorders) and frank breech (the lower extremities act as a splint, preventing flexion).

ECV should only be performed in a facility with proper equipment and staffing for emergency cesarean. One commonly used routine follows.

> *Obtain informed consent.* The patient should inform the operator if pain occurs or if the maneuvers seem too forceful.

FIGURE 14-2. External cephalic version demonstrating an alternative to the successful "forward roll."

Sonographically verify presentation, flexion of the fetal head, appropriateness of size, and adequacy of amniotic fluid. If not previously performed, rule out fetal congenital anomalies and uterine abnormalities.

A *nonstress test* is conducted and must be reactive to proceed. A *Kleihauer-Betke test* is drawn to rule out fetomaternal hemorrhage.

Determine if the *uterus is sufficiently relaxed* to allow the procedure without tocolysis. Although uterine tone may be the most important predictor of success when selecting candidates for ECV, other useful criteria are uterine irritability and contractions. If further relaxation is necessary administer *ritodrine hydrochloride, 0.15 mg/min IV for 15 min.* Analgesics and anesthetics are not generally used.

Using both hands on the patient's abdomen, *gently "disengage"* the fetal lower pole by moving it toward the fundus as well as laterally toward the fetal back. Simultaneously, pressure is exerted on the fetal head downward and contralateral to the direction of the lower pole. In sum, this is positioning the fetus in a *forward roll.* If that is unsuccessful, a back flip may be attempted. If unsuccessful, the ECV may be reattempted at a later time.

Sonographic or electronic fetal monitoring is used during and after to monitor fetal well-being and ascertain the success of ECV.

Following ECV, the *nonstress test and Kleihauer-Betke tests* are repeated. Signs of fetal compromise (e.g., electronic fetal monitoring criteria, fetomaternal hemorrhage) are treated accordingly (usually immediate cesarean) and if the Kleihauer-Betke is positive and the mother is Rh-negative, *Rh immune globulin* is given to prevent sensititization.

In the absence of worrisome findings in this screening, the spontaneous onset of labor is routinely monitored by outpatient care.

The overall success of ECV is reported to be as high as 66%, with 33%–50% success for nullipara and 45%–75% success for multiparas. Although successful ECVs may return to breech prior to delivery, this generally happens in <10%. Women with successful ECV have approximately the same cesarean rate as those with primary cephalic presentations. Although ECV may afford the individual patient the opportunity for a cephalic vaginal delivery, it would reduce overall cesarean rates by only ~1% if universally applied. *Complications of ECV* also include: intrauterine fetal demise secondary to umbilical cord entanglement (<1%), emergency cesarean (<1%), abruptio placenta, premature rupture of membranes, preterm labor, umbilical cord prolapse, fetomaternal hemorrhage, and uterine rupture.

Planned Vaginal Delivery

Health providers contemplating a *vaginal breech delivery* must be both trained as well as experienced in the process and procedure. Adequate support must be available, including: an experienced obstetrician to assist with delivery, and anesthesiologist and a pediatrician capable of providing total resuscitation and care of the newborn. Anesthesia is usually kept to a minimum, although epidural anesthesia has proven useful. The additional support personnel (e.g., nursing, respiratory therapy) and facilities must be prepared to deal with these patients as part of a comprehensive team.

Factors predisposing to fetal injury during labor and delivery of a breech presentation include: greater incidence of umbilical cord prolapse, a higher incidence of cord compromise during labor, increased incidence of placental separation, entrapment of the head by the cervix, injury to the head and neck by more rapid descent through the birth canal, injury of the head and neck by the mode of delivery, and a greater chance of injury to the upper extremities.

Thus, attempting vaginal delivery is usually reserved for patients meeting rather stringent criteria (Table 14-1).

Using such criteria, 10%–15% of all candidates will meet the criteria. Of those, ~70% will deliver vaginally, but nulliparas are only ~50% likely to succeed whereas ~75% of multiparas will be delivered vaginally. The most common indications for cesarean section are labor disorders or nonreassuring fetal heart rate patterns. Recently, induction of labor in patients with a breech presentation and an unripe cervix using proglandin ripening has been reported to be efficacious (vaginal delivery of ~50%) and safe. The use of oxytocin for labor abnormalities remains controversial.

Umbilical cord blood acid–base values for uncomplicated, term, vaginal breech deliveries differ significantly from those of uncomplicated cephalic vaginal delivery. The differences suggest a *greater*

TABLE 14-1
CRITERIA FOR ATTEMPTING VAGINAL DELIVERY

Fetal criteria
    Frank breech presentations (although selected cases of
        complete or footling breech are considered in certain
        centers)
    Gestational age of ≥34 weeks
    Estimated fetal weight of 2000–3500 g
    Flexed fetal head
Maternal criteria
    Informed consent
    Adequate maternal pelvis (many authorities believe this
        should be obtained by x-ray pelvimetry, whereas
        others believe a clinical evaluation is sufficient; data
        are inadequate to indicate this improves perinatal
        outcomes)
    Absence of maternal contraindications to labor
    Absence of maternal or fetal indications for cesarean
        section
Special circumstances
    Presentation in advanced labor with no fetal or maternal
        compromise; a controlled vaginal delivery may be
        safer in these circumstances than a hastily executed
        cesarean section
    Previable fetus
    Lethal fetal congenital anomalies

degree of acute cord compression with vaginal breech delivery. This suggestion is furthered by breech vaginal deliveries (compared to elective cesarean) having a greater risk of low Apgar scores (as high as 15-fold more). Additionally, there are *significantly more neonatal intensive care admissions for vaginal breech deliveries* (>1.5-fold).

Planned Cesarean Section Delivery

Given the risks of cord prolapse with rupture of the membranes, as well as the risks of early labor, most planned cesarean deliveries are electively scheduled at ≥38th week. One set of criteria for these cases follows (Table 14-2).

Singleton breech cesarean deliveries have lower birth weight-specific neonatal morbidity and mortality compared to vaginal births. Approximately 30% of patients anticipating a vaginal delivery will have cesarean section delivery for signs of fetal compromise or abnormalities of labor.

INTRAPARTUM

As noted previously, patients with breech presentations should come to the *hospital as soon as possible when rupture of the membranes*

TABLE 14-2
CRITERIA FOR PLANNED CESAREAN SECTION DELIVERY

Fetal criteria
  Estimate fetal weight of >3500 g
  Deflexed fetal head
  Prolonged rupture of membranes
  Unengaged presenting part
  Premature fetus (gestation of 25–34 weeks)
  Most complete or footling breech presentations >25
    weeks without detectable lethal congenital anomalies
  Variable heart rate deceleration on electronic monitoring
Maternal criteria
  Informed consent
  Contracted or borderline pelvic capacity
  Elderly primigravida
  Infertility problems or poor obstetric history
  Dysfunctional labor

or labor occurs. A *repeat sonography* is accomplished with specific attention to position, attitude, and location of fetal extremities. A *full history and physical examination* are accomplished. *Pelvic examination* is conducted, with specific attention to station and whether cord is presenting or palpable. *Fetal monitoring* is performed and fetal well being assessed. Reappraisal of the mode of delivery is performed. The *preparations necessary for delivery* are conducted (see above).

If a vaginal delivery is anticipated, the screening for fetopelvic disproportion is reassessed and the necessary preparations for vaginal and cesarean delivery are conducted. *Continuous monitoring is performed to screen for fetal compromise. Labor's progress is carefully evaluated* by monitoring dilatation and descent of the presenting part. *Artificial rupture of the membranes is avoided until the presenting part is well applied.* At the time of membrane rupture, the patient is examined vaginally to check for potential cord prolapse. As *little analgesia and anesthesia* as possible is used, with epidural anesthesia being the choice should mild analgesia and local anesthesia not be adequate. Abnormalities of labor are regarded for their potential indication of cesarean section necessity. The second stage of labor is interfered with as little as possible.

DELIVERY

Cesarean Section

The cesarean incision is chosen to be as atraumatic to the fetus as possible. A *vertical incision* in the lower uterine segment (which frequently extends into the lower fundus) is chosen when the *presenting part is higher in the uterus, if there is an indication that the fetus will require more room for delivery, and for many premature deliveries.* A *transverse lower uterine segment incision* is performed when the *lower uterine segment is well developed, the presenting part is well down in the uterus,* and there are *no special fetal requirements.*

Once the uterus is opened, the breech is *delivered by total breech extraction* (see below). If most expeditious, the fetus is grasped (as with vaginal delivery) over the hips with the thumbs on the sacrum and the fetus gently extracted at a moderate rate. In some cases, delivery is facilitated by first delivering the legs. This may be accomplished by either directly grasping the feet or by flexing the knees to facilitate grasping and delivering the feet. At the level of the shoulders, the arms are swept out of the uterus by pressure along the anterior portion of the humerus. *Care is taken not to overextend the neck.* Gentle pressure on the uterus (by the assistant) immediately above the head, while the obstetrician supports the body, facilitates delivery of the head. The cord is immediately clamped.

Vaginal Delivery of the Breech Presentation

Vaginal delivery is facilitated by: a generous episiotomy, allowing the fetus to be expelled to the level of the umbilicus before manipulation, loosening and drawing down a short loop of cord when the umbilicus come through the introitus, and having the assistant support the body while the head is being delivered.

Delivery of the Body

There are three methods for breech delivery of the body. *Total breech extraction* involves grasping both of the lower extremities initially, and then the pelvis when it is available, to literally extract the fetus from the uterus and birth canal. This is the most hazardous method of vaginal delivery. *Spontaneous expulsion* is simply allowing full delivery of the body without manipulative interference and is intermediate in fetal hazard. The safest vaginal breech delivery is *assisted breech delivery*. In this case, the fetus is spontaneously expelled to the level of the umbilicus and the remainder of the fetus is extracted by gentle pressure on the pelvis with the obstetrician's thumbs over the sacrum.

While an assistant supports the body, the obstetrician rotates the fetus as it descends so that the spine is in the midline directly under the symphysis pubis. Gentle downward pressure on the pelvis brings both scapulas under the symphysis. Rotation of the body brings the right shoulder beneath the pubic symphysis. The operator (using the right hand) locates the right humerus and exerts gentle pressure on the anterior surface until the arm is delivered. The left arm is likewise delivered (Fig. 14-3).

Delivery of the Head (Figs. 14-4 and 14-5)

As the body is rotated back to the mid position, delivery of the head is commenced. During this time, *fundal pressure by an assistant* keeps the head flexed and the body is gently lifted upward. Usually the *head delivers spontaneously* over the perineum. When assistance for delivery of the head in breech births is necessary, it can be accomplished manually or with forceps. The *Mauriceau-Smellie-Veit maneuver* involves the obstetrician placing the index and middle finger of one hand over the maxilla as the body rests of the forearm. Two fingers of the operator's other hand are applied on either side of the neck with gentle traction. As the body is elevated, this allows controlled delivery of the mouth, nose, and brow.

Piper forceps, the second method of assisted breech delivery, are specifically designed for breech birth. Moreover, their routine

FIGURE 14-3. Assisted breech delivery of the fetal body.

FIGURE 14-4. Initial operator and assistant positioning for the Mauriceau-Smellie-Veit maneuver.

utilization has been reported to improve neonatal outcomes in 1000–3000 g fetuses. The prerequisites for using Piper forceps include: operator expertise, a completely dilated cervix, and engagement of the head in the pelvis. Preferably, the head is in the direct

FIGURE 14-5. Final operator and assistant positioning for the Mauriceau-Smellie-Veit maneuver for breech delivery of the fetal head.

occiput anterior position. As the assistant supports the body, the operator gently inserts the Piper forceps on each side of the head. Keeping the body close to the forceps allows gentle traction, applied as the forceps are rotated anterior to accomplish a controlled delivery (Fig. 14-6).

Complications of Vaginal Breech Delivery

One of the most immediate and feared complications of vaginal delivery is *cervical entrapment of the head.* Without prompt delivery, severe *asphyxia leads to fetal injury or death.* Entrapment of the head is most likely to result when the incompletely dilated cervix affords passage of the body, but not the head. Thus, this complication most frequently occurs in those fetuses the least well prepared to tolerate any trauma, the premature breech presentation. *Gentle downward shoulder traction with combined fundal pressure* (by the assistant) may afford delivery. If this fails, *deep anesthesia* (halothane has been classically used) to afford cervical relaxation may be useful. Failing with the first two options, *Duhrssen's*

FIGURE 14-6. Piper forceps for breech delivery of the fetal head indicating assistant support of the fetal body.

incisions (hystrostomatomy) may preserve fetal life. These are simply incisions made into the cervix. Most recommend starting at 6 o'clock and then making additional incisions if necessary at 2 and 10 o'clock. With delivery, the incisions may extend upward into the lower uterine segment and result in hemorrhage. Fortunately, Duhrssen's incisions are rarely necessary.

There are also *a number of other potential complications of vaginal delivery of breeches.* Umbilical cord prolapse is associated with 15% of footing, 5% of complete, and only 0.5% of frank breech presentations. Direct birth trauma as the result of difficult delivery has been said to be >10-fold more common in breech vaginal deliveries compared to vertex. The arms may slide behind the neck (nuchal arms) and obstruct delivery and/or be injured by attempts at displacement.

PROGNOSIS

Breech fetuses may be neurologically different from cephalic in otherwise healthy pregnancies. *There is a negative association between breech presentation and cognitive outcomes regardless of delivery.* In the absence of birth injury, the higher risk of cerebral palsy among term breech presentation may relate more to the small for gestational status of the breech than to mode of delivery. Short-term data (see previous discussion) for cord blood acid–base studies, Apgar scores, and neonatal intensive care admissions all indicate that *vaginal delivery has more short term effects than cesarean,* but there are studies indicating that vaginal delivery in carefully selected patients is an acceptable alternative.

Overall, breech presentation remains a high-risk pregnancy with a lasting impact on the parents. Even parents undergoing cesarean for breech presentation have been found to have lower subsequent pregnancy rates (than vertex). This most probably relates to decisions not to reproduce.

OTHER MALPRESENTATIONS

TRANSVERSE LIE

Transverse lie is a position where the fetal long axis lies at right angles to the maternal long axis. Although more frequent in earlier gestation, transverse lie *occurs in <0.5% of term singleton pregnancies.* With higher order gestations, there is a marked increase in malpresentations. In singleton pregnancies the most common associations are *increasing multiparity* (relaxation of the abdominal wall and uterus), *placenta previa, fetal abnormalities, and contraction of the bony pelvis.* Perinatal mortality is markedly increased with transverse lie, exceeding 10%.

Diagnosis most often suggested by *Leupold's maneuvers* and finding the fetal heart (auscultation or Doppler) in an unexpected area. Confirmation is achieved by sonography. Moreover, *full sonographic evaluation is warranted to exclude fetal anomalies.* This evaluation will also detail whether the fetal *back is "down"* (inferior in the uterus) *or "up"* (superior in the uterus). The latter is even more hazardous for cord prolapse should the membranes rupture. *Corrective maneuvers have not proven useful and the presentation is not amenable to delivery. Thus, cesarean section is recommended when the fetus is mature.*

Lesser angulations of axis disalignment are termed "oblique lies." When vertex, these usually spontaneously convert, but warrant close follow-up.

SHOULDER DYSTOCIA

Shoulder dystocia is an obstetric emergency occurring in cephalic presentations when the shoulders fail to deliver despite the performance of routine obstetric maneuvers. Characteristically, the head delivers and remains near transverse, the final phase of external rotation (the head reassuming the position it originally emerged) does not occur; the chin is tightly applied to the perineum and the face become progressively cyanotic. The anterior shoulder is impacted behind the symphysis pubis and the posterior shoulder is lodged against the bony pelvis at an angle precluding further descent.

Although shoulder dystocia may occur with any term fetus, and *50%–90% of cases occur in normally grown fetuses,* it increases with increasing fetal size. *Any antecedent of macrosomia* (see p. 219) *places a gravida at increase risk of shoulder dystocia* with delivery, including: maternal diabetes (odds ratio 1.7) or gestational diabetes, obesity, previous macrosomic fetus, maternal birth weight >8 lb, maternal weight gain of >20 kg during pregnancy, and abnormal fetal growth factors or syndromes. Occurrence data detail the relationship of shoulder dystocia to fetal size in pregnancies not complicated by diabetes and the enhancement in those complicated by diabetes: 0.15% of deliveries >2500 g, 3% of deliveries >3500 g, 5.2% (12.2% with diabetes) of deliveries 4000–4250 g, 9.1% (16.7% with diabetes) of deliveries 4250–4500g, 14.3% (27.3% with diabetes) of deliveries 4500–4750 g, and 21.1% (34.8% with diabetes) of deliveries 4750–5000 g.

Shoulder dystocia is increased by more than a third in vacuum or forceps assisted births (to between 4.6%–45%). If the fetus is >4000 g, and there is a prolonged second stage and midpelvic instrumentation, shoulder dystocia has been reported to be as high as 23%. Conditions that create larger and/or more rigid shoulders or fetal disproportion (most notably diabetes) increase the incidence of shoulder dystocia. This may account for the increase in shoulder dystocia with *postdate pregnancies and in recurrent shoulder dystocia.* Additional correlates of shoulder dystocia include induction of labor (odds ratio 1.3). *However, the majority (>50%) of shoulder dystocia occurs without identifiable risk factors.*

Although there is an *increased risk of maternal morbidity* (e.g., extended epiosotomy, vaginal or cervical lacerations, other trauma associated with delivery, and excessive blood loss) with shoulder dystocia, the *major risks are to the fetus.* Indeed, up to *50% of neonates with this complication have been reported to have birth asphyxia or traumatic injury.* Birth asphyxia may include nothing more severe than metabolic acidosis, or may involve shock, central nervous system depression, seizures, long-term central nervous system damage, organ failure, and death. The traumatic neonatal injuries include fractures of the clavicle or humerus and brachial plexus trauma. In the absence of other complications, the fractures generally heal without incident. Most brachial plexus trauma resolves with minimal or no neurological deficit (particularly with proper rehabilitation), but avulsion of nerves may lead to Erb's palsy.

Prevention, the ideal treatment, is thwarted by shoulder dystocia's unpredictability (50% of cases do not have predisposing signs). Even the ability to detect macrosomia (see p. 219) by ultrasound or clinical means is limited. Although many authorities recommend cesarean section for fetuses with estimated birth weights >5000 g, performing a cesarean for every fetus suspected to be macrosomia has not proven medically or cost effective. Moreover, reports of labor induction for antenatally predicted fetal macrosomia indicate a marked increase in cesarean section without significant reduction in shoulder dystocia or fetal injury.

There should be an *enhanced level of vigilance for shoulder dystocia when the pregnancy is complicated by diabetes mellitus, when there are labor abnormalities* (protraction disorders, arrest disorders, or a prolonged second stage of labor), *if mid-pelvic instrumentation is necessary, and in macrosomic fetuses.* Preventative measures at the time of delivery include *suprapubic pressure* applied by an assistant as the head delivers and maximally flexing the maternal legs at the hips *(McRoberts maneuver).*

In unavoidable cases, management requires clinical judgment and individualized care. Time is of the essence. The fetus is at risk of asphyxiation, because it cannot expand the chest to breathe and umbilical cord circulation is compressed within the birth canal. Clinicians are encouraged to have a *careful, methodical series of maneuvers designed to dislodge the shoulder from behind the pubic symphysis so that delivery may occur.* Operator experience and case individualization mandates using the maneuvers in the order most likely to be effective; therefore, the following should not be interpreted as being in any recommended order.

- *Summon the additional assistance necessary* for the emergency (e.g., anesthesiology, neonatal resuscitation, additional physicians, or nursing staff).
- *Create (or extend) an episiotomy* allowing sufficient room for vaginal maneuvers. This may require proctoepisiotomy.
- Perform the *McRoberts maneuver.*
- Exert *suprapubic pressure* (Rubin's maneuver).
- Perform the *Wood's maneuver,* which is to place two fingers against the anterior surface of the posterior shoulder and apply gentle, but firm, pressure while attempting rotation.
- *Attempt to deliver the posterior arm.*

In those uncommon cases (probably <2%) not corrected by these maneuvers, a series of extraordinary maneuvers have been suggested, but all carry significant risk. *Fracture of the clavicle* will relieve the shoulder rigidity and is best accomplished by pressure away from underlying structures if a finger can be hooked behind the clavicle in the mid portion of the supraclavicular space. Fracture toward the underlying structures as well as attempting to *cut the clavicle with scissors* places both great vessels and nerves at risk. The *Zavinelli maneuver* entails deep anesthesia for uterine relaxation and sufficient pressure on the fetal head to replace it within the upper vagina or uterus, where cesarean can then be performed to complete delivery. Because the need for this is rarely encountered, it is difficult to maintain operator proficiency and the infectious complications are high. *Symphysisotomy* is utilized in many developing countries and appears to have relatively low morbidity and few sequelae. Again, it is difficult to maintain operator proficiency in this country.

There is *significant recurrence risk for gravidas who have had prior shoulder dystocia* (14×, 1% increased to 14%) *and traumatic birth* (3-fold increase). Should cesarean not be employed, patients in the latter two categories should be aware of their increased risk with attempting vaginal birth.

UMBILICAL CORD PROLAPSE

Cord prolapse occurs when the presenting part does not fill the lower uterine segment and impinge on the cervix (Fig. 14-7). This allows the cord to enter this space and lie alongside (occult) or lower (overt) than the presenting part. The overt form is far more serious and is highly associated with malpresentation, as reflected by the incidence with the following conditions: transverse lie (20%), footling breech (15%), complete breech (5%), and frank breech (0.5%).

OVERT CORD PROLAPSE

The incidence of overt cord prolapse with singleton gestations has been variously reported from *0.1%–0.5%. About 50% of cases occur with breech* presentations, and another *10% with transverse presentations,* whereas *40% occur with vertex presentations.* Nearly *two thirds of overt cord prolapse occurs in multiparas.* Due to increased instability and malpresentations, the incidence is *higher with twins (accounting for 25% of all cord prolapses)* and still higher with higher order multiple gestations. Overt cord prolapse occurs more frequently with *low birth weight infants,* in contrast to occult prolapse of the cord.

When the cord is presenting, it may be palpated through the membranes if there is cervical dilatation. Complete prolapse of the umbilical cord is associated with rupture of the membranes. The patient may feel the cord slide through the vagina and over the vulva after the membranes rupture. When the cord is first compressed, there may be violent fetal activity. The cord may be seen or palpated and the fetal heart tones will reflect fetal compromise.

More than 15% of these patients present with an intrauterine fetal demise. These cases are managed conservatively by allowing delivery to proceed. When the fetus is viable and there is complete cord prolapse, the patient should be placed immediately in the *knee-chest or deep Trendelenburg position.* A *sterile gloved hand is used to put pressure upward on the presenting part* to relieve cord compression. Attempts at *cord reposition* are nearly fruitless, but the cord is *palpated for viability* and fetal heart tones are monitored continuously. *Oxygen* is administered to the mother. *Delivery is accomplished as quickly as possible.* The mode of delivery depends on the cervical dilatation, but nearly all will be delivered by cesarean section.

Perinatal mortality, even in modern centers, exceeds 35% and morbidity of survivors is variously reported.

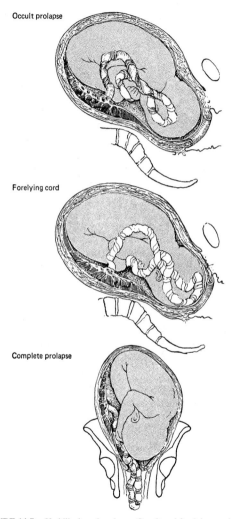

FIGURE 14-7. Umbilical cord prolapse. Occult and forelying cords occur with intact membranes, while complete cord prolapse occurs with membrane rupture.

OCCULT CORD PROLAPSE

The vast majority of occult cord prolapse is only diagnosed by electronic *fetal monitoring criteria and there is no consistent physical finding.* The fetal heart varies in relation to a contraction with a characteristic pattern in occult cord prolapse. Early and late in the contraction, when there is only enough pressure to impinge on the venous circulation, the fetal heart will accelerate as a measure of decreased venous return. With increasing pressure, there is arterial impingement, initiating a baroreceptor response causing a marked fall in fetal heart rate.

It is uncommon for cord impingement to be severe enough to result in *persistent severe variable decelerations.* When this occurs, however, it should be viewed as a *sign of true fetal compromise* for there may be *hypoxia, metabolic acidosis, and subsequent morbidity or mortality.* A pelvic examination is conducted to rule out overt cord prolapse, and the *patient's position changed* (often to the Sims or Trendelenburg). *Oxygen* is administered and the monitoring is closely observed. In the majority, the cord impingement is successfully resolved and labor proceeds without incident. Only occasionally will cord impingement as a result of occult cord prolapse require cesarean section for fetal compromise.

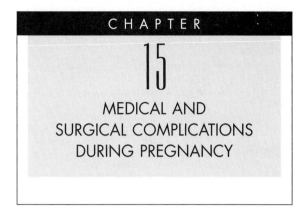

15

MEDICAL AND SURGICAL COMPLICATIONS DURING PREGNANCY

CARDIOVASCULAR DISEASES

CARDIAC ARREST

Cardiac arrest is cessation of heart action. Ventricular standstill *(asystole) and ventricular fibrillation are the immediate causes,* but the underlying etiologies are most frequently *acute myocardial hypoxia or alteration in conduction or both.* In obstetrics and gynecology, cardiac arrest occurs during *induction of anesthesia* and during *operative surgery* or *instrumented delivery. Cardiovascular disease increases the risk of cardiac arrest, and hypoxia and hypertension are contributory causes.* Cardiac arrest may follow shock, hypoventilation, airway obstruction, excessive anesthesia, drug administration or drug sensitivity, vasovagal reflex activity, myocardial infarction, air and amniotic fluid embolism, and heart block.

Cardiac arrest occurs in ~1:800 to 1:1000 operations and is apt to occur during minor surgical procedures as well as during major surgery. It occurs in *~1:10,000 obstetric deliveries,* usually operative, complicated cases. Fortunately, it is possible to *save at least 75% of patients* when cardiac arrest occurs in the well-managed and well-equipped operating or delivery room.

CARDIOPULMONARY RESUSCITATION (CPR)

CPR is used for treatment of asphyxia or cardiac arrest (Fig. 15-1).
Phase I: First Aid (Emergency Oxygenation of the Brain)
Basic life support must be instituted within 3–4 min for optimal effectiveness and to minimize permanent brain damage. Do not wait

(1) Open airway by positioning neck anteriorly in extension. Inserts show airway obstructed when the neck is in resting flexed position and opening when neck is extended.

(2) Rescuer should close victim's nose with fingers, seal mouth around victim's mouth, and deliver breath by vigorous expiration.

(3) Victim is allowed to exhale passively by unsealing mouth and nose. Rescuer should listen and feel for expiratory air flow.

FIGURE 15-1. Technique of mouth-to-mouth insufflation.

for confirmation of suspected cardiac arrest. Call for help, but do not stop preparations for immediate resuscitation.

Step 1: Place patient *supine on a firm surface* (not a bed).

Step 2: Determine whether the patient is *breathing*. If the patient is not breathing, take immediate steps to *open the airway*. In unconscious patients, the lax tongue may fall backward, blocking the airway. Tilt the head backward and maintain it in this hyperextended position. Keep the mandible displaced forward by pulling strongly at the angle of the jaw. **If victim is not breathing continue with the following.**

Step 3: *Clear mouth and pharynx* of mucus, blood, vomitus, or foreign material.

Step 4: *Separate lips and teeth* to open oral airway.

Step 5: If steps 2–4 fail to open airway, forcibly *blow air* through mouth (keeping nose closed) or nose (keeping mouth closed) and inflate the lungs 3–5 times. Watch for chest movement. If chest movement does not occur immediately and if pharyngeal or tracheal tubes are available, use them without delay. Tracheostomy may be necessary.

Step 6: *Feel the carotid artery for pulsations.*

a. If carotid pulsations are present

Give *lung inflation by mouth-to-mouth breathing* (keeping patient's nostrils closed) or mouth-to-nose breathing (keeping patient's mouth closed) *12–15 times per min*—allowing about 2 sec for inspiration and 3 sec for expiration—until spontaneous respirations return. Continue as long as the pulses remain palpable and previously dilated pupils remain constricted. If pulsations cease, follow directions in step 6b.

b. If carotid pulsations are absent

Alternate cardiac compression (closed chest cardiac massage, Fig. 15-2) *and pulmonary ventilation* as in step 6a. Place the heel of one hand on the sternum just above the level of the xiphoid. With the heel of the other hand on top of it, apply firm vertical pressure sufficient to force the sternum about 4–5 cm (2 inches) downward (less in children) about 80–100 times/min. After 5 sternal compressions, alternate with 1 quick, deep lung inflation. Repeat and continue this alternating procedure until it is possible to obtain additional assistance and more definitive care. Resuscitation must be continuous. Open heart massage should be attempted only in a hospital. When possible, obtain an ECG, but do not interrupt resuscitation to do so.

FIGURE 15-2. Technique of external cardiac massage. Heavy circle in heart drawing shows area of application of force. Circles on supine figure show points of application of electrodes for defibrillation.

Phase II: Restoration of Spontaneous Circulation

Until spontaneous respiration and circulation are restored, there must be no interruption of artificial ventilation and cardiac massage while steps 7–13 are being carried out. The physician must make plans for the assistance of trained hospital personnel, cardiac monitoring and assisted ventilation equipment, a defibrillator, emergency drugs, and adequate laboratory facilities. Three basic questions must now be considered. *What is the underlying cause, and is it correctable? What is the nature of the cardiac arrest? What further measures will be necessary?*

Step 7: Provide for intubation, administration of 100% oxygen, and mechanically assisted ventilation. A cutdown for long-term IV therapy and monitoring should be established as soon as possible. Attach ECG leads and take the first of serial specimens for arterial blood gases and pH. Promote venous return and combat shock by elevating legs, and give IV fluids as available and indicated. The use of firmly applied tourniquets or military antishock trousers (MAST suit) on the extremities may be of value to occlude arteries to reduce the size of the vascular bed.

Step 8: If a spontaneous effective heartbeat is not restored after 1–2 min of cardiac compression, have an assistant give *epinephrine, 0.5–1 mg* (0.5–1 mL of 1:10,000 aqueous solution) *IV every 5 min as indicated.* Epinephrine may stimulate cardiac contractions and induce ventricular fibrillation that can then be treated by DC countershock (see step 11).

Step 9: If the victim is pulseless for more than 10 min, give *sodium bicarbonate solution, 1 mEq/kg IV,* to combat impending metabolic acidosis. Repeat no more than one-half the initial dose every 10 min during cardiopulmonary resuscitation until spontaneous circulation is restored. Monitoring of arterial blood gases and pH is required during bicarbonate treatment to prevent alkalosis and severe hyperosmolar states.

Step 10: If asystole and electromechanical dissociation persist, continue *artificial respiration and external cardiac compression, epinephrine, and sodium bicarbonate.* Monitor blood pH, gases, and electrolytes.

Step 11: If ECG demonstrates ventricular fibrillation, maintain cardiac massage until just before giving an *external defibrillating DC shock* of 200–300 J for 0.25 sec, with one paddle electrode firmly applied to the skin over the apex of the heart and the other just to the right of the upper sternum. Monitor with ECG. If cardiac function is not restored, resume massage and repeat shock at intervals of 1–3 min.

Step 12: Thoracotomy and open heart massage may be considered (but only in a hospital) if cardiac function fails to return after all of the above measures have been used.

Step 13: If cardiac, pulmonary, and central nervous system functions are restored, the patient should be observed carefully for shock and complications of the precipitating cause.

HEART DISEASE

Congenital heart disease is the principal cardiovascular problem complicating pregnancy in the United States. Rheumatic heart disease is less a problem today than 40 years ago because of better rheumatic fever prophylaxis, improved health care, and advances in cardiovascular surgery. Syphilitic carditis has all but disappeared in pregnancy. Women with *collagen disorders* (e.g., Marfan's syndrome) or those with *prosthetic heart valves* are prone to cardiac problems during pregnancy. Reported incidences of heart disease vary from *0.5% to 2%* of obstetric patients but probably are lower in the general population because only referral centers are likely to report their experience. Manifestations of coronary heart disease are rare during pregnancy. Similarly, pericardial disorders are very infrequently seen. Hypertrophic obstructive or nonobstructive cardiomyopathy in pregnancy is rarely complicated by pregnancy and delivery.

Heart disease is a major cause of maternal death, but maternal and perinatal mortality rates are only slightly increased if the disability is minimal.

FUNCTIONAL CLASSIFICATION OF HEART DISEASE

For practical purposes, the *functional capacity of the heart is the best single measurement of cardiopulmonary status.*

Class I: Ordinary physical activity causes no discomfort.
Class II: Ordinary activity causes discomfort and slight disability.
Class III: Less than ordinary activity causes discomfort or disability; patient is barely compensated.
Class IV: Patient decompensated; any physical activity causes acute distress.

Eighty percent of obstetric patients with heart disease have lesions that do not interfere seriously with their activities (classes I and II) and usually do well. About 85% of deaths ascribed to heart disease complicating pregnancy occur in patients with class III or IV lesions (20% of all pregnant patients with heart disease). Nevertheless, much can still be done to improve the prognosis for the mother and infant in these unfavorable circumstances.

PATHOLOGIC PHYSIOLOGY

The effects of pregnancy on certain circulatory and respiratory functions are reviewed in Chapter 4. Understanding gestational cardiovascular and hemodynamic adaptations is key in preventing or managing cardiac complications during pregnancy.

Three major burdens on the heart are associated with pregnancy: cardiac output is increased by ~40%, the heart rate is accelerated by 10–15 beats per minute (bpm), and the plasma volume is expanded by 45%–50%. These unavoidable stresses must be considered in appraising the patient's ability to undergo pregnancy, delivery, and the puerperium.

By the 12th week of pregnancy, increased physiologic factors, especially blood volume increase, may produce *systolic flow murmurs.* These, together with the *third heart sound* often noted during pregnancy, can lead to a false diagnosis of heart disease. *Cardiac arrhythmias* (e.g., atrial fibrillation or flutter), *common in women with mitral valve or congenital heart disease, may be a serious sign of cardiopathy.*

In addition to these physiologic burdens, there are avoidable or treatable *medical liabilities* (e.g., anemia, obesity, hyperthyroidism, thyroid disease, infection, and emotional and physical stresses). Youth, adequate functional cardiac reserve, stability of the cardiac lesion, and an optimistic, cooperative attitude are important assets that do much to improve the cardiac patient's chances for a successful confinement.

Labor, delivery, and the early puerperium impose the following specific physiologic burdens on the maternal heart.

DURING LABOR AND DELIVERY

The *heart rate slows with each contraction and returns to the resting level between contractions.* The alteration is less in the lateral recumbent as compared to the supine position. *Oxygen consumption increases intermittently with uterine contractions,* approaching that of *moderate to severe exercise. Tachycardia during the second stage may result from distention of the right atrium* and ventricle by blood from the uterus and from the effect of straining.

DURING THE PUERPERIUM

Cardiac output increases slightly for ~1 week after delivery. Elimination of the placenta, contraction of the uterus, and reduction of the pelvic circulation suddenly make more blood available to the heart. A *decrease in plasma volume (and increase in hematocrit) occurs for about 12 h after delivery.* A second *marked decrease in plasma volume,* with an accompanying reduction in the amount of total body water, *persists for 7–9 days.* These changes are due to postpartal diuresis.

TREATMENT

Determine the functional cardiac status (class I–IV) before the third month if possible and again at 7–8 months. *Obtain consultation* with a cardiologist for all class II–IV patients early in pregnancy. *Restrict physical activity* to necessary duties only, with fatigue as a limiting factor. Acertain that the *patient obtains assistance* with essential household duties (child care, laundry, cleaning, and marketing). Assist the patient and her family to understand the medical problem and allay her fears, anxiety, and tension. *Periods of maximal cardiac stress occur at 14–32 weeks, during labor, and, particularly, during the immediate postpartum period.* Especially good rapport and medical control must be maintained at these times.

General Medical Measures

Anemia, hyperthyroidism, and obesity are corrected as indicated. In pregnant cardiac patients, *sodium restriction may be necessary after 8–12 weeks.* Warfarin anticoagulant therapy is avoided during pregnancy because of teratic effects. *Cardiac complications, such as congestive failure, pulmonary edema, infective endocarditis, and arrhythmia, are treated as in the nonpregnant patient.* Diuretics may be necessary, but *should not be used to the point of hyponatremia. Hypokalemia is also to be avoided.* Preeclampsia-eclampsia is prevented or treated. All infections must be treated specifically, promptly, and vigorously. *Intercurrent respiratory, gastrointestinal tract, or urinary tract infections can be serious.*

Therapy by Classification

Class I-II
The great majority of these patients who are asymptomatic or who have only mild distress with their usual activities can *continue in pregnancy with minimal restriction or intervention other than close medical supervision.* Severe activity-induced symptoms indicate cardiac decompensation, in which case, hospitalization, treatment for cardiac failure, and bedrest until delivery are necessary.

Class III
In selected cases, pregnant patients with mitral stenosis who develop marked cardiac symptoms with average activity may be candidates for mitral valvulotomy up to the eighth month. Generally, in the absence of an operable lesion, severe activity limitation or bedrest until term is recommended.

Class IV

All gravidas up to about the 14th week of pregnancy with severe functional incapacity at rest, who do not have an operable cardiac abnormality, should *consider abortion.* If the lesion is not correctable, sterilization should also be considered. In some cases, *cardiac surgery during pregnancy may be necessary.* If the incapacity takes place in late pregnancy, it may be possible to prolong the pregnancy by maximal medical intervention to a premature but viable delivery.

Specific Delivery Measures

Vaginal delivery is preferred for patients with heart disease, except where there are obstetric indications for cesarean section. However, *coarctation or aneurysm of the aorta contraindicates vaginal delivery,* and numerous other patients will also require cesarean section on an individualized basis. The *third stage of labor is managed carefully to limit postpartum bleeding.* Ergot preparations, which have a pressor effect, should not be used, but oxytocin may be utilized by slow intravenous infusion. Some recommend using it after delivery as prophylaxis for uterine atony. Lowering the patient's legs promptly after delivery (or deliver with the legs down) reduces drainage of peripherally pooled blood into the systemic circulation. Some patients who have experienced no cardiac symptoms during pregnancy or labor may go into shock or acute cardiac failure immediately after delivery because of sudden engorgement of the splanchnic vessels. These patients require treatment for hypovolemic shock and acute cardiac failure.

Class I or II patients may breastfeed. Cautious, brief, early ambulation of class I–III patients may be useful, provided the medical course is otherwise uncomplicated. Class II–IV patients must remain in the hospital after delivery until cardiovascular function is stable. Before discharge, it is prudent to ascertain that the patient is returning to a controlled home situation where adequate rest in a nonstressful milieu will be possible. *Contraception and sterilization* should be discussed, particularly for class II–IV patients with continuing disease or life-threatening conditions.

Surgical Measures

Therapeutic *abortion may be indicated in 5%–8% of cases of heart* disease complicating pregnancy. Patients who have had *cardiac failure in a previous pregnancy will usually have failure again* with another pregnancy, and should consider abortion or sterilization or both. *Abortion is seldom beneficial after the fourth month* but may be considered. If the cardiac lesion is severe enough to warrant abortion and if surgical treatment is not feasible, sterilization probably is indicated. If the patient is not sterilized, strict pregnancy prevention must be employed. *Mitral valvotomy is indicated in patients with severe stenosis of the mitral valve who have insufficient cardiac reserve,* even with ideal supportive therapy, to withstand the stress of pregnancy. In general, such patients will have had cardiac decompensation in a previous pregnancy despite the best care.

Surgical and other interventional therapies have materially altered the prognosis of pregnant women with valvular heart disease. Although heart valve replacement of young women remains controversial, it is uncontrovertibly safer in some circumstances than not having the procedure. Generally, because of maternal and fetal risks, *open heart surgery is undertaken only when other possibilities have more morbidity and mortality.*

PROGNOSIS

Maternal Death
Cardiovascular disease is the sixth leading cause of maternal death (after infection, preeclampsia-eclampsia, hemorrhage, trauma, and complications of anesthesia). The maternal mortality rate for all types of heart disease is *0.5%–2%* in large medical centers in the United States, and heart disease accounts for *5%–8% of all maternal deaths.*

Perinatal Mortality
The perinatal mortality rate (including fetal deaths due to therapeutic abortion) largely depends on the functional severity of the mother's heart disease. Approximate rates are shown.

Mother's Functional Disability	Perinatal Mortality Rate
Class I	~5%
Class II	10%–15%
Class III	~35%
Class IV	>50%

Perinatal Morbidity
The *incidence of congenital defects is greater among infants delivered of women with congenital and syphilitic heart disease* than among those delivered of women with normal hearts, but rheumatic and other types of heart disease do not (without other factors) increase the incidence of fetal anomalies. Other forms of perinatal morbidity depend on the circumstances of the pregnancy and delivery and may include the sequelae of hypoxia and acidosis.

PERIPARTUM CARDIOMYOPATHY

This uncommon myocardial disorder *usually presents as cardiac failure 1–5 months postpartum, but may present during pregnancy.* Peripartal cardiomyopathy has an *unknown etiology.* It is potentially critical and most often affects *multiparas* with no evidence of prior heart disease. It seems *predisposed by multiple gestation and preeclampsia-eclampsia.* It must be distinguished from other cardiac disorders.

Dyspnea and chest pain with usual activity are the most common initial symptoms, but it may present as *pulmonary edema.* A *holosystolic murmur (mitral insufficiency) develops.* Cardiac catheterization reveals *cardiomegaly (ventricular dilatation) and low output cardiac failure with pulmonary hypertension.* Pericardial effusion is never present.

Therapy includes digitalis, treatment of pulmonary edema, medical consultation, extended bedrest, and possibly anticoagulant therapy (to minimize embolization). Patients who respond and whose heart size returns to normal within 6 months have a good prognosis but should be aware that peripartum cardiomyopathy may recur with subsequent pregnancy. Indeed ~50% *of patients with peripartial cardiomyopathy recover nearly completely.* For those who *do not respond within 6 months, the disease is all too frequently fatal.* Cardiac transplantation may be lifesaving in some patients. Postmortem findings include focal myocardial degeneration and mural thrombi but no coronary disease.

TRAUMA DURING PREGNANCY

Physical trauma, especially that involving automobile accidents, affects thousands of pregnant women yearly in the United States. The *primary diagnostic concerns are to differentiate traumatic shock from drug or substance abuse and from posteclamptic coma, and to ascertain that there is not injury to the pregnant uterus or its contents.* The physiologic changes of pregnancy may mimic symptoms of shock in gravid accident patients (e.g., increased respiratory rate, hyperventilation, increased pulse rate, and potentially, lower blood pressure). Moreover, because of the physiologic anemia of pregnancy, a slightly low HCT may not be a good indication of blood loss. Obviously, it is impossible to detail therapy for the many trauma situations that might complicate pregnancy. However, certain elements of managing the pregnant trauma patient warrant emphasis.

EMERGENCY AND
SUPPORTIVE TREATMENT

Resuscitation, ensuring the airway, and administering oxygen if the patient is unconscious, is accomplished just as in the nonpregnant. *Pregnant women are prone to regurgitation with aspiration of gastric contents.* Thus, consider insertion of a nasogastric tube with suction if the patient is obtunded to avoid gastric fluid aspiration. *Vital signs are monitored, and examination for central nervous system, abdominal, or other injuries conducted. Shock must be treated* very aggressively as (it is poorly tolerated by the fetus). While *blood studies* are being done, the patient is being *assessed,* and *IVs* are being started, an *autotransfusion may be achieved by wrapping the legs with elastic bandages and elevating the legs.* In late pregnancy, it must be ascertained that the inferior vena caval syndrome is not compounding the problem. Although the problem may be temporarily solved by lateral displacement of the uterus, longer term solutions include elevating the right hip or placing the patient in a lateral recumbent position. *Administing IV fluids is crucial.* The *cystalloid of choice is usually lactated Ringer's solution.* Even transient hypovolemia should be avoided because it poses special fetal risk.

Ascertaining fetal well-being is important, regardless of gestational age. An electronic fetal monitoring device will assist in determining fetal well-being as well as assessing uterine contractions. Additional information may be obtained by a BPP. Real-time sonography is necessary in even the earliest gestations to ascertain the fetal status and detail any potential problems (either preexisting or secondary to the trauma). Consideration of patient transfer to a perinatal center may be useful. Anesthesia or cesarean section may further jeopardize the accident victim. *However, prompt abdominal delivery may be necessary to save the mother with a ruptured viscus or internal hemorrhage. Additionally, an uncontrollably distressed fetus will require immediate rescue, if there is fetal viability.* The tissue thromboplastin released from blunt trauma all too frequently leads to initiation of the clotting cascade, with development of *abruptio placentae.* Thus, careful observation of any mother with trauma is necessary for *24–48 h to ascertain that abruptio placentae is not occurring.* Best results are achieved in trauma patients by a *team approach.* Thus, in pregnant patients, consultation with a trauma surgeon, neonatologist, and other necessary specialists may improve outcomes.

HEMATOLOGIC DISORDERS

ANEMIA

The physiologic alterations discussed in Chapter 3 and certain of the pathologic changes possible during pregnancy make the determination of anemia difficult. Not only do blood values during pregnancy differ from those in the nonpregnant patient, but these factors also vary as a function of the length of pregnancy.

In every evaluation of clinical and laboratory data, the following questions must be answered.

- Is anemia present?
- Is there evidence of iron deficiency?
- Are megaloblasts present in the blood smear?
- Are there signs of hemolysis?
- Is there bone marrow deficiency?

Anemia remains the single largest medical problem complicating pregnancy in both developed and under-developed countries. Moreover, the perinatal implications of anemia are sizable, particularly because of the association between preterm birth and anemia.

IRON DEFICIENCY ANEMIA (IDA)

IDA is the most common anemia in pregnancy. About *95% of pregnant women with anemia have IDA*. IDA is also the most likely anemia of undetermined type, regardless of cell morphology. IDA is rampant simply because *dietary iron intake* in both developed and under-developed countries *is inadequate to meet the needs of fertile women*. Recent studies indicate the dietary iron intake in fertile women is 9 mg/day, whereas the estimated daily requirement is 12–18 mg/day. Moreover, the demand for absorbed iron increases from 0.8 mg/day in early pregnancy to 7.5 mg/day in late pregnancies.

Of ~*1 g (4–5 mg/dL) of elemental iron needed during pregnancy, 300 mg is for the fetus and placenta and 700 mg is added to the maternal hemoglobin.* About 200 mg of iron is lost in bleeding during and after delivery. Fortunately, some 500 mg of iron from leftover (metabolized) maternal RBCs is returned to iron stores postpartum. Therefore, the *mother loses about 500 mg of iron with each viable pregnancy. Thus, an iron reserve of >500 mg is considered the minimum in women starting pregnancy.* A recent report indicates that only 20% of fertile women have such an iron reserve; 40% will have iron stores of 100–500 mg and 40% have virtually no iron stores. Although iron absorption increases with pregnancy, it is not enough to prevent *iron deficiency anemia in at least 20% of women not taking supplemental iron.* Additionally, repeated pregnancies, especially with a short interval between, can result in severe iron deficiency.

The *symptoms (and signs) of iron deficiency anemia increase in direct relation to the severity of the anemia.* Additionally, the symptoms may be subtle because physiologic accommodations have occurred to the relatively chronic state. Thus, patients may complain of *tiredness, weakness, lassitude, anorexia, exercise intolerance, shortness of breath, or mental depression. Pallor* is most evident in the mucous membranes, the conjunctivae, the nail beds and the palmar surface of the hands. With more severe cases, *tachycardia as well as tachypnea* may result.

Laboratory Findings
Laboratory findings commonplace in IDA include Hgb ≤5g/dL, RBC ≤2.5 million/μL, mean corpuscular volume (MCV) ≤80 mm^3 (microcytosis), mean corpuscular Hgb concentration ≤93 (hypochromia), serum iron ≤60 mg/dL, total iron-binding capacity ≥300 mg/dL, transferrin saturation ≤15%, and bone marrow with faint stain or negative for iron.

Differential Diagnosis
The differential diagnosis of IDA includes *microcytic anemia* (thalassemia) or *anemia of chronic debilitating disease* (e.g., sprue).

Complications
The perinatal complications of uncorrected IDA include *maternal infections and low-birth-weight infants.* Severe IDA is associated with *increased maternal and perinatal morbidity.*

Treatment
The treatment of IDA is *iron. Oral iron supplementation is recommended for all pregnant women.* Ferrous sulfate 325 mg tid (180 mg elemental iron per day) is a reasonable source.

For women with intolerance to oral iron or poor absorption, parenteral iron is advised. Iron dextran (InFeD) may be give IM or IV and dosage is based upon both the severity of the iron deficiency as well as the patient's size.

Prognosis
The symptomatology of the IDA will resolve with correction of the anemia. *Improvement following the use of parenteral iron is usually only slightly more rapid than with oral medication.*

Prevention
The total pregnancy iron requirements of 800 mg cannot be met by adequate diet alone. Therefore, daily elemental iron prophylaxis for all gravidas of at least 65 mg/day is recommended from at least the 20th week of gestation. Ferrous rather than ferric iron is preferable because the former is better absorbed and is less expensive. Iron-treated pregnant women have greater iron reserves, higher Hgb, and lower prevalence of IDA. Additionally, their offspring have higher serum ferritin levels. A selective approach to treatment requires screening with serum ferritin in early pregnancy to identify women who do not need iron therapy.

FOLIC ACID DEFICIENCY ANEMIA (PERNICIOUS OR MEGALOBLASTIC ANEMIA OF PREGNANCY)

Pernicious anemia of pregnancy is caused by folic acid—not vitamin B_{12}—deficiency. Unusual in the United States, the reported incidence of folic acid deficiency anemia (FADA) abroad is *1:400–1:1200 deliveries.* Folic acid deficiency is most common in multiparas >30 or in individuals on inadequate diets. Other predispositions to FADA include multiple pregnancy, preeclampsia-eclampsia, sickle cell anemia (whose bone marrow requirements for folic acid are increased), and epileptics on prolonged treatment with primidone (Mysoline) or phenytoin (Dilantin), both antifolate drugs.

The usual symptomology (and signs) includes lassitude, anorexia, and mental depression. Pallor may not be marked. Glossitis, gingivitis, emesis, or diarrhea may occur, but there are no abnormal neurologic signs.

Laboratory Findings
Serum folate is low. Increased segmental PMN leukocytes are prominent. The Hgb may be ≤4–6 g/dL and the RBCs may be ≤2 million/dL. The MCV is normal or increased. Bone marrow hyperplasia with megaloblasts is typical. Serum iron levels are high and serum vitamin B_{12} levels are normal.

Differential Diagnosis
FADA is uncommon in the reproductive years, but vitamin B_{12} anemia is not. Both disorders evoke *megaloblastosis.* Strict vegetarians may develop vitamin B_{12} anemia but not FADA. In FADA, serum vitamin B_{12} values and gastric HCl are normal, but they are low in true pernicious anemia.

Complications

Secondary infections, placental separation, and bleeding often occur with FADA. Increased maternal morbidity and perinatal mortality are recognized, although the fetus does surprisingly well even when the mother's anemia is severe.

Treatment

Treatment of FADA involves *supplemental folic acid, 5–10 mg/day* orally or parenterally, until a hematologic remission is achieved. Megaloblastic anemia of pregnancy does not usually respond to vitamin B_{12}, even in large doses. Administration of *iron may also be necessary, as well as a high-vitamin, high-protein diet.* Transfusions are rarely necessary, and therapeutic abortion and sterilization are not indicated for FADA. As noted elsewhere, *the prophylactic use of supplemental folic acid prior to and early in pregnancy is recommended because of the known beneficial effect on open neural tube defects.* As this practice becomes widespread, it is anticipated to also have a beneficial effect on the incidence of FADA.

Prognosis

FADA during pregnancy is not likely to be severe unless it is associated with systemic infection or preeclampsia-eclampsia. If the diagnosis is made at least 4 weeks before term, treatment often can raise the hemoglobin level to normal or nearly normal. *The outlook for mother and infant is good if there is adequate time for treatment.* Spontaneous remission usually occurs after delivery. Anemia usually recurs only when the patient becomes pregnant again.

DRUG-INDUCED HEMOLYTIC ANEMIA

Drug-induced hemolytic anemia during pregnancy or the puerperium may occur in individuals with the *inborn error of metabolism, glucose-6-phosphate dehydrogenase deficiency (G6PD)* in erythrocytes. This *X-linked trait affects 12% of black men and 3% of black women.* The trait is *sex-linked and of intermediate dominance.* Whites, mainly of Mediterranean or Middle East origin, may develop either an acute or a chronic hemolytic anemia due to G6PD in which both the RBC and WBC lack the enzyme.

This anemia commonly *develops after diabetic acidosis, viral or bacterial infections, ingestion of fava beans, exposure to naphthalene (moth balls), or after treatment with oxidant drugs* (including primaquine, nitrofurantion, or sulfonamides). The anemia may affect either mothers or their neonates and is *self-limited, acute, moderately severe, hemolytic anemia.*

Prevention
Education of those likely to be predisposed to induced hemolytic anemia will avoid or decrease the problem.

Laboratory Tests
The diagnosis of G6PD drug-induced hemolytic anemia is made by *a G6PD test.*

Treatment
It is important to discontinue the drug or toxic substance triggering the episode. If infection is present, it must be treated vigorously. A useful adjunct of therapy is iron supplements. Transfusion is rarely necessary.

Prognosis
Recovery with proper therapy is likely.

SICKLE CELL DISEASE

Sickle cell anemia is an autosomal recessive disorder in which the *homozygous individual (sickle cell anemia) has a preponderance of Hgb S* (as contrasted to the usual Hgb A). Hemoglobin S is less soluble in deoxygenated form, and the erythrocytes sickle (deform) at low oxygen tension and especially at low pH. Heterozygous carriers (sickle cell trait) have both Hgb A and Hgb S. Those with sickle trait have RBC sickling in vitro (a useful test) but do not manifest the sickling in vivo (with rare exception), as do those with sickle cell anemia (homozygous individual). Sickle cell disease occurs almost exclusively in blacks. In the United States, *8%–10% of African Americans have sickle cell trait, and 1:500 has sickle cell anemia.*

The substitution of only a single amino acid, valine, for glutamic acid at the sixth position on each of two hemoglobin β chains distinguishes the sickle cell hemoglobin molecule from Hgb A. The *oxygen-carrying capacity and survival time of the sickle cell RBCs are adversely affected* by this anomaly. In vivo, the tendency for the RBCs to sickle depends primarily on the state of Hgb oxygenation, temperature, levels of non-S hemoglobin, and intraepithelial Hgb concentration. With sickle cell disease, intravascular sickling begins with oxygen saturation of <85% and is almost complete at 38% oxygen saturation. Patients with sickle cell trait (Hgb A and Hgb S) show no sickling until the oxygen saturation is <40%.

Sickled cells are more rigid and may block the blood flow in the microvasculature. This causes resistance to blood flow, impeding RBC passage. Adherence of RBCs to vascular endothelium and vascular stasis causes further deoxygenation and platelet aggregation, local hypoxia, worsening acidosis, accelerated sickling, and, eventually, tissue infarction occurs. All organs can be involved, especially those with turbid flow and high oxygen extraction (e.g., the spleen, bone marrow, and placenta). *Pain and edema are common in ischemic tissue* (vasoocclusive crisis). Until the RBC has become irreversibly sickled because of a damaged membrane, the sickled erythrocyte can return to its rounded shape when hypoxic or acidic conditions are neutralized. Sickle cell crises, often precipitated by infection, dehydration, fever, or exposure to cold, may last for hours or days.

With sickle cell disease during gestation, *anemia is accelerated* (a complication in ~50%) and often has a *folic acid overlay,* the frequency of *painful crises is increased, urinary tract infections and pyelonephritis are increased, and thrombosis or visceral or orthopedic pain* is quite frequent. Other complications include *hematuria, leg ulcers, bone infarction, osteomyelitis, cholecystitis, and cardiopathy.* Overtreatment with iron may result in hemochromatosis. Acute sequestration of sickled RBC is evidenced by a rapidly falling Hgb, even ≤3 g/dL. Marrow aplasia may be a sequel to a crisis.

Sickle cell disease is inimicable to pregnancy. *The fetus is at considerable risk because of the maternal complications. Moreover, genetic counseling is crucial.* For example, if both parents have sickle cell trait, the offspring's chance is 1:4 of having sickle cell anemia, and one half of offspring will be carriers. If one parent has sickle cell disease and the other has only Hgb A, all of the offspring will have sickle cell trait.

Laboratory Findings
The Hgb may fall to 7–8 g. The reticulocyte count will be elevated. Population screening for sickling is useful for carrier detection but does not differentiate between the *different hemoglobins that may be involved (S, C, or D)* or separate sickle cell trait and sickle cell disease. The definitive test is *hemoglobin electrophoresis.*

Treatment
Obstetric patients in sickle cell crisis should be referred to a tertiary hospital, where *automated erythrocytopheresis* is available, as soon as feasible. This technique removes both Hgb S-containing RBCs and irreversibly sickled cells by extracorporeal differential centrifugation. The patient's own plasma, including leukocytes, platelets, and clotting factors, is simultaneously returned together with buffy coat-poor, washed donor RBCs. All of this can increase Hgb A concentration rapidly, and hypovolemia is minimized.

To avoid crisis antenatally, *a high hemoglobin must be maintained.* The concentration of Hgb S should be <50% to prevent crisis. Thus, transfusions are often necessary. Indeed, if erythrocytopheresis is not available for crisis, partial exchange transfusion will interrupt a sickle cell crisis during pregnancy. This temporarily diminishes erythropoiesis, improves oxygen-carrying capacity of the circulating blood, and reduces the concentration of Hgb S by substituting Hgb A-containing RBC for Hgb S-containing cells.

Patients with sickle cell disease should be offered maximal obstetric care. If this is unavailable, strict contraception is recommended until their circumstances can be maximized. Cesarean section should be performed on obstetric indications.

Prognosis

Before modern treatment modalities, maternal mortality was as high as 25% in sickle cell anemia but should be <5% *today*. Transfusions decrease the severity of pain during crises and benefit the fetus indirectly. Perinatal growth retardation is common. *Almost half of all pregnancies of women with sickle cell anemia end in perinatal death unless maximal obstetric care is given.*

THROMBOEMBOLIZATION

Thrombophlebitis and Phlebothrombosis

Thromboembolization (TE) is a common complication of pregnancy antepartum (0.2%), postpartum (0.6%). and following cesarean section (1%–2%). Unfortunately, *pulmonary embolism (15% mortality) occurs in about half of those with documented deep vein thrombosis (DVT), and only 5%–10% are symptomatic before the pulmonary embolism!* Fortunately, *DVT is uncommon without predisposing factors, including postpartum endomyometritis (or other severe infection), previous TE, severe superficial thrombophlebitis, major venous varicosities, operative delivery, difficult or prolonged labor, anemia, hemorrhage, heart disease, obesity, heavy smoking, enforced bedrest (e.g., a fracture), and cancer.*

The pregnant woman's predispositions to TE include *stasis, vascular damage, and hypercoagulability.* Venous thrombi usually develop in relatively small veins and then extend centrally (they are almost always in the lower extremities or pelvis) as far as the inferior vena cava. *The usual symptoms and signs* (erythematous, tender, firm vein) *are usually absent with DVT.* If larger proximal veins are involved, however, *swelling of the affected leg, pain, tenderness, local cyanosis, and fever may occur.* If the iliofemoral system is involved, there is acute swelling of the leg, pain about the hip, vaginal bleeding, and possibly, pain over the femoral triangle. Homans' sign is of little value.

Compression stockings or pantyhose are of some preventive value. In those at risk, however, prophylaxis is best accomplished using *heparin 5000 units bid to tid* (depending on the patient's size and stage of pregnancy—one third more is required from the beginning of the third trimester through delivery). Preoperatively, subcutaneous heparin (5000 units 2 h before surgery, repeated 12 h after surgery, then bid until the patient is ambulatory) is preventive.

If the condition is even considered, initiate diagnostic studies: directional Doppler ultrasound, venography, or various tests for thrombosis. Superficial venous thrombophlebitis is treated with limb elevation, moist heat, and nonsteroidal anti-inflammatory agents.

Heparin is the drug of choice for acute therapy of DVT; 25,000–30,000 units/24 h may be given IV (continuously or intermittent bolus) or intermittently subcutaneously. This therapy must be monitored carefully because bleeding is a major side effect (5%). Other side effects include thrombocytopenia, fat necrosis, and (over the long term) osteoporosis.

Monitoring heparin's activity is primarily accomplished by *activated partial thromboplastin time (the goal is 1.5–2 times the control),* but coagulation time, thrombin clotting time, and heparin assay may be useful. Heparin should not be administered if the platelets are ≤50,000 μL. *Protamine* (1 mg/100 units of heparin) will rapidly counteract heparin's effects.

Oral anticoagulants (warfarin) usually are contraindicated during pregnancy because of possible teratic effects (nasal hypoplasia, skeletal abnormalities, and multiple central nervous system problems). It is concentrated in the breast milk and is thus problematic to the newborn but may be useful for long-term postpartum therapy in the nonbreastfeeding mother.

Septic Pelvic Thrombophlebitis (SPT)

SPT occurs in 1 in 2000 deliveries and is defined as clotting in pelvic veins due to infection. It is predisposed by infection (e.g., prolonged rupture of the membranes), operative delivery, malnourishment, and systemic disease. It most commonly occurs 2–3 days to 6 weeks postpartum. Even with modern therapy, the *mortality approaches 10%.*

The usual clinical presentation is a *picket-fence fever* (from normal up to 41°C) *in spite of adequate and anaerobic and aerobic organism antibiotic coverage.* The pelvic examination is usually normal, but about *one third of patients will have palpable veins* in the vaginal fornices or parametrial or lower abdominal areas. The pulse and the respiratory rate may be rapid. In untreated cases, *30%–40% will have septic pulmonary embolism.*

The differential diagnosis includes pyelonephritis, appendicitis, meningitis, SLE, TB, malaria, typhoid, sickle cell crisis, and adnexal torsion. *Treatment is heparin and broad-spectrum antibiotics.* Within 48–72 h, the fever should resolve, but heparin should be continued for 7–10 days. *Surgery is only indicated if medical management fails, if septic emboli occur during therapy, if the patient has puerperal sepsis and pulmonary infarction, or if medical therapy is contraindicated.* In such cases, percutaneous placement of a vena caval filter often is all that is necessary. Occasionally, however, it is necessary to ligate the ovarian veins.

LEUKEMIA, LYMPHOMA, AND HODGKIN'S DISEASE

Leukemia affects the leukopoietic tissues (lymphatic, myeloid, or monocytic) and may be acute or chronic. Lymphomas affect the lymphoreticular system and are subdivided into Hodgkin's disease and non-Hodgkin's lymphoma. All types usually occur after the childbearing age, so these conditions are an uncommon pregnancy complication.

A normochromic, normocytic anemia occurs in leukemia and Hodgkin's disease. Moderate thrombocytopenia and marked leukocytosis must be expected. Bleeding and premature delivery are common. The perinatal mortality rate is high and may depend on the necessary maternal therapy. Several cases of possible transfer of leukemia or Hodgkin's disease to the offspring have been reported and mandate careful follow-up. Approximately 85% of Hodgkin's relapses occur <2 years. Thus, if another pregnancy is planned, it is recommended to defer it until the mother's stability is determined. Definitive discussion of these unusual conditions is beyond the purpose of this text.

RENAL DISEASES

URINARY TRACT INFECTION

ASYMPTOMATIC BACTIURIA, CYSTITIS, AND SYMPTOMATIC LOWER URINARY TRACT INFECTION

The urinary tract is especially vulnerable to infection during pregnancy because of ureteral dilatation, urinary stasis, and ureterovesical reflux. Moreover, pregnancy enhances the progression rate from asymptomatic to symptomatic disease. The trauma of labor and delivery and urinary retention after delivery may also initiate or aggravate infection in the urinary system. However, one of the most important predispositions remains urethral catheterization. Maternal urinary tract infections contribute significantly to postpartum hospital stay if not aggressively managed.

Escherichia coli is the offending organism in ~80% of cases. Certain clinical events correlate well with what organism may be anticipated. *E. coli* may be anticipated in women who have not had prior urinary infections, have not had urinary catheterization, have not had antibiotics, and who have not been hospitalized. In patients with these conditions the microbial spectrum may be different and if *E. coli* is the offending organism, it is less sensitive to most antibiotics. Thus, ascertaining if these events (prior urinary infections, urinary catheterization, antibiotic therapy, and hospitalization) have occurred may alter therapy.

Asymptomatic bacteriuria occurs in at least 3% of all pregnant women, and intercurrent pyelonephritis can be expected in >30% of these patients without prophylactic treatment. By way of contrast, symptomatic urinary tract infection will develop in only 1%–2% of pregnant women without antecedent bacteriuria. Up to an additional 5% will develop urinary tract infections after delivery. Chronic pyelonephritis, a major contributor to death in older women, often follows recurrent acute urinary tract infections during successive pregnancies. Symptomatic urinary tract infection is associated with a considerable increase in the incidence of premature rupture of the membranes and premature delivery and its resultant morbidity and mortality.

The diagnosis of urinary tract infection should be based on analysis of a catheterized or clean-catch specimen of urine. The long utilized clinical screening tool of urinalysis (detection of *microscopic pyuria*) has been supplemented by two additional screening tools. The *Uriscreen* is a rapid diagnostic test based on the detection of urine catalase. The *dipstick screening* is based on leukocyte esterase and nitrite determinations. Table 15-1 briefly compares the efficacy of these screening methods (nonpregnant patients) to urine culture. It has been suggested that the high sensitivity and negative predictive value (as well as ease of use, rapidity, and low cost) of the Uriscreen and Dipstick methods may obviate the need for some cultures in ruling out the diagnosis of urinary tract infection.

If the culture reveals >100,000 colonies/mL, treatment is required. Sensitivity tests to determine response to the various antiinfective agents are desirable. Initial urinary infections in women are usually treated with nitrofurantoin (100 mg orally qid) or

TABLE 15-1
COMPARISON OF SCREENING TESTS FOR URINARY TRACT INFECTIONS

Screening Method	Sensitivity (%)	Specificity (%)	Negative Predicative Value (%)	Positive Predicative Value (%)
Urinalysis	89	88	95	76
Uriscreen	100	69	100	56
Dipstick	97	83	99	69

trimethoprim-sulfamethoxazole, although ciprofloxacin (500 mg PO once a day to bid) is increasing in usage. Initial cure rates are 88%, 93%, and 81%, respectively, for the three drugs. Change to other drugs is dictated by the results of laboratory studies. The length of treatment may be more important than which drug is used. Treatment for >7 d yields a better cure rate than <7 d regardless of the drug used. Repeat urinary tract infection screening, if not urinary culture, after completion of therapy is useful to ascertain therapeutic effectiveness.

In addition to the antibiotic therapy, adjunctive therapy may be useful in the acute stage for symptomatic relief. For urgency and frequency, give pyridium 100 mg qid. Force fluids (if indicated) and acidify the urine (vitamin C or cranberry juice). Give analgesics, laxatives, and antipyretic drugs as indicated.

If obstruction is present, urethral or ureteral catheterization may be necessary. Ureteral obstruction usually resolves after delivery, but if it is permanent, surgical repair may be required. If response to chemotherapy and ureteral catheterization is inadequate, nephrostomy may be necessary, particularly during the second trimester and before fetal viability.

PYELONEPHRITIS (UPPER URINARY TRACT INFECTIONS)

Pyelonephritis is generally caused by *E. coli,* but diabetes, prior infections, instrumentation, indwelling cathethers, calculi, and immunosuppression add a spectrum of other causative organisms. Renal damage is not always found with pyelonephritis, but is predisposed by delay in diagnosis, ineffective antibacterial therapy, and obstruction.

In many centers, *pyelonephritis is treated with very short hospitalization (even day care) during which the sepsis is treated with parenteral antibiotics, intravenous fluids are given to replace those lost as well as to maximize urinary flows, and the elevations of temperatures are controlled.* Once the acute episode is managed, therapy may continue as an outpatient with home care. Ceftriaxone and gentamycin are cost-effective parenteral once daily therapy.

GLOMERULONEPHRITIS

An initial attack of acute glomerulonephritis is rare during pregnancy. Most obstetric problems leading to glomerulonephritis involve chronic forms of the disease. There is no evidence that pregnancy aggravates glomerulonephritis.

Infertility, abortion, premature delivery, fetal death in utero, premature separation of the normally implanted placenta, and placental dysmaturity occur more frequently in women with glomerulonephritis than in normal women. Nephritis causes hypertension, predisposes to preeclampsia-eclampsia, and is associated with a high incidence of perinatal mortality and morbidity. Fetal growth and activity must be carefully monitored.

The medical treatment of glomerulonephritis is the same whether or not the patient is pregnant. Corticosteroids may be harmful, and antibiotics are ineffective. Therapeutic abortion may be justified for acute, severe exacerbations of glomerulonephritis with renal insufficiency. Glomerulonephritis may be an indication for cesarean section when placental dysmaturity or preeclampsia-eclampsia occurs.

URETERAL STONE

Ureteral stone is more common during pregnancy than otherwise because hypercalciuria occurs during pregnancy when calcium and vitamin D are supplemented, the renal pelvis and ureter dilate in response to high levels of steroid sex hormones, and minor (physiologic) obstructive uropathy is characteristic of pregnancy. Small, previously retained stones are, thus, permitted to enter the proximal ureter. Most ureteral stones are passed in the urine, albeit painfully. Others become impacted. Sudden, agonizing pain in the costovertebral angle and flank with radiation to the lower quadrant and vulva, urinary urgency, and hematuria without (initially) pyuria or fever are characteristic of ureteral stone. Intravenous urography may demonstrate partial obstruction and the stone.

Symptomatic therapy with analgesics and antispasmodics is always indicated and may be best given parenterally. Retrograde catheter manipulation may dislodge the stone and permit it to pass, or the stone may be extracted transurethrally. If such efforts are unsuccessful and progressive hydronephrosis develops, remove the stone by extraperitoneal ureterolithectomy irrespective of the patient's obstetric status. *Lithotripsy during pregnancy is contraindicated.*

GASTROINTESTINAL DISORDERS

PEPTIC ULCER

Pregnancy generally exerts an ameliorating effect on peptic ulcer, but hemorrhage or perforation may occur during or shortly after pregnancy. Pregnancy offers no protection to aggravation of peptic ulcer by anxiety. Exacerbation of peptic ulcer in the puerperium may be a result of a rise in gastric acidity during lactation.

Medical treatment is the same as for the nonpregnant woman. Treatment of *Helobacter pylori* is accomplished with multiple therapy (e.g., Prevacid, amoxicillin, and Biaxin). Cimetidine and other histamine receptor antagonists are pregnancy class B drugs (use only if clearly needed, as there are promising animal studies but no well-controlled studies in pregnant women). Surgery is rarely necessary except in the most severe emergencies.

HIATAL HERNIA

Hiatal hernia, or partial protrusion of the stomach or esophagus (or both) through the diaphragm, develops in patients with a weakened or congenitally widened diaphragmatic crux because of increases in intraabdominal pressure during pregnancy. With gestation, there is progressive enlargement of the uterus with elevation of the stomach by the uterine fundus. *Hiatal hernia occurs more frequently in multiparas and in older or obese pregnant women. About 15% of all pregnant women develop symptomatic hiatal hernia.*

Persistence of nausea and vomiting beyond midpregnancy, progressive pyrosis, and eructation during recumbency are typical findings. The sensation of substernal pressure may be severe and is relieved by erect posture but aggravated by lying down.

Conservative treatment is usually adequate to carry the patient through pregnancy and delivery: a bland diet, small meals, antispasmodics, antacids (calcium products are preferred), and cautions against lying flat or exercising immediately after eating or drinking. It may also be useful to prevent unnecessary increases in intraabdominal pressure by prescribing laxatives for constipation, by restricting lifting, and by the use of low forceps delivery so that the patient will not have to bear down during the second stage of labor. The patient should sleep in a semireclining position. Obese women should not gain extra weight. The great majority of hiatal hernias resolve soon after delivery, with dramatic relief. Thus, surgery is rarely necessary.

BOWEL OBSTRUCTION

Mechanical obstruction of the intestine (most frequently the small bowel) *occurs in about 1:6000 pregnancies.* About one quarter of cases occur during the *second trimester,* when the enlarging uterus displaces the bowel sufficiently to stretch adhesions. Mechanical obstruction should be considered as a cause of ileus in women with one or more abdominal scars. Other causes of obstruction include incarceration of a loop of intestine in an external or internal hernia, volvulus, and intussusception. Symptoms of bowel obstruction include *nausea, vomiting, and persistent abdominal pain.*

Laparotomy is indicated without delay. The maternal mortality rate may be as high as 10% if treatment of septic closed-loop obstruction is delayed. Fluid and electrolyte imbalance must be corrected early. (Note: Hypokalemic alkalosis can cause convulsions that may be confused with eclamptic seizures.) Broad-spectrum antibiotics should be given parenterally if infection occurs.

ADYNAMIC ILEUS

Mild adynamic ileus may be present for 1–3 days, even after normal delivery, or longer after cesarean section. Other obstetric and gynecologic conditions that may cause adynamic ileus are intraperitoneal or retroperitoneal hemorrhage and infection, pyelonephritis, nephroureterolithiasis, torsion of the adnexa, bladder atony, and hypokalemic acidosis. Older women seem more prone to adynamic ileus than young ones.

Adynamic ileus in obstetric and gynecologic patients almost always responds to withholding oral food and fluids, correction of fluid and electrolyte imbalance by means of parenteral fluids, intestinal (nasogastric) decompression, and evacuation of the rectosigmoid colon by enemas. In more difficult cases, gastric suction usually will suffice. If ileus is marked, a long intestinal tube (Werner, Miller-Abbott) should be inserted to decompress the small bowel.

APPENDICITIS

Appendicitis occurs in about 1:1200 pregnancies (Fig. 15-3). Management is more difficult than when the disease occurs in non-pregnant persons because the appendix is carried high and to the right, away from McBurney's point. Hence, *the traditional localization of pain does not usually occur. The distended uterus displaces the colon and small bowel, uterine contractions prevent abscess formation and walling-off, and the intestinal relationships are disturbed.* An additional confounder is pregnancy related leukocytosis. In at least 20% of obstetric patients with appendicitis, the correct diagnosis is not made until the appendix has ruptured and peritonitis has become established. Delay may lead to sepsis, premature labor, or abortion.

FIGURE 15-3. Diagram showing the level of the appendix at the various months of pregnancy (Baer).

(From A.C. Beck and A.H. Rosenthal, *Obstetrical Practice,* 7th ed. Williams & Wilkins, 1957.)

If early appendectomy is indicated, the use of *antibiotics should be carefully individualized to minimize morbidity.* If the diagnosis is made during labor or near term, cesarean section and appendectomy should be done to minimize peritonitis. Therapeutic abortion is not indicated. If drains are necessary, they should be transabdominal, never transvaginal.

With early diagnosis and appendectomy, the prognosis is good for the mother and infant, but if intraabdominal abscesses occur, labor may cause subsequent rupture, even after lengthy delays and appropriate antibiotics, with massive sepsis. Given current imaging (sonography, MRI), the detection of intraabdominal abscesses is less difficult and should they be present, cesarean section is warranted.

INFLAMMATORY BOWEL DISEASE

The cause of this group of diseases (regional enteritis or Crohn's disease, ulcerative colitis, and granulomatous colitis) remains unknown. *Young women are most commonly affected, and the peak incidence is in the second and third decades.* In the absence of pelvic abscesses, fertility is unaffected. Crohn's disease increases abortion by 25%, but ulcerative colitis and granulomatous colitis do not enhance the rate of abortion. *In general, pregnancy is not contraindicated.* Pregnancy does not generally exert an untoward influence on inflammatory bowel disease. *When conception coincides with active ulcerative colitis, however, 50%–75% of patients will suffer a severe relapse during pregnancy or in the puerperium.* When colitis has its onset during pregnancy, more than half of the patients will suffer a hectic course, and a few will die. When colitis has its onset during the puerperium, most patients will have a very severe, often protracted course.

In severe, fulminating cases, colitis induces intractable bloody diarrhea, fever, fluid and electrolyte imbalance, collapse, toxicosis, and death. When the disease becomes chronic, malnutrition and invalidism are associated with remissions and exacerbations of diarrhea.

There is no specific treatment. Dietary, symptomatic, and supportive medical measures, corticosteroids, and sulfasalazine are usually employed during pregnancy. Although, the last two are possible teratogens, that small risk is usually preferable to acute exacerbations. Sulfasalazine may cause neonatal hyperbilirubinemia, and if it is used, maternal folic acid should be administered.

BILIARY AND HEPATIC DISORDERS

CHOLEDOCHOLITHIASIS AND CHOLECYSTITIS

Severe choledocholithiasis and cholecystitis are uncommon during pregnancy despite the fact that the smooth muscle relaxation of pregnancy (due to progesterone) is predisposing and women have an increased tendency to form gallstones (one third of all women >40 have gallstones). When acute gallbladder inflammation or biliary colic does occur, it is usually in late pregnancy or, more often, in the puerperium. About 90% of patients with cholecystitis have stones.

When cholecystitis occurs, *treatment with antibiotics, IV fluids, and nasogastric drainage may be all that is required.* Meperidine or atropine is effective in alleviating pain and ductal spasm.

Gallbladder surgery in pregnant women should be attempted only in extreme cases (e.g., obstruction) *because it greatly increases the perinatal mortality rate (up to about 15%).* Cholecystostomy and lithotomy may be all that is feasible during advanced pregnancy, with cholecystectomy deferred until after delivery. On the other hand, withholding surgery when it is definitely needed may result in necrosis and perforation of the gallbladder and peritonitis. The same precautions noted previously (see p. 448) should be utilized for diagnosis and management of cases with intraabdominal abscesses. Intermittent high fever, jaundice, and right upper quadrant pain may indicate cholangitis due to impacted common duct stone.

CHOLESTATIC JAUNDICE OF PREGNANCY

Cholestatic or recurrent jaundice of pregnancy is an uncommon disorder of successive pregnancies that is caused by *an inherited deficiency in liver metabolism.* Hepatic excretory insufficiency is apparently provoked by estrogen. Cholestatic jaundice of pregnancy is characterized by itching, gastrointestinal complaints, and jaundice during the last trimester of pregnancy. The symptoms disappear within 2 weeks after delivery but tend to recur in subsequent advanced pregnancies. The levels of most liver enzymes are only slightly elevated, and the results of hepatic function tests are normal.

The diagnosis of cholestatic jaundice of pregnancy requires the exclusion of other liver disorders (e.g., viral hepatitis, drug toxicity, and cholecystitis). A history of jaundice during a previous pregnancy or with use of oral contraceptives is most helpful diagnostically. *Treatment is symptomatic.* Jaundice and itching may be reduced by administration of ion exchange resins, which absorb bile salts.

Cholestyramine may be beneficial. However, it absorbs fat-soluble vitamins and may even induce bleeding due to malabsorption of vitamin K. Thus, vitamin K supplementation should be given to both mother and newborn. This disorder is limited to the duration of pregnancy (or estrogen therapy).

ACUTE FATTY LIVER OF PREGNANCY

This rare (1:13,000) disease in the past had maternal and perinatal mortality of 75%–85%, but this is currently down to ~20%. It is a maternal multisystem disorder with hepatitis a prominent manifestation and usually occurs >35 weeks and does not tend to recur with subsequent pregnancy. The symptoms include severe nausea, vomiting, hematemesis, abdominal pain, jaundice, stupor, and progressive hepatic insufficiency. Disseminated intravascular coagulation or renal failure may be associated late problems.

Acute fatty liver must be differentiated from toxic or viral hepatitis, cholestatic liver dysfunction, cholecystitis, and pancreatitis. Effective supportive therapy is the only known treatment.

VIRAL HEPATITIS

Three types of viral hepatitis (A, B, and C) affect females of all ages. The incidence is 0.2% in pregnancy when manifestations, although similar, may be more severe and prolonged (especially in advanced pregnancy). Maternal and perinatal prognosis is quite different in the three types. Table 15-2 details characteristics of the three types.

Treatment for all three generally consists of *supportive medical measures* as for the nonpregnant patient. Certain other generalizations may be useful. Operative intervention is to be avoided, if possible. Anesthetics, analgesics, and sedatives that may be hepatotoxic must be avoided. A very low prothrombin concentration may lead to hemorrhage, which should be treated with oral or parenteral vitamin K. The *maternal and fetal risks are low* (except as noted later) *if adequate nutrition is maintained.* Terminate pregnancy only in case of impending or actual hepatic coma. Deterioration may justify cesarean section for the viable infant.

If obstetric care is good, the maternal mortality rate is approximately that of nonpregnant women with viral hepatitis. It is wise to *allow more than 1 year to elapse between hepatitis and subsequent*

TABLE 15-2
CHARACTERISTICS OF VIRAL HEPATITIS

	Hepatitis A	Hepatitis B	Hepatitis C (non-A, non-B)
Virus	RNA (27 nm)	DNA (42 nm)	RNA (30–50 nm)
Incubation (days)	15–50	45–160	18–100
Source	Enteric (fecal-oral), close family or contacts	Parenteral (body fluids), blood, saliva, vaginal secretions, semen	Parenteral (body fluids)
Laboratory diagnosis	HA Ab (1gM, 1gG)	HBsAG, HBcAb, HBsAB, HBeAg	HCAb
Perinatal transmission	Low	Active 0–28 weeks <10% 29–40 weeks 65% Carrier HBeAG+ 75%–95% HBeAg− <5% HBcAg+ <5%	Unknown
Newborn	Rare 14–30 days	Active 30–120 days Mild disease Carrier 30–120 days Severe disease (death possible)	Unknown
Carrier development (maternal)	0	5%–10%	50%
Carrier development (infant)	None	Frequent	Unknown
Sequelae	None	Chronic active hepatitis	Chronic active hepatitis

pregnancy. By this time, liver function tests should return to normal values unless serious complications have developed. The fetal effect of chronic active hepatitis depends on the extent of maternal disease (loss is high with poor liver function or esophageal varices). Treatment with immunosuppressants and corticosteroids does not preclude pregnancy.

Hepatitis A (infectious hepatitis) is usually quite benign during pregnancy, with only enteric isolation, supportive treatment, and careful monitoring of liver enzymes being necessary. Hepatitis A antibody is useful for detection. The rate of perinatal (fetal or neonatal) transmission is low, and maternal and perinatal morbidity is little affected in developed countries, although there is enhanced loss in undeveloped areas. Gamma globulin prophylaxis is effective protection for pregnant women exposed to hepatitis A. A hepatitis A vaccine is available with recommendations to be used in those with exposure risk.

Hepatitis B (serum hepatitis) occurs in about 1:500 pregnancies. Vertical transmission may be prevented by hepatitis B immune globulin and hepatitis B vaccine. Detection is by screening with hepatitis B surface antigen (HBsAg) and the hepatitis B surface antibody (HBsAb). HBsAb indicates a noninfectious state. HBsAg without HBsAb is the chronic carrier state, with a high likelihood (75%–95%) of vertical transmission. When HBsAg is detected, it is imperative to ascertain if the e antigen is present. *The maternal course is unaltered, but prematurity is increased.* Care must be taken not to infect the newborn at delivery. When the mother is HBsAg positive and HBsAb negative, the neonate should have HBsAg and HBsAb studies drawn and receive both hepatitis B immune globulin and the hepatitis B vaccine immediately. If antigenicity studies can be obtained rapidly, hepatitis B vaccine may be delayed up to 7 days of age. If the baby is HBsAg negative, the original dose is given and is then repeated 1 month later. The third dose is given 6 months after the original dose.

Hepatitis C virus (HCV) currently infects ~2% of the U.S. population, making it *the most common chronic blood borne infection.* About 40% of chronic liver disease is HCV related, and HCV is estimated to cause 8000–10,000 deaths per year in the United States. End-stage liver disease caused by HCV is the most common current indication for liver transplantation in the United States. Moreover, because HCV currently is ~3-fold higher among those 30–49 years old, the health care burden as well as deaths from HCV related liver disease will increase as much as 4-fold over the next 10–20 years.

Most HCV infections are acquired by direct percutaneous exposure to blood. Known acquisitions account for ~90% of all HCV infections: intravenous drug use (60%), sexual exposure (20%), known exposures (occupational, hemodialysis, household, perinatal—10%). The remaining 10% of individuals with HCV have no demonstrable source of infection, but the majority are of low socioeconomic status (a risk factor). In recent studies, up to 77% of intravenous drug users have HCV infections.

Acute HCV infection has been thought to progress to chronic hepatitis in ~85% of cases. However, recent studies indicate that healthy individuals who become HCV infected are at less risk for progressive liver disease than previously thought. Thus, although chronic hepatitis C increases risk for cirrhosis and hepatocellular carcinoma, there is controversy about the amount of risk and the time required for this progression. Current best estimates are that ~20–30% of infected individuals will develop fibrosis and cirrhosis. Of those with fibrosis and cirrhosis, ~20% will progress to liver decompensation and 10%–20% to hepatocellular carcinoma. The time required for the progression is 20–30 years. Risks of enhancing the progression include: alcohol intake, male sex, age >40 years at infection, and coinfection with HIV or hepatitis B virus.

Although sexual transmission of HCV occurs, to what extent is unknown. The literature suggests: HCV presence in seminal fluid, HCV presence in vaginal secretions, a higher rate of HCV infections in the sexually promiscuous (2%–12%), and molecular biologic evidence of sexual transmission. Confounding evidence is that monogamous sexual partners of HCV infected individuals have a low rate (2.5%) of interspousal transmission despite long duration of sexual exposure. Thus, the use of condoms is currently only recommended in cases of multiple partners and for those at high risk of transmission.

Mother to infant transmission of HCV is ~5%, and is restricted to infants whose mothers are viremic. If the mother is coinfected with HIV, the rate is higher. Currently, there is no data to indicate that the rate of perinatal HCV infection is influenced by the mode of delivery or by breast feeding. Pregnancy is not contraindicated in women infected with HCV.

Most who develop chronic HCV infections many not be aware that they have been infected, for the onset is so mild. Additionally, the chronic infection is asymptomatic and the duration of the disease is prolonged. Although the personal objects (razors, toothbrushes, nail clippers) of an HCV infected person should not be shared, eating utensils have not been incriminated in infections. Sexual partners should be tested for anti-HCV. HCV positive individuals should not donate blood, organs, or tissue. HCV patients with active disease should refrain from alcohol.

Interferon for 12 months is the current standard therapy for individuals with chronic HCV and elevated ALT levels, but rates of sustained virologic response are only 15%–20%. However, combination therapy (alpha interferon and ribavirin) is emerging as more efficacious, and therapy is rapidly evolving.

ABDOMINAL HERNIAS

As pregnancy advances, the enlarging uterus fills the lower abdomen, displacing the intestines, so that nonadherent bowel may recede from an inguinal aperture. Pregnancy permanently enlarges umbilical and incisional hernial rings. The uterus also shields incisional and other weak points from herniation. Hence, many abdominal hernias reduce spontaneously during pregnancy. A few irreducible (adherent) ones become incarcerated. Femoral and pelvic hernias are uncommon but are often overlooked in obstetric patients.

The patient with a large hernia should not strain in labor or delivery. Low forceps usually suffice, and cesarean section is not indicated for delivery. Elective surgery for repair of an abdominal hernia should be delayed until after pregnancy, but emergency operation for the relief and correction of an incarcerated hernia may be performed during pregnancy.

DERMATOLOGIC COMPLICATIONS

Pregnancy has a sparing effect on most dermatoses. With few exceptions, skin disorders during pregnancy and the puerperium are similar to those in nonpregnant women.

Dermatologic disorders induced by pregnancy include abnormalities of pigmentation (e.g., chloasma), herpes gestationis, noninflammatory pruritus of pregnancy, angiectids or vascular spiders, and erythema palmare. Dermatologic disorders usually aggravated by pregnancy include *Candida* vulvovaginitis, acne vulgaris (early in pregnancy), erythema multiforme, dermatitis herpetiformis, granuloma inguinale, condylomata acuminata, pemphigus, neurofibromatosis, and systemic lupus erythematosus. It is unlikely that malignant melanoma is aggravated by pregnancy. Pregnancy is likely to have a beneficial effect on acne (late in pregnancy), psoriasis, and seborrheic dermatitis.

CHLOASMA (MELASMA)

Chloasma consists of blotchy, petal-shaped, yellowish brown pigmented patches symmetrically distributed over the forehead, nose, and malar prominence. These become confluent to form the mask of pregnancy. Chloasma usually fades soon after delivery. Only cosmetic treatment is required. Hydroquinone cream (Eldoquin) 2% applied nightly may limit the development and speed the clearing of chloasma, but skin may develop a grayish color.

HERPES GESTATIONIS

This serious disease affecting about 1:4000 (1:1700–50,000) gravidas is *the most common skin disorder that affects the fetus.* The cause of herpes gestationis is unknown, but it may be a variation of dermatitis herpetiformis. It is not related to the herpesvirus, and the nomenclature is unfortunate. The *intensely burning, pruritic, occasionally painful urticarial papulovesicular eruption* involving the buttocks, extensor surfaces of the arms and legs, back, and upper abdomen begins during or after the fifth month of pregnancy. Occasionally, it is noted early postpartum. Fetal death may occur during any period. The fatal pathophysiologic sequence is unexplained.

Grouped vesicles on inflammatory bases are typical. The bullae of herpes gestationis form an annular pattern around the edge of the lesions, in contrast to those of erythema multiforme, which has bullae that are centrally located. The lesions leave small pigmented scars on healing. A high eosinophil count in blood and vesical fluid is usual. Biopsy shows subepidermal bullae, increased eosinophils, and deposits of complement in the basement layer of the skin with immunofluorescent staining. Herpes gestationis is marked by a complement fixing HG factor in the serum.

Herpes gestationis *tends to recur with subsequent pregnancies,* but the extent of the recurrence is not related to the extent of the disease in the index case. There is a genetic predisposition to herpes gestationis and the disease appears to be mediated by an IgG specific for a 180-kD component of hemidesmosomes. The maternal prognosis is good, with the process usually abating in the nonpregnant state. Perinatal outcomes are less well understood, with reports variously ranging from minimal risk to intrauterine growth retardation or perinatal death. An occasional newborn of an affected mother may manifest herpes gestationis lesions. Some authorities believe the skin manifestations are merely a reflection of a primary immunologic event taking place in the placenta.

The differential diagnosis of bullous lesions includes nonimmune as well as autoimmune lesions. Nonimmune causes of similar lesions include: contact dermatitis, bullous reactions to drugs or insect bites, and infections. Autoimmune mucocutaneous bullous (blistering) diseases includes herpes gestationis, toxic epidermal necrolysis, and erythema multiforme. Crucial elements in distinguishing among the potential causes are morphology and lesions distribution, presence or absence of mucosal lesions, and scarring. Corticosteroids are useful but not curative.

NONINFLAMMATORY PRURITUS OF PREGNANCY

The cause is not known. No cutaneous lesions can be seen, but the patient experiences intense itching all over the body. Areas excoriated by scratching may become infected.

A papular pruritic dermatosis of pregnancy with a high fetal mortality rate, associated with abnormally elevated hCG levels, has been described and must be differentiated from the benign noninflammatory pruritus of pregnancy. Symptomatic therapy is advised for the latter.

Pruritus may result from cholestatic jaundice of pregnancy (p. 451). In this condition, no rash develops but minute bilirubin deposits in the skin cause itching.

ERYTHEMA PALMARE

This benign disorder is a dusky thenar and hypothenar vascular engorgement of the skin of the hands noted 4–6 weeks after the onset of pregnancy. The erythema disappears during the early puerperium. It is based on genetic predisposition and provoked by hyperestrogenism (as are vascular spiders).

VASCULAR SPIDERS OR SPIDER ANGIOMAS

These are small, red, pulsating (arteriolar) telangiectatic points in the skin over the face, neck, thorax, and arms. Most vascular spiders develop during the second and third trimesters of pregnancy and fade almost to invisibility after delivery. They reappear during subsequent advanced pregnancies. In most instances, these angiomas have only minor, temporary cosmetic significance, but the possibility that cirrhosis and hereditary hemorrhagic telangiectasia (and their complications) may be related must be kept in mind.

PRURITIC URTICARIAL PAPULES AND PLAQUES OF PREGNANCY

This *intensely pruritic cutaneous eruption of late pregnancy is of unknown origin.* Symptoms include numerous erythematous urticarial papules and myriads of minute plaques that first appear on the abdomen and then spread to involve the thighs and, at times, the buttocks and arms. Tissue biopsy of the lesions aids in the differential diagnosis, which includes herpes gestationis, prurigo gravidarum, and papular dermatitis of pregnancy. Corticosteroid therapy is moderately beneficial, but the dermatitis improves rapidly after delivery. Occasional patients have slight subsequent itching of the hands, sometimes during menses. The infants are free of skin abnormalities. Although only a small number of patients have been followed, the probability of recurrence of the disorder in subsequent pregnancies appears to decline.

CONNECTIVE TISSUE DISORDERS

RELAXATION OF THE PELVIC JOINTS

Considerable relaxation of the pelvic joints, the result of increased steroids and relaxin, is normal during pregnancy, but about 1:100 suffers from pelvic joint pain and ~1:1500 is seriously incapacitated (Pregnancy Pelvic Arthropathy). Normally, considerable separation of the pubis (allowing vertical movement with ambulation) and instability of the sacroiliac joint occur with some instability and, occasionally, pain. This joint relaxation is progressive during the second trimester and early part of the third trimester. Undue mobility persists until after delivery. Joint stability may not return to normal until several months postpartum.

Pelvic arthropathy is presumed to be due to an exaggeration of this normal alteration of elasticity of connective and collagen tissues. The extent of disability, however, is not always directly related to the degree of joint instability. This condition is most frequently associated with obesity or multiple pregnancy. Occasionally, it may be simply an unmasking of a previously underlying disorder.

The usual symptoms include *extreme pain in the sacroiliac and pubic joints on standing, walking, and turning.* Prolonged sacroiliac backache may be a sequela to sacroiliac arthropathy of pregnancy. Orthopedic (and occasionally neurologic) consultation is useful to ascertain that other conditions have been excluded or properly managed.

Treatment for pelvic arthropathy consists of limitation of activities, analgesics, and a sturdy, fitted girdle that gives support by snug encirclement of the sacrum, symphysis, and greater trochanters. Every precaution must be taken to avoid exaggerated positions, marked traction, and sudden movement of the patient during delivery.

SYSTEMIC LUPUS ERYTHEMATOSUS

Systemic lupus erythematosus (SLE) affects principally females and develops most frequently during the childbearing years. It is an uncommon but often *extremely serious complication of pregnancy. Pregnancy does not consistently influence the course of this disorder:* ~50% remain unchanged, a few cases improve, but the rest have exacerbations (especially during the puerperium). If comparable time intervals are contrasted with nonpregnant patients with acute SLE, however, the probability of an exacerbation is 1–3 times greater in the first half, 1–2 times greater in the second half of pregnancy, and *>600 times during the puerperium.*

Moreover, SLE patients have a *marked increase in pregnancy wastage. Spontaneous abortion is increased about threefold.* Active renal disease plays a marked role in fetal loss, whereas maternal hypertension is directly related to preterm delivery. *Premature labor (and delivery)* is further directly increased by the necessity for increasing doses of corticosteroids. The incidence of *preeclampsia-eclampsia* also increased in those suffering from the disease. The incidence of *intrauterine growth retardation (IUGR)* is increased and recently it has been observed that the risk of IUGR is 50% in patients who have low serum complement activity during the pregnancy. The placental pathology is marked by decidual vasculopathy and infarction.

There is an enhanced possibility of the newborn having *congenital heart block.* Maternal anti-52 kD SSA/Ro by immunoblot is a risk predictor for neonatal congenital heart block. *Neonatal congenital heart block recurrence in subsequent pregnancy is 12%–16%.* The childhood morbidity of the SLE heart block is high, with nearly two thirds of requiring pacemakers.

Corticosteroids may relieve the symptoms and reduce the number and intensity of acute exacerbations. Prednisone, 30–50 mg (or equivalent) daily orally in 4 divided doses, may be required for treatment of an acute attack. After improvement has occurred, the drug dosage may be gradually reduced to withdrawal or to a maintenance dose of 10 mg/day. Even prolonged use during pregnancy and the puerperium has not demonstrated teratic activity sufficient to preclude usage. Occasionally, antineoplastics may be necessary. Patients must avoid overactivity and exposure to the sun and other sources of ultraviolet light. Pigmented emollient cosmetic lotions opaque to ultraviolet light may be applied over facial lesions. Analgesics and physical therapy may be given for musculoskeletal discomfort. Recently, the use of immunoadsorption therapy and cyclosporin A has been reported in pregnancy, but further study is necessary.

The *maternal mortality rate is approximately 20% and the perinatal mortality rate is about 30% in acute disseminated SLE.* The mortality rates in chronic SLE depend on the duration and severity of the disease. *The postdelivery period may be the most critical.* Thus, corticosteroids should not be discontinued too early. Pregnancy rarely exacerbates SLE so severely that therapeutic abortion is justified. Cesarean section should be performed only for obstetric indications.

Barrier-type contraception is usually recommended. *Oral contraceptives may trigger an exacerbation of SLE.* With steroids, the likelihood of infection is increased with intrauterine devices. Surgery may induce exacerbation of SLE, and this must be weighed when considering sterilization.

NEUROLOGIC DISEASES

The effect of neurologic diseases on pregnancy is rarely critical. For example, pregnancy is not an absolute contraindication to urgent neurosurgery for the evacuation of a subdural hematoma, removal of an intracranial tumor, or treatment of an intracranial aneurysm. Neurologic disorders are only rarely so serious as to require interruption of pregnancy; however, certain neurologic diseases may be aggravated by pregnancy (e.g., chorea gravidarum or Sydenham's chorea, severe nonspecific polyneuritis, and herniation of an intervertebral disk).

Consider sterilization only when the woman's life and health will be jeopardized by subsequent pregnancy or when there is a significant likelihood of transmission of serious hereditary disorders.

EPILEPSY

Epilepsy has no demonstrable effect on the clinical course of pregnancy, but recurrent attacks of grand mal or petit mal epilepsy and psychomotor seizures may be activated or intensified during pregnancy. They are more frequent during the last trimester in women who are hypertensive, proteinuric, and edematous. Convulsive seizures may be associated with alkalosis, fluid and electrolyte imbalance, cerebral hypoxia, cerebral edema, hypoglycemia, or hypocalcemia. Epilepsy may be difficult to differentiate from eclampsia, but an accurate history of seizures in the nonpregnant state is most helpful. However, the burden of proof is on the physician who claims that convulsions in the third trimester of pregnancy do not indicate eclampsia.

When seizures occur for the first time in a woman during pregnancy, a careful neurologic examination, including electroencephalographic studies, is indicated.

Proper management of the acutely seizing patient is crucial. This may be accomplished by the following. *Prevent aspiration of gastric contents* by placing the patient on her side (never on her back). Extend the head and hold the tongue out to *ensure a clear airway.* Slip an *oral airway* (or soft mouth gag) between her jaws so that she will not bite her tongue. *Gently restrain* the patient to prevent injury.

If convulsions continue, give *diazepam (Valium), 5–10 mg IV* initially (repeated if necessary at 10–15 min intervals to a maximum dose of 30 mg), or phenytoin (Dilantin), 150–250 mg IV at a rate not exceeding 50 mg/min. Sodium amobarbital IV also may be used, but rapid administration should be avoided because pulmonary edema and right heart failure may result in the patient with eclampsia. (Caution: Because of their depressive central nervous system effects, do not administer narcotics or general anesthetics unless absolutely necessary to control repeated seizures.)

Longer-term management of epileptic women during pregnancy includes avoiding fluid retention and adequate anticonvulsant therapy. Acetazolamide (Diamox) may be used as a diuretic. The most commonly used anticonvulsant, *phenytoin (Dilantin) may be mildly fetotoxic.* Thus, its use during pregnancy must be weighed against the risk. Other alternatives include phenobarbital, diazepam (Valium), and chlordiazepoxide (Librium).

Idiopathic epilepsy has a hereditary pattern. *The risk of having an infant with epilepsy is 2%–3% if one parent has epilepsy. It is 20%–25% if both parents are afflicted.*

HERNIATED INTERVERTEBRAL DISK

Herniation of the nucleus pulposus of a lumbar intervertebral disk is more frequent during pregnancy because the estrogens, progestogens, and relaxin cause the intervertebral disk's fibrous rings to weaken and swell the nuclei pulposi, hypervascularization of the back and pelvic nonosseous tissues contributes to relaxation of back support, and the equilibrium of the lumbosacral joint is disturbed during pregnancy by the increase in volume and weight of the abdominal contents. There are no obstetric complications due to disk hernia but disability and, even paralysis, may occur in extreme, neglected cases.

Temporary or permanent relief usually follows medical management: bedrest, traction, sedatives, and analgesics. Back strain or injury should be avoided during pregnancy and the puerperium, and obese patients should lose weight. Severe, recurrent, or progressive pain and incapacity may require surgery, but this is rarely necessary during pregnancy.

CEREBROVASCULAR ACCIDENTS

The *higher incidence of vascular accidents during pregnancy* than in the nonpregnant state may be partially explained by collagen changes in the blood vessels during pregnancy. Recurrent subarachnoid hemorrhage may be an indication for abortion or cesarean section. Hypertension of preeclampsia-eclampsia, IV administration of ergot (pressor) preparations, and increased intracranial pressure with straining during the second stage of labor may account for rupture of congenital cerebral aneurysms, arteriovenous malformations, or thrombosed cerebral veins.

MULTIPLE SCLEROSIS (MS)

The incidence of MS is 2–3:1000 pregnancies. Physiologic changes during pregnancy do not influence the development or the course of multiple sclerosis. Multiple sclerosis per se does not affect the course of pregnancy (including labor). However, sequelae (e.g., bladder dysfunction and stasis with subsequent infections) are frequent. Spinal anesthesia should be avoided when spinal cord disease is present. Vaginal delivery is preferred. Pregnancy is not contraindicated after several years remission.

MYASTHENIA GRAVIS

Myasthenia gravis is a metabolic disorder involving acetylcholine use at the myoneural junction. It affects motor function, causing muscle weakness, particularly of the face, tongue, throat, neck, arms, and respiratory muscles. The peak prevalence of myasthenia gravis is at ~25 years. Pregnancy may complicate the disorder, although some patients undergo remission during pregnancy. With proper management, most myasthenic patients complete pregnancy safely, and congenital myasthenia gravis is rare.

Infections may precipitate onset or relapse and must be treated aggressively during pregnancy. Symptoms of relapse include easy fatigability, intermittent double vision, drooping of the upper eyelids, facial muscle weakness, and in more serious cases, upper arm weakness and breathing difficulty. Neostigmine (Prostigmine) is beneficial. If edrophonium chloride (Tensilon) is used, it should be given cautiously IV. Because edrophonium may precipitate uterine contractions, however, it is (if possible) avoided.

Myasthenic patients usually tolerate labor well. Meperidine is the obstetric analgesic of choice. Local anesthesia is preferred. If general anesthesia is required, nitrous oxide, oxygen, and cyclopropane usually are the best combination. Oxytocin may be given, but *muscle relaxants are contraindicated.* Myasthenic patients must be carefully supervised postpartum because *relapses often occur during the puerperium.*

An *occasional newborn may have myasthenia gravis and require neostigmine* treatment for 1–2 months. Complete recovery is the rule.

CHOREA GRAVIDARUM

Sydenham's chorea (St. Vitus' dance) that recurs or develops for the first time in young women during pregnancy is *often associated with acute rheumatic fever.* Although very rare, it may be a serious complication of pregnancy. It usually appears early after the first missed period and, curiously, often vanishes following termination of pregnancy. Treatment is similar to that of Sydenham's chorea in the nonpregnant patient.

ENDOCRINE AND METABOLIC DISEASES

DIABETES MELLITUS

DEFINITION, INCIDENCE, ETIOLOGY AND IMPORTANCE

Diabetes mellitus is a metabolic disorder affecting carbohydrate, protein, and fats, with the potential for long-term degenerative alterations. It is one of the three (along with anemia and urinary infections) most frequent medical complications of pregnancy and so adversely affects pregnancy as to be an important contributor to maternal and perinatal morbidity. Although *maternal death is rare* with modern treatment, the *perinatal mortality rate may be as high as ~5%.*

Pregnancy is diabetogenic. Manifestations of this include gestational diabetes, intensification of overt diabetes, increased insulin requirements, and the enhanced occurrence of metabolic complications (e.g., ketoacidosis).

There are *two major types of diabetes mellitus.* Type 1, insulin-dependent diabetes, is usually of juvenile onset and is associated with deficient insulin secretion. The insulin deficiency is from destruction of the pancreatic beta cells. The pathogenesis may be autoimmune or multifactorial. Type 2 diabetes is generally late onset and has elevated serum insulin levels, and tissue insensitivity to insulin (insulin resistance), impaired insulin secretion, and inappropriate hepatic glucose secretion. Type 2 also has a strong hereditary component, usually developing in adults who are overweight or pregnant.

"Gestational diabetes mellitus" (GDM) is carbohydrate intolerance of varying severity, with onset or first recognition during pregnancy. It is characterized by insulin resistance as well as impaired insulin secretion. This decade has witnessed significant controversy relative to GDM diagnosis, management, and influence on outcomes. GDM is greatest in women >35 years old, when prepregnant weight is <49 kg or >65 kg, and in women with chronic hypertension.

Clinically, many have found it useful to classify (especially for purposes of management and counseling) diabetics according to the system of White (Table 15-3). Recently, the World Health Organization as well as various national diabetes groups have recommended various changes to their longstanding diagnostic criteria and classification, including:

- Diagnostic fasting plasma (blood) glucose is >7.0 mmol/L (126 mg/mL).

TABLE 15-3
CLASSIFICATION OF PREGNANT DIABETIC WOMEN

Class	Characteristics
A	Diabetic based only on an abnormal glucose tolerance testing
B	Onset of diabetes after age 20; duration of diabetes 10–19 years; no vascular disease
C	Onset of diabetes between ages 10–19; duration of diabetes 10–19 years; no vascular disease
D	Onset of diabetes age <10; duration of diabetes ≥20 years; vascular disease, including calcification of leg vessels
E	Same as group D, plus calcification of pelvic vessels
F	Same as group E, plus nephropathy (often Kimmelstiel-Wilson intercapillary nephrosclerosis)
H	Coronary artery disease
R	Malignant proliferative retinopathy

After J. Hare and P. White, Gestational diabetes and the White classification. *Diabetes Care* 3:394, 1980.

- Impaired glucose tolerance (IGT) allows for the new fasting level.
- A new category of impaired fasting glycemia (IFG) encompasses values above normal, but below diabetes (plasma >6.1 to <7.0 mmol/L, whole blood >5.6 to <6.1 mmol/L.
- GDM include gestational impaired glucose tolerance as well as previous GDM.
- Classifications define both process and disease stage.

There is considerable variation in incidence of all types of diabetes from ethnic group to ethnic group. There is also variation within ethnic groups related to familial predisposition, exposure to toxins, obesity and exercise. In heterogenous U.S. populations, the incidence of preexisting type, 1 diabetes during pregnancy is - between 1:125 to 1:350 and gestational diabetes probably occurs is *1%–5% of gestations,* but reports have varied from 0.15%–20%.

Pregnancy poses a risk to diabetics with renal compromise or retinopathy and these functions merit preconceptional evaluation. Women with GDM are at increased risk of diabetes, usually type 2. There is a significant association between elevated mean glycosylated hemoglobin (HBA1c) at 16–20 weeks gestation and preeclampsia in IDDM pregnancies. Women with GDM who again become pregnant are at a greater risk for subsequent diabetes. This is further enhanced by multiparity, obesity, an earlier diagnosis during pregnancy, insulin requirement for control, a shorter interval (<24 months) between pregnancies and a larger weight gain between pregnancies (>15 lb). The incidence of diabetes does not appear to be increased in patients with GDM who utilize low-dose progestin and estrogen combination oral contraception or who use postmenopausal hormonal therapy.

EFFECT OF DIABETES MELLITUS ON PREGNANCY AND DELIVERY

Infertility and abortion are increased (2–3 times) in poorly controlled diabetics. Rigid control of the glucose removes these risks. Maternal fluid and electrolyte balance is easily disrupted. Both the mother and the infant may be edematous. The incidence of *polyhydramnios is 10 times* the general incidence. *Preeclampsia-eclampsia is much more frequent (30%–50%),* especially with poor glycemic control in early pregnancy, prepregnancy vascular sclerosis, and/or hypertension.

The 3 fold increase in congenital abnormalities found in the offspring of uncontrolled diabetics is also lowered by proper glucose control. The most *common abnormalities are cardiac,* but the most increased abnormality (it almost never occurs except in diabetic pregnancies) is the caudal regression syndrome. *Premature labor and delivery* are common in the more advanced classes (>C), and the likelihood of an *excessively large fetus* (>4000 g) is greater in classes A and B. The risk of *fetal death is heightened,* particularly after the 36th week, because of maternal glucose instability (with possible acidosis) and placental insufficiency. *Dystocia and operative delivery* are more frequent, and fetal mortality and morbidity rates are consequently increased.

The incidence of early neonatal death from *respiratory distress syndrome or hypoglycemia* (due to hyperplasia of fetal islets of Langerhans) is increased. In later life, obesity and type 2 diabetes are increased in the offspring of women with GDM.

CLINICAL FINDINGS

Diabetic screening in all women is desirable but is mandatory in the following circumstances: a family history of diabetes; a previously unexplained premature, stillbirth, or hydramnios; a prior newborn weighing >4000 g (9 pounds), or a previous term-sized infant with respiratory distress syndrome. Obesity or glucosuria before the 20th week or recurrent glucosuria after the 20th week should be investigated. Recently, it has also been suggested that women who themselves had low birth weights are at increased risk for GDM, as are women with polycystic ovary syndrome (PCOS). A recent report indicates that selective screening will miss only 4% of GDM, but ~90% of pregnant women will need screening for GDM.

The *current diabetic screening* is to administer a 50 g oral carbohydrate load and draw a blood glucose in 1 h. If that level is >150 mg/mL, the test is positive and other (more definitive) testing is necessary. A better tolerated alternative to the usual 50 g glucose beverage is a comparable amount (~28) of jelly beans. A normal fasting blood glucose level does not rule out gestational diabetes. Moreover, fasting blood glucose levels may be slightly elevated or the postprandial blood glucose may be elevated in other diseases besides diabetes (e.g., liver disease). Fasting glucosuria suggests diabetes but is less reliable during pregnancy because of the lowered renal threshold for glucose. Lactose, which may give false-positive tests for glucose, may be excreted in the urine during the last 4–6 weeks of pregnancy and during the postpartum period.

When the diabetic screen is abnormal or if the signs and symptoms are suggestive, *a glucose tolerance test* is performed. The generally accepted normal values for whole blood glucose in the oral glucose tolerance test (100 g glucose load) are fasting level,

90 mg/mL; 1 h, 165 mg/mL; 2 h, 145 mg/mL; 3 h, 125 mg/mL. A glucose tolerance test containing one or more above-normal values is abnormal. Before glucose tolerance testing, place the patient on a high-carbohydrate intake for at least 48 h because carbohydrate restriction decreases tolerance.

Caution: It is unnecessary and possibly harmful to perform a glucose tolerance test on a patient whose initial blood glucose level is ≥200 mg/mL. Proceed to therapy for diabetes.

In pregnancy, the fasting blood glucose level is often slightly low, yet the oral glucose tolerance curve may be of the diabetic type. These changes are most marked after the sixth month. Following delivery, glucose tolerance tests return to nonpregnant values within 72 h. Thus, if delivery events indicate a glucose tolerance test as being desirable, it should be done <48 h of delivery.

TREATMENT

Emergency Measures

Diabetic Acidosis and Coma
Admit the patient to a hospital and obtain medical consultation. Determine blood glucose, pH, CO_2 combining power, serum electrolytes. Treat with insulin as for any patient with diabetic acidosis or coma.

Insulin Shock
If the patient is comatose and it is not possible to rapidly differentiate between diabetic coma and insulin shock, treat first for insulin shock by giving 20–40 mL of 50% glucose in water slowly IV. Determine the cause and make the necessary adjustments of insulin or glucose.

ANTENATAL CARE

Ideally, the patient is evaluated as a candidate for pregnancy *before conception* and both *health care and diabetic control optimized.* Fingerstick dextrose determinations are obtained before breakfast, lunch, dinner, and bed. It is inappropriate to attempt to regulate pregnant diabetics (because of their special and rapidly changing status) with urine testing. Blood glucose should be maintained with a *mean of 100 mg/ml ±10 mg/mL.* The maximum must not exceed 120 mg/mL.

Diet is adjusted to the ideal nutritional state depending on the patient's height, weight, and build. The goal is not weight reduction but prevention of both fasting and postprandial hyperglycemia.

Diet is usually according to the American Diabetic Association (ADA) guidelines. Generally, diabetics should have 35 kcal/kg unless obese, in which circumstances no less than 30 kcal/kg should be given. There are innumerable formulas for calculation of the distribution of calories, but it is important to have ~50% carbohydrates, at least 100 g of protein, and the rest fat. For example, a woman whose ideal weight is 60 kg (132 pounds) should have a daily diet of 2100 kcal (35 × 60). The caloric value of carbohydrate and protein is 4.1 kcal/g, and that of fat is 9.3 kcal/g. Thus, a sample dietary composition follows.

- 50% carbohydrate = 1050 kcal/4.1 kcal/g = 256 g
- 25% protein = 525 kcal/4.1 kcal/g = 128g
- 25% fat = 525 kcal/9.3 kcal/g = 56 g

It is also important to divide the calories into meals that release the nutrients in a regular fashion. Currently, 2/9, 2/9, 2/9, 2/9, 1/9 is favored. Also, vitamins, minerals, and dietary supplements are individualized to the patient's needs.

In most circumstances, the patient, internist, and obstetrician should work in close cooperation. A team framework for care (with additional consultants as necessary) has been demonstrated to be effective in caring for pregnant diabetic women.

Overt diabetic women require insulin, and the insulin requirement is usually greater during pregnancy. Diet and insulin must be regulated by blood glucose determinations as noted previously. *Oral hypoglycemic agents, which are teratogenic, should not be used during pregnancy.* As a starting point, the combination of insulin is usually intermediate and short-acting, and they are usually given in 2–3 doses/day to enhance precision. The NPH/regular insulin ratio should be 2:1 in the morning and 1:1 in the evening, and the morning total should be twice the evening total. For example, a total of 90 units/day should be divided as 40 units NPH and 20 units regular in the morning, and 15 units NPH and 15 units regular in the evening. Four divided doses of insulin affords even better control in some patients. Alternative regimens with Humulin and other insulins are equally effective. Insulin pumps have been improved and now are easier, less painful, and less hazardous. A practical implantable pump and continuous glucose sensors are on the horizon, and should usher in a new era of meticulous control.

The routine evaluation of diabetic patients should include either skin testing for *tuberculosis* or a chest x-ray. The *ocular fundi* must be evaluated, *renal function* determined, and a periodic series of screening for *urinary tract infection* (increased 3 times) instituted. In the classes with vascular involvement, an *ECG* is mandatory at any age.

It has been suggested that maternal glycemic criteria be used for insulin therapy in GDM. Nonobese patients with fasting plasma glucose (by oral glucose tolerance test) of <96 mg/mL may be assigned to diet therapy and monitored for the necessity of insulin for at least two weeks. Obese women or those with fasting plasma glucose >95 mg/mL (on OGTT) should receive insulin therapy immediately.

FETAL SURVEILLANCE

Sonography is used to determine gestational age, fetal viability, and possible defects as soon as pregnancy is confirmed, then at 4–6 week intervals until biophysical profile monitoring is undertaken. *Fetal cardiac septal thickness is increased in diabetic pregnancies.* Indeed, fetuses of even well-controlled diabetic women demonstrated septal thickening prior to an alteration in cardiac function. There is a higher rate of *polyhydramnios, fetal macrosomia, and fetal anomalies* in fetuses of diabetic women.

NST or BPP monitoring for fetal well-being is initiated at 27 weeks. Recently, *fetal heart rate variability* and *umbilical artery peak systolic velocity* have been suggested as markers for fetal cardiovascular homeostatsis. *Amniotic fluid insulin levels* (obtained by amniocentesis) may identify the hyperinsulinemic fetus prior to delivery. This information is particularly useful for intensification of maternal insulin therapy (to decrease the incidence and severity of diabetic fetopathy) or allowing normoinsulinemic fetuses to continue to the onset of labor.

LABOR AND DELIVERY

It is appropriate to consider elective delivery when the LS ratio and Pg indicate *pulmonary maturity*. Nearly all may have vaginal delivery if the vertex is presenting and other details are favorable. *Cesarean section is indicated if the fetus weighs >4000–4500 g* or if *presentation is abnormal.* When signs of fetal compromise develop, terminate pregnancy by the most expeditious means. If the pulmonary maturity testing does not indicate fetal maturity, the decision to deliver the infant or continue observation becomes a calculated risk. The usual insulin dose is not given on the day of delivery, and insulin by infusion is used to treat the hourly monitored blood glucose.

NEONATAL CARE

A neonatologist or pediatrician should be present at delivery. At the time of delivery the *cord should be clamped immediately* to avoid hypervolemia. It is usually appropriate to obtain *cord blood for pH, blood gases, and glucose. Cord blood insulin may be useful in the assessment of diabetic control in late pregnancy.* In brief, the correlation between status neonates with cord blood insulin follows: <20 microU/mL are normal, 20–50 microU/mL have mild fetopathy, and those >50 microU/mL have marked fetopathy.

Immediate care (including resuscitation) should be the same as any other delivery, with special attention to respiration, cardiac, neurologic, drying, warming, and getting to a controlled environment as soon as possible. Most babies of diabetic mothers are admitted to an observation nursery. *Frequent blood sugar determinations* are performed (q 30–60 min) in the first 2–3 h, with continued blood sugar determination before feedings for the first 12–24 h. Blood glucose <45 mg/dL is defined as hypoglycemia, and oral feeding, preferably with milk should be administered. Immediate IV glucose therapy is required for hypoglycemia <30 mg/dL or if the hypoglycemia is not rapidly responsive to the oral glucose load.

Respirations are observed, the infant is turned frequently, and breathing is stimulated when necessary. The newborn is observed for tremor or convulsive movements. These may be due to *hypocalcemia,* in which case give 10% calcium gluconate, 100 mg/kg slowly IV, after a blood specimen is drawn for calcium and glucose determinations.

POSTPARTUM MANAGEMENT

Careful evaluation of the mother's diabetic status is maintained during the puerperium because extraordinary changes occur. For example, one third of the late pregnancy dose of insulin is usually all that is needed the day after delivery.

PROGNOSIS

Joint management in a team approach will result in lower maternal and perinatal mortality and morbidity. The maternal mortality rate with modern therapy should be <0.2%. Deaths are due to diabetic coma, preeclampsia-eclampsia, infection, nephropathy, cardiac complications, dystocia, and embolism. Neglect and improper treatment are the main contributory causes of virtually all maternal deaths. An increase of diabetic retinopathy and nephropathy occurs in most patients during pregnancy. Insulin dependent diabetics who experience a pregnancy are at increased risk of postpartum thyroiditis.

Women who experience GDM during their pregnancy should have an oral glucose tolerance test 6–8 weeks postpartum. Additionally, certain abnormalities precede the development of type 2 diabetes in these high-risk women: regulation of glucose clearance, glucose production, and plasma free fatty acid concentrations as well as defects in pancreatic beta cell function.

Factors influencing fetal survival are the severity of diabetes, control of diabetes during pregnancy, placental function, placental bleeding, preeclampsia-eclampsia, polyhydramnios, and interruption of pregnancy <34th week or after the 38th week of gestation. The perinatal mortality rate even with modern therapy is <5%. Fetal anomalies occur in ~4% of infants but are more frequent when polyhydramnios is present. In general, vaginal delivery is safer than cesarean section for the fetus (except for the macrosomic fetus). Glucose control in the immediate preconception interval as well as the first trimester may have a greater influence on birth weight than does glycemic control in later pregnancy.

Pregnancy termination may be justified in certain instances of diabetic retinopathy, retinitis proliferans, severe vascular (usually cerebral or coronary) disease, or Kimmelstiel-Wilson disease.

The offspring of women with type 1 diabetes are at significant risk of childhood obesity.

Thoughtfully organized preconception counseling for women with diabetes has been demonstrated to: beneficially influence outcomes, reduce resource utilization, and substantially reduce costs. All too frequently, however, diabetic women's pregnancies remain unplanned. Thus, diabetic women frequently start pregnancy with suboptimal glucose control. Moreover, pregnant women with pre-existing diabetes have greater anxiety and hostility (compared to nondiabetic women), but this is not associated to level of glycemic control. In part, this may be due to these patients perceiving negative messages about pregnancies and/or becoming pregnant without optimal planning. Thus, there appears an opportunity to improve communication by *carefully constructed nonjudgmental dialogue and materials concerning:* self-monitoring of glycemic control, prepregnancy information, modifiable risk factors, target glucose levels, target HgAlc levels, support services, utilization of health care, and anticipated outcomes.

Additionally, this may represent an opportunity to discuss recommendations concerning *other aspects of ambulatory diabetic care* including: diabetes testing (fasting plasma glucose is adequate) every 3 years for those >45 years of age, more frequent or earlier testing for those with risk factors, benefits of close metabolic control to achieve optimal glucose levels, importance of diligent glucose self-monitoring, and attention to lifestyle, diet, exercise, and appropriate therapies.

THYROID DISORDERS

IN GENERAL

Thyroid changes related to pregnancy involve: immunological modifications with increased risk of antithyroid autoantibodies, potential alterations in iodine supplies and metabolism (increased glomerular filtration), specific hormonal changes related to pregnancy, hCG's mild thyroid stimulating activity, and certain pregnancy complications' association to hyperthyroidism. *Pregnancy's hormonal effect creates an overall increase in thyroid activity.* This includes the following: hCG's mild thyroid stimulating activity, a 2- to 3-fold increase in thyroxine-binding globulin concentrations, a 30%–100% increase in total triiodothyronine and thyroxine concentration, increased serum thyroglobulin and increased renal iodide clearance. The *two specific pregnancy complications* related to hyperthyroidism are gestational trophoblastic disease and hyperemesis gravidarum. Additionally, *both hyperthyroid and hypothyroid states do occur during pregnancy.*

Thyroid hormones do not cross the placental barrier after several weeks gestation. *Antithyroid drug, iodine, and autoantibodies do cross the placenta.* Thus, assessment of thyroid function during pregnancy should carefully integrate: symptoms, TSH, and free thyroid hormones. If Graves' disease or Hashimoto's thyroiditis is suspected, thyroid autoantibodies may also be useful. Evaluation of thyroid nodules during pregnancy is limited. Technetium scintigraphy is not advisable prior to the fourth month of pregnancy and 123-iodine should not be used for the entire pregnancy. Needle aspiration may be used during pregnancy, but full exploration is limited because of scintigraphy's restrictions.

The *incidence of thyroid cancer is probably higher during pregnancy.* Potentially, the course of thyroid cancer is enhanced by the hCG's TSH-like effect(s). Treatment with radioactive iodine cannot be initiated in pregnancy because of fetotoxic effects.

HYPERTHYROIDISM (THYROTOXICOSIS)

Thyrotoxicosis does not increase the hazard of spontaneous abortion or fetal anomalies but does *increase the incidence of premature delivery, postpartum hemorrhage, cardiovascular complications secondary to myocardial stress, psychosis, liver damage, and thyroid storm.* Preeclampsia-eclampsia may occur slightly more often in women with toxic goiter. Overtreatment of thyrotoxicosis during pregnancy may result in maternal and fetal hypothyroidism and may cause maldevelopment and goiter in the infant.

TREATMENT

Emergency Measures
All pregnant patients with moderate or marked thyrotoxicosis should be hospitalized at bedrest and given propranolol and possibly, sedatives.

Specific Measures
Individualize treatment according to the degree of toxicity and the duration of pregnancy. Toxic goiter during pregnancy may require antithyroid drug therapy (e.g., propylthiouracil or equivalent, 0.1 g PO tid or qid). To avoid resultant hypothyroidism, levothyroxine (Synthroid) should be given. Subtotal thyroidectomy must not be attempted until the patient has become euthyroid following medical treatment and is rarely necessary during pregnancy. Iodides are used before surgery but can damage the fetal thyroid gland. Therapeutic abortion is almost never required. Toxic goiter is not an indication for labor induction or cesarean section.

Treatment of Complications
Levothyroxine (Synthroid) should be administered whenever hypothyroidism develops, immediately before and for several weeks after thyroidectomy, or when the patient receives a thiourea compound.

Neonatal
If a congenitally athyroid or markedly hypothyroid infant does not receive thyroid or one of its analogs promptly, followed by continuation of the maintenance dose to ensure euthyroidism, normal mental and physical development cannot be expected.

PROGNOSIS

The prognosis is excellent for mother and fetus if normal thyroid function can be achieved promptly and then maintained.

HYPOTHYROIDISM

Slight thyroid deficiency is common, and although replacement therapy is not harmful, it seldom is indicated. More *severe deficiency*

causes abortion, premature labor, and congenital fetal anomalies.
Hashimoto's disease is by far the most common cause of hypothyroidism in the general population. Women with moderate to severe degrees of hypothyroidism are relatively infertile, and sterility is the rule in myxedema. Maternal hypothyroidism raises the risk of fetal hypothyroidism, requiring careful management because of the perinatal risks of mental sequelae and compressive goiter.

TREATMENT

Pregnant women with early hypothyroidism may be treated initially with relatively large doses of thyroid supplement, levothyroxine (Synthroid). Doses are started at 0.05–0.1 mg/day, and increase weekly to the limit to tolerance (~0.3 mg/day), adjusting to maintain the optimal effect. The optimal dosage may be estimated on the basis of the serum T_3 and T_4, but clinical judgment is often very accurate. Thyroid overdosage causes nervousness, tremors, tachycardia, insomnia, sweating, vomiting, diarrhea, and weight loss.

The nonspecific use of thyroid medication must be condemned.

PROGNOSIS

With prompt, adequate, and continued thyroid replacement, the *prognosis is excellent for mother and infant.* If a hypothyroid infant does not receive prompt replacement therapy, irreversible mental and physical retardation is to be expected.

AUTOIMMUNE THYROID DISEASE

Autoimmune mechanisms are responsible for only about 10% of all clinical thyroid disorders. However, they play a major role in two thirds of the most serious thyroid diseases: *Graves' disease and Hashimoto's disease or thyroiditis.* Autoantibodies do not appear to play a role in the development of thyroid cancer.

Predisposition to autoimmune disease is inherited (50% concordance in identical twins, about 10% in fraternal twins or siblings). Autoimmune disease never appears at birth, and its appearance follows a random distribution over time. Currently, there is no effective method of antigenically treating autoimmune thyroid disease. All one can do is to correct the hyperthyroid or hypothyroid state and maintain normality. Additionally, because the autoantibodies do cross the placenta, the perinate must be carefully evaluated.

Postpartum transient autoimmune thyroiditis (of Amino) is an interesting variant. In the last trimester of pregnancy, there usually is an amelioration of the autoimmune process followed by a rebound (thyrotoxicosis) after delivery. Antithyroid drugs should control the problem but contraindicate breastfeeding.

PARATHYROID DYSFUNCTION AND TETANY

Pregnancy normally causes a slight (secondary) hyperparathyroidism. Severe, chronic hyperparathyroidism causing osteitis fibrosa cystica is rare during pregnancy, except in patients with longstanding renal disease. The most serious problems relating to parathyroid dysfunction during pregnancy are hypoparathyroid tetany and muscle cramps. Tetany is usually associated with a calcium deficiency, phosphate excess, or lack of vitamin D and parathyroid hormone. In established hypoparathyroidism, hypocalcemia is a dilutional phenomenon during pregnancy. The requirements for vitamin D and calcium in parathyroid disease may be greater than in nonpregnant women.

Tetany may follow infection or the hypocalcemia that sometimes occurs during lactation, or it may be seen during the latter months of pregnancy if calcium supplements are inadequate. Of course, hyperventilation during labor may precipitate tetany.

Tetany of the newborn is unusual in breastfed infants but may occur transiently if the infant's phosphate intake is excessive (e.g., if too much cow's milk rather than formula is given or as a result of relative hypoparathyroidism in the neonatal period).

INFECTIOUS DISEASES

All systemic infectious diseases of the mother, if severe enough, can complicate pregnancy by causing fetal injury, death of the fetus, or premature labor and delivery. High fever, septicemia, and toxicosis are usually responsible. Most maternal infectious diseases (e.g., pneumonia, scarlet fever, and typhoid fever) are not responsible for fetal anomalies. However, the so-called TORCH infections (toxoplasmosis, rubella, cytomegalovirus disease, herpes simplex) and syphilis may be devastating to the fetus.

TOXOPLASMOSIS

Toxoplasmosis, a multisystem disease caused by the protozoan *Toxoplasma gondii*, is a serious threat to the fetus. Serologic evidence of *T. gondii* infection is present in almost 25% of women in the United States. Most cases are chronic and probably pose little risk to the fetus. The acute case may lead to fetal infection with marked sequelae.

The major vector in the United States remains unclear. The infection may be obtained from consumption of undercooked meat. Cats have been overemphasized as a vector. Only about 1% of cats hunting and consuming rodents harboring *T. gondii* are infected. If infection occurs, the cat sheds oocytes in the feces for only about 2 weeks. During this time, human inoculation must occur by hand-to-mouth contact of cat fecal material.

Toxoplasmosis, usually asymptomatic in adults, resembles cytomegalovirus disease in the infant. *Severe perinatal toxoplasmosis is associated with growth retardation, microcephalus or hydrocephalus, microphthalmia, chorioretinitis, central nervous system calcification, thrombopenia, jaundice, fever, and death.*

Routine antenatal screening for antibodies to *T. gondii* has been recommended. The Sabin-Feldman dye test and the indirect immunofluorescence test are diagnostic of toxoplasmosis. Both tests give positive results 2–3 weeks after infection and for years thereafter. Thus, without sequential tests, an acute infection cannot be distinguished from a chronic one. The diagnosis of toxoplasmosis in a newborn is supported by elevated IgM in cord blood.

Treatment of toxoplasmosis during pregnancy is problematic. Pyrimethamine currently is the drug of first choice against *T. gondii*. This drug, however, may be teratogenic, especially during the first trimester. If the newborn is treated with pyrimethamine, folinic acid supplementation will be required to reduce the toxicity of the drug. Sulfadiazine often is used additionally. Sulfonamide therapy is effective but must be discontinued before delivery. Sulfonamide drugs have a greater albumin-binding affinity than bilirubin, which may rise after delivery to critical levels. Even exchange transfusion of the newborn may be necessary to avoid kernicterus.

A cat should not be a hazard if minimal precautions are taken—frequent handwashing and occasional soaking of litter boxes with ammonia solution. Pregnant women should cook meat well or freeze meat for at least 4 h before consumption to destroy *T. gondii* tissue cysts. Women at high risk for toxoplasmosis (e.g., veterinarians, butchers, or those with many cats) should be screened periodically for the disease.

The outlook for the neonate with congenital toxoplasmosis is serious to grave. Encysted (intramuscular) focus of *T. gondii* cannot be eradicated and may cause recrudescence of the disease. If a woman has an affected child, subsequent progeny probably will be unaffected.

TABLE 15-4
EXANTHEMATOUS DISEASES IN PREGNANCY

Disease	Effect of Disease on Pregnancy	Effect of Disease on Offspring
Rubeola (measles)	Abortion; premature labor if disease is severe	May be born with rash
Varicella (chickenpox)	Severe, disseminated epidemic type may be fatal to mother due to necrotizing angiitis	Virulent infection may cause fetal death in utero; newborn may be born with pocks
Rubella (German measles)	Occasional early abortion	Congenital anomalies if disease occurs during first trimester

EXANTHEMATOUS DISEASES

Most of the exanthematous diseases are caused by viruses, which invariably gain access to the fetus via the placenta (Table 15-4).

The effect on pregnancy and the fetus depends on the virulence of the virus, the mother's resistance to the disease, and the stage of fetal development. Fetal immunity depends largely on maternal active immunity (e.g., rubella) or passive immunity (e.g., immune serum globulin administration). High fever or toxicosis may cause increased uterine contractility and loss of the pregnancy. Viral placentitis and viremia followed by fetal death in utero may lead to abortion or premature delivery.

RUBELLA (GERMAN MEASLES)

The rubella virus is extremely teratogenic. Many infants are abnormal and maldeveloped if the mother contracts rubella during the first trimester of pregnancy. Excluding patients affected during epidemics, the risk of congenital anomalies occurring during the first 3 months of pregnancy declines from almost 50% (first month) to about 10%. After the first trimester, the danger of anomalies is negligible, but vision or hearing defects or both are common.

Fetal defects include *cataracts, congenital heart disease, dental dysplasia, deafness, and mental retardation.* It may take 1–2 years to be certain of the extent of infant defects. There is some evidence that an abnormal child may be born of a mother who has previously been vaccinated but contracts a subclinical form of the disease when reexposed during pregnancy. Thus, *rubella screening titers* (specific serum hemagglutinating antibody) *are considered routine in antenatal care* to demonstrate the susceptibility to rubella.

Prophylactic immune serum globulin may prevent the rash but not the viremia of rubella, even when given before exposure to the disease. Therefore, the virus remains a significant threat to the fetus. This has led to the recommendation that immune serum globulin is rarely indicated in pregnancy.

Attenuated rubella virus vaccine will confer active immunity for a prolonged but uncertain period. Because the vaccine can potentially infect the fetus, it is recommended that immunization should be carried out in women only if they are not pregnant and pregnancy can be avoided for 3 months after vaccination. Although this remains a good guideline, *when vaccination has occurred during pregnancy, there have been few, if any, demonstrable teratic effects.* Reactions to the vaccine may include mild fever, local soreness at the site of injection, and arthralgia. Spread of the virus to others is not a problem.

CYTOMEGALOVIRUS (CMV) DISEASE

Most cases of CMV disease are *clinically inapparent.* In some adults, the symptoms are like those of infectious mononucleosis. The disease may be *sexually transmitted.* During pregnancy, the only sign may be mild leukorrhea. Specific virus-neutralizing and complement-fixing antibody reactions indicate that most women have (at some time) sustained this infection. About 20% of adults do not have neutralizing antibody to cytomegalovirus and thus are considered susceptible for acute infections.

There is now evidence that CMV is much more prevalent during pregnancy than was thought and causes severe anomalies in ~10,000 infants in the United States per year. CMV is recovered from 15%–20% of women examined in public health clinics and from the semen of men who have had numerous sexual partners. The virus can be cultivated from the salivary glands of 10%–25% of healthy individuals, from the cervix of 10% of healthy women, from the urine of 1% of all newborns, and sometimes from breast milk. This carrier state probably explains subsequent cases occurring in the same family.

Cytomegalovirus disease is usually acquired by the fetus during early intrauterine life. In the newborn, the disease produces *erythroblastosis and thrombocytopenia that lead to scattered hemorrhages.*

Chorioretinitis, periventricular necrosis with calcification, micro-cephaly, and sclerosis of the bones are often noted at birth. Early jaundice beginning on the first or second day, melena, hematemesis, and hematuria develop. The antemortem diagnosis can be made by identification of cytomegalic inclusion cells in the gastric washings, cerebrospinal fluid, or fresh urine. Culture of CMV is proof of the diagnosis. The direct and indirect serum bilirubin are elevated, but the Coombs' test is negative. Death may occur soon after birth as a result of interstitial pneumonitis, focal hepatitis, or adrenocortical failure.

There is no cure. Corticosteroids and supportive therapy together with immune serum globulin may be helpful. When the obviously infected infant survives, marked developmental and psychomotor deficiencies and hepatosplenomegaly usually are present. Hearing loss is frequent in the more numerous cases of clinically inapparent CMV.

SEXUALLY TRANSMITTED DISEASES

Herpes simplex (p. 577), syphilis (p. 688), and gonorrhea (p. 684) are discussed on the pages indicated.

POLIOMYELITIS

Poliomyelitis, which exerts an unfavorable effect on pregnancy and the puerperium, has been virtually eradicated in the United States, but it is still a serious problem in developing countries. *Pregnant women have a greater incidence of poliomyelitis than nonpregnant* women of comparable ages. Approximately 67% of pregnant women who contract poliomyelitis are between ages 20 and 29, and ~75% are parous.

Pregnancy aggravates poliomyelitis, and the disease in turn increases the risk of abortion and fetal loss. Rare congenital anomalies are ascribed to poliomyelitis. The infant may show growth retardation if the mother contracts poliomyelitis in the early months of pregnancy. The fetus may contract poliomyelitis during its passage through the birth canal.

Salk vaccine contains killed virus. Sabin vaccine is an attenuated live virus preparation. Either can be given whether the patient is pregnant or not, but it is preferred to give the vaccine to nonpregnant women. Immune serum globulin may assist in protecting the exposed infant against poliomyelitis. If the newborn survives but has acquired the disease, flaccid paralysis may be present.

The maternal mortality rate in pregnancy complicated by poliomyelitis is markedly increased. The later in pregnancy the disease is contracted, the higher the morbidity and mortality rates for both mother and infant.

PULMONARY TUBERCULOSIS

Tuberculosis of the bronchi, lungs, and pleura is not directly affected by pregnancy. Tuberculous pregnant women are slightly more *prone to spontaneous abortion and premature delivery* than other women. Tuberculous endometritis is exceptional. Interruption of pregnancy because of pulmonary tuberculosis is almost never justified now that antituberculosis drugs are available. Infants born of tuberculous mothers are no more likely to develop the disease than others provided that they are separated from the infected mother and unfavorable environment at birth.

However, it is important to discourage pregnancy in women with active tuberculosis and to maintain close medical supervision of those tuberculous women who do become pregnant. Institute follow-up study of all women with a history of treated tuberculosis, and be alert to the possibility of reactivation of tuberculosis during each pregnancy. Advise deferring pregnancy (and prescribe contraception, if acceptable) until tuberculosis has been inactive for at least 2 years if minimal, 3 years if moderately advanced, and 5 years if far-advanced.

In patients who have had tuberculosis, order chest x-rays after the fifth month, immediately after delivery, and 6 months after delivery. The management of the pregnant patient with tuberculosis requires the collaboration of the pulmonary physician and the obstetrician. The treatment of tuberculosis includes rest (physical and emotional), hospitalization if the disease is moderate or advanced, and chemotherapy. The reader is referred to other texts for details of treatment.

MALARIA

Malaria may cause infertility, abortion, or premature labor and delivery. Infants of mothers with malaria are often smaller than average. Approximately 10% of infants born of women with demonstrable parasitemia will have plasmodia in cord blood.

Malarial relapses often occur during pregnancy for unknown reasons. A renewal of attacks is common during the puerperium or after hemorrhage and infection. Labor is frequently prolonged and hazardous for obstetric patients with malaria. These women become fatigued sooner, and operative delivery is required more often. The parasite is not transmitted in the milk, but lactation should be discouraged in women with clinical evidence of malaria.

The severity of maternal malaria is reflected in the stillbirth rate, which rises as pregnancy approaches term, and the vitality of newborns who do survive is temporarily reduced.

No antimalarial drug is completely safe for use during pregnancy. If a pregnant woman must be treated for malaria, other texts should be consulted for details of treatment.

LISTERIOSIS

Maternal listeriosis may be responsible for abortion and fetal disease or death depending on the severity of the infection and the duration of pregnancy. Encephalitis and granulomatosis of the newborn are described. Pregnant women suffering from a septic form of this disease may have only malaise, but they may transmit the infection to the fetus either transplacentally or when the fetus is exposed to the organisms in the lower genital canal during birth.

A diagnosis of listeriosis during pregnancy is difficult but can be made by complement-fixation or fluorescent antibody tests of leukorrheic discharges. A positive complement-fixation test in high dilution is almost invariably present in acute maternal infection. Gram-positive rods should be sought in the meconium of the newborn to diagnose listeriosis early.

Treatment (both mother and child) consists of large doses of ampicillin or erythromycin.

16

OPERATIVE OBSTETRICS

ANESTHESIA[*]

Anesthesia management is markedly influenced by pregnancy. Pregnancy-induced physiologic alterations may be compounded by labor, pregnancy-associated conditions (e.g., pregnancy-induced hypertension), or intercurrent disease states of the mother or fetus (e.g., heart disease, pulmonary hypertension, diabetes, or isoimmunization). The pregnancy alterations most influencing anesthesia are those of the *cardiovascular, pulmonary, and gastrointestinal systems.*

At term, cardiac output is increased by 30%–40% above nonpregnant levels in the absence of aortocaval compression. Increased cardiac output speeds the onset of inhalation anesthetics. Uterine involution leads to an autotransfusion of ~500 mL. Thus, there is potential for fluid overload with volume loading.

Parturients have a diminished functional residual capacity despite increased total lung capacity, increased oxygen consumption, and diminished oxygen saturation. Little apnea may produce significant hypoxia. Therefore, supplemental O_2 is recommended with either regional or general anesthesia. There is a decrease in physiologic dead space and a decreased gradient between arterial and end-tidal CO_2 tensions. Thus, with general anesthesia, the end-tidal CO_2 levels should be maintained several torr higher than in the nonpregnant patient.

Term parturients have increased intragastric volumes, decreased gastric pH, accentuated intragastric pressure, and delay in gastric emptying. Thus, there is enhanced risk of gastric aspiration. Aspiration of gastric contents may cause maternal death.

---

[*]Modified from M.L. Pernoll and J. Mandel, Cesarean section. In: J.S. McDonald, ed. *Bonica's Text of Obstetrical Anesthesia.* 1994.

PREOPERATIVE PREPARATION

LABORATORY DETERMINATIONS

For the normal patient undergoing anesthesia, determination of Hct or Hgb is necessary, but a differential count contributes little to management. The history and physical examination are generally sufficient predictors of derangements of electrolytes and the coagulation profile. In the majority of patients, a preoperative ECG is unnecessary, and although chest x-ray carries little fetal risk, it should be obtained only if the history and physical examination suggest its necessity.

The population of patients requiring cesarean section includes a higher proportion of high-risk pregnancies than those delivered vaginally. *For operative patients, individualized studies are required.* For example, diabetic women will need a serum glucose determination. Preeclamptic women may exhibit coagulation defects in the coagulation cascade and platelet function, and assessment may require the usual platelet count, fibrinogen, prothrombin, and partial thromboplastin times as well as more specialized testing.

For the anticipated cesarean section patient, *blood is usually typed* for ABO/Rh *and screened* for unexpected significant antibodies. Patients who have active bleeding (e.g., placenta previa or abruptio placentae), preeclampsia, overdistention of the uterus, coagulopathy, or prolonged labor or who required oxytocin stimulation are at risk of hemorrhage and should have at least 2 units of packed red cells available. In response to concerns about HIV, many obstetricians advise gravidas to have 1–2 units of blood drawn during pregnancy, usually in the late second or early third trimester and stored for autotransfusion if necessary.

FASTING

The practice of maintaining patients *NPO past midnight before elective cesarean section or major anesthesia* should lower intragastric volume and raise pH, thus reducing the risk of gastric aspiration.

INTRAVENOUS HYDRATION

Fasting, emesis, or insensible loss may directly diminish intravascular volume, aortocaval compression may cause inadequate venous return in parturients, and complications (e.g., toxemia and hemorrhage) may be present. Therefore, volume repletion is an important part of anesthetic management of any parturient. This is even more pressing if the use of sympatholytics is anticipated.

The use of glucose in volume expansion has been controversial. Addition of 25 or 57.5 g of dextrose produces a significant rise in maternal and cord glucose concentrations, with a noticeable increase in fetal insulin levels and decrease in fetal glucagon levels. These changes are accompanied by a significant incidence of neonatal hypoglycemia at 2 h of age and an increase in the incidence of neonatal jaundice. Use of 7.5 g of dextrose was not associated with such effects and neither was administration of glucose at rates <6 g/h. It seems prudent not to deprive the parturient of maintenance glucose infusion but not to use solutions containing 5% dextrose for acute volume loading. Dextrose administration of <6 g/h or 7.5 g acutely should be considered safe.

ACID ASPIRATION PROPHYLAXIS

Acid aspiration prophylaxis is *mandatory for a gravida undergoing a general anesthetic*. The nonparticulate antacid, sodium citrate, when given <1 h preoperatively, is effective in raising gastric pH >2.5. Although cimetidine and ranitidine—type 2 histamine (H_2) antagonists—also are capable of raising gastric pH, sodium citrate is the treatment of choice because of the simplicity of use and lower cost.

PREMEDICATIONS

With the exception of acid prophylaxis, premedication of obstetric patients is rarely necessary or desirable. Anticholinergics are also used for obstetric premedication because these drugs blunt bradycardic responses to succinylcholine, diminish oral secretions, and possibly decrease gastric volume. Atropine 0.01 mg/kg and glycopyrrolate 0.005 mg/kg do not significantly affect the fetal heart rate, but with administration of larger doses of atropine, tachycardia may occur. Glycopyrrolate produces antisialagogic effects with less maternal tachycardia and sedation. Hence, it may be preferable.

MISCELLANEOUS

Informed consent for the procedure must be obtained before the patient receives medication. Establish a secure, large-bore *IV route* (preferably with a ≥18-gauge needle) preoperatively.

For cesarean section, place an *indwelling catheter* in the bladder. *Surgically prepare the abdomen* after administration of a regional anesthetic but before administration of a general anesthetic. To control blood loss immediately after delivery, have sufficient *oxytocin* available for rapid infusions and to add to subsequent IV solutions.

CHOICE OF ANESTHETIC TECHNIQUES

Which anesthetic technique should be used is *determined by many factors,* including the procedure to be done, the length of time anticipated for the procedure, the discomfort the procedure is likely to evoke, the effect of anesthetic agents on the mother and fetus, the urgency for the procedure (e.g., cesarean section), the contraindications, and patient preference. The question of the best anesthesia for cesarean section is further clouded because studies of maternal and fetal outcome with general and regional anesthesia have not provided unequivocal evidence of superiority of any technique. It is impossible to conclude that one anesthetic technique will be optimal for all situations. The patient's desire for or against a given anesthetic is an important determinant. Most patients prefer to be awake during delivery. Thus, epidural anesthesia is used in about 40% of cesarean sections in the United States.

Epidural anesthesia benefits intervillous blood flow. This increases with the sympathetic block to the point of hypotension. When hypotension occurs, however, intervillous blood flow declines precipitously. Nonetheless, maternal stress response should not be a problem with epidural anesthesia to T6. Although genital herpes may not affect epidural anesthesia administration, administration of an epidural through an area of active lesions or to a patient with active HSV-2 viremia is contraindicated because of consequences of herpetic encephalitis. Contraindications to epidural or spinal anesthesia include coagulopathies and intercurrent infection. When maternal demise occurs with regional anesthesia, it is usually from errors in technique, vascular or subarachnoid injection, inadequate volume repletion, or unsuspected cardiac disease. When emergency cesarean section is indicated, time considerations may prevent the use of epidural anesthesia.

General anesthesia is more commonly employed in emergencies because it *takes less time.* However, general anesthesia (because of aspiration) is associated with a greater incidence of maternal mortality and may be responsible for slightly more blood loss than regional anesthetics. *A 20% reduction in intravillous blood flow occurs with induction of general anesthesia in healthy parturients.* No disease state provides an absolute contraindication to all forms of general anesthesia, however.

Anesthetics cannot be compared by fetal effects. Cord pH may be lower after regional anesthesia, but the fetus may exhibit higher Apgar scores and shorter times to sustained respiration. There is little difference in neonatal neurobehavioral outcome after epidural vs. general anesthesia, except in cases of maternal hypotension. A prolonged interval from induction to delivery is associated with poorer fetal outcome under general anesthesia. This is not the case with subarachnoid anesthesia.

EPIDURAL ANESTHESIA

The single greatest risk of epidural anesthesia is hypotension. The incidence is ~30% with labor and 36% without labor, and the hypotension occurs from aortocaval compression and sympathetic block. Hydration and left uterine displacement do not entirely eliminate hypotension. Except for those patients who are at risk for volume overload, preloading with approximately 1000 mL of crystalloid will materially decrease hypotension. A patient may appear to be in no distress while significant hypotension is developing. Thus, the blood pressure must be monitored carefully following induction of epidural anesthesia.

The toxicity of local anesthetics may be influenced by numerous factors in the gravida undergoing epidural anesthesia. Pregnancy has been demonstrated to diminish the dose of bupivacaine necessary to produce cardiovascular collapse, and hypoglycemia diminishes the dose of bupivacaine necessary for cardiovascular collapse. Indeed, the risks of bupivacaine have materially decreased obstetric utilization (see the discussion that follows). Cimetidine but not ranitidine has been shown to interfere with hepatic clearance of lidocaine. Thus, ranitidine is recommended for parturients who undergo epidural anesthesia when H_2 blockade is desired. Because propranolol interferes with lidocaine and bupivacaine metabolism, exercise caution in administration of multiple doses of lidocaine (or bupivacaine) to patients receiving this medication. Preeclampsia also diminishes lidocaine clearance.

Greater safety may be obtained by slow induction of epidural anesthesia. Time permitting, an initial dose is administered, with an interval of at least 10 min before a subsequent injection. This technique also allows for assessment of the adequacy of catheter placement.

Fetal toxicity of local anesthetic agents is affected by the same factors influencing maternal toxicity. Fetal acidosis (e.g., from maternal hypotension, hypoxia, or uteroplacental insufficiency) increases fetal local anesthetic levels by ion trapping. Thus, the relative merits of available anesthetic techniques need careful evaluation.

Various local anesthetic agents have been used extensively for epidural anesthesia: bupivicaine, lidocaine, 2-chloroprocaine, and mepivacaine. Recently, the safety of the first three drugs has been questioned.

Epidural 2-chloroprocaine has been associated with persistent neural blockade and adhesive arachnoiditis. Since 1983, the FDA has recommended that 0.75% concentration of bupivacaine not be used in obstetrics because it had been associated with toxic reactions, including maternal deaths. Therefore, it is advised that ≤5 mL of any bupivacaine solution be injected in the period required to manifest premonitory signs of a toxic reaction (30–60 sec). The use of epinephrine in obstetric epidural anesthesia is controversial.

Epidural administration of narcotics has become almost routine practice in many institutions. Fentanyl 50–100 fg added to the local anesthetic can improve both quality and duration of anesthesia. Fetal depression has not followed these small doses.

It is imperative that the ability to deliver oxygen under positive pressure, suction, and the equipment and drugs necessary for tracheal intubation be available at the location where any anesthetic is administered. Standards of monitoring adhered to in the operating room should apply to the patient undergoing epidural anesthesia, including an ECG and blood pressure monitor.

Generally, the *left lateral recumbent position* to displace the uterus favorably is preferred for initial catheter placement and induction of anesthesia, although the sitting position is also acceptable. Place obese patients in a slightly head-up position during induction, but do not inject such patients in the sitting position.

Special training and detailed technical knowledge are necessary to undertake epidural anesthesia. The exact location of an epidural catheter is uncertain (e.g., 3–10/10,000 are subarachnoid). Thus, before administration of the therapeutic dose, employ a test dose of the anesthetic. Usually the test dose consists of a combination of epinephrine and local anesthetics to detect intravascular and subarachnoid catheter placement, respectively.

Management of Complications

Unintended dural puncture occurs in 1%–3% of obstetric epidurals. Following this event, the incidence of *postlumbar puncture headache is 30%–78%.* Instillation of 30–60 mL of preservative-free saline or 5 mL of the patient's blood through a subsequent successful epidural catheter is suggested.

The first preventive or therapeutic measure for *hypotension* is left uterine displacement or left lateral recumbency. Adequate volume repletion with crystalloid should rapidly follow. Should this fail, ephedrine is the agent of choice because it is cardiotonic and does not depress uterine blood flow.

Subarachnoid injection of local anesthetic in quantities intended for the epidural space has been associated with significant morbidity and mortality. Such occurrences are rare, but the absence of cerebrospinal fluid flowing from the epidural needle does not guarantee it is extradural. If an impending total spinal or convulsion is suspected, withdraw the needle immediately. Rapidly institute supportive measures, for example, cardiopulmonary resuscitation. The airway must be assured, preferably by endotracheal intubation. The patient is ventilated with 100% O_2 while the circulation is supported with positioning, fluids, and ephedrine as needed. Cardiac status must be ascertained (EKG) and appropriately managed.

Toxic levels of local anesthetics may occur by either cumulative absorption of local anesthetics injected into the epidural space or by unintended intravascular injection. Toxicity is usually manifested by *generalized seizures,* but *cardiovascular collapse* may follow bupivacaine administration. The toxic reaction is often accompanied by *prodromal symptoms* (e.g., tinnitus and perioral numbness). If these are noted, *oxygen* should be immediately administered. A small dose of *thiopental* (50–100 mg) may prevent seizures. *Consider immediate induction of general anesthesia* if prodromal symptoms intensify. CPR must be promptly begun if a generalized seizure or cardiovascular collapse occurs.

Likewise, *fetal status demands promptly assessment.* If the fetus is delivered immediately, local anesthetic levels may be elevated due to ion trapping. Hence, cardiopulmonary resuscitation and supportive measures for the neonate may also be necessay.

Almost *20% of patients will experience some discomfort while undergoing cesarean section with epidural anesthesia.* This can almost always be predicted by careful assessment of the quality of the block. Reassurance and emotional support may be adequate, but if unsuccessful, give general anesthesia. Nitrous oxide in concentrations below 50%, and fentanyl (1 fg/kg) should be safe adjuncts.

Droperidol is effective in ameliorating nausea and vomiting after spinal and epidural anesthesia. Metaclopromide, 0.15 mg/kg, given immediately after umbilical cord clamping, also significantly reduces nausea without sedation.

Shivering frequently occurs in patients undergoing epidural anesthesia. This may be controlled by warming IV and local anesthetic solutions and applying radiant heat to the gravida's face and chest. If that fails, give meperidine 25–50 mg for relief.

SUBARACHNOID ANESTHESIA

Subarachnoid anesthesia is *more likely to create supine hypotension* than epidural anesthesia, probably due to the greater extent and speed of onset of the sympathetic block. The fall in cardiac output and blood pressure may be corrected by positioning the patient in the left lateral decubitus or by left uterine displacement. Either of these is essential in the safe conduct of subarachnoid anesthesia. As with epidural anesthesia, the laboring patient undergoing subarachnoid anesthesia is at lower risk for hypotension than one not in labor. This is due to the transient autotransfusion with uterine contractions.

Volume preloading can only reduce the risk of hypotension. It may be more effective when combined with uterine displacement, however. As with epidural anesthesia, the only exceptions to volume preloading are those patients at risk for volume overload. Preloading is accomplished with ~1000 mL of crystalloid. Despite these measures, up to 50% of patients will manifest significant hypotension and should be treated with IV ephedrine.

Because of the much lower dosages involved, local anesthetic toxicity and placental transfer of local anesthetics are not problems with subarachnoid anesthesia. Although frequently used for subarachnoid anesthesia, tetracaine may result in inadequate anesthesia. Combining tetracaine with procaine (instead of glucose) yields a solution of greater baricity, resulting in greater patient comfort and reduced supplemental analgesia requirements. Bupivacaine has been used as 0.5% isobaric, 0.5% hyperbaric, and 0.75% hyperbaric solutions, but analgesia may be incomplete in hyperbaric 0.5% doses of <12.5 mg.

Hyperbaric lidocaine provides rapid onset but relatively brief duration of anesthesia. It also carries a high incidence of dysphagia due to high blockade; thus, subarachnoid lidocaine (especially for cesarean section) has been discouraged. The duration of tetracaine and bupivacaine is adequate for virtually all cesarean sections. Hence, the addition of epinephrine is usually unnecessary. With single-dose subarachnoid anesthetic, control of spread is achieved by baricity, volume of injection, and patient position. Cerebrospinal fluid dynamics are altered at term, particularly during labor, due to engorgement of the epidural veins, and hyperbaric solutions should be used for obstetric subarachnoid anesthesia. The anesthetic may be induced with the patient in right lateral decubitus position if she is turned to the left in approximately 1 min. When technical considerations prevent this, the sitting position may be used, but anesthetic onset will be delayed.

Management of Complications

The complications of spinal anesthesia are similar to those of epidural anesthesia. Postlumbar puncture headache is greater, even when using 25-gauge needles. Treatment is as noted previously. Hypotension and high levels of blockade also occur more frequently. However, with reduced dosage, local anesthetic toxicity is rarely seen. Treatment for hypotension and high blockade levels is as with epidural anesthesia.

GENERAL ANESTHESIA

Adequate maternal and fetal oxygenation are the most important physiologic considerations in both induction and maintenance of general anesthesia. Intubation, while perhaps more difficult, is even more critical because of the risks of aspiration. *General anesthesia during pregnancy should not be undertaken without endotracheal intubation.*

Induction Agents

Thiopental is used extensively for induction of anesthesia for cesarean section. However, it is well recognized that smaller doses must be used for the pregnant patient. Doses of 4–7 mg/kg are not associated with diminished Apgar scores, but with larger doses, neonatal depression may occur. Pregnant patients eliminate thiopental faster than nonpregnant women, whereas neonatal elimination is significantly slower than in normal adults.

Breast milk and feeding should not be affected by a single dose of 5 mg/kg thiopental for anesthetic induction.

Muscle Relaxants

Muscle relaxants are used for both induction and maintenance of general anesthesia. Induction of general anesthesia implies rapid sequence induction. Therefore, it is useful to provide light anesthesia and allow surgical exposure. The commonly employed agents may all be given safely before cord clamping. However, several factors conspire to make pregnant women more susceptible to muscle relaxants.

In the first 10 weeks of pregnancy, plasma cholinesterase activity falls rapidly and remains low, putting >10% of patients at risk for prolonged duration of succinyldicholine-induced muscle relaxation. Prolonged paralysis occasionally occurs with succinyldicholine. Magnesium sulfate administration renders parturients particularly susceptible to muscle relaxants. Therefore, monitoring the degree of neuromuscular blockade should be performed even after a single intubating dose.

Administration of depolarizing agents may have a number of unpleasant side effects (e.g., muscle fasciculations, myalgias, and increased intragastric pressure), and preadministration of a small dose of nondepolarizing muscle relaxant is often used in nonpregnant patients as a preventative. However, pretreatment is not recommended for pregnant patients because the advantage is less and they are more likely to develop drug complications.

Although succinyldicholine continuous infusion was used widely for maintenance of muscle relaxation during cesarean section, it has largely been replaced by the *short-acting nondepolarizing agents, atracurium and vecuronium*. Pancuronium has been used for maintenance of muscle relaxation in cesarean section. An umbilical venous/maternal venous ratio of 0.22 has been determined for this drug. However, this value increases with prolongation of the incision-to-delivery interval. Fortunately, neonatal depression associated with pancuronium is rare. Atracurium provides good maintenance of muscle relaxation in cesarean section with minimal neonatal effects at doses of ~0.3 mg/kg. It does not cross the placenta in significant quantities. It may become acceptable as an induction agent when succinylcholine is contraindicated.

The maternal venous/umbilical venous ratio for maintenance vecuronium is 0.11, and its neonatal half-life is 36 min. Maternal clearance is increased in pregnancy; thus, there is rapid blockade resolution. In doses of 0.04 mg/kg, adverse neonatal effects are not found for vecuronium or pancuronium (by Agpar or neuroadaptive scores). After further study, this drug may become acceptable when succinyldicholine must be avoided. Placental transfer of curare may occasionally cause neonatal depression.

Maintenance Agents—Narcotics

All narcotics cross the placenta. Thus, narcotics were discouraged for obstetric anesthesia. Newer, short-acting narcotics, such as fentanyl 1 fg/kg administered within 10 min of delivery, produce no appreciable neonatal effect, however. Attenuation of the hypertensive response to intubation in pregnancy-induced hypertension may be achieved by fentanyl 200 fg plus droperidol 5 mg or alfentanil 10 fg/kg administered 1 min before induction of general anesthesia.

The practice of administering small doses of narcotics during induction of general anesthesia should be reserved for those patients in whom the benefits of diminution of cardiovascular response to intubation outweigh the risks of a depressed neonate. Ensuring the availability of naloxone and staff capable of managing the apneic newborn is essential if narcotics are used. Following delivery, there is no contraindication to the administration of narcotics, and fentanyl in doses up to 5 fg/kg permits diminution of the inhalational anesthetic.

Inhalational Agents

Inhalational agents cross the placenta as a function of time and concentration. However, inhalational agents permit adequate anesthesia at lower concentrations of nitrous oxide. This permits the use of a higher Fio_2 and provides greater safety.

Halothane, enflurane, and isoflurane are all used for maintenance of cesarean section anesthesia, have an acceptable incidence of maternal recall, and are not associated with depression of uterine blood flow. However, all three agents cause dose-dependent depression of uterine contractility. Currently, isoflurane is used most frequently.

Nitrous oxide crosses the placenta rapidly, with a fetal/maternal ratio of 0.8 after 3 min. Prolonged administration of high concentration nitrous oxide has been associated with poor perinatal outcome. Therefore, it is recommended that *concentrations of nitrous oxide be limited to 50%*. If delivery has not been effected within 15 min, nitrous oxide should be discontinued. Also, nitrous oxide should be avoided in the severely compromised fetus.

Agents for Control of Blood Pressure

The treatment of hypotension usually involves: prevention using prehydration, relieving aortocaval compression, restoring intravascular volume, and using ephedrine when necessary.

Hypertension, most frequently a problem during intubation, is brief and not serious for the normal parturient. When acute, either due to pregnancy-induced hypertension or coexisting cardiovascular disease, consider short-acting narcotics. These attenuate the response to intubation but may induce hypoventilation in the neonate. Nitroglycerine infusion obtunds the hypertensive response without adverse neonatal effects. However, this must be used with caution because of increased intracranial pressure. Nitroprusside has been used without cyanide toxicity for the acute management of transient hypertension. Discontinue nitroprusside if the patient is resistant to the drug or if tachyphylaxis develops.

Technical Considerations

Rapid sequence induction is the induction of choice for general anesthesia for pregnant patients. Since cricoid pressure is an accepted practice in such cases and preparation for the management of regurgitation is routine, the only distinction between the rapid sequence and the deliberate sequence is the avoidance of positive pressure mask ventilation. Positive pressure ventilation by mask may produce gastric distention and regurgitation. Nevertheless, application of cricoid pressure prevents gastric inflation, assuring no airway obstruction.

Pulse oximetry is routinely used. For those parturients exhibiting desaturation during induction of general anesthesia, apply gentle (<35 cm H_2O) ventilation by mask and cricoid pressure.

We favor the following procedure for cesarean section. Routinely administer sodium bicitrate 30 mL before induction. Following preoxygenation, perform rapid sequence induction with thiopental 1.0 mg/kg and succinyldicholine 1.0 mg/kg. Accomplish intubation with a tracheal tube of appropriate size. Maintain oxygen 50%, nitrous oxide, and isoflurane 0.5%–1.0%. Following return of twitch, continue muscle relaxation with atracurium or vecuronium. After clamping of the umbilical cord, decrease isoflurane to 0.25%, or discontinue this and give fentanyl <5 fg/kg. This reverses neuromuscular blockade. Then, extubate the patient following sustained head lift and responsiveness.

Airway management during pregnancy may be complicated by edema of preeclampsia, bearing down during the second stage of labor, or weight gain in pregnancy. Do not attempt to intubate with a tube >7.0 mm. A series of smaller endotracheal tubes should be available in the event of an inability to pass the selected size endotracheal tube.

Failed endotracheal intubation is evident in the majority of avoidable maternal deaths associated with anesthesia. This applies in about 1 in 300 cesarean sections. Successful management of failed intubation requires a concerted plan of action of which mask ventilation with cricoid pressure is an accepted component.

LOCAL ANESTHESIA

Local infiltration anesthesia for major obstetric surgery (e.g., cesarean section) has never been widely used and is so rare today that few obstetricians and surgeons have learned the technique. There are few, if any, absolute contraindications to other anesthetics or absolute indications for local anesthesia. The procedure takes more time than other anesthetic techniques. Additionally, in an attempt to relieve pain, toxic levels may be reached.

CESAREAN SECTION

Cesarean section is the transabdominal delivery of a viable fetus (with placenta and membranes) through a uterine incision. If the fetus is previable, the same procedure is termed abdominal hysterotomy. Primary describes the first cesarean, and repeat cesarean section is used to describe any cesarean section after the first. The various types of cesarean section used are lower uterine segment (or low segment—incision in the lower uterine segment), classic (incision in the uterine corpus), extraperitoneal (the uterus is entered without incising the peritoneum), and cesarean hysterectomy (cesarean section followed by hysterectomy). Several other descriptive terms are used: elective (vs. mandatory), transverse (incision at right angle to the uterine long axis), and vertical (incision corresponds to the long axis of the uterus).

INCIDENCE

In 1965, the U.S. cesarean delivery rate was ~4.5%; by 1985, it was ~22.7% and has remained at or above that level. The current indications for cesarean section include ~48% repeat cesareans, ~29% dystocia, 16% fetal distress, 5% breech, and 2% other complications. Regrettably, the medicolegal climate in the United States may be largely responsible for the increasing use of cesarean section.

CONTRAINDICATIONS

There are few contraindications to cesarean section in the presence of a valid indication. These contraindications include pyogenic infections of the abdominal wall, an abnormal fetus incompatible with life, a dead fetus (except to save the life of the mother), and lack of appropriate facilities, equipment and supplies, or personnel.

INDICATIONS

Cesarean section is warranted when vaginal delivery imposes risks exceeding that of cesarean section to the mother or fetus. The indications may be absolute or relative and are summarized in Table 16-1.

OPERATIVE PROCEDURES

Lower segment cesarean section is the procedure of choice because there is less blood loss, the scar is less likely to rupture in a subsequent labor (and delivery), and there is less chance of bowel adhesions to the incisional site. The classic cesarean section is only employed for specific indications. Extraperitoneal is a more problematic variation of the lower segment cesarean section and is rarely used today. Vaginal cesarean section has been abandoned. Cesarean hysterectomy is also only used for very specific indications.

TABLE 16-1
COMMON INDICATIONS FOR CESAREAN SECTION

Repeat cesarean section
Dystocia
  Fetopelvic disproportion (Passage insufficiency)
    Bony pelvis
      Pelvic inlet (usually anterior-posterior <10 cm)
      Midpelvis (usually ischial spines <9.5 cm)
      Outlet (very unusual and then almost never seen in
        the absence of other pelvic contractures)
    Soft-tissue obstruction
      Low-lying placenta (especially posteriorly
        implanted)
      Uterine leiomyomas
      Ovarian tumors
      Other genital tract neoplasia (rare)
  Fetal complications (the Passenger)
    Normal fetus
      Macrosomia (>4000 g)
      Malposition and malpresentation
      Breech unfavorable for vaginal delivery
      Deflexed head
      Transverse or oblique lie
      Brow
      Posterior mental position
      Shoulder presentations
      Compound presentations
    Anomalous fetus
      Meningomyelocele
      Hydrocephalus
      Sacrococcygeal teratoma
      Miscellaneous fetal anomalies
  Abnormalities of labor (the Powers)
    Primary uterine inertia
    Prolonged latent phase (unusual, but >20 h in a
      nullipara and >14 h in a multipara)
    Protraction disorders
      Protracted active phase dilatation (nulligravida
        <1.2 cm/h, multigravida <1.5 cm/h)
      Protracted descent (nulligravida <1 cm/h,
        multigravida <2 cm/h)

TABLE 16-1
(Continued)

Arrest disorders
Prolonged deceleration phase (nulliparas ≤3 h, multiparas ≤1 h)
Secondary arrest of dilatation (no dilatation for ≥2 h)
Active phase arrest of descent (≥1 h)
Failure of descent in the deceleration phase or second stage (≥1 h)
Uterine inertia due to fetopelvic disproportion
Failed induction
Fetal compromise
Uteroplacental insufficiency
Cord accidents
Metabolic acidosis
Obstetric hemorrhage (maternal or fetal or both)
Abruptio placentae
Placenta previa
Ruptured uterus
Vasa previa
Multiple gestation
Twins
Twin A any presentation except vertex
Twin B not suitable for vaginal delivery
Failure of intrapartum external version
Fetal distress (even if Twin A has been delivered vaginally)
All monoamniotic twins
Triplets or greater number
Infections
Severe chorioamnionitis
Active maternal genital herpes
Some cases of genital condylomata acuminata
Maternal and/or fetal complications potentially adversely influenced by labor or vaginal delivery or both
Antepartal testing indicative of labor intolerance
Cervical dystocia
Medical
Fulminant preeclampsia-eclampsia
Diabetes (only occasionally indicated)
Erythroblastosis

(Continued)

TABLE 16-1
(Continued)

Severe maternal heart disease
Other debilitating conditions
Surgical
 Cervical or uterine scarring of extent that may
  rupture with labor (e.g., extensive myomectomy,
  trachelorrhaphy)
 Cervical cerclage
  All abdominal cervical cerclages
  Certain vaginal cerclages (e.g., cannot remove)
 Serious maternal problems (e.g., vesicovaginal or
  rectovaginal fistula)
 Prior extensive vaginal plastic operations
Carcinoma of the cervix

SURGICAL PRINCIPLES

The principles of hemostasis, accurate tissue apposition, avoidance
of tissue necrosis, minimizing suture material, reducing operating
time, and avoiding infection will influence outcome beneficially.

ELECTIVE PROCEDURES
WITH CESAREAN SECTION

Carefully consider elective procedures coincident with cesarean section. These include operating time, need for transfusion, infection
potential, and so on. Tubal ligation is the most frequent coincident
procedure and rarely is medically contraindicated. Incidental appendectomy (the second most common elective procedure with
cesarean section) may be accomplished safely if the appendix
is readily accessible and there are no other complicating factors.
Pedunculated myomas can be ligated and removed, but excision of
other myomas nearly always leads to hemorrhage.

ABDOMINAL INCISIONS

*The choice of abdominal incision for cesarean section is predicated
on the type of uterine incision planned and whether or not access
to the upper abdomen is necessary.* To perform a lower uterine segment cesarean section, enter the abdomen through a lower abdominal transverse (Pfannenstiel) or a vertical abdominal incision. There

is a better *cosmetic result with the transverse incision,* and the patient may wear a bikini swimsuit without the scar showing. In addition, healing proceeds faster, the incision is less painful, and there is less risk of hernia formation (the action of the abdominal muscles tends to pull the incision together, not apart). The primary advantages of the vertical incision are more rapid performance than for a transverse incision and better access to the upper abdomen.

Transverse Abdominal Incisions

For best cosmetic results, make the symmetric incision about 2 cm superior to the symphysis pubis to curve slightly cephalad laterally. Divide the subcutaneous tissues similarly and obtain hemostasis. After transversely incising the rectus fascia, grasp the midline raphe and separate the underlying tissues by sharp dissection. Retract the rectus muscles (and pyramidalis, if present) laterally and enter the attenuated posterior fascia and parietal peritoneum transversely or vertically by sharp dissection.

To close the peritoneum, begin the transverse incision closure with a running 0 or 00 polyglycolic suture. Approximate the rectus muscles in the midline and close the fascia with interrupted or running 0 to 00 polyglycolic suture. Approximate the subcutaneous tissues and close the skin appropriately.

Vertical Abdominal Incision

The abdomen is usually entered through a low vertical midline incision, although a transverse abdominal incision occasionally may be used for a classic cesarean section. The midline incision usually follows the linea nigra and extends from the umbilicus to the symphysis pubis. After incision of the subcutaneous tissues, sharply incise the midline raphe and enter the parietal peritoneum by sharp dissection.

The vertical incision is usually closed with the peritoneal layer sutured with a 0 to 00 polygycolic suture. The fascial tissues are closed with interrupted 0 absorbable or nonabsorbable sutures. Following reapproximation of the subcutaneous tissue, the skin is closed.

LOWER SEGMENT CESAREAN SECTION

After the peritoneum is entered, identify the veriscouterine peritoneal fold and incise the uterine peritoneum transversely ~1 cm from the bladder attachment. Remove the areolar connections between the bladder and the lower uterine segment for 3–4 cm by blunt dissection, and retract the bladder toward the symphysis pubis, exposing the lower uterine segment. The lower uterine segment is an anatomic area extraordinarily influenced by late pregnancy and labor (e.g., without labor, it is located far down in the pelvis, but after full dilatation, it may be one-third the distance to the umbilicus). Thus, judgment is necessary to properly locate the uterine incision. Carefully enter the lower uterine segment transversely by sharp dissection. Extend the incision laterally, curving cephalad with bandage scissors. Visualize and avoid the uterine vessels just beyond the limits of the incision.

Use a vertical incision in the midline of the lower uterine segment for more access to the uterus. The major problem with this incision is extension into the myometrium of the uterine corpus.

Next, deliver the fetus, the placenta, and membranes. Explore the uterine cavity with a laparotomy pad over the gloved hand to ensure the removal of the placenta and membranes. Close the uterine incision in two running or interrupted layers using 0 or 00 absorbable suture (e.g., polygycolic). Replace the bladder over the area of the incision. Close the visceral peritoneum using a running suture with 000 or 0000 absorbable suture.

CLASSIC CESAREAN SECTION

The indications for classic cesarean section are placenta previa, transverse or oblique fetal lie, and when rapid delivery is essential.

The classic cesarean section is the simplest to perform. Make a vertical incision in the lower portion of the uterine corpus (above the vesicouterine fold) through the visceral peritoneum into the myometrium. After the uterine cavity is entered, extend the incision caudally and cranially using bandage scissors. Effect the delivery of the infant, the placenta, and the membranes. Repair the incision with three layers of absorbable suture (e.g., polyglycolic). Close the two deeper layers with a running or interrupted 0 or 00 and the superficial layer with a running (or baseball) 00 or 000 suture.

EXTRAPERITONEAL CESAREAN SECTION

Extraperitoneal cesarean section avoids entering the peritoneal cavity. This procedure may have had advantages before extensive use of antibacterial agents but it is rarely used today.

CESAREAN HYSTERECTOMY

The indications for cesarean hysterectomy include inability to control bleeding (e.g., from uncontrollable atony, from the placental implantation site of a previa), rupture of the uterus (with repair impractical), *placenta accreta, massive infection of the uterus involving tissue necrosis, and uterine or cervical tumors* (e.g., uterine leiomyomas, cervical carcinoma in situ). Subtotal hysterectomy (i.e., leaving the cervix) is reserved for cases (usually hemorrhage) in which the patient's well-being is threatened by the significant operative time and risk of total hysterectomy.

Cesarean hysterectomy is technically the same as other hysterectomy except for the size of the uterus, the friability of tissue, and the extraordinary vascularity. Over two thirds of cesarean hysterectomy patients require transfusion, and morbidity remains high.

INTRAOPERATIVE CONTROL OF BLEEDING

The blood loss from an average vaginal delivery is ~500 mL, whereas that from an uncomplicated cesarean is ~1200 mL. The effect of this on the gravida may be appreciated by noting the Hct on the third postpartum day when the early hemodynamic alterations have begun to stabilize. The vaginally delivered patient will have increased her Hct by about 3, whereas the average postcesarean patient will have decreased her Hct by approximately 3.

Intraoperative blood loss may be decreased by meticulous surgical hemostasis, exteriorization of the uterus (through the abdominal incision) for removal of the placenta (and membranes) or repair of the uterine incision, and postdelivery administration of oxytocin. Administer the latter slowly IV (5–10 IU) immediately after delivery of the newborn or immediately after delivery of the placenta. Then, add 10–20 IU to each liter of fluid until the uterus is well contracted.

COMPLICATIONS

MATERNAL MORTALITY

The maternal mortality rate of cesarean section is 40–80/100,000, which is >25 times that of vaginal delivery. Indeed, *infectious morbidity and mortality are 80 times higher than that of vaginal delivery.* However, those having cesarean delivery may be at higher relative risk because of factors necessitating the procedure. Anesthetic complications contribute 10% to the overall maternal mortality. However, both low-risk patients and high-risk patients may be affected. Thus, anesthesia has consistently remained the fifth or sixth cause of maternal mortality.

INTRAOPERATIVE MATERNAL MORBIDITY

Intraoperative surgical complications with cesarean section are >11% (~80% minor and 20% major). *Major complications include bladder injury, laceration into cervix or vagina, laceration in the corpus uteri, laceration through the isthmus into the broad ligament, laceration of both uterine arteries, intestinal injury, and trauma to the infant with sequelae.* Complications are higher in emergency (~19%) than in elective (~4.2%) cases. Minor complications include blood transfusion, injury to the infant without sequelae, minor laceration of the isthmus, and difficulty in delivering the infant.

The risk factors in emergency cesarean section, but not in elective cesarean, include station of the fetal presenting part (very low or very high), labor before surgery (no labor or very lengthy labor enhances risk), low gestational age, rupture of fetal membranes (with labor) before surgery, previous cesarean section, and skill of the operator. Although uncommon, massive venous air embolus may complicate cesarean section. Measures to decrease the possibility of venous air embolus include adequate prehydration and avoidance of extreme Trendelenburg position.

POSTOPERATIVE MATERNAL MORBIDITY

Postoperative morbidity following cesarean section is ~15%, of which ~90% is infectious (endometritis, urinary tract and wound sepsis). *Complications are more likely after emergency (~25%) than elective cesarean section (~5%).* Predispositions to postoperative morbidity are duration of ruptured membranes before surgery, duration of labor before surgery, anemia, and obesity.

Factors most significantly associated with the risk of postoperative infection include rupture of the membranes for ≥8 h, labor for ≥12 h with cervical effacement and dilatation to ≥4 cm, multiple vaginal examinations, low socioeconomic status, and complicating medical conditions. The use of prophylactic antibiotics materially decreases infectious morbidity and mortality. In <2% of postcesarean patients, infections will become life-threatening because of septic shock, pelvic abscess, or septic pelvic thrombophlebitis.

Other factors enhancing risk due to infection include a lack of prenatal care, maternal age (the very young are at increased risk), malnutrition, lower gestational age, longer preoperative hospital stays, and systemic illnesses (e.g., diabetes, systemic lupus erythematosus, or chronic renal disease). The number of vaginal examinations that place the patient at risk for infection may be 3–7. There are conflicting data about the effect of intrauterine catheter monitoring on the risk of postcesarean section infectious morbidity.

Common noninfectious cesarean postoperative complications (<10% of the total) include paralytic ileus, intraabdominal hemorrhage, bladder paresis, thrombosis, and pulmonary disorders (e.g., pneumonia).

PERINATAL MORTALITY AND MORBIDITY

Cesarean section carries less risk for the infant than a complicated vaginal delivery, and thus, by inference, perinatal mortality and morbidity are decreased. This may apply to certain conditions. There is no proof, however, that the current high cesarean section rate has generally enhanced mental performance or reduced the overall incidence of neurologic abnormalities of those delivered by cesarean section.

Iatrogenic prematurity from elective repeat cesarean has been a major concern. Nonetheless, with currently available means of fetal assessment, including ascertaining gestational length (e.g., early pregnancy testing, early ultrasound examination) or defining fetal pulmonary maturity (e.g., LS ratio, phosphatidylglycerol) before elective cesarean section, iatrogenic prematurity has been markedly decreased.

PROPHYLACTIC ANTIBIOTICS

Prophylactic antibiotics with all cesarean sections may lower the infectious morbidity. However, ~20% of women will still require systemic antibiotic therapy for postoperative uterine infection, and some serious postoperative pelvic infections still occur. Yet even using current risk criteria, ~50% of cases that become infected will not have been identified. Finally, although prophylactic antibiotics do significantly reduce febrile morbidity and endomyometritis, the data are less conclusive for wound and urinary infections. Nonetheless, the use of prophylactic antibiotics for the risk groups is well accepted.

Preoperative maternal antibiotics may result in therapeutic levels in the fetus. This complicates the evaluation of the newborn at risk for sepsis. Thus, except in extreme cases, antibiotics are usually administered IV after the cord is clamped or after the uterine wound and peritoneal cavity are lavaged with an antibiotic solution.

The usual microorganisms involved in postcesarean endometritis are group B streptococci, aerobic gram-negative bacilli, anaerobic gram-positive cocci, and anaerobic gram-negative bacilli.

Prophylactic antibiotics should be effective for the contaminating organisms, inexpensive, nontoxic, and clinically effective. Prophylactic antibiotics should not be one of the few antibiotics reserved for the treatment of specific severe infections or a drug used against bacterial pathogens with acquired resistance. Although many antibiotics have been studied for their prophylactic efficacy, first- and second-generation cephalosporins are probably the best. If more than one agent is used, they should be tailored to cover both anaerobic and aerobic organisms. There is no single agent or combination of agents that can be designated the treatment of choice.

PREVENTION OF UNNECESSARY CESAREAN SECTION

Although cesarean section delivery rates continue to rise, there are increasing reports of methods that could decrease the number of cesarean sections. These include *vaginal birth following cesarean section, use of active management of labor, antepartum external version to decrease the number of breech presentations, vaginal birth for selected breech presentations, and the selective use of forceps.* Particularly noteworthy are increasing trends for vaginal birth after cesarean (VBAC), which has been demonstrated to be both effective and relatively safe. It may be anticipated that two thirds of those women who had a prior cesarean section will undertake a trial of labor if it is offered, and ~80% will achieved a vaginal delivery. With vaginal birth, there will be less maternal morbidity due to uterine dehiscence (~2%) or uterine rupture (0.3% with repeat cesarean and 0.5% with VBAC). Hence, if there is no urgent or continued indication for cesarean section, vaginal delivery should be chosen, and the policy of "once a cesarean section, always a cesarean section" should be abandoned.

17

GYNECOLOGIC HISTORY AND EXAMINATION

HISTORY

It is common practice to obtain much of the history by paramedical personnel, interactive computer activities, or a patient questionnaire completed before seeing the physician. Hence, the patient–physician interaction can be *focused with emphasis on the patient's concerns.* Additionally, important positive and negative findings may be reviewed with the patient before the physical examination.

AGE, MARITAL STATUS, GRAVIDITY, AND PARITY CHIEF COMPLAINT

The *patient's main problem(s) in her own words* listed in her order of seriousness comprise the chief complaint.

PRESENT ILLNESS

The patient's *health at the onset of illness and the symptoms in sequence of development form the present illness.* As much detail (e.g., facts, dates) as is possible is included, documenting what, where, when, why, how, and to what degree each complaint affects her.

PAST HISTORY

MENSTRUAL HISTORY

The age and character of the *menarche (or menopause) should be described.* The last menstrual period *(LMP),* previous menstrual period *(PMP),* and last normal menstrual period *(LNMP),* if relevant, should be recorded. Also, the regularity, duration, amount of bleeding (number of perineal pads or tampons), pain, mucous discharge, and intermenstrual or postcoital spotting should be recorded.

GYNECOLOGIC HISTORY

Record the following. *Gravida (G), the number of previous pregnancies; para (P), the number of previous term pregnancies; abortions (Ab), the number of pregnancies terminated (spontaneously or electively) before 20 weeks gestation or 500 g; premature deliveries (Pre), the number of pregnancies terminated between 21–35 weeks gestation or 500–2499 g; living children (LC),* the number of children currently living, with *twins noted in parenthesis* at the end of the sequence. Often, this is recorded in a summary with just the numbers in the sequence noted; [e.g., 4,2,1,2,4 (Twins 1 pr.) would mean the woman had been pregnant 4 times, had 2 term pregnancies, had 1 abortion, had 2 premature births, and has 4 living children (here, the twins were premature but survived)].

In some patients, a more detailed obstetric history is indicated, including dates of all pregnancies; their duration, character, and duration of labor; and method of delivery (with type of uterine incision if cesarean birth). Complications, weight and gender of infant(s), stillbirths, abortions, neonatal complications, and current status of living children should be noted also.

MEDICAL AND SURGICAL HISTORY

Record *medical allergies* (e.g., penicillin, iodine, horse serum) as well as important nonmedical allergies (e.g., shrimp). Record any excessive bleeding potentially indicative of a *coagulopathy.* A summary of the patient's *childhood and later illnesses* in chronologic order together with complications and the treatment prescribed for each is important. Record *operations and injuries,* with dates and outcome. Record all *medications* (prescription, proprietary) as well as *alternative health care* (medications, acupuncture, etc.).

FAMILY HISTORY

Age, health, and cause and date of death of first- through third-degree relatives (often a brief pedigree is the best demonstration of this material) should be recorded. Also note *familial or hereditary abnormalities, diseases, bleeding tendencies, occurrence of cancer, tuberculosis, diabetes mellitus, heart disease, hypertension, and nervous or mental disorders.*

SEXUAL HISTORY

Current and past contraception usage should be recorded, as well as libido and the frequency of coitus. Additional notes should be made about the duration of present marriage or living arrangement, patient's assessment of the relationship, age and health of spouse/partner, former marriages or relationships (when and how long) and degree of compatibility, vaginal and pelvic infections, and sexually transmitted diseases (including HIV).

SOCIAL HISTORY

The patient's *occupation,* avocation(s), and travel (especially abroad or in the tropics) should be appraised for hazards. Reactions to others may be assessed tangentially by questions relating to successes, failures, and participation in social or religious organizations.

PERSONAL HISTORY (HABITS)

Sleep pattern, exercise habits, and alcohol, tobacco, and drug usage should be noted.

   Health maintenance parameters should be assessed: This includes the status of *age- and gender-specific screening* (e.g., last mammography, last Pap smear, fecal occult hemoglobin screening, lipoprotein screening, Tay-Sachs screening). Additionally, the status of routine immunizations must be reviewed. This includes status of adult DT (diptheria, tetanus), "flu" immunizations, as well as rubella and chicken pox (varicella).

SYSTEM REVIEW

A positive or negative comment for each portion of this category will aid in health assessment.

GENERAL

Comment on the patient's health, present weight, average weight, weight before present illness, reason for weight loss or gain, skin disorders, and change in hair pattern.

HEAD AND NECK

Pain, tenderness, swelling, restriction of neck, and trauma should be noted.

EYES

Vision with and without glasses, double vision, irritation, swelling of the lids, and prominence of eyes deserve comment.

EARS

Record pain, buzzing, discharge, and patient's assessment of hearing.

NOSE

Obstruction to nasal passages, bleeding, discharge, and change in ability to smell require recording.

MOUTH

General condition of the teeth, gums, tongue, bleeding, and chewing difficulties should be noted.

THROAT

Speech difficulties, swallowing, or voice changes are notable.

CARDIOVASCULAR

Skin color (pale, ruddy, dusky), edema, precordial or substernal pain, irregular or labored heartbeat, and shortness of breath at rest or with exercise should be recorded.

RESPIRATORY

List any of the following: cough, wheezing, sputum, hemoptysis, chest pain with breathing, chills, fever, and night sweats.

GASTROINTESTINAL

The patient's appetite, thirst, digestive difficulties (e.g., nausea, vomiting, prandial or postprandial pain, hematemesis, food intolerance), jaundice, and frequency, character, and color of stools should be assessed.

URINARY

Urinary frequency, nocturia, oliguria, dysuria, hematuria, urethral discharge, sores, swelling, and other urinary alterations should be recorded.

NEUROPSYCHIATRIC

Strength, ability to work, skin sensations, ataxia, dizziness, tremor, headaches, "spells" or "fits," acuity of memory, and strange occurrences should be explored if warranted.

PHYSICAL EXAMINATION

VITAL SIGNS

At the minimum, the patient's *weight, height, blood pressure, and pulse* are recorded. The *temperature and respirations* are also useful, but more often recorded if related to the chief complaint.

GENERAL

The patient's *appearance, state of nutrition, ability to ambulate, attitude, and color of skin* (e.g., pallor, plethora) are often recorded.

HEAD AND NECK

Skull size and shape, hair (amount, color, and texture), tumors, and tenderness may be useful.

EYES

Prominence of the eyes or lids as well as the size, shape, pupillary reaction to light, character of conjunctiva and sclera, fundi, and ocular movements should be assessed.

EARS

The external ear, external auditory canal, and tympanic membrane should be examined, and discharge, cerumen, tophi, tenderness, or other abnormalities must be noted.

NOSE

Any deformity, septal deviation, septal erosion, obstruction, tenderness, discharge, or tenderness over the sinuses requires comment.

NECK

Swelling, pulsations, tracheal deviations, thyroid, lymph nodes, retractions, and abnormal masses should be noted.

MOUTH AND THROAT

The lips, gums, tongue, dentition, tonsils, and oropharynx should be examined.

THORAX

The general size, shape, symmetry, and spinal integrity may bear notation.

BREASTS

The size, shape, equality, masses, tenderness, scars, and nipple discharge should be noted (see next section for discussion).

HEART

The point of maximal impulse at the apex, abnormal pulsations, retractions, or venous distention in the neck or in other veins should be noted. Auscultation of the heart should be accomplished.

LUNGS

Inspect the chest to reveal the equality of inspiration and expiration. Palpate to reveal muscle tone, tenderness, and tactile fremitus. Percussion should reveal resonance, cardiac silhouette, diaphragmatic exclusions, and gastric tympany. Auscultation reveals the quality and intensity of breath sound, rales, fremitus, and friction rubs.

ABDOMEN

Note the *size, shape, and abdominal contour as well as masses, visible peristaltic waves, prominent veins, and herniation.* Palpation may indicate the thickness of the abdominal wall, the liver edge, the spleen and any tenderness, rigidity, masses, hernias, and the presence or absence of a fluid wave. Percussion should confirm organ position or masses. Auscultation will reveal the presence of peristaltic tones.

BACK

The back should be checked for kyphosis or scoliosis. Costovertebral angle tenderness should be noted.

EXTREMITIES

Size, shape, color, and movements of the hands should be visualized, and condition of the fingers and nails should be noted. The size, color, condition, and movement of the legs should be assessed. The peripheral vascular system may be appraised by palpating the radial, femoral, distal pedal, posterior tibial, and popliteal arteries for thickness and resilience.

NERVOUS SYSTEM

Cerebral function, cranial nerves, cerebellar function, motor and sensory systems, and reflexes should be reported.

PELVIC EXAMINATION

A proper pelvic examination records *visual inspection and palpation of the external genitalia; Bartholin's urethral, and Skene's glands (BUS); introitus, vagina, and cervix. The bimanual examination includes palpation of the uterus, ovaries, and uterine tubal areas. The rectovaginal examination must include palpation of vagina, rectum, and rectovaginal septum as high as the cul-de-sac* (see next section for details).

IMPRESSION (ANALYSIS)

List probable diagnoses for each problem (in same order of chief complaint).

PLAN

Record a *plan for each problem* (i.e., diagnosis and therapy). Note any *tests performed in the office* (e.g., wet mount and Pap smear) and indicate *other testing the patient is to have* (e.g., mammography) and when she will be seen again. Indicate any *counseling or instructions* given to the patient.

SIGNATURE

Include time and date of notation.

GYNECOLOGIC EXAMINATION

Increasingly, obstetrician–gynecologists, nurse practitioners, physician assistants, and other health care professionals are providing the entire spectrum of *primary health care for women,* as well as taking care of their reproductive needs. Thus, it is proper to *determine if the patient is being seen for a specific issue, or if she is expecting her entire health care to be met with this exchange.* The depth of the general workup and health care advice may then be appropriately detailed. For example, if the patient wishes to be seen for gynecologic complaints only and is already under the care of another primary physician, the gynecologic examination will be the focus of the visit.

The *gynecologic evaluation devotes particular attention to examination of the breasts, abdomen, and pelvis.* The general examination and appropriate laboratory studies should be performed. An appraisal of other body systems should be done more frequently than the usual standards when indicated by the history or unusual physical findings.

BREAST EXAMINATION

The breast examination has three components: *breast self-examination (BSE), physician examination, and mammography.*

BREAST SELF-EXAMINATION (BSE)

After age 20 years, BSE is recommended on a monthly basis for all women. Women who do BSE as recommended discover breast disease significantly earlier, and death from breast cancer can be avoided or delayed by early diagnosis and prompt therapy. Moreover, BSE is simple, costs nothing, and is painless. Despite these advantages, only approximately one third of women perform BSE monthly, and of those, only about half do this correctly.

Since BSE is more often and better performed if taught by a nurse or a physician, *the time of examination is an ideal opportunity to teach BSE and discuss its significance.*

Most information will be gained in a menstruating woman *immediately after menses* when hormonal changes in the breast are at a minimum. In nonmenstruating women, it is often most convenient to choose a time when there is another monthly duty (e.g., paying bills) to trigger remembering to do BSE.

The examination is begun in the upright position with good direct light. Looking in a mirror, the patient *inspects the breasts carefully, first with her arms at the sides, and then raised above her head.* She is seeking abnormalities of contour or symmetry, skin changes, masses, retraction, or nipple alterations.

Palpation of the supraclavicular and axillary regions is performed next. She is looking for changes from previous examinations, masses, nodes, or other abnormalities.

Next, the patient *reclines,* with a towel or small pillow beneath the back on the side of the breast being examined (to rotate the chest so that the breast may be symmetrically flattened against the chest wall). Next, using the flat of her fingers, she *systematically palpates each quadrant of the breast by pressing against the chest wall.* Finally, the *areola and the area beneath the nipple should be palpated* and the *nipples compressed* for evidence of secretion. Again, she is looking for changes from previous examinations, lumps (masses), and any other abnormalities. Should anything raise concern, the patient should immediately *consult her physician.* Many women find keeping a simple sketch as a record of the findings from month to month to be a useful way to detect change.

PHYSICIAN BREAST EXAMINATION

A complete physician breast examination is recommended every *2–3 years for women age 20–40* (Figs. 17-1, 17-2, and 17-3). *Women >40 should have at least annual examinations.* The physician should proceed as follows.

With the patient sitting in good light with her arms at the side, a *visual inspection* is performed. The patient is asked to press her hands on her hips (*tensing the pectoralis muscles*), and the inspection continued. With her *arms raised above her head,* both breasts and axillae are examined. Finally, the patient is asked to bend forward from the erect position to reveal irregularities or dimpling when the breasts fall forward. The health provider must look for the same abnormalities as the patient (i.e., asymmetry, masses, nipple retraction, skin retraction, or other changes). Often, oblique light is helpful to confirm surface dimpling.

With the patient sitting, the patient is asked to extend her arms 60°–90°. Careful *palpation of each axilla* is performed using the flat

FIGURE 17-1. Inspection of breasts. Observe breasts with patient sitting, arms at sides and overhead, for presence of asymmetry and nipple or skin retraction. These signs may be accentuated by having the patient raise her arms overhead. Skin retraction or dimpling may be demonstrated by having the patient press her hand on her hip in order to contract the pectoralis muscles. (From J.L. Wilson. In: J.E. Dunphy and L.W. Way, eds., *Current Surgical Diagnosis & Treatment,* 4th ed. Lange, 1979.)

of the fingers of the right hand for the left axilla and the left hand for the axilla. Both the *supraclavicular and infraclavicular areas are carefully palpated* for masses. With the patient leaning forward, *bimanual palpation of each breast* is performed using the flat of the

FIGURE 17-2. Palpation of axillary and supraclavicular regions for enlarged lymph nodes.

(From A.E. Giuliano. In: L.W. Way, ed., *Current Surgical Diagnosis & Treatment,* 6th ed. Lange, 1983.)

fingers. Both side-to-side and upper-to-lower palpation may be necessary depending on the configuration of the breasts.

With the patient supine and arms above the head, the breasts are again inspected. The axilla are reassessed with the patient's arms

FIGURE 17-3. Palpation of breasts. Palpation is performed with the patient supine and arm abducted.

(From A.E. Giuliano. In: L.W. Way, ed., *Current Surgical Diagnosis & Treatment,* 6th ed. Lange, 1983.)

extended. The breasts are palpated between the examining fingers. Finally, with the woman's arms relaxed at the sides, *careful palpation of each breast quadrant* is performed by compression against the chest wall. One breast at a time is palpated by holding the fingers flat against the breast and carefully feeling with gentle pressure. Gentle compression of the areas beneath the areola and nipple with the thumb and index finger will detect masses and express fluid. Should a nipple discharge be present, it should be smeared on a slide and fixed for *cytologic examination.*

The breasts are observed for consistency, thickened areas, irregularities, areas with dissimilar consistency, cordlike duct structures, as well as shotty or nodular masses. It is determined whether masses are fixed to the skin or chest wall.

When a breast mass is identified, the presumptive diagnosis is usually established by *mammography.* It may be necessary to *aspirate a cyst or biopsy* to confirm the diagnosis.

MAMMOGRAPHY

High-quality *mammograms* may be obtained with ≤0.3 rad exposure. This technique has been demonstrated to correctly identify ~89% of cancers (41.6% of which were not detectable clinically). The American Cancer Society guidelines for mammographic screening of asymptomatic women are widely accepted.

- Baseline mammogram for all women age 35–40 years
- Mammography at 1–2 year intervals from age 40 to 49 years
- Annual mammograms for women ≥50 years

High-risk women (e.g., previous breast cancer, mothers or sisters with bilateral or premenopausal breast cancer, and those with histologic abnormalities associated with subsequent breast cancer—Chapter 18) *should have biannual examinations and annual mammography.* Such a screening program will identify >6 cancers per 1000 asymptomatic women. Moreover, the tumors will be detected earlier (80% have negative axillary nodes vs. 45% not screened). Approximately 40% of early breast cancers can be discovered only by mammography, and ~40% can be detected only by palpation. Thus, both modalities are crucial.

ABDOMINAL EXAMINATION

The abdomen is observed with the patient sitting, and then examine in the dorsal recumbent position with knees slightly flexed to improve abdominal relaxation. The contour is noted (flat, scaphoid, or protuberant), and inspection of the abdomen conducted for respiratory movement, prominence or enlargement of internal organs, asymmetry, scars, and significant skin changes (e.g., striae, rashes). The escutcheon pattern is noted, as well as other hair distribution. Auscultation is performed in each of the quadrants.

The abdomen is palpated gently for evidence of tenderness, herniation, or masses. Deeper palpation will reveal deep masses or sensitivity, especially over the cecum, colon, and bladder. The liver is identified by percussion and the edge is palpated. Upper abdominal palpation screens the gallbladder, epigastrium, and spleen. Muscle guarding and abdominal rigidity may indicate infection. *Gentleness is essential. Progressing from areas of less tenderness to the areas of discomfort facilitates examination.* With hematoperitoneum, the guarding increases as the pressure of palpation is increased. Rebound tenderness is a sign of peritoneal irritation and must be investigated further.

PELVIC EXAMINATION

With the patient in the lithotomy position and appropriately draped, the examination usually begins with the health provider seated. Surgically clean gloves are used. It is desirable to have a female attendant present as a chaperone and assistant. The pelvic examination consists entirely of inspection and palpation.

INSPECTION

Observation of the external genitalia identifies labial development, hair distribution, and abnormalities. Gentle lateral traction separates the labia majora and facilitates inspection of the clitoris as well as both labia minora. The glans may be exposed by slight traction on the foreskin. Separation of the labia minora allows visualization of the urethral meatus. The vaginal orifice is observed for vaginal discharge and the status of the hymen. Inflammation, cysts, or tumors may be seen in the region of Bartholin's glands. The fossa navicularis may reveal discharge, scars (e.g., episiotomy), or lesions (e.g., condylomata). Further inspection and palpation over the perineum, thighs, mons veneris, and perianal region may reveal skin changes, masses, and tender areas. Any discernible external genital lesions (e.g., inflamed, hypertrophied, atrophied, or ulcerated areas) are recorded.

SPECULUM EXAMINATION

Warming the speculum with tap water serves to further patient comfort as well as to lubricate the instrument. Other lubricants may confuse vaginal cytology, bacterial smears or cultures, and wet preparations for *Trichomonas, Candida,* and *Bacterial vaginosis.* A good light source, preferably daylight or a blue-white spotlight facilitates the examination. A single-blade speculum is advantageous to view the vaginal surface (e.g., searching for a vesicovaginal or rectovaginal fistula). The Kelly air vaginoscope is especially useful for examination of the very young or when the introitus is atrophic (Fig. 17-4).

One method to facilitate speculum insertion, is to ask the patient to *relax* and then to bear down slightly as with a bowel movement. This reduces muscular resistance to introduction of the speculum. Spreading the labia with the gloved fingers of one hand, and inserting the gloved index finger of the same hand slightly into the

Graves vaginal speculum   Pederson vaginal speculum

Sims vaginal retractor   Kelly air vaginoscope
                                (cystoscope) for children

FIGURE 17-4.   Vaginal specula and vaginoscope. These come in various sizes.

vagina, to slightly depress the perineum while asking the patient to relax the muscles being pressed on, may also facilitate relaxation.

The speculum is most easily inserted by holding the blades slightly obliquely to the axis of the vagina while directing them downward and inward at approximately 45° to avoid the urethra. The vaginal canal may be visualized while inserting and opening the speculum. To avoid a traumatic encounter with a vaginal obstruction, mass, or friable lesion, observation is continued as the speculum is advanced. As the blades of the bivalve speculum approach the cervix, opening the instrument allows the blades to slip into the anterior and posterior fornices, fully expose the cervix. The blades may be fixed in the open position by tightening the screw lock.

The *cervix merits careful examination* (i.e.: color, size, contour, surface characteristics, and the squamocolumnar junction). Lacerations; displacement; size and configuration of the external os; distortion or ulceration; type and amount of discharge, blood, or fluid present in the cervical canal; and the character of the endocervix (through a patulous os) are all notable.

Before digital examination, *a clean scraping of the squamo-columnar junction and the endocervix are obtained.* In some cases, *vaginal mucus from the posterior vaginal fornix and from the cervical canal* may also be obtained for cytologic examination. The smear on the slide is fixed immediately. By touching or gently wiping ulcerations or friable lesions with a cotton-tipped applicator contact bleeding may be determined. *Suspicious lesions may be biopsied.* Topical treatment of common lesions (e.g., condylomata) is usually deferred until after bimanual examination.

Slowly removing the speculum while *observing the vaginal surfaces* facilitates inspection. Notable features include: the color, the presence or absence or rugae, the apparent thickness of the mucosa, and any abnormalities (redness, ulceration, or tumors). When *cystocele, rectocele, or descensus is suspected, the insertion of a single blade of the speculum* and having the patient bear down assists in demonstrating the degree of relaxation or herniation. The single blade is placed in the posterior of the vagina to demonstrate anterior defects, and anteriorly to demonstrate apical and posterior defects. *Striping Skene's glands and the distal urethra (distally)* after removal of the speculum facilitates determination of infection in these areas. Smears or cultures (or both) of expressed discharge is helpful in determining the responsible agent to select appropriate therapy.

PALPATION

Digital examination is easiest with the patient in the lithotomy position and the examiner standing with one foot on a step or low stool and the elbow on that knee to brace the examining arm and hand. The gloved, lubricated index finger is gently inserted into the vagina by applying slight downward pressure at the fourchette and asking the patient to relax. After a pause to enhance relaxation, the middle and forefinger of the examining hand may be inserted into the vagina.

Palpation of Structures of Introitus

Tenderness, masses, and thickening at the introitus *may be palpated between the thumb and forefinger.* With the thumb external and the palm turned downward, enlargement and/or sensitivity of Bartholin's glands may be appreciated. Direct palpation of the lower vaginal wall may detect abnormalities. Similarly, the urethra and base of the bladder may be palpated to detect relaxation, local dilatation, masses, and tenderness.

Palpation of Cervix

Lightly *outlining the cervix* with the fingers determines its size, position, contour, consistency, and dilation. Gently *moving the cervix* stretches the uterosacral and transverse cervical ligaments, thus, revealing the degree of freedom of the cervix. Additionally, cervical motion will usually elicit tenderness if there is an inflammatory process in the upper genital tract.

Palpation of Bladder Base

Feeling *beneath the bladder* determines sensitivity, relaxation, or masses. Slight tenderness and a suggestion of thickening over the normal ureter at or near its insertion into the bladder are normal.

Bimanual Examination

The foregoing procedures require only one unaided hand. In bimanual examination, the other hand is used on the abdomen to outline the deeper pelvic structures. The abdominal hand is held palm down on the abdomen with the fingers together and slightly flexed, but using the flat of the fingers against the abdominal wall. Generally, the *vaginal fingers are used to elevate structures for palpation through the abdominal wall.* Ideally, first one hand and then the other are used in the bimanual examination because masses in the right pelvis may be palpated more easily with the right hand, and vice versa. If the patient, with mouth open, takes shallow, rapid breaths, it assists to avoid tensing the abdominal wall.

Palpation of Uterus

If the uterus cannot be outlined by elevation, the fundus may be depressed with the abdominal hand while the fingers of the hand in the vagina are resting against the cervix and lower portion of the corpus. Relaxation of the vaginal walls and fornices may permit palpation of much or all of the cul-de-sac and of the posterior aspect of the uterus. A normally free uterus usually can be brought well downward and forward by the abdominal hand. This makes possible vaginal palpation of both the anterior wall and the uterine fundus. *The uterine position, size, consistency, contour, and mobility as well as the patient's discomfort on manipulation are all notable.* Gentle exploration of the posterior fornix and uterosacral ligaments may reveal masses, fullness, fluctuation, and sensitivity, but acute tenderness in this region may inhibit examination.

Palpation of Adnexa

By turning the fingers in the vagina so the palm is upward, the two examining fingers may be positioned slightly posteriorly but high into one of the lateral fornices. By sweeping the abdominal examining hand downward over the vaginal fingers, the *ovary may be palpated between the examining fingers.* Recall that the ovary may not be palpable in the postmenopausal woman, in women on oral contraceptives, prior to adolescence, in the obese, and in women with abdominal scarring.

The ovary usually lies just lateral to the uterus near its midportion. If the ovary is not felt initially, it may be found in the cul-de-sac, the lateral pelvic wall, or the space anterior to the uterus. In these sites, if the ovary is not readily movable it may signal adhesions between the ovary and tube and adjacent structures. The ovary is normally sensitive (tender), distinguishing it from nontender masses, such as fecal material within the bowel. *Rectovaginal examination may permit the best delineation of the ovary.* The position, size, consistency, contour, and mobility of each ovary, as well as any unusual tenderness are notable.

Ordinarily, the uterine tube is not sensitive, and is so delicate that *a normal tube cannot be palpated.* Tenderness, swelling, or a cordlike thickening between the ovary and the uterus indicates tubal disease. Inflammation or tumor may also convert the tube into an enlarged mass that is easily mistaken for an ovarian tumor.

Salpingitis, endometriosis, or cancer may involve one or both adnexa so extensively that these structures and the uterus become a single mass filling the entire true pelvis. The cul-de-sac may be filled or obliterated, thus altering gynecologic landmarks.

Rectovaginal Examination

Rectovaginal examination should be performed routinely even though all of the internal genital structures have been palpated properly on vaginal evaluation. Anal abnormalities, lesions of the rectovaginal septum, and even sacral masses may be felt only on rectovaginal examination. This examination is invaluable in children, virgins, and elderly women, in whom the vaginal introitus is so small that only a single finger can be inserted. Rectovaginal examination is much preferred to rectal examination only because the second finger reaches farther when the first finger is in the vagina, and rectovaginal septal abnormalities may be discovered.

With the patient and the examiner positioned as for bimanual vaginal examination, the lubricated second finger of the examining hand is used for the anal portion of the examination. Inserting the distal half of the middle finger into the anal canal is facilitated by the patient bearing down slightly to relax the anal sphincter. When the examining finger has been inserted a short distance, the forefinger may be introduced into the vagina. The perineal body will then be between the two fingers. Patient relaxation is aided by adopting a *gentle, slow, deliberate manner.* Finally, by reaching as high as possible in the pelvis with the tips of both the vaginal and rectal fingers, bimanual palpation may be conducted, just as with the vaginal examination. By sweeping the rectal finger about the circumference of the bowel with the patient bearing down, *up to 50% of all large bowel polyps and cancers may be located.*

To demonstrate a *rectocele,* the rectal finger is brought back to the perineal body, removing the vaginal finger. As this is done, the rectal pouch will be entered, and its protrusion into the vagina may be evident at the introitus. The patient may be able to see a rectocele herself, or have it demonstrated if she holds a mirror at the appropriate angle.

Feces from the rectal examination may be *tested for the presence of occult blood.* This is particularly important in women ≥45 years of age, when rectal carcinoma becomes more prevalent.

LABORATORY STUDIES

SMEARS OR CULTURES

BACTERIA

Obtaining specimens for *bacterial smears or cultures may be accomplished by using a sterile cotton-tipped applicator.* Fluid exudates may be obtained from the urethral meatus, Skene's and Bartholin's ducts, the vaginal walls, the posterior vaginal fornix, and the cervical os.

Using bacteriologic technique, the applicator is directly applied to the culture medium or to a transfer medium. Avoid heating and drying the sample. When gonorrhea is suspected, a sterile chocolate agar or blood agar plate is inoculated. An alternative is the use of Transgrow medium. Smears are prepared by spreading the discharge in a thin layer on a clean glass slide. For staining, the slide may be air-dried. If it is to be used for other techniques (e.g., immunofluorescent identification of herpesvirus or *Chlamydia*), it must be handled according to the methods recommended for that technique.

TRICHOMONAS VAGINALIS

Wet mount preparations for *T. vaginalis* may be obtained from the posterior fornix, the cervical os, and the urethral meatus. A clean cotton-tipped applicator moistened with normal saline is used to swab the site of exudation or discharge. A drop of the exudate is transferred to a polished slide and a clean cover slip applied. Immediate microscopic examination (while still warm) is most effective in detection of trichomonads. This technique is also useful for examining other pathogens in a wet mount (e.g., *Bacterial vaginosis*). If these organisms are not identified in the wet smear, careful inspection of the stained exfoliative vaginal cytologic smear (Papanicolaou) generally will reveal their presence. It is rarely necessary to prepare cultures. Should culture be necessary, however, an aerobic methodology with Trichosel or Difco's hash medium (B-1016T, a modified trypticase medium, not requiring addition of serum) is most effective.

CANDIDA ALBICANS

For demonstration of *Candida,* the technique is similar to that for trichomonads, but 1–2 drops of *10% aqueous potassium hydroxide* is added to the discharge to be viewed on the slide. This dissolves the epithelial, inflammatory, and red blood cells. The mycelia, hyphae, and spores are usually prominently displayed. The material most likely to show mycelia is the white plaque of vaginal thrush, which must be rubbed from the mucosa with a moist cotton applicator. In questionable cases of *Candida,* it is necessary to culture vaginal fluid on Sabouraud's or Nickerson's medium.

URINE

A *midstream, clean-catch urine specimen* (or catheterize the patient if necessary) in a sterile container is used to screen for urinary tract infection. Sterile technique and equipment after thoroughly cleansing the urethral meatus with a mild antiseptic solution affords the best opportunity for an uncontaminated specimen.

CYTOLOGIC EXAMINATION

The cytologic examination (Papanicolaou or Pap smear) is a *cancer screening technique* that is a well-established portion of preventive health care for women. The purpose of the Pap smear is to detect precursor lesions as well as invasive cervical carcinoma. When cytology is positive for premalignant or malignant cells, further diagnostic procedures (e.g., colposcopy, cervical biopsy, conization, endometrial biopsy, or D&C) must be performed to determine the diagnosis. However, a positive cytology is ~95% accurate in the diagnosis of cervical carcinoma.

The patient should not have douched for >24 h before obtaining a cytologic specimen and must not be menstruating. During the speculum examination when the cervix is first exposed, a specially designed small plastic or wooden spatula is used to *lightly scrape the squamocolumnar junction. Endocervical cells are obtained separately, often using a small brush within the endocervix.* Exfoliated cells from the vaginal pool contained in the posterior vaginal fornix may be obtained by spatula. The material from each site is immediately placed on separate slides, and a preservative spray or solution is applied.

BETHESDA PAP SMEAR SYSTEM

Most laboratories currently report findings to the physician using the *Bethesda Pap Smear system* (1991 revision). This system defines the Pap smear request as a medical consultation. The report includes: an assessment of specimen adequacy, smear reading containing determination of epithelial changes, and clinical recommendations. Squamous cell abnormalities are classified according to biologic potential.

- Low-grade squamous intraepithelial lesions (LGSIL) include grade I cervical intraepithelial neoplasia (CIN), also termed mild dysplasia, and human papillomavirus lesions.
- High-grade squamous intraepithelial lesions (HGSIL) include moderate and severe dysplasia (CIN II and III).
- Atypical squamous cells of undetermined significance (ASCUS) identifies cells that need further studies to identify if they are reactive or neoplastic.
- Similarly, atypical glandular cells of undetermined significance (ACGUS) require additional qualification as to reactive or neoplastic nature.

ACGUS is perhaps the *most controversial category of the Bethesda Pap Smear System:* there is not enough agreement on diagnostic cytologic criteria, there is a high number of false-negative diagnoses, and interobserver agreement in reclassification is poor. There is also increasing evidence that the frequency of serious histologic changes is much greater in ACGUS than in ASCUS; *>45% of ACGUS patients will have cervical intraepithelial neoplasia, invasive cervical cancer, or endometrial cancer.* Fortunately, ACGUS is uncommonly encountered (<0.2% of all Pap smears). By contrast, *ASCUS is the most common abnormal diagnosis, occurring in ~3.5% of all Pap smears.* Because of a high correlation with histologic high-grade cervical neoplasia, most authorities recommend that all minimally abnormal Pap smear diagnoses (LGSIL, ASCUS, and ACGUS) be investigated.

How frequently cervical cytologic screening should be obtained is currently debated. However, *yearly evaluations are generally recommended.* More frequent examination is indicated for women with previously abnormal cytologic studies, women with more than one sexual partner (or an uncircumcised partner), women with a history of sexually transmitted disease, and those with genital condylomata or herpes. In addition to premalignant and malignant changes, the cytologic smear is useful for the detection of viral infections (e.g., herpes simplex, condylomata acuminata) and folic acid and vitamin B_{12} deficiencies.

Pap smear screening and subsequent treatment of the detected lesions has proven effective in reducing the incidence and mortality of cervical cancer. However, *a pitfall of the Pap smear is the public perception that it is highly accurate for the individual,* while there is a *false-negative rate of at least 5%.* Currently, Pap smears remains a *screening test* and, as is the case with all screening tests, *Pap smears should only assign a probability of disease in an individual.*

Despite these limitations, Pap smears should be encouraged. *Regular smears at intervals based on individual risk remains the best method of cervical cancer detection.* However, the constraints of the Pap smear require patient education concerning value and test limitations, as well as treatment or follow-up of all abnormal smears (based on clinical and cytologic findings).

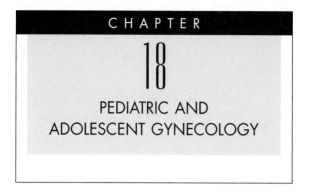

The reproductive tract in pediatric and adolescent patients differs from that of the adult, requiring special techniques and equipment for examination. The gynecologic problems addressed in children and adolescents may differ markedly from those of adult women but may be no less serious. Both the anatomy and physiology of the reproductive tract will change from the hormone-stimulated state of the newborn to the relatively estrogen-free state of the young child to the blossoming of womanhood during adolescence.

ANATOMIC AND PHYSIOLOGIC CONSIDERATIONS

NEWBORN

The newborn female reproductive tract has experienced *prolonged stimulation by transplacentally acquired maternal hormones.* With transection of the umbilical cord, these hormone levels fall, with slow reversal of their effects over the first month of life. Breast buds are present in most female newborns, and some will produce milk if massaged. Breast massage should be avoided to prevent infection or continued milk production.

At birth, the clitoris is prominent, with a clitoral index of <0.6 cm² (clitoral index = length in centimeters × width in centimeters). The labia minora are large and may protrude through bulbous labia majora. The hymen is prominent and red, protecting a vagina that averages 4 cm long. A whitish vaginal discharge of mucus and exfoliated cells with an acid pH may be prominent. The uterus may be enlarged (4 cm long), with cervical eversion present. The endometrium may slough and vaginal bleeding may occur within a few days after birth. Parents can be reassured that the *bleeding will stop by 10 days of age.* The ovaries have not descended from the abdomen and cannot be palpated if normal.

YOUNG CHILD (UNDER 7 YEARS)

With little estrogen stimulation, the external genitalia have involuted from birth. The labia majora are flat, and the labia minora are thin, as is the hymen. The clitoris is no longer prominent, but the *clitoral index remains unchanged.* The mucous membranes are pink and only slightly moist. The diameter of the hymenal opening is ~0.4 cm. The vagina is ~5 cm long, and its secretions have an alkaline pH. Vaginal fornices do not develop until puberty. Therefore, the cervix is appositioned against the vaginal vault and is difficult to see or palpate. If seen, the cervical os is a small slit. The regressed uterus does not return to the size of the newborn until 6 y. The ovaries have many follicles that decrease in number until menarche. During this time, the ovaries begin their descent into the true pelvis.

OLDER CHILD (7–10 YEARS)

As estrogen stimulation returns, the mons pubis thickens, the labia majora fill out, and the labia minora become more rounded. The hymen thickens, and the opening enlarges to 0.7 cm. The vaginal mucosa thickens, and the vagina elongates to 8 cm. The body of the uterus enlarges primarily by myometrial proliferation. The endometrium gradually thickens. The ovaries enlarge and descend lower into the pelvis. The follicles enlarge, although none will participate in ovulation, then gradually regress in size. *Breast buds may appear.*

YOUNG ADOLESCENT (10–13 YEARS)

During this phase of development, the *external genitalia continue to approach adult appearance.* Bartholin glands begin to produce mucus immediately before menarche. The hymenal opening enlarges to about 1 cm. The vagina lengthens to adult size (10–12 cm), and vaginal secretions become acidic. The vaginal fornices develop. The body of the uterus becomes twice as long as the cervix. The ovaries descend further into the true pelvis. Breast development continues, with buds progressing to small mounds. *Other secondary sex characteristics develop* (pubic and axillary hair), the body becomes more rounded, and the adolescent growth spurt begins.

GYNECOLOGIC EXAMINATION

NEWBORN

Because internal examination usually is unnecessary and difficult at this age, *examination is usually limited to the external genitalia.* Assessment includes the overall appearance, and looking for anomalies in addition to ambiguity of sex differentiation. An abnormal or enlarged clitoris may suggest congenital adrenal hyperplasia. The hymen is inspected for patency (to rule out imperforate hymen or vaginal agenesis). Rectal examination may detect the cervix, but normally no other reproductive organs will be palpable.

CHILD

Avoiding the use of stirrups often enhances the child's cooperation. An adequate view of the genitalia can be obtained with the child in the frog leg position (knees flexed, legs fully abducted) on the examination table or in the mother's lap. Enlisting the child's cooperation is often facilitated by direct conversation and explanation during the examination. After a general examination, including inspection and palpation of the breasts, attention may be directed to gentle palpation of the abdomen. Ovarian tumors in this age group usually occur in the low to midabdomen.

Evaluation of the external genitalia includes evidence of proper hygiene as well as lesions of the skin, inflammation, tumors, excoriations, or vaginal discharge. The labia minora should be separate posteriorly. Ascertaining the presence of a vaginal opening is usually accomplished by direct visualization. Digital rectal examination must be gentle.

If visualization of the upper one third of the vagina is necessary (e.g., foreign body, abnormal bleeding, screening for in utero DES exposure, or penetrating injury), a vaginoscope, cystoscope, or laparoscope may be used and *examination under anesthesia may be necessary.* In the younger child, a 0.5 cm instrument can be used. In the older child, an 0.8 cm instrument usually can be passed through the hymenal orifice.

YOUNG ADOLESCENT

At this age, the girl may be very sensitive about the changes in her body. She should be an active participant in the history and examination process. She should be asked whether or not she wishes her mother to be present, and a *female assistant should be present* if the mother is not. It is important to reassure her that she may be embarrassed or somewhat uncomfortable but that the examination will not be painful and her hymen will not be damaged. Sufficient time must be available to allow for an unhurried examination and full explanation of each procedure.

Explaining and teaching breast self-examination during the breast examination helps to establish this preventive measure. Stirrups usually are accepted in this age group. After examination of the external genitalia, the cervix and vagina may be inspected using a long-bladed Huffman-Graves vaginal speculum. If the hymenal opening is of sufficient size, bimanual palpation may be accomplished with a single finger in the vagina. If not, the uterus and ovaries may be palpated using the rectal approach.

After the examination, it is crucial to discuss the findings with the patient and address her concerns. *Patient–doctor confidentiality should be maintained.* If there is some problem of which the parents should be made aware (e.g., pregnancy), advising the patient and serving as a supportive advocate may assist her in the necessary communication(s).

CONGENITAL ANOMALIES OF REPRODUCTIVE TRACT TYPICALLY DIAGNOSED BEFORE MENARCHE

ABNORMALITIES OF THE HYMEN

There are so many normal variations in the appearance of the hymen (e.g., size and number of orifices, thickness) that essentially the only true anomaly is *imperforate hymen.* The solid membrane of the imperforate hymen is thought to be a persistent portion of the urogenital membrane formed whenever the mesoderm of the primitive streak abnormally invades the urogenital portion of the cloacal membrane.

Obstruction of the vaginal outlet by the imperforate hymen causes a *buildup of vaginal secretions,* initially a *mucocolpos,* and later (postmenarche) a *hematocolpos.* The mucocolpos may be seen as a flat or mildly protruding, thin, shiny membrane. The vagina is distended and may fill the pelvis. Sonography will distinguish between this condition and vaginal agenesis. Hematocolpos is diagnosed in an amenorrheic adolescent with a bulging purplish red hymenal membrane and distended vagina. Blood may fill the uterus (hematometra) and spill from the uterine tubes into the peritoneal cavity.

Imperforate hymen is corrected surgically at the time of diagnosis. In the newborn, the procedure involves simple excision without sutures. In the postmenarchal patient, the membrane must be excised or incised as sutured because simple incision and drainage are likely to result in spontaneous closure and recurrence of hematocolpos.

In some cases, an apparently imperforate hymen has very tiny openings and is termed *microperforate hymen.* Treatment is similar to that for imperforate hymen. A septate vagina may have a single thick median ridge at the hymenal orifice separating the two halves, leaving a double hymenal opening. Surgical correction is necessary if obstruction of vaginal drainage is evident or if it will interfere with intercourse.

VAGINA

VAGINAL SEPTUM

A vaginal septum may be transverse or longitudinal. The *transverse septum* is the result of faulty canalization of the embryonic vagina and may occur at any level. Septa in the upper portion usually are patent, whereas those in the lower portion of the vagina may be imperforate and result in mucocolpos or hematocolpos. Incomplete septa may be followed until menarche, when complete excision can be performed more easily. *A complete transverse septum should be incised at diagnosis* to allow drainage to occur until menarche, when complete excision of the remaining septum along with the attached dense, subepithelial connective tissue can be performed.

A *longitudinal vaginal septum* results from improper fusion of the distal ends of the mullerian ducts. The septum is fibrous, with an epithelial lining that divides the vagina into two. There may be an *accompanying bicornuate uterus with one or two cervices.* Treatment is necessary only if there is obstruction of drainage from one side of the vagina, if dyspareunia is present, or if it would interfere with vaginal delivery. *Rarely, a double vagina,* complete with two separate muscle layers, occurs and may be accompanied by double vulva, bladder, and uterus.

AGENESIS

Nearly all patients presenting with an absent vagina have one of four circumstances: the Mayer-Rokitansky-Kustner-Hauser syndrome,

Kallmann's syndrome, male pseudohermaphroditism, and testicular feminization. In the two syndromes, the individuals are genetically female (46,XX), whereas in the latter two circumstances, the individuals are genetically male (46,XY). Numerically, although still rare, *the Mayer-Rokitansky-Kustner-Hauser syndrome is by far and away the most common.*

Vaginal agenesis when associated with absence of the cervix and complete or partial uterine absence (and possibly the uterine tubes) is the Mayer-Rokitansky-Kustner-Hauser syndrome (also called the Rokitansky sequence). This condition is the result of embryologic failure of the mullerian ducts to make contact with the posterior portion of the urogenital sinus. Defects of the urinary tract (45%) and spine (10%) are common, as is hearing deficiency. On examination, a dimple is noted where the hymenal opening should be, with the remainder of the external genitalia appearing normal. Imaging (sonography, CT, or MRI) usually confirms the absence of, or rudimentary internal genitalia, with normal ovaries. Almost all of Mayer-Rokitansky-Kustner-Hauser syndrome patients will have a 46,XX karyotype, but *male pseudohermaphroditism and testicular feminization must be ruled out* via karyotypic documentation. Treatment of the Mayer-Rokitansky-Kustner-Hauser syndrome patient usually involves only the development of a neovagina (see below).

Kallmann's syndrome (KS) is the association of olfactory deficit with irreversible, congenital gonadotrophin deficiency (IHH). There are several variants, and it occurs in both sexes. In at least one of the male syndromes there is spontaneous endogenous gonadotrophin secretion recovery in later life (the Bauman variant). The nongonadal manifestations of Kallmann syndrome vary: unilateral renal aplasia, coloboma of iris, deafness, midline anomalies, oculomotor apraxia, and Moebius anomalad. Most (but not all) patients have low serum levels of basal gonadotrophins, testosterone, or estrogen, and had a poor response to LHRH stimulation. Gene mutations that affect hypothalamic, pituitary, and gonadal function include: three genes that cause inherited hypogonadotropic hypogonadism, gene mutations for the beta-subunits of FSH and LH have been characterized, and both activating and inactivating mutations have been identified for the gonadotropin receptor genes. Treatment includes exogenous sex hormone replacement and psychological support, with long-term follow-up to ensure normal sexual development, normal bone mass, and psychosocial outcome, with fertility induction when indicated.

The evaluation of *pseudohermaphroditism and testicular feminization* necessarily involves detailed psychologic evaluation for gender acceptance before initiating therapy. Therapy must be highly individualized and is probably best performed in one of the national centers experienced in dealing with these complex problems.

The *treatment of vaginal agenesis involves the creation of a vagina* when the patient is contemplating sexual activity. This can be accomplished without surgery by having the patient use a series of *progressively larger dilators to exert pressure* in the dimple where the hymen should be for 20–30 min daily for several months. If this is unsuccessful, a *vagina may be created surgically.* Currently, three surgical procedures are popular for creation of the neovagina: *Abbe-McIndoe* (performed vaginally using a split thickness skin graft over a stint), *Vecchetti* (a combined vaginal and laparascopic approach), and the *use of a portion of sigmoid* (requires laparotomy and bowel surgery).

The ovaries function normally in the Mayer-Rokitansky-Kustner-Hauser syndrome and pregnancies have been reported by in vitro fertilization with use of a surrogate. Transvaginal ovum recovery is materially easier in those cases where the neovagina was created by pressure.

Partial vaginal agenesis, usually only the lower one third, is believed to result from failure of the urogenital sinus epithelium to invade the vagina at 4–5 months gestation. The upper vagina, uterus, and tubes are normal. *Visual examination externally is the same as total vaginal agenesis, but sonographic examination confirms the presence of internal genitalia.* Rectal examination may reveal a distended upper vagina (especially if postmenarchal), and renal anomalies may be present.

Treatment of partial vaginal agenesis requires *drainage of the obstructed upper vagina,* usually by creation of a lower vagina.

UTERUS

Most uterine anomalies are not diagnosed until after menarche unless other abnormalities of the reproductive tract are present (see Fig. 18-1 and Chapter 22).

URETHRA

Epispadias is the term used to describe the female urethra that opens cephalad to a bifid clitoris as the result of *failure of normal fusion of the anterior wall of the urogenital sinus.* This may be accompanied by exstrophy of the bladder and defects in the abdominal wall as well as the pelvic girdle. Urological reconstruction is performed in infancy, but gynecologic repair usually is delayed until adolescence.

**COMPLETE BILOCULAR
UTERUS**

**BILOCULAR UNICERVICAL
UTERUS**

**BICERVICAL UTERUS
BICORNIS**

**UNICERVICAL UTERUS
BICORNIS**

UNICORNUATE UTERUS

UNILATERAL ATRESIA

FIGURE 18-1. Congenital uterine abnormalities.
(From B. Pensky, *Review of Medical Embryology.* Macmillan, 1982.)

GYNECOLOGIC DISORDERS IN PREMENARCHAL CHILDREN

VULVOVAGINITIS

Vulvovaginitis is likely the *most common gynecologic problem in childhood.* The susceptibility of young girls to infection is high because of the thin, atrophic vaginal mucosa (lack of estrogen stimulation), contamination by feces (poor hygiene), and relatively impaired immune mechanisms of the vagina. The history, physical examination, and cultures and laboratory tests should be conducted keeping in mind the possibility of sexual assault.

Nonspecific vulvovaginitis is a polymicrobial infection associated with disturbed homeostasis, usually secondary to poor hygiene or foreign body. Vulvovaginitis due to secondary inoculation results from blood borne or contact inoculation of the vagina with pathogens infecting other areas of the body (e.g., urinary tract infection, upper respiratory tract infection). *Specific vulvovaginitis* is primary infection by such organisms as *Neisseria gonorrhoeae, Bacterial vaginosis, Treponema pallidum, and herpes simplex.*

The *vaginal discharge* (mucopurulent or purulent) from acute vulvovaginitis may be minimal or profuse. If the thin mucous membrane of the vulva or vagina is denuded, there may be a blood-tinged appearance to the discharge. The odor may be very foul. The patient may experience only mild discomfort or severe perineal pruritus and burning, with itching so intense that the child scratches to excoriation with bleeding. The inflamed area may burn when urine passes over it, suggesting urinary tract infection (UTI) when indeed the urinary tract is uninvolved. In these cases, a clean-catch specimen cannot diagnose UTI because leukocytosis and contamination from the vagina are difficult to eliminate.

Examination of the perineal area reveals erythema or soreness that may be localized or extending to the anus and thighs. A *rectal examination* is essential to evaluate the pelvic organs. *Vaginoscopy* should be performed if the infection is recurrent or refractory to treatment, especially if a foul-smelling bloody discharge (associated with foreign body) is present. The most common foreign body is toilet paper, although various small objects, such as beads and toys, can be found. Radiographs are not reliable for diagnosis because most objects are not radiopaque. Objects in the lower third of the vagina can be flushed out with warm saline or removed with bayonet forceps, but vaginoscopy is necessary to ensure that no objects remain higher. Recurrent placement of foreign bodies is not unusual.

VAGINAL BLEEDING

The *source* of vaginal bleeding may be *uterine* (endometrial) in origin or localized to the *vulva/vagina*. If bleeding is *endometrial* in origin, disorders of sexual maturation should be investigated. Otherwise, such lesions as vulvovaginitis, foreign body, vulvar skin lesions, urethral prolapse, trauma, botryoid sarcoma, and adeno-carcinoma of the cervix or vagina should be considered.

URETHRAL PROLAPSE

When the urethral mucosa protrudes through the meatus, it forms a hemorrhagic, tender vulvar mass. A short course of *estrogen cream* is therapeutic when there is *no urinary retention* and the *mass is small*. If the *mass is large or urinary retention is present* (or both), *surgical resection* of the prolapsed tissue is required under anesthesia with postoperative urinary catheterization for 24 h.

TRAUMA

Although most injuries to the genitalia of children are accidental, an *index of suspicion must be maintained* to avoid missing evidence of child abuse or sexual abuse. The description of the accident should fit the injury produced.

Injury to the vulva usually results in *hematoma* formation that requires no specific therapy other than cold compresses, unless the urethra is obstructed or the hematoma is large and continuing to increase in size. If the urethra is obstructed, the bladder must be drained, usually by the suprapubic approach. A large hematoma should be incised and drained, with ligature of the bleeding points. Continued bleeding necessitates packing with gauze for 24 h and prophylactic antibiotics. *Radiographs* of the pelvis may be advisable to rule out fracture.

If the *hymen is lacerated,* bleeding may be minimal, but a penetrating injury must be suspected and vaginoscopy performed even if the patient is asymptomatic. Although most vaginal injuries involve the lateral walls with little bleeding and little pain, *a lesion extending to the vaginal vault requires pelvic exploration* to rule out extension into the broad ligament or peritoneal cavity. Small intravaginal hematomas require no therapy. Large intravaginal hematomas should be incised and drained, with ligature of the bleeding point.

LICHEN SCLEROSUS

Lichen sclerosus (hypotrophic dystrophy) of the vulva is seen most commonly in postmenopausal women but may be seen in young children. Histologic findings are the same in both groups, with no malignant potential in children. Whitish plaques or papules are seen no further than the middle of the labia majora and do not encroach into the vagina. Because this lesion is susceptible to infection and bruises easily, vulvar irritation, pruritus, dysuria, and bleeding from scratching are typical.

Treatment consists of *good hygiene* and *short-term use of hydrocortisone creams* to stop the pruritus and allow healing. About 80% will improve significantly with onset of puberty.

LABIAL ADHESION

Labial adhesion, which is common in prepubertal children, is believed to be related to the thinness of the skin over the labia minora as the *result of low estrogen levels.* Local irritation can lead to scratching, with injury and adherence in the midline. Most adhesions are asymptomatic and undiagnosed unless interference with urination occurs. Dysuria, pruritus, irritation, and vulvovaginal infections may result. Rarely, total occlusion causes *urinary retention.*

Treatment of symptomatic adhesions consists of 7–10 days of *Premarin* cream once or twice a day. If medical treatment is unsuccessful, surgical separation may be necessary. Recurrence is common until puberty, when spontaneous resolution will occur.

GENITAL TUMORS

Although uncommon, about 50% of the genital tumors of children are either malignant or premalignant and must be considered when any of the following findings are present: chronic genital ulcer, nontraumatic swelling of the external genitalia, tissue protruding from the vagina, abdominal pain or enlargement, bloody foul discharge, and premature sexual maturation.

BENIGN TUMORS

The common benign genital tumors of children are *teratomas, hemangiomas, simple cysts of the hymen, retention cysts of the paraurethral ducts, granulomas,* and *condylomata acuminata.* Small cysts usually require no therapy. Larger cysts require excision and marsupialization of the remaining wall to prevent recurrence. Teratomas require surgical excision. Capillary hemangiomas usually regress spontaneously, but cavernous hemangiomas may bleed extensively if traumatized and must be evaluated for removal or ablation.

MALIGNANT TUMORS

Botryoid Sarcoma (Embryonal Carcinoma of the Vagina)

Botryoid sarcoma is seen most often in girls less than 3 years. It is a rapidly growing tumor arising in the submucosal tissues of the vagina but may involve the cervix as well. The vaginal mucosa protrudes from the vagina in polypoid growths. Biopsy is required for diagnosis. Six months of *chemotherapy* is followed by *surgical removal,* radical hysterectomy, and vaginectomy without oophorectomy. Further chemotherapy for 6–12 months follows. If the tumor cannot be removed, *radiation therapy* is given to shrink the tumor.

Other Malignant Tumors

Endodermal carcinoma, mesonephric carcinoma, and clear cell carcinoma of mullerian origin (associated with in utero DES exposure) are seen in children or adolescents. Virtually all genital tumors seen in adult women have been reported in children, and the treatment is similar.

SEXUAL MATURATION

NORMAL

Before adolescence, the normal pulsatile release of gonadotropin-releasing hormone (GnRH), does not occur. With the onset of this hypothalamic activity, the pituitary releases FSH, and the process of ovarian stimulation leads to the production of estrogen. The end-organ response to gradually increasing estrogens and finally progesterone determines the alterations that occur during adolescence and result in puberty. Although the age of onset of puberty is influenced by genetic as well as environmental factors, the secondary sexual changes leading to sexual maturity occur over 3–5 years (most within 2–4 years), *usually between ages 9–14.*

Early in the process leading to puberty, the genital system undergoes marked alterations. The external genitalia gradually assume the adult appearance. The vagina develops progressively thicker mucosa and, while becoming more distinct from the cervix, reaches its adult length (10–12 cm). It also is more distensible and progressively more moist and acidotic with the reappearance of lactobacilli. *The uterine corpus enlarges to twice the length of the cervix, and the ovaries descend into the true pelvis.*

Late premenarche is marked by *accelerated somatic growth and* often *rapid changes in secondary sexual characteristics.* The body habitus begins to assume more feminine characteristics, with breast buds appearing and gradually increasing in size. *Thelarche,* breast development, is the earliest adolescent change toward puberty, preceding regular ovulation by ~2 years. Pubic hair (*pubarche*) and axillary hair appear later. The method of classifying adolescent secondary sexual development through puberty proposed by *Marshall and Tanner* (Table 18-1) has become widely accepted. Although puberty is technically defined as the maturation of endocrine and gametogenic function to the point of reproductive capability, it is not uncommon for menarche (the first menses) to be used nearly interchangeably. This is unfortunate, for the first few cycles (generally up to a year) are usually anovulatory. *The average age of menarche in the United States is 12.8 years.*

TABLE 18-1
**TANNER CLASSIFICATION OF ADOLESCENT
DEVELOPMENT IN THE FEMALE**

Breast Development	Public Hair Development	Stage
Papillae elevated (preadolescent), no breast buds	None	I
Breast buds and papillae slightly elevated	Sparse, long, slightly pigmented	II
Breast buds and areolae confluent, elevatd	Darker, coarser, curly	III
Areolae and papillae project above breast	Adult-type pubis only	IV
Papillae projected, mature	Lateral distribution	V

DISORDERS OF SEXUAL MATURATION

ACCELERATED SEXUAL MATURATION (PRECOCIOUS PUBERTY)

Sexual precocity is defined as the onset of sexual maturation ≥2.5 SD earlier than the normal age (i.e., onset of secondary sexual characteristics <8 years or menarche <10 years). Accelerated sexual maturation may be *complete or incomplete,* depending on whether one or all of the secondary sexual changes are occurring. The *work up is similar* in both circumstances and is geared to determining whether there is *gonadotropin production* and if there is a *detectable underlying disorder* causing the condition. In the majority of cases there will be *maturity of the hypothalamic–pituitary–ovarian axis.*

A complete medical, family, and social history is essential. Pubertal development staging (Tanner) and plotting growth provide *quantifiable data for comparison to the norm.* Complete *physical examination and pelvic examination* will assist in guiding the proper utilization of further diagnostic tests. Frequently *imaging* (ultrasound, CT, or MRI) will be useful. *Hormonal analyses* (most commonly FSH, LH, and estradiol) are often useful. In cases of early pubertal development, *an interval of observation* assists to ensure that sexual maturation is continually progressive, as some cases will spontaneously regress.

INCOMPLETE ACCELERATED SEXUAL MATURATION

PREMATURE THELARCHE

Isolated development of breast tissue (one or both breasts) *before age 8 years* (excluding the newborn period) is considered premature thelarche and *frequently occurs between 1 and 3 years.* Although there may be no change in bone growth and no estrogen effect documented in the vagina, girls with premature thelarche have significantly *higher estradiol levels* than normal prepubertal girls. Thus, premature thelarche does not involve increased sensitivity of breast tissue to estrogens. Breast biopsy should not be performed, and generally *no specific therapy* is indicated.

PREMATURE PUBARCHE

Isolated development of pubic or axillary hair before age 8 years may be idiopathic and of no clinical significance. However, this hair growth may be a sign of excess androgen production from an inborn error of metabolism (congenital adrenal hyperplasia from steroid enzyme deficiency) or tumor. *Excess androgen production must be excluded* before idiopathic premature pubarche is diagnosed.

PREMATURE MENARCHE

Isolated cyclic vaginal bleeding before age 10 years is considered premature menarche. In the past, it was thought that estrogen levels were not increased and that bleeding resulted from endometrial sensitivity to low level estrogens. More recently, *higher levels of estradiol* have been identified. *Other causes of vaginal bleeding should be excluded.* There is no adverse effect on growth, future fertility, or menstrual pattern. No therapy is advocated.

COMPLETE ACCELERATED
SEXUAL MATURATION

MATURE HYPOTHALAMIC–PITUITARY–OVARIAN AXIS (GONADOTROPIN PRODUCTION)

These young females experience the orderly process of *puberty at an earlier age than normal,* typically close to the expected age of puberty but possibly as early as 2–3 years of age. On occasion, CT scan of the brain may reveal a small *hamartoma in the hypothalamus.* Precocious puberty may also be the result of other central nervous system (CNS) lesions (e.g., *tumors, previous fractures, meningitis, or encephalitis*). It is believed that irritation of the hypothalamus begins the maturation early, but the overall process may be very prolonged (years).

Treatment is directed toward the *CNS lesion,* if it is treatable. In idiopathic cases of incomplete accelerated sexual maturation, complete accelerated sexual maturation, or cases without a treatable CNS condition, *recent therapy* has been gonadotropin releasing hormone agonists *(GnRHA).* Currently, most authorities recommend GnRHA utilization from diagnosis until the projected onset of the normal adolescent growth spurt (11–12 years). The long-term use of GnRHA has been supplemented in some trials by the use of growth hormone to treat any potential retardation of attaining full height. The combination, while promising for those of short stature, is still under investigation. The potential osteopenia associated with long-term GnRHA use has been reported to respond to concurrent supplemental calcium administration.

Uterine bleeding during GnRHA treatment for precocious puberty is common, and may be massive and recurrent. However, most episodes resolve spontaneously and necessitate no further treatment. Thus, pretreatment counseling concerning this potential complication (to those being treated as well as to their families) may assist in avoiding unnecessary anxiety and achieving better compliance.

IMMATURE HYPOTHALAMIC–PITUITARY–OVARIAN AXIS (NO GONADOTROPIN PRODUCTION)

Early feminization may result from either *ingestion of exogenous estrogens or prolonged use of estrogen-containing creams.* Additionally, it has occurred with utilization of hair products containing placental extracts. Once estrogen or other product usage is established, immediate discontinuance is advised.

Early endogenous estrogen production is most likely of *ovarian origin.* Large *follicular cysts, teratomas, granulosa cell tumors, or cystadenomas* of the ovary may either produce estrogen or stimulate estrogen production. Nonovarian estrogen may be produced by adrenal adenomas, but both are rare. Autonomous secretion of gonadotrophin by a tumor is even more rare, but has been reported.

The largest single association with precocious puberty in the absence of gonadotropin production is the *McCune-Albright syndrome.* This condition, consisting of polyostotic fibrous dysplasia, irregular cutaneous pigmentation, and precocious puberty, holds an unfavorable prognosis. The precocious puberty usually occurs at a very early age and results in short stature from early epiphyseal closure and pathologic fractures. Many affected girls are infertile, with menstrual abnormalities. The *cause is unknown,* and *no specific treatment is available.* Recently experimental therapy for this form of gonadotropin independent precocious puberty (which is resistant to therapy with GnRH analogues) has included ketoconazole. Additionally, some authorities recommend the addition of growth hormone.

SEQUELAE OF ACCELERATED SEXUAL MATURATION

For reasons not yet clear, *precocious puberty predisposes* young women *to subsequent (postpubertal) hyperandrogenism.* Indeed, about two thirds of young women who have precocious puberty will develop hirsutism, the first sign of hyperadrogenism in young women. Although *hirutism* poses an esthetic problem, it is usually a progenitor of *infertility* and the *polycystic ovarian syndrome.*

The work up of hirsutism and hyperandrogenism frequently includes: *testosterone, androstenedione, dehydroepiandrosterone sulphate, 17 alpha-hydroxyprogesterone (basal and after ACTH), luteinizing hormone, and FSH. Imaging* (i.e., pelvic sonography) may be useful. Therapy will depend upon the results of the diagnostic work up. (See p. 721)

Additionally, girls with precocious puberty are at *increased risk for anovulation* during late (but not early) adolescence onward. At particular risk are those with a low weight at birth and/or a high 17-hydroxyprogesterone response to ACTH at prepubertal diagnosis of accelerated sexual maturation.

DELAYED SEXUAL MATURATION

As with accelerated sexual maturation, a *complete history,* including a three generation pedigree, is the starting point in the work up. The absence of onset of puberty beyond 2.5 SD of the normal age is considered delayed. *Absence of thelarche by 13 years or menarche by 15 years* warrants investigation, and evaluation may be initiated earlier if there is concern. Patients with delayed sexual maturation may be classified into one of three categories: *delayed menarche with adequate secondary sexual development, delayed puberty with inadequate or absent secondary sexual development, or delayed puberty with virilization.* Delayed puberty in females is a *rare condition.* The majority of delayed puberty is associated with a genetic disorder or hypothalamic–pituitary–ovarian problem. Of course, anatomic abnormalities of the ovaries, uterus, or lower genital tract are rare but important considerations.

Obtaining a complete medical, family, and social history is essential, as are plotting growth and performing pubertal developmental staging (Tanner criteria). A complete physical examination and pelvic examination will assist in guiding the proper utilization of further diagnostic tests. Frequently *imaging* (ultrasound, CT, or MRI) will be useful. Hormonal analyses (most commonly *FSH, LH, and estradiol*) are often useful.

Complete workup and differential studies are described in Chapter 25.

PREGNANCY IN CHILDREN AND ADOLESCENTS

Precocious or juvenile pregnancy occurs in girls with precocious puberty and has been reported at less than 6 years of age. Most cases involve sexual abuse or incest. There is an increased incidence of premature onset of labor, pregnancy-induced hypertension, and spontaneous abortion. If the patient is under 9 years of age, abnormal labor occurs in ~50% and neonatal loss may approach 35%.

Adolescent pregnancy is increasing at an alarming rate. The attitudes and expectations of the teenager regarding pregnancy and motherhood usually are far from realistic. Prenatal care and nutrition often are suboptimal. The incidence of cigarette smoking, drug abuse, and sexually transmitted disease is high. Preeclampsia-eclampsia, premature delivery, and intrauterine growth retardation occur more frequently in adolescents than in adult women, making adolescent pregnancy, in general, high risk. Although adolescents may have a lower rate of gestational diabetes mellitus than adults, it still occurs. Thus, the incidence of screening for gestational diabetes mellitus in adolescents may be modified by the risk of their ethnic group or other risk factors.

Perhaps the best hope for preventing or improving the outcome of adolescent pregnancy lies in *early sex education, conscientious contraceptive counseling, and emphasis on prenatal care.*

BREAST PROBLEMS OF THE CHILD OR ADOLESCENT

The child or adolescent presenting with a breast complaint is evaluated just as is the adult female (see Chapter 19). A thorough history, a detailed physical examination, and a careful sonography is sufficient to obtain the correct diagnosis in most cases. Mammograms are difficult to interpret because of the dense glandular breast tissue and almost never reveal microcalcifications, even in the presence of breast cancer.

Fortunately, breast carcinoma is very rare before age 20. Indeed, if malignant tumors are seen in children or adolescents they are more likely to be metastatic (or secondary) than primary to the breast. Thus, the spectrum of breast malignancy encountered in children or adolescents is composed of relatively uncommon tumors, with rhabdomyosarcoma and hematolymphoid tumors being the most frequent. Sarcomas may arise in cystosarcoma phyllodes, or more rarely, from other structures. Primary breast carcinoma must be ruled out.

Nearly all breast problems encountered in children and adolescents are benign. The majority of patients present because of "a lump," and the vast majority of these are fibroadenomas. Cystosarcoma phylloides is more commonly encountered than fibrocystic breast disease and intraductal papilloma. When patients present with breast pain or discharge, they are evaluated as adults (see Chapter 19).

Although surgical care of any lesion has a primary objective of complete excision of the lesion, biopsies of the developing breast should also aim to protect the breast bud, nipple, and areola. Special breast surgical problems of the child or adolescent requiring extraordinary operative approaches are gynecomastia and macromastia.

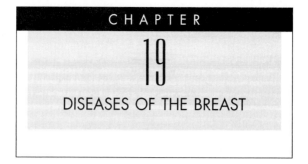

CHAPTER

19

DISEASES OF THE BREAST

At some time in their lives nearly all women experience a problem with their breasts. Although these afflictions range from totally benign to highly malignant, the majority of problems are self-limited or readily treatable (Table 19-1). Indeed, the most common problems encountered in multidisciplinary care settings are a question of a *mass* (~65%), *pain* (~15%), *nipple problems* (including discharge, ~10%), or a question concerning *family history or other symptoms* (~10%). However, the very real specter of breast cancer makes preventive care (screening), early detection, thorough evaluation and complete care of every case a compelling medical necessity.

Moreover, the high incidence and potential seriousness of breast disorders combine to cause *breast problems to be one of the most frequently encountered problems in health care for women.* Patient expectations are not confined to just answering concerns relative to their chief complaint. They also appreciate rapid and comprehensive response(s) to detected problems, education, prevention, and a resource for learning more about breast problems. Thus, to meet the expectations of their patients, providers of female health care need a *thoughtful, well-organized, and carefully conducted plan for management of breast diseases.* One measure of not meeting patient expectations concerning breast problems is that failure to diagnose breast cancer in a timely manner is the most common reason for malpractice litigation in the United States.

Diagnosis may be accomplished in breast problems by using standard techniques: *a careful history, physical examination of the breasts, documentation, and imaging* (usually mammography, possibly sonography). The history should establish how long the problem has existed, whether any other changes have been observed, any risk factors, and whether there is a history of biopsy or breast cancer. The physical examination aims to identify those features distinguishing malignant from benign changes and should involve axillae and periclavicular areas as well as the breasts.

TABLE 19-1
TYPES, INCIDENCE, AND PEAK YEARS OF BENIGN BREAST DISEASES

Type	Incidence (%)	Peak (Years)	Symptoms
Mammary dysplasia	~50	30–50	Bilateral, painful, solid or cystic masses with cyclic variability
Fibroadenoma	2–3	20–40	Usually unilateral (10% –15% bilateral), firm, discrete, solitary, nontender mass
Intraductal papillomas	3–5	45–55	Bloody, serous, or turbid nipple discharge from a duct without palpable mass
Fat necrosis	>5	Any age	Half give a history of trauma, ecchymosis, skin retraction, or local tenderness
Mammary duct ectasia	~1	50–60	Tender, bilateral masses, possible nipple retraction, enlarged axillary glands
Macromastia	<0.1	Puberty	Diffuse enlargement with continued growth
Galactocele		Perilactation	Cystic ductal dilatation
Breast abscess	~2	Lactation	Unilateral, localized inflammation, fever, pain, tenderness, segmental erythema,

TABLE 19-1
(*Continued*)

Type	Incidence (%)	Peak (Years)	Symptoms
			caused by *Staphylococcus aureus;* in absence of lactation, must be biopsied

Mammography often details even occult masses and assists in clarifying the nature of masses. *A second level of evaluation, which depends on the results of the primary investigation, may be necessary to establish a proper diagnosis of any lesions that are discovered.* In some cases, sonography may be an alternative to fine-needle aspiration for distinguishing a cyst from a solid mass. When *doubt remains as to whether a mass is benign or malignant, a biopsy in mandatory.* Fortunately, that is increasingly possible using fine-needle aspiration or needle core biopsy, either may be clinically or image-guided.

A crucial issue in management of all breast problems is their *psychological impact.* Many forces combine to make these problems one of the most psychological charged areas in medicine. Examples of the psychological stress inducers include: the physical symptoms, prior conditioning, breast cancer risk perceptions, societal emphasis of breasts, and breasts linkage to feminine body image. Thus, caring for a woman's breast problems involves a great deal more than caring for just breast cancer.

The preventive aspects of breast disease, [i.e., breast self-examination (BSE), physician breast examination (PBE), and mammography, are discussed elsewhere (see p. 512)]. This type of preventive-screening program will identify >6 cancers per 1000 asymptomatic women. In these cases, the tumors are detected earlier (80% have negative axillary nodes vs. 45% not screening). About 40% of early breast cancers can be discovered only by mammography and ~40% can be detected only by palpation; thus, both modalities are crucial.

COMMON BENIGN
BREAST DISEASES

FIBROCYSTIC BREAST DISEASE (MAMMARY DYSPLASIA, FIBROCYSTIC MASTOPATHY, CHRONIC CYSTIC MASTITIS)

Mammary dysplasia is the most common breast disorder, ~50% of women between 30 and 50 years of age are affected, but it is uncommon in postmenopausal women. Fibrocystic breast disease (FCBD) is characterized by *bilateral, painful, usually multiple breast masses.* Fluctuation in mass size and discomfort occur rather quickly and are usually related to the menstrual cycle, with the most pain and largest size occurring during the premenstrual interval. Indeed, it is the pain, size fluctuation, and multiplicity of masses that are most useful in distinguishing this process from carcinoma and fibroadenoma.

The etiology of FCBD remains unknown. In some manner, *estrogenic stimulus* seems associated because after menopause the condition almost inevitably improves. Other associations have been the *consumption of methylxanthines and saturated fats.* Recently, however, an as yet unconfirmed report indicated *Trichomonas* (some *T. tenax* and some *T. vaginalis*) positive cultures from surgical specimens.

Mammography is often used for the clinical diagnosis and women ≥25 years with FCBD should have baseline mammography. *Biopsy may be necessary* for suspicious lesions or if the breasts are too dense to adequately visualize the lesions. *Sonography is very useful in differentiation between cystic and solid lesions.*

Microscopically, cysts (both macroscopic and microscopic) are derived from terminal ducts and acini. Papillomatosis, adenosis, fibrosis, and ductal epithelial hyperplasia may occur. Because estrogen promotes growth of mammary ducts and periductal stroma, estrogen is presumed to be a causative factor. The improvement normally seen during pregnancy and lactation suggests that progesterone may help to alleviate the disorder. Although not necessarily part of the process, if epithelial dysplasia occurs, it is more likely to lead to breast cancer.

Treatment is largely symptomatic. Patients are advised to perform *monthly breast self-examination.* It is useful for her to keep a *schematic representation of the lesions,* so that if changes other than those of the mammary dysplasia occur, she can promptly report this to her physician. The patient should *avoid trauma* (e.g., apply good support while jogging) and wear a *supportive and protective brassiere both night and day.* Analgesics may assist in relief of pain. In some patients, lowering body weight may be useful and it seems largely beneficial to *minimize saturated fats.* Long-term restriction of dietary *methylxanthines* (e.g., caffeine) may relieve some women. Unconfirmed reports suggest that vitamin E may help to alleviate symptomatology.

Breast cysts occasionally reach a size or complexity requiring aspiration under local anesthesia. The aspirated fluid should be examined cytologically, for the presence of macrocystic disease multiplies (3- to 4-fold) the risk of cancer. If no fluid is obtained or if the fluid is bloody or if a mass persists, biopsy is indicated.

In the past, low-dose androgens were used for therapy of the disorder, but undesirable (virilizing) side effects often developed. *Medroxyprogesterone acetate* 5–10 mg orally daily for 5–10 days at the end of each cycle may be beneficial. Similarly, *low-dose oral contraceptives* may give relief but no cure. *Danazol* often gives marked relief, but objectionable side effects may develop. *Tamoxifen* 10 mg bid by mouth may be useful. *Bromocriptine* (a dopamine-receptor agonist that inhibits prolactin secretion) 2.5 mg bid may relieve the mastalgia.

FCBD virtually disappears at menopause. However, the prognosis until that time must be guarded and vigilance maintained to rule out breast carcinoma. Therefore, these patients must be followed carefully and indefinitely.

A benign condition that must be included in the differential diagnosis of *FCBD* and *fibroadenoma* of the breast is focal fibrosis. *Focal fibrosis* usually presents as an enlarging solid mass or developing density on mammography or as an oval mass on sonography. Focal fibrosis will account for up to 10% of lesions coming to imaging-guided core biopsy and usually does not require further therapy.

FIBROADENOMA OF THE BREAST

Fibroadenoma of the breast is a common (accounting for ~50% of breast biopsies), *benign, usually unilateral* (10%–15% bilateral), *solid* (firm), *discrete, usually solitary, and nontender mass that commonly develops at 20–40 years of age.* Fibroadenomas generally are 1–5 cm in diameter. This tumor is more frequent and tends to occur at an earlier age in blacks than whites or Asians. Fibroadenomas are *composed of both fibrous and glandular tissue.* Tumor *growth is stimulated by pregnancy, and regression* (often with calcification) *occurs postmenopausally.*

In the past, it was thought that fibroadenomas must be differentiated from mammary dysplasia and breast carcinoma by excision.

Advances in imaging technology (x-ray, sonography, and MRI) as well as less invasive (fine needle aspiration) and directed biopsies have afforded a more conservative approach and are effective in distinguishing fibroadenomas from breast cancer. Recent reports utilizing a conservative approach indicate that *most fibroadenomas remain static or regress when conservatively managed* and that transformation from fibroadenoma to cancer is rare. It is now speculated that most fibroadenomas stop growing when ~20 mm, after which they remain static or regress. Thoughtful clinical examination, mammography, sonography, and fine needle aspiration or core biopsy remain necessary to confidently separate fibroadenoma from carcinoma as well as cystosarcoma phyllodes.

Cystosarcoma phyllodes (giant mammary myxoma) may clinically and histologically resemble a breast fibroadenoma with unusually proliferative cellular stroma. It may grow rapidly to large size. *Cystosarcoma phyllodes may be malignant (5%), but is more likely to be intermediate (12.5% of cases) or benign (82.5%). Recurrences occur in ~10% of those initially treated by simple excision.* When the surgical margins are not clear, revision is indicated. Until recently, wide excision was employed for recurrences; however, borderline and malignant tumors may warrant a more aggressive surgical approach. Local recurrence of any grade tumor is usually followed by further recurrences. In addition to local recurrence, poor prognostic indicators include tumor size and histological grade.

INTRADUCTAL PAPILLOMA

Intraductal papillomas characteristically occur in the *perimenopausal interval with a bloody, serous, or turbid nipple discharge.* Although a tumor is rarely palpable, it frequently is possible to determine the involved duct by palpably initiating the discharge. The initial workup includes *mammography and cytological examination of the fluid. Definitive imaging* may be achieved by the retrograde injection of dye into the involved ductal system (galactography) by duct cannulation. The accuracy of galactography is ~88% for papillomas, ~85% for cancer, and ~77% for other benign lesions. Sonography may be a complementary diagnostic tool to galactography in patients with a discharging breast. Another alternative is to do MR imaging and/or an MR galactograph. The differential diagnosis must include galactorrhea and breast cancer. *Treatment generally is excisional biopsy of the involved duct.* Histologically, intraductal papillomas vary from the clearly benign to the anaplastic with invasive tendencies.

MASTODYNIA

Mastodynia (or mastalgia) is the pain and breast enlargement caused by edema and engorgement of the vascular and ductal system, generally in response to the luteal phase of the menstrual cycle. It is a diagnosis of exclusion and is reserved for cases of nearly intolerable symptoms with no palpable abnormalities save tenderness and generalized tissue thickening. It must be differentiated from neoplasms (usually painless except for fibrocystic breast disease) and mastitis (rare except in postpartum patients).

General therapy usually consists of *breast support, avoidance of methylxanthines* (in case of some fibrocystic breast disease component), *avoidance of excessive salt, occasional diuretics, and perhaps vitamin E* (1200–1800 U/day). Specific therapy may be low-dose *testosterone* (5 mg every other day when symptoms are present) or *danocrine* 100–400 mg/day for up to 6 months. Should virilization begin to appear with use of testosterone, discontinue the therapy immediately.

OTHER NONPUERPERAL BENIGN BREAST DISEASE

Fat necrosis is presumably related to trauma, although only about one half of patients with fat necrosis recall an injury. Ecchymosis, skin retraction, or local tenderness may or may not be present. The mass is usually tender. Generally, the mass resolves slowly, and only occasionally is biopsy required to rule out malignancy.

Mammary duct ectasia usually occurs in the fifth decade. It is characterized by ductal dilatation, inspissation of breast secretions, and chronic intraductal and periductal inflammation, with plasma cell predominance. Nipple retraction from scarring may occur, and enlarged axillary glands are frequent. Once differentiated from breast cancer, no therapy is necessary.

Galactocele is cystic dilatation of a duct with thick, inspissated milky fluid, present during or shortly after lactation. Galactocele indicates ductal obstruction. Diagnosis is facilitated by mammography, and needle aspiration is usually curative.

Macromastia, occasionally unilateral, has its onset at puberty, although it may develop with pregnancy or even after menopause. The cause of macromastia is unknown. The disorder does not predispose to cancer. Therapy includes tamoxifen or surgical reduction (often not curative).

Breast abscess in the nonlactating woman is very rare. Thus, biopsy of any indurated tissue is prudent.

Benign breast diseases are summarized in Table 19-1.

PUERPERAL MASTITIS

Puerperal mastitis is usually marked by *unilateral, often localized inflammation, with fever, localized pain, tenderness, and segmental erythema.* Often a fissured nipple (entry site of the bacteria) still exists. The usual causative agent is hemolytic *Staphylococcus aureus.* Hence, penicillinase-resistant antibiotic therapy (e.g., oxacillin, cephalothin) must be used for a minimum of 10 d. Primigravidas are more often affected. Puerperal mastitis tends to occur in *two epidemiological types, epidemic and sporadic.* In the epidemic type, the infection often can be traced to a carrier, and this type tends to fulminate. Therefore, intensive therapy is required. Weaning, prolonged antibiotic therapy, suppression of lactation, cold packs to the breast, and a brassiere worn day and night are recommended.

In the sporadic type of puerperal mastitis, *the infant (the most frequent source of the infecting organism) may continue to nurse.* By decreasing engorgement, the likelihood of abscess formation is decreased. A nipple shield may assist in controlling discomfort. Antibiotic therapy is the same as for the epidemic type.

In either type, if antibiotic therapy is initiated before suppuration, the infection is usually controlled within 24 h. If the infection advances to form an abscess, surgical drainage will be required.

CARCINOMA OF THE BREAST

One of every 9–11 American women will develop breast cancer at some time during her life. The mean and median age of breast cancer occurrence is 60–61 years. While the direct etiology remains unknown, a number of associations or risk factors for breast cancer, based largely on the patient's past and family history, are listed in Table 19-2.

Breast cancer *risk is partially explained by founder mutations identified in certain cancer predisposing genes,* notably BRCA1, BRCA2, and TP53. Those at increased risk on this basis have a strong family history of breast and ovarian cancers, but little evidence of significantly increased cancer risk at other sites. Longitudinal studies of such families reveal that the susceptibility varies by subset, from autosomal dominant, to low penetrance genes, to purely environmental. The Ashkenazic Jewish ethnic group has been indicated to be at higher risk for breast and ovarian cancers on the BRCA1 and BRCA2 basis. This again, however, is confined to families with

TABLE 19-2
RISK FACTORS IN BREAST CANCER

High risk factors
  Previous breast cancer
  Breast cancer in mother or sister
Moderate risk factors
  Age >40 years
  Menarche <12 years
  Menopause >50 years
  First pregnancy >35 years
  Nulliparity
  Cancer of the endometrium or ovary
  Severe mammary dysplasia (when accompanied by
    proliferation changes, papillomatosis, or atypical
    hyperplasia)
  Breast cancer in aunt or grandmother
Symptoms indicating risk
  Lump in breast
  Nipple discharge
  Ulceration of the nipple
  Recent onset of pain in one breast

the mutation(s) and the overall incidence of breast or ovarian cancer risk is no higher among Ashkenazic Jewish women compared with non-Jewish Caucasians. Thus, individuals from any racial or ethnic population may have deleterious mutations. Currently, *known mutations leading to cancer predisposition likely account for only ~3%–10% of breast cancer* in the general population.

Another potential genetic predisposition to breast cancer may involve *variant genotypes at other loci,* which confer a relatively smaller degree of cancer risk, but which are carried by a larger proportion of the general population. This class of predispositions, likely necessary to understand the genetic basis for breast cancer in the general population, requires understanding the complex interactions of the genes with one another and with the environment. To date, these are less will studied or understood. Indeed, in large twin studies based on genetic modeling, *inherited genetic factors account for 18%* (95% CI, 4%–32%) of overall breast cancer risk. *Nongenetic factors shared by twins account for 7%* (0%–16%) and *unique exposure or environmental factors for 75%* (65%–85%). Thus, while up to one-third of breast cancer may be attributed to a genetic predisposition, current knowledge indicates that environment retains a substantial role.

TABLE 19-3
HISTOLOGIC TYPES OF BREAST CANCER[a]

Type	%
Infiltrating ductal (not specified)	70–80
Medullary	5–8
Colloid (mucinous)	2–4
Tubular	1–2
Papillary	1–2
Invasive lobular	6–8
Noninvasive	4–6
Intraductal	2–3
Lobular in situ	2–3
All others	<1

[a]After A.E. Giuliano, The breast. In *Current Obstetric and Gynecologic Diagnosis and Treatment,* 6th ed., M.L. Pernoll and R.C. Benson, eds. Appleton & Lange, 1987.

Unopposed estrogen may increase the risk for breast cancer, but the oncotic effect is not as well correlated as it is for endometrial carcinoma. *Oral contraceptives do not appear to enhance the risk of breast cancer.*

Most breast carcinoma arises from the epithelial lining of the breast ductal system. If the origin of the cancer is the large or intermediate-sized ducts, it is termed ductal (~90%); if it arises from the epithelium of the lobular terminal ducts, it is termed lobular. Several histological subtypes of breast cancer have been identified (Table 19-3). However, 70%–80% are nonspecific infiltrating ductal carcinomas, and the *histologic type has little bearing on prognosis,* as projected by tumor staging. *Breast cancer is multicentric;* (i.e., more than one malignant focus can be identified in the same breast in 40% of patients and in the opposite breast in ~2% of patients). There is a 5%–8% incidence of cancer occurring later in the opposite breast.

Breast cancer occurs in the upper outer quadrant in ~45% of cases, in the central zone (periareolar or subareolar) in ~25%, in the upper inner quadrant in ~15%, in the lower outer quadrant in ~10%, and in the lower inner quadrant in ~5%. Lymphatic dissemination is the rule, with the axillary regional lymph nodes involved about twice as frequently as the internal mammary nodes. Unfortunately, hematogenous spread of breast cancer frequently occurs, most often to bone, liver, or lungs. Nodal metastases are present in ~1% of patients with noninfiltrating cancers.

CLINICAL FINDINGS

SCREENING

The screening processes of self-examination, physician examination, and mammography are discussed in Chapter 17.

SYMPTOMS AND SIGNS

About 90% of breast abnormalities are discovered by the patient, and about 10% are found during a physical examination for other reasons. The initial finding, in the great majority of breast cancers *(66%), is a firm or hard, nontender, fixed mass with ill-defined margins* (due to local invasion). In about 11%, a painful breast mass is the presenting sign. Nipple discharge (9%), local edema (4%), nipple retraction (3%), and nipple crusting are the other usual presentations. Initial symptomatology involving ulceration, itching, pain, enlargement, redness, or axillary adenopathy is infrequent.

SPECIAL CLINICAL FORMS OF BREAST CANCER

Paget's carcinoma accounts for 1%–3% of all breast cancers. It usually occurs as a pruritic or burning eczematoid ulceration of the nipple, although the nipple may not be grossly involved, and nipple discharge is only occasionally present. Paget's carcinoma is a particular form of intraductal carcinoma arising in the main excretory ducts of the breast. It usually is well differentiated and multicentric, with extension to the skin of the nipple or areola. Although in about two thirds of patients the underlying carcinoma may be palpated, there is great danger that this lesion may be treated as a dermatologic lesion, with the usual risk of metastases and the harm of delaying treatment.

Inflammatory carcinoma is the most virulent type and accounts for ~3% of breast cancers. It occurs as a rapidly enlarging, usually diffuse, and sometimes painful mass, with induration of the surrounding tissues. The overlying skin is often red, warm, and possibly edematous due to infiltration of malignant cells in subdermal lymphatics. The disease is rarely curable because metastases occur early and are widely distributed.

Breast cancer during pregnancy or lactation accounts for only 1%–2% of all breast cancers and complicates approximately 1 in 3000 pregnancies. However, it is difficult to diagnose (secondary to the physiologic changes), and the overall survival rate is low when compared to nonpregnant rate. Axillary metastases are present at diagnosis in 60%–70%, and for them the 5-year survival is 30%–40%. However, if the cancer is confined to the breast, the 5-year survival is ~70%. Delay posed by pregnancy and lactation must be avoided to preserve the mother's life.

LABORATORY FINDINGS

With extensive metastases, expect an elevated sedimentation rate. *Hypercalcemia is a frequent observation in advanced breast cancers.* Liver or bone metastases cause *elevated alkaline phosphatase* levels. *Carcinoembryonic antigen (CEA) may serve as a marker* for recurrent breast cancer. CA153 may be a useful marker in monitoring pregnant breast cancer patients.

MAMMOGRAPHY AND OTHER IMAGING TECHNIQUES

Mammography has greatly increased the diagnosis of small, even occult, cancers (see also Chapter 16). Mammography may identify some breast cancers up to 2 years before they reach palpable size. The *primary limitations* of mammography are that it may not reveal clinical cancer in a very *dense breast* (e.g., the young woman with mammary dysplasia) and that it may *not reveal medullary type* cancer. The indications for mammography are summarized in Table 19-4. Recent studies indicate that MRI may play a useful role in the cases where mammography is limited.

Because of the incidence of early metastases, radiographs of the chest, lumbar spine, pelvis, and skull should be part of a breast cancer workup. Additionally, bone scans may be necessary in some cases and may be a part of follow-up.

Ultrasound scanning may be useful in visualizing palpable focal masses in women <30 years (thus reducing the need for radiation). Ultrasound is also helpful in the differentiation of cystic from solid masses and in demonstrating potentially malignant solid tissue adjacent to or within a cyst.

TABLE 19-4
INDICATIONS FOR MAMMOGRAPHY

- To screen at regular intervals (see Chapter 17)
- To assess a questionable or ill-defined breast mass or other suspicious breast change
- To evaluate each breast at intervals when a diagnosis of potentially curable breast cancer has been made
- To search for an occult breast cancer from an unknown primary in women with metastatic disease in the axillary nodes or elsewhere
- To appraise women with large breasts that are difficult to examine
- To reassure women with cancerophobia

DIFFERENTIAL DIAGNOSIS

The *differential diagnosis of breast cancer* includes (in decreasing order of frequency) *fibrocystic breast disease, fibroadenoma, intraductal papilloma, duct ectasia, and fat necrosis.*

SPECIAL PRETHERAPY WORKUP

BIOPSY

The definitive *diagnosis of cancer requires analysis of tissue.* Thus, mammography cannot be a substitute for biopsy. The indications for breast biopsy include a *persistent breast mass, bloody nipple discharge, exzematoid nipple changes, and suspicious or positive mammography results.* About 30% of cases considered strongly suggestive of cancer will be found to be benign on biopsy. In contrast, about 15% of abnormal foci thought to be benign will be diagnosed as malignant on biopsy.

Needle biopsy (under local anesthesia) may be used to aspirate tumor cells or obtain a small tissue core. *False-negative needle biopsies occur in 15%–20% of cancers. Open biopsy is more conclusive* and preferably is performed as a separate procedure (often under local anesthesia) before definitive therapy, and there has been no demonstrable adverse effect from a 1–2 week delay. Occasionally, when mastectomy is contemplated for a very suspicious lesion, the

TABLE 19-5
INDICATIONS FOR OPEN BREAST BIOPSY

- Suspicious mammographic abnormalities
- Clinically suspicious mass, regardless of mammographic findings
- A cystic mass that does not completely collapse on aspiration or contains bloody fluid
- Serous or serosanguineous nipple discharge that is not galactorrhea

open biopsy may be assessed by frozen section and definitive therapy immediately performed under the same anesthetic. The indications for open breast biopsy are summarized in Table 19-5.

HORMONE RECEPTOR SITE ANALYSIS

Estrogen and progesterone receptor assays are usually obtained at the time of initial diagnosis. This information is *valuable for hormonal management of patients with recurrent or metastatic disease* and may even provide some prognostic assistance. For example, with recurrence or metastases, ~60% of patients with estrogen receptors in their original cancers will respond to hormone therapy, whereas <10% of estrogen receptor-negative patients will respond. Patients with estrogen receptors in their tumors have a more favorable course following mastectomy than those with estrogen receptor-negative tumors. Postmenopausal patients have a higher incidence of estrogen receptor-positive tumors (~60%) than do premenopausal patients (~30%).

The synthesis of progesterone receptors is estrogen-dependent, and progesterone receptors have been found in ~40% of estrogen receptor-positive tumors. When both types of receptors are present, ~80% of patients with recurrent or metastatic disease respond to hormone therapy.

There is no significant relationship between hormone receptor site activity and chemotherapy responsiveness.

STAGING

Clinical and histologic staging are of great prognostic significance and are used in designing the treatment plan. Table 19-6 details staging and crude 5-year survival.

TABLE 19-6
CLINICAL AND HISTOLOGIC STAGING OF BREAST
CARCINOMA AND RELATION TO SURVIVAL

Clinical Staging (American Joint Committee)	Crude 5-year Survival (%)
Stage I	85
Tumor <2 cm in diameter	
Nodes, if present, not believed to contain metastases	
Without distant metastases	
Stage II	66
Tumor <5 cm in diameter	
Nodes, if palpable, not fixed	
Without distant metastases	
Stage III	41
Tumor >5 cm or	
Tumor any size with invasion of skin or attached to chest wall	
Nodes in supraclavicular area	
Without distant metastases	
Stage IV	
With distant metastases	10

Histologic Staging	Crude Survival (%)	
	5 years	10 years
All patients	63	46
Negative axillary lymph nodes	78	65
Positive axillary lymph nodes	46	25
1–3 positive axillary lymph nodes	62	38
>4 positive axillary lymph nodes	32	13

SOURCE: From A.E. Giuliano. In *Current Obstetric and Gynecologic Diagnosis and Treatment,* 7th ed. M.L. Pernoll, ed. Appleton & Lange, 1991.

TREATMENT

Direct therapeutic options include *surgery, radiation therapy, chemotherapy, endocrine therapy, and combinations of these methods.*

SURGERY

The major surgical procedures and the extent of each are summarized in Table 19-7.

Radical mastectomy, which is effective for local control of cancer, is disfiguring. Moreover, it may not offer an advantage over less radical surgery combined with radiation therapy. Following any of the more radical surgeries, physical therapy is advisable, principally to limit edema of the arm. Additionally, incision placement, tissue volume removal, and nodal removal are critical determinants of cosmetic and functional outcomes. The BRCA founder mutation is not an independent predictor of survival. The mutation status should not influence decisions regarding adjuvant therapy. However, those with

TABLE 19-7
SUMMARY OF SURGICAL TREATMENTS
FOR BREAST CANCER

Procedure	Extent of Surgery
Radical mastectomy	En bloc removal of the breast, pectoral muscles, and axillary nodes
Extended radical mastectomy	In addition to the above also includes the internal mammary nodes
Modified radical mastectomy	En bloc removal of the breast, underlying pectoralis major fascia (but not muscle), and axillary lymph nodes
Simple mastectomy	Removal of the entire breast
Segmental mastectomy	Removal of the area involved, e.g., partial mastectomy, quadrant excision, or lumpectomy (often combined with axillary node sampling)

BRCA founder mutations are at increased risk for breast cancer after breast conservation.

RECENT THERAPEUTIC DIRECTIONS

Conservative surgical therapy for breast cancer, often characterized as "lumpectomy" *and adjuvant therapy* (may include radiation and/or chemotherapy), *is now accepted as a portion of the therapeutic armamentarium.* Ipsilateral breast cancer recurrence in the 10 years following conservative surgery and radiation for early stage invasive cancer is ~15%. This is even higher if the original surgical excision has positive margins. Thus, optimal local control of early invasive breast cancer maximizes long-term survival.

Tamoxifen is currently the most important anti-breast cancer drug in clinical use and also has the *potential to be an important chemopreventive breast cancer agent.* The long-term usage side effects include approximately 50% of women having *adverse endometrial effects.* The benign effects include: extensive endometrial senile cystic atrophy, endometrial hyperplasia, and endometrial polyps. The malignant effect is that *tamoxifen doubles the risk for developing endometrial cancer in postmenopausal women.* This worrisome effect is time of use dependent. Fortunately, screening patients with breast cancer for endometrial abnormalities while they are taking tamoxifen is readily accomplished (e.g., outpatient hysteroscopy) and can assist in prevention of both benign and malignant side effects. Currently, *if long-term tamoxifen is planned, the following endometrial screening may prove prudent.*

- Pretreatment uterine assessment is accomplished by transvaginal sonography and/or outpatient hysteroscopy.
- Symptom-free women with normal pretreatment uterine cavity should undergo annual screening with transvaginal sonography (some indicate this may be initiated from 2–3 years after onset of treatment).
- The only acceptable transvaginal sonographic finding is a thin rectilinear endometrium.
- Hysteroscopy or saline infusion sonography should be utilized for evaluation of any endometrial symptoms or any transvaginal sonographic abnormality (including endometrial thickening).

The management of *early non-high-grade breast cancer in the elderly by complete local excision and tamoxifen* alone has been utilized. The rationale for this approach is that standard therapy for younger women (axillary dissection, radiotherapy, and chemotherapy) has a morbidity that may not be well tolerated in the elderly (>70 years). Yet ~30% of all breast cancers occur in elderly women. Therefore, a more conservative approach for early non-high-grade breast cancers may avoid axillary dissection and radiotherapy. Preliminary results appear promising, and further study may lead to wider application of this, or a variant of this, conservative management.

Some advocate *prophylactic mastectomy for women with BRCA1 or BRCA2 gene mutations.* The rationale for this approach is that the current level of screening technology and the rudimentary state of chemoprevention do not assure that breast cancer will be detected at an early, curable stage in young women. Prophylactic mastectomy is usually combined with cosmetic reconstruction. Certainly, careful discussion of all options is essential in management of these high-risk patients. Further study will likely establish or deny the validity of this aggressive prophylaxis.

Other potentially useful procedures includes *sentinel node biopsy.* The rationale is that breast cancer metastasizing through the lymphatics will initially reach one or a few nodes in the corresponding lymph basin. Thus, the status of these nodes will predict the status of all the other nodes in the basin. The nodes are detected by dye or radioactivity injected about the tumor. Several studies have validated the concept. *Detection rates of 66%–100% and false-negative rates of 0%–17%* have been reported. Obviously, before recommended for widespread clinical use, false-negative rates of no more than 2%–3% should be achieved.

Although not yet recommended for cancer, recent studies have reported beneficial experience with *endoscopic extirpation of benign breast tumors* via an extramammary incision.

RADIATION THERAPY

Although initially radiation therapy was used after surgery when the axillary nodes were positive, it is now increasingly employed as *part of primary therapy for small tumors in conjunction with segmental mastectomy and axillary node sampling.* For patients with small primary tumors, less than total mastectomy combined with radiotherapy may be as effective as the more radical operations.

Usually 4500–5000 rad are delivered by external beam to the breast and anterior chest wall (including the internal mammary chain). If lymph nodes are positive, the ipsilateral supraclavicular and axillary nodes also are irradiated. When more radiation is necessary to a localized area, the site may be enhanced with interstitial iridium-192. Major complications of such therapy (arm edema or weakness, radiation pericarditis, and soft tissue necrosis) occur in ~2% of patients.

CHEMOTHERAPY

Overall, *~75% of patients with breast cancer succumb in <10 years.* Thus, the *assumption holds that many patients with breast cancer already have disseminated disease at the time of diagnosis. Therefore, chemotherapy is used as an adjunct to initial therapy,* with the objective of eliminating occult metastases responsible for late recurrences. There are several regimens currently used and still others under investigation. Such adjuvant chemotherapy improves survival (~20%) and lengthens the disease-free interval in premenopausal women, especially those with one to three positive nodes. The effect in postmenopausal women is less beneficial.

ENDOCRINE THERAPY

In the past, oophorectomy, adrenalectomy, and hypophysectomy were used to decrease or eliminate estrogen stimulation of breast cancer, especially in postmenopausal women. Although, the last two procedures have largely been abandoned, *oophorectomy is still often used to reduce estrogen exposure of the tumor* in premenopausal women. However, *tamoxifen* (an antiestrogen) is rapidly becoming the most commonly used agent in endocrine therapy. Overall, about one third of patients respond, but the response with estrogen receptors in the tumor is ~60%, and with both estrogen and progesterone receptors, the response is ~80%. By contrast, only 5%–10% of receptor-negative tumors respond to tamoxifen therapy.

PSYCHOLOGIC THERAPY

The psychological impact of breast cancer merits sensitive and thoughtful attention during workup, therapy and follow-up. Up to 80% of breast cancer patients report significant distress even during initial treatment. Psychological factors may heavily influence patient's participation in treatment decision-making, having a treatment choice, and post-treatment satisfaction. Body image is an example of a specific area warranting exploration. Although patients may participate in treatment decision-making based on survival, satisfaction with body image may be disturbed by surgery. *Cancer patients uniformly evidence an improvement in mood, coping, and adjustment as a result of psychotherapeutic intervention.* Group psychotherapy (workshop participation, treatment manual, and explanatory videotapes) for recently diagnosed breast cancer patients has been demonstrated to reduce distress among breast cancer patients. Additionally, stress-coping frameworks assist in addressing quality of life: person (demographics, current concerns, and optimism), social resources (family functioning, necessary assistance), illness-related factors (symptom distress, medial characteristics), appraisal of illness, and quality of life. Finally, current health behaviors and readiness to pursue life-style changes merit consideration.

The importance of full discussion by care providers regarding the rationale of therapy and its cosmetic and emotional effects cannot be over-emphasized. Reconstructive surgery as well as prosthetics must be considered. Support groups (e.g., The Service Committee of the American Cancer Society's program Reach to Recovery) may also be very useful.

ALTERNATIVE THERAPY

Alternative therapy, often uninitiated by and unknown to those responsible for the breast cancer care, is rapidly increasing in the United States. Indeed, ~50% of women with breast cancer use at least one type of alternative therapy and about one third used two types. Although, most therapies are used for <6 months, the type used is influenced by ethnicity. Blacks (36%) most often use spiritual healing. Caucasians use dietary methods (35%) and physical methods (e.g., massage, acupuncture—21%), whereas Chinese (22%) most often use herbal remedies. Latinos most often use dietary therapies (30%) and spiritual healing (26%). Thus, those caring for breast cancer patients should *initiate dialogues with their patients concerning the alternative therapies* they may be employing.

CURRENT THERAPY SUMMARY

Although breast cancer therapy is currently in transition and several crucial conclusions are not available, certain guidelines are useful. Potentially curable lesions may be treated by partial mastectomy plus axillary lymphadenectomy and radiation therapy or by modified radial mastectomy. If in the premenopausal patient axillary nodes are involved, adjuvant chemotherapy is prudent. Radical mastectomy should be reserved for cases of advanced local disease with tumor invading the pectoralis muscle. Extended radical mastectomy is justified for patients with medial lesions without signs of distant spread. Receptor-positive breast cancers may benefit from endocrine therapy.

FOLLOW-UP CARE

OBJECTIVES

Follow-up care should be lifelong and has two objectives: *to detect recurrence(s) and to observe the other breast for evidence of carcinoma.*

BREAST SELF-EXAMINATION, PHYSICIAN EXAMINATIONS, AND MAMMOGRAPHY

Every month, the patient should examine her own breast(s). Mammography should be obtained annually or when any change is detected. During the first 3 years, when metastases are most likely, physician examinations are performed every 3–4 months. Between 4 and 5 years, examination is performed every 6 months. After 5 years, examinations are continued at 6–12 month intervals. Women heterozygous for BRCA founder mutations require even more vigilant surveillance for they are at increased risk for contralateral breast cancer.

TUMOR MARKERS

In brief, *tumor markers are neither sensitive nor specific enough for early diagnosis of malignancy, but may be useful in postsurgical follow-up.* However, there is no unanimity concerning which tumor markers should be used in a panel for follow-up of breast cancer patients. Most recently, it appears that Ca 153 and Ca 27-29 have better correlation with clinical course of breast cancer than CEA and MCA, but obviously this is an area of intense investigation.

ESTROGEN OR PROGESTERONE AFTER BREAST CANCER

The use of estrogen or progestational agents in women free of disease after primary breast cancer therapy *remains controversial,* particularly if the primary cancer was hormone receptor positive. However, recent evidence indicates that this is not the risk previously thought and that hormonal replacement may, in some instances, be undertaken. Additionally, there is no evidence that estrogen replacement therapy increases the risk of invasive breast cancer in women with previous benign breast disease.

One of the difficulties posed by hormone replacement therapy is *mammographic density changes,* which confound interpretation and detection of small lesions. These density changes are more prevalent with certain hormone(s): estrogen plus cyproterone acetate (46%), estrogen plus medroxyprogesterone acetate (43%), tibolone users (28%), and estrogen alone (18%). Formation of breast cysts or solid tumors does not seem related to any of the hormone replacement regimens.

PREGNANCY AFTER BREAST CARCINOMA

Pregnancy following treatment of breast carcinoma carries less risk than previously indicated. Currently, particularly in stage II or I cases, some authorities are recommending deferring pregnancy for at least 2 years. If a complete evaluation is negative at that point and the patient is knowledgeable concerning the risks, pregnancy may be undertaken. It has been suggested that such a protocol does not enhance the chance of death from breast carcinoma. It seems prudent to individualize recommendations for hormonal replacement therapy or pregnancy after breast cancer following consultation with the team caring for the patient and perhaps with oncology centers.

PROGNOSIS

The mortality rate for breast cancer patients exceeds that for age-matched controls by nearly 20 years. Thus, 5-year follow-up information is less useful than in other tumors, and *10-year surveillance is necessary.*

Survival is most reliably correlated with the stage of breast cancer (Table 19-6). If the disease is localized to the breast, without regional spread (by microscopic analysis), 5-year survival may approach 90%. When breast cancer involves the axillary nodes, the 5-year cure rate is 40%–60%, and the 10-year clinical cure rate is only ~25%.

Other possible *beneficial correlations to survival include presence of estrogen and progesterone receptors and older age* (breast cancer seems to be more malignant in younger women). The least favorable anatomic site for breast cancer is the median portion of the inner lower quadrant.

Survival after breast carcinoma is significantly worse among African American women. African American women are significantly younger at the time of diagnosis, are more likely to present with advanced stage breast carcinoma, are more likely to have inflammatory, medullary and papillary histologic tumor types, and are less likely to have estrogen or progesterone receptor positive tumors. Despite these differences, race remains an independent predictor of breast carcinoma survival.

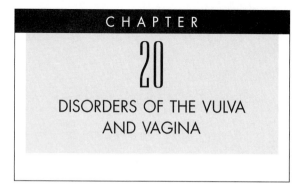

CHAPTER

20

DISORDERS OF THE VULVA AND VAGINA

COMMON VULVOVAGINAL INFECTIONS ASSOCIATED WITH LEUKORRHEA

Leukorrhea is a usually whitish vaginal discharge that may occur at any age and affects virtually all women at some time. Although some vaginal discharge (mucus) is physiologic and nearly always present, when it becomes greater or abnormal (bloody or soils clothing), is irritating, or has an offensive odor, it is considered pathologic. Pathologic discharge is often coupled with *vulvar irritation.* Commonly, the pathologic conditions are due to *infection of the vagina or cervix.* Other causes may include *uterine tumors, estrogenic or psychic stimulation, trauma, foreign bodies* (retained tampon), *excessive douching* (especially with irritating medications), and *vulvovaginal atrophy* (hypoestrogenism).

Vulvovaginal disorders constitute the major reason for office gynecology visits. These disorders are heavily influenced by the physiologic alterations summarized in Table 20-1. Estrogen and progesterone influence the nonkeratinized squamous epithelium of the vagina and vulva. Without hormonal influence, the epithelium is thin and atrophic and contains little glycogen, and the vaginal fluid has a high pH. By contrast, with adequate estrogen and progesterone, cellular glycogen content increases and the pH decreases (partially due to breakdown of glycogen to lactic acid). During their reproductive lives, most women harbor three to eight major types of pathogenic bacteria at any given time (Table 20-1).

Physiologic vaginal secretions consist mainly of *cervical mucus* (a transudate from the vaginal squamous epithelium) and *exfoliated squamous cells.* Lesser amounts are contributed by the metabolic products of the microflora, exudates from sebaceous sweat glands, Bartholin glands, and Skene glands, and small amounts of

TABLE 20-1

SUMMARY OF THE HORMONAL INFLUENCE, VAGINAL pH, AND USUAL (PREDOMINANT) VAGINAL ORGANISMS AT DIFFERENT TIMES OF A FEMALE'S LIFE

Time of Life	Hormonal Influence	Vaginal pH	Usual Predominant Vaginal Organisms	
Birth	Estrogen Progesterone	3.7–6.3	Anaerobic and aerobic	
Infant	None	6.0–8.0	Gram-positive cocci and bacilli	
Puberty–Reproductive	Estrogen Progesterone	3.5–4.5	Aerobes	(%)
			Lactobacillus	(70–90)
			Staphylococcus epidermidis	(30–60)
			Diphtheroids	(30–60)
			Alpha-hemolytic Streptococcus	(15–50)
			Group D Streptococcus	(10–40)
			Nonhemolytic Streptococcus	(5–30)
			Escherichia coli	(20–25)
			Beta-hemolytic Streptococcus	(10–20)
			Anaerobes	(%)
			Bacteroides fragilis	(5–40)
			Bacteroides species	(1–40)
			Peptococcus	(5–60)
			Peptostreptococcus	(5–40)
			Clostridium	(5–15)
			Veillonella	(10–15)
Menopause	Little or none	6.0–8.0	Gram-positive cocci and bacilli	

572

endometrial and oviductal fluid. When there is little hormonal stimulation (e.g., prior to puberty and postmenopausally), vaginal secretions are scant and the genital tract is less resistant to infection. Physiologic events enhancing the amount of cervical mucus and vaginal discharge occur as a result of sexual or other emotional stimulation, ovulation, pregnancy, and with the excessive estrogen produced by feminizing ovarian tumors.

The normal vaginal flora is most likely to be interrupted during *nonphysiologic conditions* with the symptomatology noted. The most common organisms causing leukorrhea include *Trichomonas vaginalis (protozoon), Candida (yeast), Gardnerella (or a combination of organisms collectively known as Bacterial Vaginosis) and Chlamydia (bacterial).* Helminths (e.g., *Oxyuris*) may cause leukorrhea in children. Leukorrhea is unusual in genital gonorrhea or tuberculosis.

Investigation of vaginal discharge involves collection of *historical information* (what, when, where, why, and to what degree); *examination of the vulva, vagina, and cervix; assessment of the discharge (texture, color, odor); and preparation of a saline wet mount* (see p. 523). In the majority of infections, it is not necessary to perform a culture for confirmation of diagnosis.

TRICHOMONAS VAGINALIS

Trichomonas infection generally is *manifest as a diffuse vaginitis with varying vulvar involvement. T. vaginalis* infections result in marked pruritus with variable edema and erythema. Numerous red points (strawberry patches), which rarely bleed, may be scattered over the vaginal surface and cervical portio. The cervix, urethra, and bladder may be secondarily infected. The leukorrhea is characterized as *thin, yellow-green, and occasionally frothy, with a fetid odor.* The discharge has a pH of 5–6.5. On saline wet mount, the *unicellular flagellate* may be observed moving about in a field of many leukocytes. The trichomonads are pear shaped and smaller than epithelial cells but larger than white cells.

T. vaginalis is almost always a sexually transmitted infection. It causes 20%–25% of infectious vaginitis and is responsible for up to 3 million cases a year (United States). The source often can be traced to the male partner, who may harbor the flagellate beneath the prepuce or in the urethra or urethral prostate, yet remain asymptomatic. Moreover, ~25% of females harboring T. vaginalis are also asymptomatic, although some may have urinary frequency and dyspareunia. T. vaginalis vaginitis is frequently followed by chronic bacterial cervicitis.

The treatment for trichomoniasis is *oral metronidazole* (a single 2 g dose, 1 g q12h × 2, or 250 mg tid for 5–7 days). The side effects of metronidazole include nausea, occasional vomiting, a metallic taste, and intolerance to alcohol. It should not be taken during the first trimester of pregnancy. It is necessary to treat both partners. Men usually are treated with metronidazole 2 g PO or 1 g q12h × 2. In cases of sensitivity to metronidazole, topical clotrimazole is used.

CANDIDA ALBICANS

Candida albicans and related pathogens, *Candida glabrata* and *Candida tropicalis,* are *natural fungal inhabitants of the bowel and are also found on the perineal skin.* Thus, vaginal contamination from these sources is common. *C. albicans* is also found in the vaginal flora of ~25% of asymptomatic women. Candidal infections occur when vaginal flora abnormalities take place (e.g., a decrease in lactobacilli), and 80%–95% are caused by *C. albicans.* With *Candida* infections, there is *generally more vulvar pruritus than with Trichomonas* infections but less burning. The usual symptomatology includes vaginal discharge, vulvar pruritus, burning, and dyspareunia. *Candida* vaginitis commonly leads to dermatitis of the vulva and thighs. Symptomatology generally begins in the premenstrual phase of the cycle, but *~20% of women with Candida are asymptomatic.* Unlike bacterial or protozoal vaginitis, *Candida* infections are not considered a sexually transmitted disease and are not commonly associated with mixed infections or sexually transmitted diseases. At particular risk for developing candidiasis are *diabetics, oral contraceptive users,* those who have recently taken *antibiotics, and pregnant women.*

Vaginal discharge due to *Candida* infection has a *cottage cheese appearance, usually without odor. White, curdlike collections of exudate* often are present, and some are lightly attached to the cervical and vaginal mucosa. When these are removed, slight oozing occurs. There may be both erythema and edema of the vulva and vagina. The discharge with Candida infection has a pH of 4–5. Mixing the secretions with a drop of *10%–20% KOH* microscopically reveals the characteristic mycelia and hyphae, with only a moderate leukocyte response. Should culture be necessary, it may be accomplished using Nickerson's or Sabouraud's medium.

The treatment for *C. albicans* infection is *topical 2% miconazole nitrate, 1 applicator or vaginal suppository at bedtime for 3–7 days.* Alternatively, clotimatzole or butoconazole vaginal suppositories or cream may be used nightly for 7–14 days. If *C. albicans* recurs (a frequent occurrence), the patient should have a glucose screening examination for carbohydrate intolerance. It is also worthwhile to inquire about the possibility of a sexual partner with *Candida* infection about the prepuce. Finally, it is crucial to recognize that *C. glabrata* and *C. tropicalis* are resistant to the imidazoles and may be the cause of recurrent infections. The discharge must be cultured, and treatment is topical gentian violet q3–4d × 2–3. Boric acid (600 mg in gelatin caps) inserted high in the vagina bid and douching every other night (to a total of three times) with dilute povidone-iodine may be useful therapeutic adjuncts.

BACTERIAL VAGINOSIS

Bacterial vaginosis (BV) is the clinical diagnosis describing an overgrowth (100–1000-fold) of certain facultative and obligate anaerobic bacteria derived from the patient's endogeneous vaginal flora. It is also known as Bacterial vaginitis, Nonspecific vaginitis, *Haemophilus vaginalis,* and *Gardnerella vaginalis.* The usual bacterial species involved are: *Bacteriodes* species, *Petostreptococcus* species, *G. vaginalis, Mycoplasma hominis,* and members of the *Enterobacteriaceae.* Although *asymptomatic in approximately one half of patients, BV occurs in 10%–25% of general obstetrics and gynecology patients.* The incidence of BV is *higher (~2/3) in patients being seen for STDs.*

The primary symptom of BV is a relatively *alkaline, malodorous (fishy), gray (dark or dull), watery, homogeneous discharge that is worse during menses and after intercourse.* Vulvar pruritis is a less frequent symptom. In addition to history and physical examination, the investigation of BV includes a vaginal pH, a "whiff" (smell) test, and a microscopic wet-mount. The wet-mount is usually characterized by: *clue cells, an abundance of bacteria of various morphologies, the absence of homogeneous bacilli (lactobacilli), and an absence or paucity of inflammatory cells.* Pap tests are not effective in the diagnosis of BV and cultures are necessary only when the discharge does not respond to treatment or overgrowth of a specific organism is suspected. The diagnosis of BV (false-positives <10%) is confirmed by 3 of the 4 following criteria:

- pH >4.5,
- Clue cells,
- Positive KOH,
- Homogeneous discharge.

Treatment may be *local* (intravaginal) *or systemic* (oral). The local regimens include: *0.75% metronidazole gel bid for 5 d, and 2% clindamycin cream once a d for 7 d.* Oral metronidazole (500 mg bid, 250 mg tid) for 7 d is >90% effective, whereas a single 2 g dose is less effective (~70%) and has a greater incidence of gastrointestinal upset. *Recurrences occur with vexing frequency.* Although treatment of partners is not recommended unless BV is recalcitrant to therapy, this remains a controversial area. The higher association of BV and STDs should heighten the practitioner's suspicion concerning gonorrhea, chlamydia, syphilis, hepatitis and HIV.

BV may be associated with *furthering the incidence of* a number of gynecological complications, including: *PID, postabortal infections, and posthysterectomy vaginal cuff cellulitis.* Although not completely proven, treatment of the BV appears to decrease the incidence of these complications and provides at least part of the rationale for prophylactic antibiotic therapy in these circumstances.

Additionally, BV has been incriminated in *increasing the incidence of preterm delivery, premature rupture of membranes, amnionitis, chorioamnionitis, and postpartum endometritis.* Thus, it is currently recommended that BV screening be considered during pregnancy in risk patients, but data supporting low-risk screening has not emerged. There is also no common agreement on therapy or rescreening. During pregnancy, 2% clindamycin intravaginal cream may be used once a d for 7 d, but may be less effective. Alternatively, clindamycin 300 mg bid for 7 d may be used. Finally, metronidazole oral therapy may be used after the first trimester.

CHLAMYDIA TRACHOMATIS

Chlamydial infections are caused by the obligate intracellular bacterium, *Chlamydia trachomatis.* Other closely related infections are lymphogranuloma venereum, inclusion conjunctivitis, urethritis, cervicitis, salpingitis, proctitis, epididymitis, and pneumonia of the newborn. *C. trachomatis infection may be the most prevalent sexually transmitted disease in the United States, affecting >3 million persons annually. It is often asymptomatic (~60%–80% of infected women and ~10% of infected men).* The organism is best detected by enzyme-linked amino acids in a fluorescein-conjugate monoclonal antibody test. The infections usually begin as mucopurulent, often odorous or pruritic discharges, and the *principal site of infection is the cervix.* Chlamydia can be eradicated from the vagina and cervix by *tetracycline or erythromycin 500 mg PO qid for 7 days.*

COMMON VULVOVAGINAL VIRAL INFECTIONS

HERPES SIMPLEX VIRUS (HSV)

HSV infections of the genital tract are a sexually transmitted disease. Type 2 HSV accounts for ~90% of infections, and 10% are type 1. This DNA virus has an *incubation period of 3–22 days,* and *even primary attacks may be asymptomatic,* although most patients complain of *fever, malaise, anorexia, local genital pain, leukorrhea, dysuria, or even vaginal bleeding.* Typical genital lesions are multiple *vesicles that progress to shallow ulceration often surrounded by redness or erythematous patches.* Painful bilateral inguinal *adenopathy* is usually present during the primary infection. If the urethra or bladder is affected, dysuria or urinary retention may result. The lesions gradually heal without scarring (7–10 days) unless bacterial superinfection occurs.

The *diagnosis is usually made on the typical appearance* of vesicles and ulcers. *Cytologic smear* of the ulcers or vesicles demonstrates classic multinucleated giant cells with acidophilic intranuclear inclusion bodies. *Definitive culture* may be obtained from the fluid of unruptured vesicles using Hanks medium. However, false-negative cultures are frequent. *Serologic diagnosis* is possible, and use of the gamma globulin or macroglobulin response may determine if the attack is recurrent or primary.

Affected individuals harbor the virus indefinitely. Recurrent lesions may be triggered by emotional distress, exposure to the sun, or a variety of other stimuli. After the primary lesion, the patient frequently develops paresthesias in the affected region before a recurrence (the virus resides in specialized nerve endings during latent intervals). Recurrent lesions account for much of the morbidity but are not as painful as the primary lesions.

Genital herpes during pregnancy is hazardous to the fetus. Serial cultures for the detection of asymptomatic viral shedding have been very disappointing as a diagnostic technique during pregnancy. *It is recommended that an infant not be delivered through the birth canal with active lesions.* Although cesarean section does not guarantee that the infant will not be infected, it may be undertaken if it is <4 h after rupture of the membranes. Delivery through an infected birth canal with active lesions poses ~50% chance of the neonate developing neonatal herpes. Of those infected, ~50% die and ~25% have permanent neurologic sequelae. Additionally, HSV type 2 has been suggested (but not proven) as etiologic in cervical dysplasia.

Currently, there is *no cure for herpes simplex viral infections.* Symptomatic measures include hot sitz baths, douching with Burrow's solution, and oral or parenteral acyclovir. Local or oral acyclovir may shorten the course of an initial attack but has little effect on recurrences. Valacyclovir may also be used for treatment of an initial infection (1 g bid PO for 10 d, started <72 h after onset of symptoms), treatment of recurrances (500 mg bid PO for 5 d, started <24 h after onset of symptoms) or for suppression (1 g PO a day, limited to <1 yr of use). Another suppressive agent is famciclovir.

General rules for prevention of dissemination include covering small lesions situated away from the oral or vaginal orifices with occlusive dressing during sexual contact, the use of condoms, and the application of contraceptive cream or foam. A partner may become infected despite these precautions. If a regular partner has had genital herpes or has not been infected despite prolonged exposure, precautions are probably not necessary.

HUMAN PAPILLOMAVIRUS (HPV)

A member of the Papovavirus group, *human papillomavirus causes condylomata acuminata.* The virus is *sexually transmitted, commonly affects both partners, and affects the same age group as other venereal diseases.* This DNA virus causes easily discernible, raised, papillomatous lesions of the vulva as well as less discernible lesions of the vagina and cervix. The lesions are much more *florid in* patients who are *diabetic, pregnant, taking oral contraceptives, or immunosuppressed.* The most common complaints concern the lesions themselves, but vaginal discharge or pruritus may be present.

The vaginal or cervical lesions are occasionally exophytic or papillomatous (wartlike) but may also be flat, spiked, or inverted. The flat condylomata are white lesions with a somewhat granular surface and a mosaic pattern (some with punctuation) on colposcopy. The papillomatous condylomata is a raised white lesion with fingerlike projections, often containing capillaries. The spiked condyloma is a hyperkeratotic lesion with surface projection and prominent capillary tips. Inverted condylomata grow into cervical glands and, thus, do not occur in the vagina.

Subtypes 6 and 11 are primarily responsible for genital warts. Cytologic smear or biopsy of vaginal or cervical lesions reveals *koilocytes,* which are superficial or intermediate cells characterized by an enlarged perinuclear cavity that stains only faintly. Biopsy often is necessary to distinguish cervical condylomata from dysplasia.

Treatment in nonpregnant patients generally consists of weekly applications of *podophyllin (25% in tincture of benzoin)*. If after 4–6 weeks this is not successful, *cryosurgery, electrocautery, or laser therapy* may be necessary. Podophyllin should not be used during pregnancy, and if it is used within 6 weeks of biopsy, the pathologist must be notified because bizarre changes occur that could alter the diagnosis. *During pregnancy, cryosurgery is most commonly used for therapy* of condylomata. If vaginal or introital lesions are present, consider cesarean section because of the possibility of bleeding from the very friable lesions as well as the possibility of the fetus acquiring laryngeal papillomatosis (infection of the vocal cords by papillomavirus) during the birth process.

MOLLUSCUM CONTAGIOSUM

Molluscum contagiosum is an autoinoculable virus with an incubation period of *1–4 weeks*. Asymptomatic pink to gray, discrete, umbilicated epithelial skin tumors <1 cm in diameter develop generally on the vulva. The histologic picture is that of *numerous inclusion bodies in the cell cytoplasm*. Each lesion must be treated by desiccation, freezing or curettage, and chemical cauterization of the base.

OTHER VULVOVAGINAL INFECTIONS

BARTHOLIN DUCT CYST AND ABSCESS

The Bartholin duct is susceptible to infectious occlusion because of its length and narrowness. Infectious organisms (often *Neisseria gonorrhoeae* with secondary streptococci, staphylococci, or *Escherichia coli*) become pocketed within the passage to form an abscess. The inflammation usually resolves, but permanent occlusion of the distal duct causes *retention of mucus* produced by the gland, and a *cyst develops.* The process is usually unilateral and occurs in *up to 2% of women.* The gland is almost never seriously involved with the ductal infection, but in older women acquiring a mass in the Bartholin area, carcinoma (see p. 592) must be excluded.

Clinical manifestations include *acute pain, tenderness, and dyspareunia.* Surrounding tissues (at the junction of the mid and lower thirds of the labia minora) become inflamed and edematous. The introitus may be distorted, and a fluctuant mass usually is palpable.

FIGURE 20-1. Marsupialization of Bartholin cyst.

Rarely are systemic symptoms reported or signs of infection noted. Smears and cultures may reveal a specific bacteriologic diagnosis. By the time the process is seen, however, the culture usually will not be reliable.

The differential diagnosis includes inclusion cysts, large sebaceous cysts, hidradenoma, congenital anomalies, primary malignancy, and metastatic cancers. *Treatment consists of drainage* of the infected cyst or abscess, preferably by *marsupialization* (Fig. 20-1). This procedure best affords permanent fistula formation. Other procedures (e.g., simple incision and drainage) frequently lead to recurrence. Marsupialization is feasible under local anesthesia, and fine interrupted chromic catgut or polyglycolic acid sutures are generally employed. If considerable surrounding inflammation is present, *broad-spectrum antibiotics* should be given until appropriate antibiotics for organisms in the abscess pus (determined by culture at the time of surgery) can be determined. Bedrest, local dry or moist heat or both, and analgesics should be used as indicated. Prognosis is good with marsupialization. With other treatment, recurrent infection and cystic dilation are likely. Rarely, it is necessary to surgically excise the entire gland. Although in all cases it is desirable to biopsy an area for pathologic section, this becomes crucial in the perimenopausal or postmenopausal woman because of the risk of Bartholin carcinoma.

HIDRADENITIS

Hidradenitis is a *refractory infection of the apocrine sweat glands usually caused by staphylococci or streptococci*. It is analogous to cystic acne, and symptoms are soreness and local swelling, edema, cellulitis, and suppuration of the groin. Involvement of apocrine glands establishes the diagnosis. Treatment consists of hot, wet packs, drainage, and specific antibiotics chosen on the basis of culture and sensitivity testing. Excision may be necessary, but the wound must be allowed to heal by secondary intention.

TOXIC SHOCK SYNDROME (TSS)

Toxic shock syndrome generally occurs in previously healthy women of childbearing age (usually 12–24 years). The incidence is currently ~5/100,000 menstruating women per year. TSS is characterized by abrupt *onset of high fever (102°F); a diffuse macular erythematous rash (sunburnlike) over the face, trunk, and proximal extremities; and hypotension (systolic <90 mm Hg).* Additionally, there is involvement of three or more of the following systems: gastrointestinal (vomiting and watery diarrhea), muscular (tenderness), mucous membranes (nonpurulent conjunctivitis, sore throat), renal (failure), hepatic (failure), hematologic (thrombocytopenia), and central nervous system (nuchal rigidity, headaches, confusion). Renal failure and cardiac failure are manifestations in severe cases and generally occur within <48 h of onset.

Coagulase-positive Staphylococcus aureus has been isolated from the vagina of victims, but blood cultures are negative. The cause is *most likely an exotoxin (exfoliatin)* produced by some strains of staphylococci. *TSS begins (95% of cases) within 5 days of the onset of menses in which tampons are used, and superabsorbent tampons appear to be linked to causation.* Other potential sources of TSS include delivery, diaphragm usage, surgery, soft-tissue abscess, pyelonephritis, and osteomyelitis.

The *laboratory workup* must include a CBC with differential count, electrolytes, UA, BUN, creatinine, liver function studies, blood culture, throat culture, and vaginal culture. A lumbar puncture should be performed if signs of meningitis are present, and the CSF should be analyzed and cultured. The *differential diagnosis* includes Kawasaki disease (in children), scarlet fever, Rocky Mountain spotted fever, leptospirosis, gram-negative sepsis, and measles.

Treatment includes removal of a tampon if present (as well as culture for penicillinase-producing *S. aureus*), admission to a critical care unit for intensive (often invasive) monitoring, correction of fluid and electrolyte deficiencies (sizable deficits occur from third spacing), corticosteroid therapy (methylprednisolone 30 mg/kg or dexamethasone 3 mg/kg as a bolus, repeated q4h prn), antistaphylococcal antibiotics (beta-lactamase-resistant antibiotics, e.g., nafcillin, oxycillin, or methicillin 1 g IV q4h or vancomycin 500 mg IV q6h if penicillin allergy exists), and management of renal and cardiac insufficiency. It may be necessary to give blood and blood products (packed RBCs, fresh frozen plasma, platelets). Corticosteroids shorten the fever duration and reduce the severity of illness. Dopamine infusion may be necessary (2–5 μg/kg/min) if fluids do not correct hypotension. Naloxone may be used in persistent hypotension for its antiendorphin activity. Since gram-negative sepsis is in the differential diagnosis, an aminoglycoside should be given until gram-negative sepsis is ruled out. For both vancomycin and the aminoglycoside, drug levels must be carefully monitored.

Complications include adult respiratory distress syndrome (ARDS), intractable hypotension, and hemorrhage from disseminated intravascular coagulation, any of which can be fatal. Mortality from TSS is 3%–6%. Desquamation, especially of palms and soles, occurs 1–2 weeks after onset of TSS. There is a *30% recurrence rate,* especially in the first 3 months after the attack. The recurrences are reduced to ~5% by administration of antistaphylococcal antibiotics in the initial episode. If a woman recovers from TSS, she should forego the use of tampons until cervicovaginal and nasal cultures for *S. aureus* are negative twice at 4-week intervals and then avoid tampon use at night.

FURUNCULOSIS

Furuncular abscesses caused by staphylococcal infections are termed furunculosis or boils. Symptoms usually include throbbing pain and regional tenderness. Pustular areas require incision and drainage, with culture of the pus. Treatment includes segregation, topical moist heat periodically, and systemic antibiotics (e.g., cephalosporin).

TUBERCULOSIS

Vulvovaginal tuberculosis, rare even in developing countries, is manifest by chronic, minimally painful, exudative sores that are reddish, raised, moderately firm and nodular, with central apple jelly-like contents. Later, ulcerative, undermined, necrotic, discharging lesions develop. There is some tendency toward healing with heavy scarring, but induration and sinus formation are common in the scrofulous type of infection. The differential diagnosis includes cancer and sexually transmitted diseases. Demonstration of *Mycobacterium tuberculosis* is necessary for diagnosis. Treatment consists of antituberculosis chemotherapy.

VULVAR INFESTATIONS

PEDICULOSIS PUBIS

Pthirus pubis (crab louse) is transmitted by sexual contact or from bedding or clothing. The eggs are laid at the base of the pubic, axillary, or scalp hair. When the eggs hatch, the lice attach to the skin and cause intense itching. Close observation reveals minute, pale brown insects and their ova attached to hair shafts near the skin. The treatment consist of 1% gamma benzene hexachloride cream/lotion or shampoo (not recommended for pregnant or lactating women) or pyritherans applied to the infestation and adjacent hair areas. Retreatment may be required in 1 week. It is necessary to treat all contacts and sterilize infected bedding and clothing.

SCABIES

Sarcoptes scabei causes intractable itching and excoriation of the surface in the vicinity of minute skin burrows where the parasites have deposited ova. The mite is transmitted directly from person to person. Treatment is 1% gamma benzene hexachloride cream/lotion from the neck down overnight, washing off thoroughly after 8 h, or 10% crotamiton cream or lotion applied from the neck down twice nightly and washed off thoroughly after the second application. With this infestation, contacts must be treated, and all infected clothing and bedding must be sterilized.

ENTEROBIASIS (PINWORMS)

Enterobius vermicularis is a short, spindle-shaped roundworm that commonly infects children. The usual symptomatology is nocturnal perianal itching, which leads to excoriation. The usual diagnostic technique is a short strip of cellophane pressure-sensitive tape applied to the perianal region and then spread on a slide. This reveals the adult worms or ova in >90% of cases. Therapy is a single oral dose of mebendazole 100 mg.

BENIGN VULVAR LESIONS

ECZEMA

Eczema is a *nonspecific, common, pruritic, moist dermatitis characterized by excoriation and crusting with later lichenification.* Eczema is often a contact dermatitis caused by irritants in soap, bath oils, or deodorant medications, dyes in clothing, or allergy to wool or silk. Sensitivity tests and the exclusion of other dermatitis aid in diagnosis. General treatment depends on elimination of the irritant. Therapy is Burrow's solution followed by steroid creams (e.g., 0.5% hydrocortisone bid).

PSORIASIS

Pruritic, reddened, slightly elevated lesions (without the typical silvery scale seen on elbows and knees) are seen in body folds. The elbows and knees are frequently affected by the scaly lesions, however. Psoriasis is a chronic, often familial, disorder of unknown etiology. Exacerbations often occur in winter, and treatment includes improving hygiene and 0.5% hydrocortisone cream applied bid. More extensive lesions require dermatologic consultation.

BENIGN NEOPLASIA

A number of benign tumors may involve the vulvovaginal area. These are generally characterized as either *cystic or solid.* The cysts include *epidermal cysts, sebaceous cysts, and apocrine sweat gland cysts.* A cyst of epidermal origin may arise from trauma or occlusion of pilosebaceous ducts. These tend to be small, solitary, lined with squamous epithelium, and filled with sebaceous material as well as desquamated epithelial cells. Most are asymptomatic.

Cysts of the sebaceous or sweat glands are frequently multiple and almost always involve the labia majora. They are asymptomatic unless infection develops. Apocrine sweat glands become functional after puberty. Then, occlusion of the ducts results in an extremely pruritic, microcytic disorder, *Fox-Fordyce disease.* Should the apocrine glands become infected by streptococci or staphylococci, the process termed *hidradenitis supprativa* occurs.

Less common cysts or pseudocysts include Skene duct cysts, urethral diverticula, inguinal hernia, occlusion of a persistently patent vaginalis (canal of Nuck), dilation of mullerian duct vestiges, and supernumerary mammary tissue.

The most worrisome benign vulvar solid tumors are pigmented nevi. Because nearly all vulvar nevi are of the junctional type, they may give rise to *malignant melanomas.* Thus, vulvar pigmented nevi should be viewed more cautiously than elsewhere on the body. All small pigmented lesions of the vulva are suspect and should be removed with a 0.5–1 cm margin. Other benign solid tumors usually are incidental findings and, like the cystic tumors, usually are provisionally diagnosed by clinical examination. If therapy is required, excisional biopsy is usually sufficient.

An *acrochordon* (or skin tag) is a small, flesh-colored, polypoid tumor composed of fibrous epithelial elements and is never malignant. *Mesodermal vulvar tumors are infrequent,* although leiomyomas arise from the round ligament and fibromas and lipomas also occur. *Neurofibromas* are usually small lesions that arise from the neural sheath and are of little consequence unless associated with general neurofibromatosis (von Recklinghausen disease).

VULVAR DYSTROPHIES

Disorders of vulvar epithelial growth and nutrition produce numerous nonspecific gross changes collectively termed vulvar dystrophies. These abnormalities are divided into *hypertrophic, atrophic, and mixed types.* Generally, the lesions are circumscribed or diffuse white lesions of the vulva and do not have a uniform microscopic appearance throughout. Therefore, *multiple biopsies* are necessary. The toluidine blue test and colposcopy may assist in detailing areas most suitable for biopsy. *The malignant potential of vulvar dystrophies is <5%.* Table 20-2 is the International Society for the Study of Vulvar Disease classification of vulvar dystrophies.

Treatment of atrophic dystrophies is *topical* 2% testosterone proprionate in petrolatum bid for 1 week, then daily, gradually decreasing to one to two applications per week. Androgenic side effects may occur—thus the amount used should be minimal. Control of itching is accomplished by removal of any source of irritation (e.g., nylon panties, use of strong soaps), intermittent Burrow's solution wet dressings (bid or tid), and topical fluorinated corticosteroid (e.g., 0.025%–0.1% triamcinolone acetonide) bid for 1–2 weeks. Because these latter compounds may cause vulvar atrophy and contracture, the dose must be decreased as symptoms subside. *Surgical repair* is indicated in cases of lichen sclerosis with severe constriction of the vulva at the posterior fourchette.

TABLE 20-2

CLASSIFICATION OF VULVAR DYSTROPHIES ADOPTED BY THE INTERNATIONAL SOCIETY FOR THE STUDY OF VULVAR DISEASE

	Clinical Features	Histologic Features
Lichen sclerosis	Pruritic, thin, parchment-like atrophic area; introital stenosis	Thin, loss of rete homogenization; inflammatory infiltrate
Hyperplastic[a]	Pruritic, thick, gray or white plaques on skin or mucosa	Acanthosis, hyperkeratosis, inflammatory infiltrate
Mixed[a]	Areas compatible with both forms may be present at the same time	(See above)

[a]Atypia may accompany hyperplastic dystrophy and is graded as mild, moderate, or severe.

HYPERTROPHIC DYSTROPHIES

Chronic vaginal infection or other chronic irritation may cause benign *epithelial thickening and hyperkeratosis*. In the acute phase, this lesion may be red and moist, often with evidence of secondary infection. Following subsequent epithelial thickening and maceration, a raised white lesion (lichen simplex chronicus or neurodermatitis) often develops, which may involve any of the external genital area. Diagnosis is afforded by multiple biopsy assessment. Characteristically, hyperkeratosis and acanthosis with thickening of the epithelium and elongation of the rete pegs occur. If advancement to atypical hyperplasia or carcinoma in situ occurs, expect pleomorphism and loss of epithelial cellular polarity. The patient must be reexamined periodically to rule out advancement to frank cancer. *Surgical excision of more advanced lesions is indicated.*

ATROPHIC DYSTROPHIES

Lichen sclerosis et atrophicus (LSA) is a cutaneous degenerative disorder of unknown cause. The vulva is most frequently affected, but the skin of the back, axillas, beneath the breast, neck, and arms also may be affected. The topical disease can occur in most age groups but is *most common in white women >65 years.* In the perineal area, LSA classically involves the vulvar, perineal, and perianal areas in an hourglass pattern. The skin is white, thin, and wrinkled, and there may be surface atrophy of the labia minora and majora. The chief symptom is *pruritus.*

Microscopically, LSA is distinguished by hyperkeratosis, epithelial atrophy, and flattening of the rete pegs. Beneath the epidermis is a homogeneous, collagenous, acellular, pink-staining zone. Below this lies a concentration of plasma cells. Cellular pleomorphism and loss of epithelial cell polarity are typical. Although the lesion appears atrophic, the rate of cellular turnover is higher than in normal skin or many hypertrophic lesions. Thus, there is an *enhanced rate of malignancy.*

Treatment of hypertrophic and atrophic lesions involves eliminating infection and the cautious use of estrogenic creams or topical corticosteroids and testosterone (e.g., 1% hydrocortisone and 2%–3% testosterone tid to qid). Treat carcinoma in situ or invasive cancer in a dystrophic area definitively. Lesser vulvar intraepithelial neoplasias (VIN I or mild dysplasia, VIN II or moderate dysplasia) should be treated conservatively to relieve symptoms. However, arrange close follow-up for signs of progression.

VULVAR CARCINOMA IN SITU

SQUAMOUS CELL CARCINOMA

A vulvar carcinoma in situ (CIS) is diagnosed when the *full epithelial thickness is replaced by hyperchromatic cells* with poorly defined cellular boundaries. Increased cellular density, abnormal mitoses, multinucleated cells, and increased nuclear/cytoplasmic ratios may also be noted. Chronic infections, granulomatous disease, and the vulvar dystrophies have long been associated with enhanced susceptibility to vulvar CIS. There is increasing evidence that papillomavirus infections may play a major role in the etiology of vulvar intraepithelial neoplasia (VIN). VIN is most often found in women >40 years of age. However, with evidence of papillomavirus, the median age falls to ~31 years. *The progression rate from VIN to carcinoma appears to be low.*

CIS of the vulva is likely to be located *posterior to the vaginal orifice* in the vulvar and perineal areas. VIN III (severe dysplasia and CIS), like the vulvar dystrophies and VIN I and II, is most frequently *multifocal, and contiguous areas may be affected.* For example, with vulvar CIS the following may be affected: anus (22%), clitoral glans (18%), vagina (10%), and urethral meatus (2%).

The *symptoms of vulvar CIS usually are nonspecific* (e.g., mild irritation or itching). The gross appearance of the vulva with CIS is *variable* (white patches, reddish nodules, dystrophic areas, pigmented nevi). Biopsy is mandatory to establish the diagnosis. Because the lesions are usually discrete and multifocal, the toluidine blue test or colposcopy or both are helpful to identify the correct area(s) for sampling. Colposcopic examination will not reveal the characteristic tissue and vascular patterns often found on the cervix, but it is useful in identifying white or pigmented lesions for biopsy.

The *toluidine blue test,* which stains nuclei in the superficial epithelium, is not diagnostic of CIS, but the dye is a useful adjunct. Aqueous 1% toluidine blue is applied to the vulva, and after drying for >1 min, the excess is gently removed with a cotton swab moistened with 1% acetic acid. The areas retaining a blue color are the ones to be biopsied. Although exfoliative cytology may be useful in ulcerated lesions, it is of much less value for vulvar than for cervical lesions because the thick keratinized skin does not shed cells readily.

Biopsy is easily accomplished using a 4–5 mm Keyes dermal punch after local anesthesia has been administered. The dermal thickness is penetrated, the specimen is elevated, and the underlying stroma is incised. Bleeding may be controlled using pressure or Monsell's solution (ferrous subsulfate) or silver nitrate.

Therapy for CIS requires the removal of all vulvar VIN together with any condylomata acuminata. Currently, the therapeutic modalities include laser vaporization, topical 5-fluorouracil (5-FU), and surgery. Carbon dioxide laser treatment allows healing in 2–3 weeks without scarring. Ablation is usually to a depth of 3–4 mm under local or general anesthesia. More than one therapy session may be necessary for very extensive lesions. The use of 5-FU will successfully eliminate CIS in ~75% of patients, but it causes vulvar edema, and severe pain may be reported for ~6 weeks. Wide local excision has all but been replaced by laser therapy. Should surgical therapy be necessary, wide local excision, a skinning vulvectomy (i.e., removal of the superficial vulvar skin and replacement with a split-thickness graft while preserving the clitoris) and simple vulvectomy are options. Prognosis for patients with CIS is good with all modes of therapy.

PAGET'S DISEASE

This *rare vulvar intraepithelial lesion,* which most often affects postmenopausal Caucasian women, is associated with other vulvar disorders (31%) or more distant carcinoma or CIS. The latter group approaches 30% of cases and includes the breast, cervix, rectum, urethra, and skin. Therefore, *identification of vulvar Paget's disease mandates a thorough search for other cancers.*

Vulvar Paget's disease may be confused with other chronic pruritic vulvar lesions. Paget's disease is typically a *velvety, red skin discoloration* that comes to resemble eczema with secondary maceration and the development of white plaques. It is *slowly growing* but may spread to the perineum, perianal area, or thighs. The primary *symptom is pruritus. Biopsy is mandatory,* and Paget cells on microscopy are pathognomonic (it is equivalent to Paget's disease of the breast).

Extramammary Paget's disease is an in situ lesion that warrants *simple vulvectomy* with careful pathologic examination, including the surgical margins. *Local recurrence* is a major problem, and repeated local surgical excisions may be necessary. However, *progression to adenocarcinoma is rare.* Women with vulvar Paget's disease posttherapy should have an annual breast evaluation (Chapter 17), vulvar evaluation, cervical cytologic study, and screening for malignant gastrointestinal disease.

CANCER OF THE VULVA

Cancer of the vulva occurs primarily in postmenopausal women. There is usually a long history of *vulvar irritation, with itching, local discomfort, and possibly bloody discharge.* Whereas early lesions may appear as chronic vulvar dermatitis, the late lesions appear as nodules, exophytic lesions, or hard ulcerated areas. Diagnosis requires biopsy.

Vulvar tumors are 85%–90% epidermoid in origin. Nonetheless, cancer of the vulva may arise also from the urethra, glandular elements of the vulva, or mucosa of the lower third of the vagina. Vulvar cancers are *intraepithelial or invasive.* Vulvar cancer is the fourth most common female genital cancer (after endometrial, cervical, and ovarian cancer) and accounts for ~5% of gynecologic malignancies. The patient with vulvar malignancy is predisposed also to other malignancies; 22% will have another primary tumor (most commonly of the cervix). The average age of patients with vulvar cancer is *65, and >50% of afflicted women are >50 years.*

The cause of vulvar cancer is unknown, although HSV type 2 and HPV are possible etiologic agents. *Preexisting genital condylomata are the sites of ~5% of vulvar cancers.* Although most patients with vulvar cancer give no history of predisposing conditions, many other local disorders may be present [e.g., hypertrophic and atrophic vulvar dystrophies, chronic granulomatous disorders (especially lymphogranuloma venereum, syphilis, and granuloma inguinale), chronic irritation, extramammary Paget's disease, pigmented moles, irradiation, and intraepithelial carcinoma]. Associated etiologic factors include poor hygiene and lack of proper medical care. The mean age of patients with vulvar CIS is ~10 years less than patients with invasive cancer.

Cancers of the vulva are diagnosed most often (in order of frequency) in the *labia majora, the prepuce of the clitoris, the labia minora, Bartholin gland, and the vaginal vestibule.* Vulvar cancer usually begins as a *surface growth, with ulceration and extension downward and laterally.* Slow growth is typical, and although metastases are unpredictable, the malignant cells may remain in the regional lymph nodes for some time before further dissemination. *Eventual metastases* occur via lymphatic channels of the vulva to the superficial and deep inguinal or femoral nodes and the external iliac and obturator nodes. Since the lymphatics of the vulva cross, tumor cells may spread from one side to the other.

TYPES OF VULVAR CANCER

EPIDERMOID VULVAR CANCER

Epidermoid cancer most frequently involves the anterior half of the vulva and arises in the labia (major and minor) in 65% of patients and in the clitoris in 25%. Over one third of tumors are midline or bilateral. There is no positive correlation as to frequency of metastases between the gross appearance, exophytic (cauliflower-like), ulcerative lesions, or red velvety tumors. The primary determinant of metastases and subsequent outcome is tumor size. However, histologic grading is pertinent to potential metastasis if the tumor is <2 cm.

Typical grade I epidermoid carcinomas of the vulva are composed of well-differentiated spicule or prickle cells, many forming keratin pearls. Occasional mitoses are seen. Malignant cells invade the subepithelial tissues, and leukocytes and lymphocytes infiltrate the stroma and tissues adjacent to the tumor. Grades II and III epidermoid cancers are composed of increasingly poorly differentiated cells. Verrucous carcinoma, a variant of epidermoid cancer, grossly resembles condylomata acuminata. *Local spread is common,* but lymphatic metastasis in elderly patients is uncommon.

MALIGNANT MELANOMA

Malignant melanoma, comprising 6%–11% of all vulvar carcinomas, is the second most common type of vulvar cancer. Melanomas, extremely aggressive malignancies, usually arise from pigmented nevi of the vulva. Melanomas predominantly affect postmenopausal white women. Malignant melanomas most frequently involve the labia minora or the clitoris. Generally, malignant melanomas are single, hyperpigmented, raised, nontender, ulcerated lesions that bleed easily. All malignant melanomas spread early by the venous system. Also, local recurrences are frequent. Treatment is similar to that for squamous cell carcinomas.

BASAL CELL CARCINOMA

Basal cell carcinomas are ulcerative lesions composed of small, rounded, basophilic malignant cells derived from the innermost layer of the epidermis. The cells are arranged in irregular groups and often penetrate the underlying connective tissue. Occasional mitoses are observed, but there is no keratinization. Unlike keratinizing squamous cell carcinoma, *basal cell carcinomas metastasize infrequently and late; however, local recurrence is common.* Basal cell carcinomas account for *2%–3% of vulvar cancers,* and they almost always arise in the skin of the *labia majora.* The usual treatment, is wide *local excision* because the tumor does not metastasize readily. However, ~20% recur. One exception to therapy is the basal–squamous cell type tumor, which requires treatment similar to that for invasive squamous cell carcinoma.

BARTHOLIN GLAND CARCINOMA

Although the cure rates are the same, stage by stage, for Bartholin gland carcinoma and squamous cell carcinoma, two factors make Bartholin gland carcinomas more dangerous. Generally, the diagnosis of cancer of the Bartholin gland is delayed because it is slightly less accessible than cervical cancer and may be interpreted as a Bartholin cyst. Additionally, because the tumors have access to the lymphatic channels draining the rectum, they may metastasize directly to the deep pelvic lymph nodes. Nonetheless, therapy for Bartholin gland carcinoma is similar to that for squamous cell carcinoma.

VULVAR SARCOMAS

Sarcomas of the vulva represent <2% of vulvar cancers. The most common of these stromal cell cancers are leiomyosarcoma and fibrous histiocytoma. Adenocarcinomas of the vulva (except those of Bartholin origin) are extremely rare. Metastatic cancers to the vulva may come from other genital tract tumors or from the kidney or urethra.

CLINICAL FINDINGS

Pruritus is the most common symptom of *ulcerated vulvar cancer.* A *lump* may be present for months or years before the patient consults a physician. A sore *(ulceration), odorous discharge, and bleeding usually occur later,* but in postgranulomatous cases, these signs often occur early. *Lymphadenopathy is* always suggestive of metastasis. *Pain, a late symptom,* depends on the tumor's size and location as well as the presence or absence of infection. On physical examination, nodular, ulcerative lesions, especially those occurring in postmenopausal women and those containing granulomatous or leukoplakia changes, are particularly suggestive of vulvar cancer.

STAGING

Staging is summarized in Table 20-3.

DIAGNOSTIC PROCEDURES

In the *workup of vulvar carcinoma,* obtain CBC (with differential and HCT), BUN, AST, lactic dehydrogenase, and electrolytes. It is useful also to have a UA, chest x-ray, and IVP. An ECG should help identify patients at risk from anesthesia or operative procedures. A *repeat biopsy* should be obtained if the first is inadequate. Toluidine blue dye may be used to determine better sites for biopsy. Colposcopy

---

TABLE 20-3
STAGING OF CARCINOMA OF THE VULVA[a]

Cases should be classified as carcinoma of the vulva when the primary site of the growth is in the vulva. Tumors present in the vulva as secondary growths from either a genital or extragenital site should be excluded from registration, as should cases of malignant melanoma.

FIGO Nomenclature

Stage 0   Carcinoma in situ.

Stage I   Tumor confined to vulva—2 cm or less in diameter. Nodes are not palpable or are palpable in either groin, not enlarged, mobile (not clinically suspicious of cancer).

Stage II   Tumor confined to the vulva—more than 2 cm in diameter. Nodes are not palpable or are palpable in either groin, not enlarged, mobile (not clinically suspicious of cancer).

Stage III   Tumor of any size with (1) adjacent spread to the urethra and any or all of the vagina, the perineum, and the anus, and/or (2) nodes palpable in either or both groins (enlarged, firm, and mobile, not fixed but clinically suspicious of cancer).

Stage IV   Tumor of any size (1) infiltrating the bladder mucosa or the rectal mucosa or both, including the upper part of the urethral mucosa, and/or (2) fixed to the bone or other distant metastases. Fixed or ulcerated nodes in either or both groins.

TNM Nomenclature

1.1   Primary tumor (T)

TIS, T1, T2, T3, T4

See corresponding FIGO stages.

1.2   Nodal involvement (N)

NX   Not possible to assess the regional nodes.

N0   No involvement of regional nodes.

N1   Evidence of regional node involvement.

N3   Fixed or ulcerated nodes.

(Continued)

TABLE 20-3
(Continued)

	N4	Juxtaregional node involvement.
1.3		Distant metastasis (M)
	MX	Not assessed.
	M0	No (known) distant metastasis.
	M1	Distant metastasis present.
		Specify_____

[a]American Joint Committee for Cancer Staging and End-Results Reporting; Task Force on Gynecologic Sites: Staging System for Cancer at Gynecologic Sites, 1979.

may demonstrate the need for multiple biopsies and detail suspicious areas. *Lymphangiography* is indicated for cancer in stages II-IV (Table 20-3). *Cystoscopy, colposcopy, proctoscopy, or barium enema* is required if the symptoms suggest involvement of pelvic organs by the tumor or injury to pelvic organs during therapy. A *liver scan* is required for malignant melanoma.

TREATMENT

The primary treatment of vulvar cancer (except in those previously noted instances requiring local excision) is *radical vulvectomy and regional lymphadenectomy.* The operative extent may be modified according to the medical condition of the patient or by the site or extent of the cancer.

Lymphadenectomy may involve unilateral or bilateral deep or superficial inguinal lymph node areas. *Cloquet's node* is the highest deep inguinal lymph node beneath the inguinal ligament, and it must be submitted for a frozen section examination. If metastatic disease is present, an *ipsilateral extraperitoneal deep pelvic lymphadenectomy* should be performed eliminating the common iliac, external iliac, hypogastric, presacral, and obturator lymph nodes. *Contralateral lymph node dissections* are usually done if the ipsilateral lymph nodes are positive.

Anemia and metabolic and cardiovascular diseases should be treated intensively before surgery. Preoperatively, broad-spectrum antibiotic therapy for several days may be beneficial if local infection is present. Additionally, minidose heparin prophylaxis (5000 U SC bid or tid) started preoperatively and continued postoperatively is useful to prevent deep venous thrombophlebitis.

Topical fluorouracil (2%–5% bid) has been used for treatment of vulvar CIS. Radiotherapy is not a primary treatment but may be of great value in the treatment of a cancer recurrence, particularly basal cell carcinoma. Radiation also is useful in instances of known incomplete surgery or for palliation of inoperable cancer. Paget's disease and malignant melanoma do not respond well to radiation.

Routine *follow-up* involves examination every 3 months for 2 years and every 6 months thereafter. Five-year survival is ~60% after surgical treatment of invasive squamous cell carcinoma. With tumors 2 cm diameter, the incidence of nodal metastasis is 10%–15%, and when nodal metastasis occurs, the 5-year survival rate is 15%–30%. Operative mortality rate is ~5%, and death may be due to cardiovascular complications, primary or secondary hemorrhage, infection, or venous thrombosis.

CANCER OF THE VAGINA

Cancer of the vagina is usually asymptomatic and is most often revealed by abnormal vaginal cytology. Early in its course, there may be painless bleeding from an ulcerated tumor. In late cases, expect pain, bleeding, weight loss, or local swelling. *Squamous cell carcinoma represents ~85% of primary vaginal cancers.* The rest (in decreasing frequency) includes adenocarcinomas, sarcomas, and melanomas. Primary cancer of the vagina represents ~1%–2% of gynecologic malignancies and usually develops about 10 years after the menopause.

Two special vaginal carcinomas are noteworthy: clear cell carcinoma and sarcoma botryoides. Clear cell carcinoma of the cervix or vagina occurs in females age 10–30 years whose mother received diethylstilbestrol during early pregnancy. The tumor is multicentric but is most commonly found in the upper third of the vagina. Sarcoma botryoides occurs most frequently in young children. In all cases, however, loose connective tissue and rich vascular lymphatic circulation favor rapid growth and early cancer dissemination. Tumors of the lower vagina metastasize in the same manner as vulvar cancer, whereas those in the upper vagina spread like cervical cancer.

Painless bleeding is the initial manifestation in ~50% of cases of carcinoma of the vagina. Primary vaginal carcinoma must be distinguished from extensions of the vulvar or cervical cancer and cancer metastasis from the urinary tract, gastrointestinal tract, or ovary. Staging is summarized in Table 20-4.

The preferred treatment is *radiation. Radical surgery* (exenteration) should be reserved for vaginal cancers near the introitus, for sarcomas, and for definitely localized cancers involving the urethra

TABLE 20-4
STAGING OF CARCINOMA OF THE VAGINA[a]

Preinvasive carcinoma

Stage	0	Carcinoma in situ, intraepithelial carcinoma.

Invasive carcinoma

Stage	I	Carcinoma limited to the vaginal wall.
Stage	II	Carcinoma has involved the subvaginal tissue but has not extended to the pelvic wall.
Stage	III	Carcinoma has extended to the pelvic wall.
Stage	IV	Carcinoma has extended beyond the true pelvis or involved the mucosa of the bladder or rectum. Bullous edema as such does not permit allotment of a case to stage IV.
Stage IVA		Spread of carcinoma to adjacent organs.
Stage IVB		Spread to distant organs.

[a]American Joint Committee for Cancer Staging and End-Results Reporting; Task Force on Gynecologic Sites: Staging System for Cancer at Gynecologic Sites, 1979.

or bladder. Prognosis depends on the type, location, extent of the tumor, and treatment response. With adequate treatment, the 5-year survival in stage I and II of carcinoma is *70%–75%*. Few malignant melanomas respond to treatment. Adequate survival data are not available for sarcoma of the vagina, but the prognosis for most patients is poor.

CHAPTER

21

THE CERVIX

ANOMALIES OF THE FEMALE GENITAL TRACT

Malformations occur in nearly 10% of female genital tracts. Known genetic problems cause 20%, about 5% are due to chromosome aberrations, and approximately 10% are due to environmental causes. Multifactorial inheritance (e.g., a combination of environment and genetics) probably accounts for the rest.

Anomalies of the vulva and labia are rare. They include bifid clitoris (occurs most frequently with bladder exstrophy), congenital vaginal prolapse, and vulvar duplication (seen with duplication of the urinary and intestinal tracts). Occasionally, one labia is much larger than the other. If therapy is required, surgical excision is easily accomplished.

Anomalies of the hymen occur frequently, as it is the most variable structure of the genitalia. The variations include imperforate hymen, variation of orifice diameter, more than one orifice, thickening of the membrane, or a median ridge between two orifices. The imperforate hymen requires opening or early complications of mucocolpos or hematocolpos will occur. Later complications may include endometriosis and adenomyosis.

Vaginal anomalies include transverse and longitudinal vaginal septa. Transverse vaginal septa are discussed on pages (p. 531). Longitudinal vaginal septa are commonly associated with cervical or uterine anomalies or both. A double vagina is found in association with duplication of the cervix. When asymptomatic, these defects require no therapy. One of the more common associations of total vaginal agenesis is the Rokitansky sequence (p. 532).

Uterine anomalies usually occur as a result of failure of mullerian fusion. The potential defects include subseptate uterus, arcuate uterus, bicornuate uterus, unicornuate uterus, rudimentary uterine horn, uterus didelphys, duplex cervix, cervical atresia, and septate vagina. The most serious complications of these defects are

597

problems of reproduction. Various surgical corrections are feasible but are beyond the scope of this text.

Fallopian tube anomalies are rare. They include aplasia, atresia, and duplication (particularly distal).

The most common ovarian anomalies include *anomalous ovarian descent,* in which the ovary may be in the inguinal canal or the labia majora. Complete *ovarian agenesis* occurs if the primordial gonads do not form. Agonadism is the formation of the ovaries, followed by degeneration. These and other ovarian anomalies, including gonadal dysgenesis, are discussed in Chapter 23. In Turner's syndrome (45,XO), the patients have height and weight <3rd percentile, broad chest and small nipples, webbed neck, aortic coarctation, prominent epicanthal folds, nevi, and short fourth metacarpals. Karyotyping should be performed in all dysgenetic patients. The presence of a Y chromosome increases the incidence of neoplasia in the genital ridge.

Clinically, *most genital tract anomalies confront the physician at the time of birth or at the menarche* (Chapter 18). At birth, ambiguous genitalia or other problems of sexual identification must be resolved (Chapter 18) to obviate sexual misassignment. This is usually accomplished by careful physical examination, pelvic ultrasound, hormonal assessment, and karyotype. Some problems of sex identification may be described as female or male pseudohermaphroditism or true hermaphroditism. *Female pseudohermaphroditism* is masculinization of a female fetus in utero. The most common abnormality is clitoral enlargement, although varying labial fusion, hypospadiac urethral meatus, and a malpositioned vaginal orifice may also be present. Female pseudohermaphroditism may be fetal in origin (congenital adrenal hyperplasia) or maternal (exogenous androgens, exogenous androgenic progestins, or secondary to functional ovarian tumors or tumors of the adrenal gland).

Male pseudohermaphroditism is seen most often in the androgen insensitivity syndrome (*testicular feminization syndrome*) in which the karyotype is 46,XY but the individual appears female. This is an X-linked genetic disorder. Another possible cause (albeit rare) is *genetic mosaicism.*

True hermaphroditism (rare) occurs when there is dual gonadal development. Some of these individuals are genetic mosaics, but most are 46,XX. The degree of masculinization depends on the amount of testicular tissue present.

Intrauterine exposure to diethylstilbestrol (DES) or analogs is associated later with clear cell carcinoma of the vagina or cervix. Other vaginal abnormalities include vaginal adenosis, incomplete septa, fibrous bands, and segmental vaginal narrowing. Intrauterine *exposure to DES also causes uterine deformity* (T-shaped uterus with hysterography) and cervical abnormalities, including incompetent cervix, complete or incomplete circular sulcus, recessed areas surrounding the external os, portio vaginalis completely covered by columnar epithelium, pseudopolyp formation due to localized, eccentric hypertrophy of endocervical tissue, and rough or smooth anterior cervical lip protuberances. The end result of these defects (cancer not included) is a higher than expected reproductive wastage.

CERVICAL EVERSION

The squamous epithelial covering of the cervix normally extends to or just within the external os. Thus, *when the endocervical columnar epithelium replaces the squamous epithelium on the external cervix, it is termed an eversion.* This is a physiologic process that occurs when hormonal factors cause endocervical hypertrophy and hyperplasia. The resultant increased tissue has only the opportunity for expansion to the exterior. Although the process may enhance the amount of vaginal discharge, the columnar epithelium is not as resistant to trauma or infection as is squamous epithelium. Hence, this process contributes to cervicitis. Cervical eversion does not require topical therapy, only observation to differentiate it from an erosion or ulceration (localized loss of the cervical mucosa).

When the abnormal hormonal stimulus is not present, the condition reverts to or toward normal. However, another process of resolution is that of *squamous metaplasia of the columnar epithelium.* As this superficial epidermidization occurs, deeply infolded columnar epithelia may remain unchanged. The gland openings are often narrowed to form mucous collections, termed *nabothian cysts.* Their appearance is usually sufficient to differentiate them from the other cystic cervical lesions (e.g., mesonephric cysts or endometriosis). *Mesonephric cysts* are remnants of the wolffian duct and are present deep in the stroma external to the external os. They may reach 2.5 cm in diameter and contain a ragged cuboidal epithelium. They usually require no therapy. *Endometriosis* is manifest on the cervix as small (generally <2 mm) reddish to purple to nearly black cysts on the ectocervix. Patients with cervical endometriosis are more likely to have internal endometriosis also. Biopsy of the lesion should reveal the endometrial glands, stroma, and perhaps, old blood. Therapy is cauterization or excision.

CERVICITIS

Nonspecific chronic cervicitis probably affects at least 50% of all women at some point in life. Eversion (with trauma and infection) and puerperal lacerations are probably the two major etiologic factors, although, poor hygiene, diminished resistance to infection, and irritation (e.g., retained tampon) also may be causative. The three most common organisms cultured are *staphylococci, streptococci, and chlamydia.* However, many other vaginal organisms may cause the problem. Rarely, very unexpected organisms (e.g., *Corynebacterium diphtheriae*) cause cervicitis. The usual symptomatology is *leukorrhea* (purulent discharge, often with a disagreeable odor) or vulvar–vaginal irritation (itching or burning). Backache, lower abdominal pain, dyspareunia, dysmenorrhea, dysuria, and postcoital spotting may also occur. The clinical signs depend on the stage of the infection. When acute (hours to 2 days), the cervix is reddened, and the discharge indicates acute inflammation. During this stage, the *cervix is tender when moved.* After the acute stage, the signs of chronic cervicitis are those of chronic infection: a pus-laden cervical mucus, friable and vascular surface tissue, gland infection, and cervical hypertrophy.

The *cervical cytology may be obscured by infection,* and it is often necessary to resolve the infection before a meaningful cervical cytological study can be obtained. The *usual workup* includes investigation for the common causes of vaginitis and cervicitis (*Trichomonas vaginalis, Candida albicans,* and *bacterial vaginosis*), monoclonal immunofluorescent stains for *Chlamydia,* and culture for *Neisseria gonorrhoeae.* Both herpes simplex and human papillomavirus (see p. 577, 578) may infect the cervix.

The *differential diagnosis* of cervicitis includes an early neoplastic process, chancre, chancroid, tuberculosis, and granuloma inguinale. Specific therapy (Chapter 24) is administered for the causative organism(s). Local therapy (vaginal acidification, removal of irritants, improved hygiene) is beneficial. Local surgical therapy (incision, excision, coagulation, and conization) is infrequently applied, but cryosurgery is commonly used to treat a severe chronic infection. Complete healing generally requires 2–3 months, with reestablishment of normal mucosa. *Colposcopy is especially useful in evaluation of atypical cases or those with unusual findings.*

CERVICAL INJURIES

Cervical lacerations due to childbirth are common. Gross lacerations occur in any quadrant. These are of varying length, may bleed extensively, and can contribute to both immediate and delayed postpartum hemorrhage. They should be repaired at the time of delivery. Nonapparent submucosal separation of the fibrous connective tissue stroma may occur at the level of the internal cervical os and later become apparent as an incompetent cervix. Although nonobstetric *cervical lacerations may occur with instrumentation* (e.g., D & C), they are unusual and, except for cases of postmenopausal atrophy, chronic inflammation, or extreme fibrosis, are largely preventable.

Other cervical injuries may include *perforation* (self-induced or iatrogenic) and *ulcerations from tampons or pessaries. Annular detachment* is rare but may occur when the external os fails to dilate and the prolonged pressure of the fetal head causes vascular infarction.

Cervical stenosis may be of congenital, inflammatory, or neoplastic origin but most commonly is postsurgical (electrocoagulation, cryotherapy, laser vaporization, or conization). Dysmenorrhea may result, and complete occlusion may cause hematometra. Therapy is careful surgical dilation.

CERVICAL NEOPLASIA

BENIGN (CERVICAL POLYPS)

Cervical polyps are relatively common in the reproductive age group. There are two primary types of cervical polyps, *endocervical and ectocervical. The majority are endocervical polyps,* which are small, usually pedunculated (but occasionally sessile) tumors, composed of proliferative columnar epithelium with a vascular and connective tissue supporting structure. They originate from the endocervix and may occur at the external os as red, soft, friable tumors a few millimeters to several centimeters in diameter and on a stalk that can be 1 cm or more in length. Polyps may cause discharge or abnormal bleeding. Occasionally, a submucous uterine or cervical leiomyoma on a pedicle will occur at the cervix.

Local inflammation may play a fundamental role in the formation of cervical polyps. Occasionally, polyps arise from the cervical portio. These *ectocervical polyps are covered with squamous epithelium* and are more often sessile, fibrous, and less likely to bleed than endocervical polyps.

Local *complications of polyps* include torsion, necrosis of the tip, and infection. Although metaplasia is common, anaplasia is rare. Cervical cytology often indicates inflammatory atypia. The differential diagnosis must include products of conception, endometrial polyps (benign, adenocarcinoma or sarcoma), and a prolapsed leiomyoma. Malignant transformation of a polyp is uncommon (<1%). The usual therapy is polypectomy, which may be accomplished by avulsion (often with simultaneous torsion) or excision. The base is often curetted or electrocoagulated. Recurrence is common, not because polyps per se are recidive but because the factor(s) that caused the primary episode persist.

CERVICAL DYSPLASIA AND CANCER

The incidence of cervical cancer has decreased remarkably over the past 50 years, and it is now the *sixth most common cancer in U.S. women.* The decrease is thought to be the result of screening (cervical cytology, the Papanicolaou smear) and prevention (therapy for preinvasive disease). Nonetheless, between 1% and 2% of all women >40 years will develop cervical cancer. The *average age at diagnosis is 45–47 years,* but the disease can occur much earlier. *Squamous cell carcinoma constitutes 87% of cases,* and nearly all the rest are adenocarcinoma or adenosquamous carcinoma. Sarcomas and other malignancies are rare. Of the U.S. women developing cervical cancer, >50% have not been screened within 3 years. However, cervical cancer is a much larger problem worldwide and in many countries (e.g., Thailand) cervical cancer is the most common cancer in women.

Uterine cervix dysplasia and cancer are both etiologically linked to human papillomavirus (HPV) infections. Although HPV has a high prevalence in all human populations, it has a peak incidence at 20–24 years of age and subsequently gradually declines to ~40–45 years. HPV is a pleiomorphic virus with literally hundreds of types, subtypes or variants. *HPV DNA (as infectious virions, episomal or integrated DNA) is detected in 90% of cervical cancers and 80%–90% of cervical dysplasias.*

Although HPV infection is undoubtedly the most important etiologic agent in the development of cervical dysplasia and cancer, there are *likely other factors operative,* including: shifts in number of target cells, regeneration, microorganism infection (e.g. chlamydia), hormones, smoking, and immunity. Epidemiological risk factors for cervical intraepithelial neoplasia (CIN) include: early age at first intercourse, multiple sexual partners, oral contraceptive use, high parity, lower socioeconomic status, poor diet, immunosuppression, and promiscuous male sexual partners. Indeed, males may be a relatively symptomless reservoir.

Only a portion of infected females develop condyloma. Most condyloma are polyclonal, heterogenous, self-limited (up to 12 months) proliferative cellular responses to low grade HPV infection and are at most slightly dysplastic. However, *10%–20% of infections persist.* Although, these infections create risk of CIN, the degree of risk and the amount of time for the process to be expressed (as well as progressing to cancer) remains unknown. There is evidence in low grade squamous intraepithelial lesions (*LGSIL*) that *75% will spontaneously resolve, 19%–20% will remain unchanged, and only 5%–6% will progress within a year.* Unfortunately, there is incomplete data concerning LGSIL recurrence as well as comparable data concerning high grade squamous intraepithelial lesions (HGSIL).

Nonetheless, in patients *with CIN there is serological evidence of HPV infection years before onset of the disease.* This minority of HPV infections are marked by the simultaneous presence or subsequent development of distinctly monoclonal higher grade dysplasia and in situ or invasive cancer. Moreover, there is good evidence that *cervical neoplasia occurs in a stepwise fashion* progressing from infection to: integration of oncogenic HPV, specific genetic alterations, and eventual histological expression of the neoplasia. Several issues potentially influencing the relationship between infection and neoplasia follow.

- *Viral type.* Most genital condyloma are caused by the low risk HPV types 6 or 11. High risk HPV (usually 16 or 18) is associated with high grade dysplasia and in situ cancer.
- *Mechanisms of cellular transformation.* Mechanisms potentially capable of explaining the cellular transformation in the cervical transformation zone include clonal selection of cells with increasingly undifferentiated phenotypes and independent development of different morphological types of premalignancy.
- *A small, but susceptible target cell population.* Cells in the transformation zone targeted by HPV have the capacity for both squamous and glandular differentiation. Different HPV types appear to influence this differentiation: low risk with squamous, HPV 16 usually with squamous, and HPV 18 with adenosquamous or adenomatous.
- *Factors influencing viral-host interaction.* A variety of factors influence whether the lesions regress, persist, or progress: over expression of viral E6 and E7 genes, activity of specific HPV variants, and inactivation of TP53 (with decreased capacity for DNA repair), and host immunological competency.

Currently, research is very active in the HPV–dysplasia association. This is certainly the case for screening methods. At the present, two consensus primer systems (MY09/11 and the GP+5/+6 pairs) and a second generation hybrid capture system (HC-II) are under most extensive use and scrutiny for HPV DNA detection.

These methods have high absolute sensitivity and potential for automation. HPV seroreactivity to a given type reflects mainly type-specific HPV infection (as measured by DNA detection), but also signals past exposure to other types that may be serologically detected.

Although HPV DNA testing has demonstrated capability to improve the detection rate of HGSIL, the *exact role of HPV DNA testing to detect or follow cervical dysplasia or cervical cancer is currently being defined.* The possibilities being considered for HPV DNA testing include utilization as: a sole primary screening modality, as an adjunct to cytology, the triage of borderline and mild dysplasia, the follow-up of certain HGSIL after therapy. Two advantages of the HPV DNA testing is that it may be obtained in self-collected vaginal samples and self-collected samples are at least as good for detection as those collected by a physician. Self-collection may increase screening in settings where cytology is not readily or always performed.

The *sensitivity of HPV DNA testing for high grade CIN is 75%–95% and for cervical cancer is 93%–95%.* However, there is considerable variability of the HPV positivity rate in women with no cervical epithelial neoplasia (3%–20%). To date, HPV DNA testing compared to cytology for the detection of HGSIL has: greater sensitivity, lower specificity, and a relatively unknown false negativity rate. Additionally, cost-effectiveness of HPV DNA testing when more widely applied is still to be determined.

It is known that women with minor *cytological abnormalities who test negative for HPV have a low risk of developing high grade CIN within 3 years.* Thus, it has been suggested that using HPV DNA testing in combined screening with cytology offers the possibility of greater protection and/or longer screening intervals. However, the risk of reduced surveillance in HPV negative women has not been determined.

Recent reports indicate some *specific circumstances where HPV DNA testing may be useful including women with low-grade or borderline smears, post surveillance of CIN, and early cancer being monitored for complete excision.* An additional area where HPV testing may be useful is in the *immunocompromised.* For example, women with HIV are at increased risk of cervical neoplasia, yet cytological screening is limited by a high rate of inflammatory disease. The conjunctive use of HPV DNA testing may assist in determining those needing more aggressive follow-up and therapy.

In attempting to assess screening methods for detection of cervical dysplasia or cancer it should be borne in mind that both Pap smear collection methodologies as well as interpretations are also improving. For example, spatulas have been modified with a longer blade to collect endocervical cells. The ThinPrep® process increases detection of premalignant precursors and improved specimen adequacy. Additionally, colposcopy plays a vital role in the evaluation of any abnormalities detected by screening. Colposcopy and histology have a better concordance than cytology and histology in diagnosis of SIL.

Cervical cancer is the end result of progressive cervical epithelial alterations, most commonly (~90%) occurring at the squamocolumnar junction. The exact etiology is unknown, but risk factors for the continuum of cervical dysplasia and cancer are multiple sexual partners, early first coitus (<20 years), young age at marriage, young age of first pregnancy, high parity, lower socioeconomic status, and smoking.

CERVICAL INTRAEPITHELIAL NEOPLASIA (CIN)

The process whereby cervical cancer usually occurs begins with cervical intraepithelial neoplasia. CIN may occur soon after early sexual activity (teen years), with a *peak incidence by 25–35 years. CIN affects 1.2%–3.8% of nonpregnant women.* If CIN is untreated, carcinoma in situ *(CIS) appears at about 30–40 years.* The degree of CIN is determined by the extent to which the neoplastic cells involve the full thickness of the cervical epithelium. CIN I (mild dysplasia) indicates that the neoplastic cells are confined to the lower third of the epithelium. In CIN II (moderate dysplasia), the neoplastic cells occupy up to two thirds of the epithelial thickness, and CIN III (severe dysplasia) comprises undifferentiated neoplastic cells extending almost to the surface. CIN III also includes CIS, in which the undifferentiated neoplastic cells extend the full thickness of the epithelium. CIN may follow three courses: regression, persistence, or progression to invasive cancer. The risk of progression increases with increasing anaplasia. Spontaneous regression rarely occurs once CIS is established.

Certain gross changes (e.g., a white surface patch) may suggest CIN, but *colposcopy will often aid in the diagnosis.* Suggestive colposcopic findings include coarse mosaicism and punctation. Ultimately, diagnosis depends on *colposcopically directed biopsy* or cervical conization. At the time of biopsy or conization, a thorough endocervical curettage should be performed.

CANCER OF THE CERVIX

Although >95% of cancers of the cervix can be cured, about 80,000 women in the United States die of this disorder each year. Earlier diagnosis and proper therapy will continue to reduce this loss.

PATHOGENICITY

Most incipient *cancers of the cervix develop slowly,* passing through dysplasia to acute malignancy. It has been estimated that the transition from CIS to invasive cancer *requires approximately 7 years.* Most cancers of the cervix develop in the cellularly active intraepithelial layer at the squamocolumnar junction.

Initial stromal invasion to even 2 mm beyond the basement membrane is a localized process requiring months to years. Beyond this point, however, lymphatic or hematogenous penetration and metastases occur. Lymphatic spread of malignant disease to the regional lymph nodes (parametrial, hypogastric, obturator, external iliac, sacral) is far more frequent than spread via the bloodstream, (e.g., to the lungs or brain).

The *more pleomorphic or extensive the cancer, the more likely are nodal metastases.* If squamous cell carcinoma is confined to the cervix (stage I), pelvic lymph node metastases occur in 15%–20% of cases. Once the parametrium is involved (stage IIB), carcinoma will be present in the lymph nodes in ~35% of cases. Paraaortic lymph node inclusion of cervical cancer must be expected in about half of patients with stage III lesions.

PATHOLOGY

About 87% of cancers of the cervix are of the squamous type. The rest include adenocarcinomas, adenosquamous carcinomas, and occasional sarcomas.

Epidermoid cancers of the cervix are graded according to predominant cell type. The degree of differentiation expressed as grades 1–3 roughly parallels the malignant potential of epidermoid carcinoma of the cervix.

In grade 1, the well-differentiated carcinomas, there are many well-keratinized epithelial cells, often in pearls or clusters, with identifiable intercellular bridges and <2 mitoses per high-power field (hpf). Overall, minimal variation in the size and shape of tumor cells is evident.

In *grade 2,* there are infrequent epithelial pearls, moderate keratinization, occasional intercellular bridges, 2–4 mitoses/hpf, and moderate variation in the size and shape of tumor cells.

In *grade 3,* expect no epithelial pearls, only slight keratinization, and no intercellular bridges. More than 4 mitoses/hpf is usual, with marked variation in the size and shape of the tumor cells. Occasional small, elongated, closely packed tumor cells are present together with numerous giant cells.

Undifferentiated malignant squamous cell tumors metastasize earlier than do well-differentiated cancers, but the latter also respond well to radiation therapy. Tumor cells near or involving blood vessels increase the risk of hematogenous spread, which worsens the prognosis. In contrast, collections of lymphocytes surrounding tumor cells indicate a reduced likelihood of metastases and a better prognosis.

Adenocarcinomas of the cervix, derived from glandular elements of the endocervix, are tall, columnar, secretory cells arranged in an adenomatous pattern supported by stroma cells. An uncommon but often virulent adenocarcinoma arises from mesonephric (wolffian) duct remnants within the cervix. This tumor is composed of small cuboidal, slightly irregular cells in a poorly defined glandular pattern.

Adenocarcinomas of the cervix are graded as well-differentiated, moderately differentiated, and poorly differentiated. Considerable variability in various areas makes more precise grading impossible. Regrettably, adenocarcinomas of the cervix usually are concealed within the cervical canal and, therefore, are rarely diagnosed until they are ulcerated, (i.e., advanced).

During pregnancy, marked changes in the endocervix occur, including hypertrophy and hyperplasia of glandular cells. These changes, evident on biopsy or curettage, may be surprising. However, gestational changes should not be permitted to confuse the diagnosis of cancer.

CLINICAL FINDINGS

Signs and Symptoms

There are no signs or symptoms of noninvasive cancer of the cervix. However, periodic testing (e.g., cytologic assessment by Pap smears, colposcopy, and biopsy) and a high index of suspicion must be applied.

Postcoital spotting or blood-tinged leukorrhea is often an early sign of ulcerative cervical cancer. Hence, some form of intermenstrual bleeding is the most common symptom or sign of invasive cervical malignancy.

Bladder or rectal discomfort or dysfunction and fistulas are late manifestations of cancer of the cervix. Pain, often unilateral and radiating to the hip, may develop with advanced cervical cancer when the ureter becomes partially occluded or when the sacral nerves are involved by the tumor. *Anemia, anorexia, and weight loss are signs of advanced malignant disease.*

Staging

Staging, or the plotting of the probable extent of malignant cervical disease, is essential for treatment and prognosis. Numerous staging schemes have been suggested, and the International Classification of Cancer of the Cervix (Table 21-1) is commonly used.

TABLE 21-1
INTERNATIONAL CLASSIFICATION OF CANCER OF THE CERVIX[a]

Preinvasive carcinoma	
Stage 0	Carcinoma in situ, intraepithelial carcinoma.
Invasive carcinoma	
Stage I	Carcinoma strictly confined to the cervix (extension to the corpus should be disregarded).
IA	Microinvasive carcinoma (early stromal invasion).
IB	All other cases of stage I. (Occult cancer should be labeled "occ.")
Stage II	Carcinoma extends beyond the cervix but has not extended onto the pelvic wall. The carcinoma involves the vagina but not the lower third.
IIA	No obvious parametrial involvement.
IIB	Obvious parametrial involvement.
Stage III	Carcinoma has extended to the pelvic wall. On rectal examination, there is no cancer-free space between the tumor and the pelvic wall. The tumor involves the lower third of the vagina. All cases with hydronephrosis or nonfunctioning kidney.
IIIA	No extension onto the pelvic wall.
IIIB	Extension onto the pelvic wall and/or hydronephrosis or nonfunctioning kidney.
Stage IV	Carcinoma extended beyond the true pelvis or clinically involving the mucosa of the bladder or rectum. Do not allow a case of bullous edema as such to be allotted to stage IV.
IVA	Spread of growth to adjacent organs (i.e., rectum or bladder with positive biopsy from these organs).
IVB	Spread of growth to distant organs.

[a]American Joint Committee for Cancer Staging and End-Results Reporting: Task Force on Gynecologic Sites: Staging System for Cancer at Gynecologic Sites, 1979.

DIAGNOSIS

Biopsy and the microscopic assessment of tissue obtained are essential for the diagnosis of cancer or its elimination. Where to biopsy is especially important.

Because necrosis and inflammatory elements are present in bleeding, presumably invasive cancer of the cervix, biopsies from an ulcerative area may be useless or difficult to interpret. Therefore, *obtain biopsies from the edge of the lesion,* where normal and malignant tissue offer a contrast. This may be facilitated by the Schiller test.

Schiller Test

Aqueous solutions of iodine stain the surface of the normal cervix brown because normal cervical epithelial cells contain glycogen. Areas of cancer within the epithelium over the cervix do not contain glycogen, and these remain unstained when Schiller's solution or Lugol's solution is applied. Hence, biopsy of Schiller-positive areas as well as granular, nodular, or papillary lesions usually will confirm invasive cancer when it is present.

Colposcopy

Colposcopy may identify possible early invasive carcinoma in an area of CIN. Directed biopsies from such suspicious sites may reveal early stromal invasion. Colposcopically directed punch biopsies and light curettage of the endocervix *may obviate a more extensive cone biopsy* of the cervix. Frank invasion usually produces ulceration and bleeding, however, and colposcopy then becomes unnecessary for biopsy.

← ───────────────────────────────

TABLE 21-1 *(Continued)*

Note: The interpretation of the physical and microscopic findings is to some extent subjective, and the personal opinion of the examiner unavoidably influences the staging of various cases. This is especially true with stages II and III. Therefore, when the results of therapy for carcinoma of the cervix are being reported, all cases examined should be reported so that the reader can determine what series of cases in his or her own experience the data apply to. In reporting the results of therapy for stage II carcinoma at a given institution, the statistics for stage III should be included so that the reader may compare the reported results with a more surely comparable series of cases at another institution.

COMPLICATIONS

Metastases to regional lymph nodes occur with increasing frequency from stage I (about 15%) to stage IV (at least 60%).

Extension occurs in all directions. Most commonly, the tumor grows laterally in the base of the broad ligaments on one or both sides. The ureters often are obstructed lateral to the cervix. Hydroureter and hydronephrosis impair kidney function. Almost two thirds of patients with carcinoma of the cervix die of uremia when ureteral obstruction is bilateral. Perivascular, perineural, and lymphatic channels facilitate cancer spread.

Cervical carcinoma *may invade the uterus* by direct surface extension up the cervical canal. Downward extension often involves the *vagina.* Invasion of the *rectum* is by posterior extension from the cervix along the uterosacral ligaments. Anterior progression is followed by invasion of the *bladder* in stages III and IV.

Pain and swelling in the leg, particularly the upper thigh, may indicate lymphatic occlusion or obstruction of the venous return by carcinoma. Pain in the *back* and in the distribution of the lumbosacral plexus indicates chronic infection or neurologic involvement by extending cancer. *Metastasis to the liver is common,* but spread to lung or brain is rare.

Vaginal fistulas involving the gastrointestinal and urinary tracts are particularly discouraging. Incontinence of urine and of feces are major complications, particularly in debilitated individuals. Pelvic infections may complicate cervical carcinoma. Obstruction of the cervical canal may require drainage of a *pyometra* and chemotherapy to resolve infection. *Death due to hemorrhage occurs in about 10%–20%* of cases of extensive invasive carcinoma of the cervix. Protracted bleeding causes anemia.

DIFFERENTIAL DIAGNOSIS

Eversion and redness around the cervical os caused by infection, irritation, or hormonal imbalance are smooth, soft, and minimally irregular. Unlike carcinoma, eversion is not exudative and does not bleed easily.

The small, hard *chancre of primary syphilis* is a shallow, oval, or circular ulceration with a glistening surface and a firm edge and base. There is minimal serous discharge, and bleeding is uncommon. Treponema pallidum may be identified by darkfield examination of the thin exudate. Serologic tests for syphilis are positive.

The characteristics of *chancroid (soft chancre), granuloma inguinale, lymphogranuloma venereum, and cervical tuberculosis* are
described elsewhere.

Abortion of a cervical pregnancy results in a soft, nontender,
deep, freely bleeding cavity, usually within the cervical canal.
Biopsy of the tissue lining the cavity will usually disclose trophoblastic debris but no cancer cells.

Metastatic choriocarcinoma or other secondary cancer must be
considered in the diagnosis, as well as rare conditions, such as actinomycosis, amebiasis, and schistosomiasis.

PREVENTION

The incidence of cervical cancer should be reduced by (1) *improved
personal hygiene,* including prevention and prompt treatment of
vaginitis and cervicitis, male circumcision in infancy, precoital
washing of the penis, and habitual use of condoms; (2) *avoidance
of intercourse at an early age and limiting the number of consorts;*
(3) *regular periodic cytologic screening of all women,* especially
parous women in low socioeconomic groups and those who have
had numerous sexual partners; (4) *prompt evaluation* (colposcopy
and possible biopsy) of any abnormalities detected by screening;
and (5) *treatment of suspicious cervical lesions.*

TREATMENT OF CERVICAL DYSPLASIA

MILD OR MODERATE DYSPLASIA

As noted above (see p. 605) the majority of CIN I or II lesions regress,
some persist, and only a minority progress to CIN III ($\sim$15% and
$\sim$20%, respectively). Therefore, it is reasonable to *follow such patients with medical therapy* (to treat HPV or bacterial infections)
and serial cytologic and/or colposcopic studies every 6 months.
*Cryosurgery, laser therapy, loop electrosurgical excision procedure
(LEEP), and electrocoagulation* are the methods most often used to
treat CIN I or II.

MODERATE TO SEVERE
DYSPLASIA (CIN III)

*CIN III lesions require cryotherapy, laser, LEEP, or definitive sur-
gical therapy. If there is extension up the cervical canal, conization
is required initially.*

SEVERE DYSPLASIA (CIS)

The most effective method of treatment of CIS, and the one usually recommended for women >40, is *total abdominal hysterectomy with a wide vaginal cuff.* Whether to remove the ovaries is a decision that must be based on the patient's age, the status of the ovaries, and family history of cancer. *Cervical conization* may be considered for patients who desire pregnancy or who are reliable and can be carefully supervised. In either case, cervical smears every 6 months are recommended. *LEEP,* compared to standard (cold knife) conization provides: the same sample adequacy for histological evaluation, results in the same success rate, and enhances subsequent colposcopic surveillance.

There seems little question that *inadequate specimen margins in a conization represent potential for disease progression.* An adequate conization specimen is particularly difficult to obtain in HIV infected women. Nearly 50% will have a positive margin rate. Thus conservative management in these patients may need reevaluation.

Adjunctive maintenance intravaginal 5-FU therapy after standard surgery for HGSIL reduces recurrence in HIV infected women. Cidofovir 1% gel inhibits (partially or completely) cervical dysplasia lesion after 3 every other day administrations.

TREATMENT OF CERVICAL CANCER

EMERGENCY MEASURES

Vaginal hemorrhage originates from gross ulceration and cavitation in stage II–IV cervical carcinoma. Ligation of bleeding points and suturing are impractical. *Styptics,* such as negatol (Negatan), 10% silver nitrate solution, or acetone, are effective, although later slough may result in further bleeding. *Vaginal packing or radiation* (if tolerance permits) is helpful. *Embolization or ligation* of the uterine or hypogastric arteries may be lifesaving.

GENERAL MEASURES

A brief hospitalization for thorough study and preparation may be necessary before therapy is begun. The *basics of a cervical cancer workup* include CBC (anemia or infection), liver function tests (liver metastases or liver disease), BUN (impaired renal function or ureteral obstruction), cystoscopy (bladder invasion), sigmoidoscopy (bowel invasion), sonography (to detect tumor masses), chest x-ray (pulmonary disease or metastases), intravenous urograms (obstruction), skeletal survey (metastases), and a barium enema (bowel invasion or disease). Additionally, a pelvic and abdominal CT scan or MRI will assist in detailing local metastases.

It is imperative to eradicate infections (vaginal, urinary, or pelvic) before surgery or radiation. Additionally, anemia must be corrected, any intercurrent diseases controlled, and nutrition improved.

Pain may be controlled with such analgesics as acetaminophen with codeine 8 or 15 mg qid as necessary. *Diarrhea* is often treated with diphenoxylate (Lomotil) 2.5 mg, loperamide (Imodium) 2 mg, or paregoric 4–8 mL qid as necessary. For *urinary frequency and dysuria,* a 2–3 day course of Pyridium (100 mg q6h) may relieve symptoms.

LOCAL MEASURES

During radiation therapy, plain warm water douches may aid in comfort and hygiene.

TREATMENT ACCORDING TO STAGE

Stage IA (Microinvasive Carcinoma, Depth of Invasion <3 mm)

Total extrafascial abdominal hysterectomy with a wide vaginal cuff is current therapy. However, several limited studies have reported beneficial outcomes with cervical conization in highly selected cases. Patients with invasion <3 mm without demonstrable vascular or lymphatic invasion have 0.21% lymph node involvement whereas those >3.0 mm but <5.0 mm have 6.8% lymph node metastasis. Therefore, many authorities suggest that those with >3.0 mm, but <5.0 mm of invasion should be treated as stage IB.

Stage IB

External supervoltage *radiation* and intracavitary and forniceal cesium or radium therapy *or radical hysterectomy and pelvic lymphadenectomy* probably are equally effective in the treatment of stage IB carcinoma. The latter often is favored in young, otherwise healthy, slender patients. The ovaries need not be removed unless they are abnormal or the woman is perimenopausal. Older patients, obese patients, and those who have serious medical problems are best treated by radiation. With *Stage IB ~15% of women have regional pelvic lymph node metastasis.*

Stages IIA and IIB

With rare exceptions, stage II cervical cancer should be treated by *radiation*. In some centers, pretreatment laparoscopy or laparotomy for biopsy of paraaortic lymph nodes may be done in stage IIB patients. If the nodes are cancer-positive (~15%), paraaortic extended-field radiation therapy should increase survival, although complications may be more frequent and severe.

Stages IIIA and IIIB

Radiation therapy is used for all stage III cases. Pretreatment paraaortic lymph node sampling is important. However, these nodes will be positive in 30%–50% of patients. Hence, extended-field therapy may be beneficial.

Stage IV

Supervoltage external radiation therapy to the whole pelvis is generally utilized for almost all stage IV patients. However, if the cancer has extended anteriorly or posteriorly without spread elsewhere, anterior or posterior exenteration may be chosen as primary therapy.

Treatment must be individualized for cervical stump cancers, bulky or barrel-shaped cancerous cervices, and laterally recurrent lesions.

Chemotherapy may be an appropriate adjunct in some cases or if the patient fails to respond to conventional therapy. Neurosurgery for relief of pain may be considered in selected cases.

RADIATION THERAPY

Radiation is generally the preferred treatment for advanced invasive carcinoma of the cervix. X-ray, radium, ^{60}Co, the cyclotron, linear accelerator, or other sources of radiation may be used. All stages of cancer may be treated by this method, and there are fewer medical contraindications to radiation than to radical surgery. Optimal results have been achieved with the use of externally applied supervoltage radiation combined with intracavitary and paracervical vaginal radium.

The objectives are destruction of primary and secondary carcinoma within the pelvis and preservation of tissues not involved in the cancer. The amount of radiation required to destroy cancer varies from patient to patient. A safe cancericidal dose for cervical carcinoma is about 7000 rad to point A and about 5000 rad to point B (see p. 615) administered over a period of 4–5 weeks.

Although it is impossible to administer adequate homogeneous radiation to destroy cancer throughout the pelvis without damaging vital structures, such as the bowel, bladder, ureters, and blood vessels, the cervix can be treated intensively because it has a high tolerance to radiation. The cervix and vagina can tolerate 24,000 rad, but the bladder and ureter will be seriously injured by doses higher than 7000 rad and the bowel by doses higher than 4000–5000 rad. Major blood vessels have approximately the same tolerance to radiation as the intestine. Therefore, dosage is determined by the radiosensitivity of both cancer cells and noncancerous tissue. In practice, the experienced oncologist or radiologist applies as much radiation as possible to the cancer within a reasonable time, with particular concern for the neighboring organs.

When vaginal contractures, a cervical stump, or the patient's condition precludes radium therapy, external radiation may be used alone. Cesium or radium alone is often used when the cancer is small and medical or surgical problems contraindicate protracted external radiation therapy.

The Manchester method of radiation therapy for cervical cancer is one of the most logical and popular methods. This method emphasizes the importance of calculating the radiation dosage as delivered to two precise points in the pelvis. *Point A is defined as lying 2 cm lateral to the central canal of the cervix and 2 cm above the lateral fornix in the axis of the uterus* (approximately the point where the uterine artery crosses the ureter). *Point B lies 5 cm lateral to the central canal of the cervix and 2 cm above the lateral fornix (at the pelvic side wall).* Point B represents a lymph node focus adjacent to the iliac vessels. This point is a pelvic focus for metastatic cancer from the cervix.

Rubber applicators for carrying radium tubes in tandem are available in three lengths for the deep, average, and shallow uterus. Paracervical rubber ovoids for radium application are designed so that the distance of the radium from points A and B can be varied by changing the amount of radium used, the thickness of the three graduated ovoids, and rubber spacers. The dosage depends on the amount of radium inserted and the distribution employed. *By using both intrauterine and paracervical radium applicators, the maximal dose of radiation is applied to the area of greatest benefit and least risk.* This is far more effective than a radium tandem placed in the cervix alone or radium placed only in the vagina.

The optimal predetermined dosage from cesium or radium alone to point A is 7000 rad. This dosage is delivered in two sessions of 2–3 days each, the first preceding external radiation therapy and the second following it. Treatment is more effective if external radiation therapy is also used. An external radiation dose of 3000 rad is given through two anterior and two posterior ports to the parametrium (point B) within 4 weeks.

TREATMENT OF CERVICAL CANCER DURING PREGNANCY

Therapy of cervical cancer during pregnancy is variable and requires great individualization, but one plan is noted here.

First Trimester

Deliver 6000 rad of external radiation to the pelvis through each of four ports. Concurrently, give two courses of intracervical and paracervical radium and await spontaneous abortion.

Second Trimester

Deliver intracervical and contracervical radium. In 7–10 days, perform an abdominal (classic) hysterectomy. Two weeks after surgery, begin 6000 rad of external radiation and then give a further course of intracervical and contracervical radiation during the last week of external radiation.

Third Trimester

Perform classic cesarean section when the infant is viable. In 7–10 days, begin 6000 rad of external radiation and then give two courses of intracervical and paracervical radium 1 week apart, the first during the last 7–10 days of external radiation.

SURGICAL MEASURES (SEE ALSO TREATMENT ACCORDING TO STAGE)

Total hysterectomy with removal of a wide vaginal cuff is the surgical treatment of choice for women over age 40 with in situ carcinoma of the cervix. Deep conization of the cervix may be acceptable for younger women who wish to have more children, but this is a calculated risk even when the woman understands the need for vaginal cytologic smears every 6 months for an indefinite time.

Radical total hysterectomy (Clark-Wertheim or Okabayashi), together *with pelvic lymphadenectomy,* is performed for treatment of *stage I and stage IIA* cervical carcinoma by surgeons skilled in the technique required for this exacting procedure. The 5-year survival rate with operation is as good as that for radiation therapy in selected cases. Obesity, advanced age, and serious medical problems that are likely to complicate surgery or convalescence greatly reduce the number of candidates for elective cancer surgery. In general, the hazards of the operation exceed those of radiation therapy.

Radical total hysterectomy and pelvic lymphadenectomy often are used as definitive treatment of cervical cancer if (1) the patient is pregnant, (2) large uterine or adnexal tumors are present, (3) the patient has chronic salpingitis, (4) there are small or large bowel adhesions in the pelvis or to the abdominal wall, (5) the patient is under age 35 and wishes to keep her ovaries, or (6) she refuses or abandons radiation therapy but is a good surgical risk.

COMPLICATIONS OF THERAPY

The mortality rate due to radiation is about 1% and that due to surgery is about 2%. The morbidity rates are approximately 2% and 5%, respectively.

Radiation therapy may cause early side effects, including nausea and vomiting, weight loss, dysuria, and urinary frequency. Such complications as tissue fibrosis, hemorrhagic cystitis, small or large bowel stenosis, or fistulas may develop later.

A serious complication of radical abdominal hysterectomy is *ureteric fistula.* However, the incidence of this complication has been reduced to 3%–5% by advanced operative techniques. Other serious problems include bowel injury, hemorrhage, wound infection or dehiscence, pulmonary embolism, atonic bladder with urinary retention, and cystic lymphangioma.

PROGNOSIS

The *earlier the stage at which cancer is diagnosed, the better the prognosis.* Preinvasive cancer is commonly diagnosed in women <30 years, but most patients with invasive carcinoma are 40–50 years old at the time of diagnosis. Thus, it appears to take 5–10 years for carcinoma to penetrate the basement membrane and become invasive. Untreated patients usually die 3–5 years after invasion occurs.

Reported survival rates according to the stage at which the cancer is discovered vary widely. A composite of 5-year survival rates at major cancer centers worldwide where radiotherapy is the primary method of treatment is as follows: stage I 86%–89%, stage II 43%–70%, stage III 27%–43%, and stage IV 0%–12%.

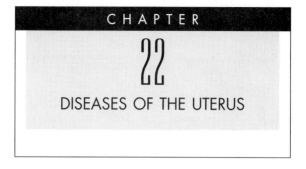

BENIGN UTERINE NEOPLASMS

LEIOMYOMA (MYOMAS, FIBROIDS, FIBROMYOMAS)

Leiomyomas are discrete, rounded, firm, white to pale pink, benign myometrial tumors composed mostly of smooth muscle with varying amounts of fibrous connective tissue. Approximately *95% arise from the uterine corpus* and ~5% from the cervix. Only occasionally do they arise from a fallopian tube or round ligament. Leiomyomas are the *most frequent pelvic tumors,* occurring in ~25% of white and ~50% of black women by age 50 years. Leiomyomas account for *~10% of gynecologic problems* and have their peak incidence in the fifth decade. Although the cause is unknown, each tumor (98% are multiple) is monoclonal, originating from a single muscle cell (whether an embryonic cell rest or blood vessel smooth muscle is unclear). They enlarge in response to estrogen. Thus, *enlargement is marked with pregnancy.* Premenarcheal leiomyomas are rare, and menopause or castration causes regression.

Uterine leiomyomas are classified by *anatomic location* (Fig. 22-1). Most commonly they are *subserous* (beneath the peritoneum), *intramural* (within the uterine wall), or *submucous* (only 5%–10% are beneath the endometrium). Leiomyomas may become pedunculated in either the subserous or submucous locations. A special variation of pedunculation is retroperitoneal extrusion between the leaves of the broad ligament (intraligamentous). Although adhesions to other organs are rare, in extreme cases pedunculated leiomyomas may derive their entire blood supply elsewhere, becoming *parasitic.*

PATHOLOGY

Only 2% of leiomyomas are solitary. They may grow to >45 kg. Each tumor is limited by a pseudocapsule, a potential cleavage plane

FIGURE 22-1. Leiomyomas of the uterus.

useful for surgical enucleation. Leiomyomas may be multinodular and are generally lighter in color than normal myometrium. On typical cut section, leiomyomas exhibit a whorled or trabeculated pattern of smooth muscle and fibrous connective tissue in varying proportions. *Microscopically,* the myocytes are mature and of uniform size, with a characteristic benign appearance. The smooth muscle cells are arranged in bundles and have interspersed fibrous tissue in direct relation to the extent of atrophy and degeneration that has occurred. Telangiectasia or lymphectasia occasionally is present.

Blood supply is generally through one or two major arteries, and the tumors tend to outgrow their blood supply with subsequent *degeneration.* Of larger leiomyomas, two thirds demonstrate some degeneration. Acute leiomyoma degeneration is relatively uncommon, but this may be *necrotic, hemorrhagic* (red degeneration), or *septic.* Chronic degeneration may be atrophic, hyaline (65%), cystic, calcific (10%), myxomatous (15%), or fatty. Leiomyosarcomas occur in ~0.1%–0.5% of patients with leiomyomas. However, it is not known if they arise from the leiomyomas.

CLINICAL FINDINGS

Symptoms and Signs

The majority (about two thirds) of women with leiomyomas are *asymptomatic.* When symptoms occur, they depend on the number, size, location, situation, and status (usually vascular supply) of the tumor(s). Gynecologic symptoms most commonly are *abnormal uterine bleeding, pressure effects, pain, and infertility.* Abnormal uterine bleeding is encountered in ~30% of patients with uterine leiomyomas. Menorrhagia is the most common abnormal uterine bleeding pattern, and although any pattern is possible, premenstrual spotting and prolonged light flow after menses often occur. Iron deficiency anemia commonly occurs as a result of the heavier menstrual blood loss. Rarely, a secondary polycythemia due to increased erythropoietin occurs with leiomyomas. The cause of this mechanism is uncertain.

The gynecologic symptoms resulting from leiomyomas exerting pressure are *variable* but most commonly include enlarging abdominal girth, pelvic fullness or heaviness, urinary frequency (from bladder impingement), and ureteral obstruction. Much less commonly encountered are large tumors, causing pelvic congestion with lower extremity edema or constipation. Parasitic tumors may cause intestinal obstruction. Cervical tumors may lead to leukorrhea, vaginal bleeding, dyspareunia, or infertility.

The *most common pain (about one third of patients have pain) caused by leiomyomas is acquired dysmenorrhea.* However, the most severe and characteristic pains with leiomyomas are associated with *degeneration* (especially, carneous or septic, in which there is a sudden onset of unremitting pain that may occur as an acute abdomen), *torsion* (usually recurrent acute pain), or *uterine contractions* while attempting to expel a pedunculated submucous tumor. *Pelvic heaviness and a sensation of bearing down* are common complaints with large tumors. Occasionally, pelvic impaction of a leiomyoma may create nerve impingement, with pain radiating to the back or lower extremities.

Uterine leiomyomas emerge as the *sole abnormality in 2%–10% of infertility patients.* The causal relationship remains unclear, but myomectomy may be indicated in long-standing infertility with no other demonstrable cause. *Abortions probably occur two to three times more frequently in patients with leiomyomas.* Thus, in recurrent pregnancy wastage with leiomyomas as the only abnormality, *myomectomy is indicated.* This results in term pregnancy rates of 40%–50%.

Pregnancy complicated by leiomyoma may lead to *abortion, premature labor, malpresentation, failure of engagement, unusual pain or tenderness, dystocia, desultory labor, and postpartum hemorrhage.* However, with no discernable correlation between size, placement, or other characteristics and outcome, there is no way to anticipate which patients will encounter difficulty. There is an increased use of *tocolytics, preterm delivery, and cesarean delivery* in women with leiomyoma complicating pregnancy.

Physical examination (abdominal and pelvic) generally reveals firm, irregular but smooth, nodular masses attached to the uterus.

Laboratory Findings

Anemia is the most common laboratory finding with uterine leiomyomas (as a result of abnormal uterine bleeding and infection). Leukocytosis as well as elevated ESR may occur if leiomyomas are complicated by endometritis or carneous or septic degeneration.

Imaging

Sonographic examination may be useful with leiomyomas to confirm the clinical diagnosis, measure the uterus and tumors, assist in diagnosis of difficult cases, and sequentially measure tumor size. Recurrent refractory shadowing in a pelvic mass strongly suggests leiomyoma. Color Doppler sonography further assists detailing the tumor vascular pattern and impedance of arterial blood flow within in around the leiomyoma. The latter findings may be useful in distinguishing leiomyoma from adenomyosis. X-ray is only diagnostic for calcific alterations or when there is urinary system impingement (IVP). Localization and detailing leiomyoma is most accurately accomplished by MRI. *MRI may be able to differentiate adenomyosis from leiomyomas from leiomyosarcomas.* Additionally, the "bridging vascular sign" on MRI is useful in the diagnosis and differentiation of an exophytic uterine leiomyoma from other adnexal masses. Finally, MRI has been advocated to assist in surgical planning and to monitor the response to medical therapy.

DIFFERENTIAL DIAGNOSIS

The uterine enlargement or irregularity caused by a leiomyoma also may be caused by pregnancy, adenomyosis, leiomyosarcoma, or solid ovarian neoplasms. On imaging studies leiomyomas may be confused with focal myometrial contraction. Other conditions to be considered include subinvolution, congenital anomalies, adherent adnexa, omentum or bowel benign hypertrophy, and sarcoma or carcinoma. Finally, there is a very rare variant of leiomyoma, benign metastasizing leiomyoma. The condition is characterized by multiple smooth muscle nodules, primarily located in the lung.

TREATMENT

The *treatment of leiomyomas obviously depends on a number of variables,* including number, size, location, symptomatology, degeneration, reproductive desires (age, parity, wish to reproduce), general health, proximity to the menopause, and potential for malignancy. With small asymptomatic leiomyomas, *conservative management* (i.e., careful follow-up but no therapy) consists of examinations (and possibly ultrasonic imaging) every 4–6 months. Indeed, the majority may be managed this way, thus avoiding surgery.

The necessity for intervention generally is based on: *bleeding* causing a *falling Hct or Hgb despite adequate iron and nutritional therapy,* a combined uterine–leiomyoma *size* such that the ovaries and masses cannot be assessed adequately on pelvic examination (about the size of a 12–14 week gestation), *untoward leiomyoma location* (e.g., cervical or leiomyoma causing ureteral obstruction), and *pain* or *signs of symptomatic degeneration.* Removal of leiomyomas during pregnancy is rarely warranted because of the extraordinary bleeding encountered. Even after delivery, surgical therapy should be delayed 3–6 months for tumor involution if at all possible.

When it is desirable to temporarily delay surgery (e.g., to correct a medical problem or to enhance hematological status), cause the tumor to decrease in size preoperatively (e.g., to facilitate surgery), or circumvent surgery entirely (e.g., near the menopause), *patients may be treated with an GnRH analog.* These compounds cause pseudomenopause with marked shrinking of the tumors. An *alternative is danazol 400 mg/d for 4 months.* The presumed mechanism of danazol is due to reduced estrogen concentrations and to antiprogesterone effects. Unfortunately, these *medical therapies can be given for only very limited time and have sufficient side effects to cause many patients to discontinue their use.*

Preoperatively, the usual gynecologic evaluations and a cytologic (Pap) smear. are required (Chapter 29). In patients with abnormal bleeding, a *differential curettage* is advisable to ascertain the endometrial status. In all women >35, in those >30 and anovulatory, and when the diagnosis is uncertain, the status of the endometrium must be known (i.e., rule out endometrial cancer). This may be established by *hysteroscopy and directed biopsies or D & C.* In the case of pedunculated submucous leiomyomas, excisional biopsy may be curative.

Definitive surgery is usually myomectomy or hysterectomy. Myomectomy is employed for patients wishing to preserve fertility and is increasingly being accomplished by laparoscopy or hysteroscopy. However, many leiomyomas are not amenable to endoscopic methods and must be removed by laparotomy. Patients must be appropriately counseled preoperatively concerning the risks, potential benefits and occasions when myomectomy cannot be performed (e.g., due to tumor situation) and hysterectomy will be necessary. Moreover, if the endometrial cavity is entered during myomectomy accomplished by laparoscopy or laparotomy, it may be prudent to deliver subsequent infants by elective cesarean section because of the hazard of uterine rupture.

The submucous, pedunculated leiomyoma can be removed vaginally by *hysteroscopy.* Symptomatic, small leiomyomas, particularly those that are subserous and pedunculated, may be easily removed by *laparoscopy.* Large leiomyomas or those with unusual placement will require *abdominal myomectomy or hysterectomy.* The ovaries should be preserved if possible (especially in those <40–45 years). However, if they are diseased or have a compromised blood supply or if the patient is postmenopausal, removal is warranted. For reasons not yet defined, within 48 h after surgery, myomectomy patients have an increased incidence of postoperative fever, as compared to hysterectomy patients.

The incidence of recurrence following myomectomy is 15%–40% even if all macroscopic leiomyomas are removed at the time of surgery. At least one half of recurrent leiomyomas require further surgical therapy. *Hysterectomy is totally curative.*

Transcatheter uterine artery embolization of symptomatic uterine leiomyomas has recently received considerable attention. The primary objectives of this technique are to decrease related symptomatology and attempt to avoid surgical intervention. The primary indications include menometrorrhaia, anemia, or pain. The procedure is reported to *reduce tumor (and subsequently uterine) volume by 20%–80% in more than 90% of patients. Pain is common in the first 24 h after the procedure* and may require IV nonsteroidal antiinflammatory drugs and narcotics. Patients undergoing this procedure report significant improvement in health-related quality of life and symptoms specifically referable to leiomyoma.

Complications of uterine artery embolization of leiomyomas include *endometritis, pyometra, uterine necrosis, sepsis, and delayed vaginal extrusion of necrotic pedunculated submucous leiomyomas.* Additionally, there are cases with minimal response and reports of *mistakenly attempting to treat adenomyosis* (which does not respond to this technique). A fatal septicemia has been reported following the procedure. The procedure is not currently recommended for women desiring continued fertility. Limited application and absence of long-term follow up precludes better definition of beneficial results, defining the incidence of complications, and detailing the impact on subsequent fertility.

ADENOMYOSIS

See Chapter 29.

ENDOMETRIAL POLYPS

Endometrial polyps are *suggested by abnormal vaginal bleeding,* most commonly menometrorrhagia or postmenopausal light staining. Polyps occur from age 29 to 59, with the *majority occurring after age 50.* The incidence of asymptomatic polyps in postmenopausal women is ~10%.

Endometrial polyps usually arise in the fundus and may be attached by a slender stalk (pedunculated) or have a broad base (sessile). Occasionally, polyps prolapse through the cervix. Grossly, endometrial polyps are velvety smooth, red to brown, ovoid masses from a few millimeters to centimeters in size. Histologically, endometrial polyps have stromal cores with marked vascular channels and endometrial mucosal surfaces that may cover glandular components. The distal polyp may show stromal hemorrhage, inflammatory cells, ulceration, and engorged blood vessels. Occasionally, multiple polyposis occurs. Another uncommon variant is the pedunculated adenomyoma (differentiated by interlacing bands of smooth muscle).

The *differential diagnosis* includes submucous myomas, retained products of conception, endometrial cancer, and mixed sarcomas. Polyps are *estrogen sensitive and may undergo malignant change,* in which case, a better prognosis is likely as compared with nonpolypoid endometrial cancer.

The diagnosis is made easily by *hysteroscopy,* and the *treatment is excision.* This may be accomplished easily by hysteroscopy followed by curettage of the stalk. A wire snare or scissors may be used to sever the base of a large polyp. It is wise to sample the endocervical canal by curettage when polyps are removed to rule out endometrial cancer. During D & C, explore the uterine cavity using an Overstreet or similar polyp forceps. Polyps tend to recur, and hysterectomy is definitive but rarely necessary for benign endometrial polyps.

TAMOXIFEN AND THE ENDOMETRIUM

Tamoxifen is already the world's most widely prescribed anticancer drug and *nonmalignant indications for usage are increasing.* The compound has *antiestrogenic activity* and generally exerts beneficial effects. Most notably, *tamoxifen improves the overall survival and decreases recurrences of breast cancer while beneficially influencing bone density and lipid profiles.* Marring these striking effects are some *unpleasant side effects and a distinct effect on the endometrium.*

The endometrial effect of tamoxifen, most often used in postmenopausal breast cancer patients, merits comment. Sonography will reveal nearly *60% of these patients to have an inhomogeneous endometrium of >5 mm.* Histologically, while the overlying epithelium is atrophic, tamoxifen induces specific *subepithelial endometrial alterations consisting of cystically dilated glands lined with atrophic epithelium and periglandular stromal condensation.* These changes occur in the endometrium as well as in endometrial polyps. Other long-term consequences of these changes are not known, but there is a significant increase in the development of endometrial carcinoma.

Thus, although the overall benefits may outweigh the risks, patients taking tamoxifen should be aware of the risk and the symptoms of endometrial cancer, promptly report any alterations to their physician, and be prospectively carefully monitored.

ENDOMETRIAL HYPERPLASIA

Endometrial hyperplasia is an extremely important lesion because of its probable correlation with the majority of endometrial cancers. In occasional older patients, a less well-differentiated endometrial cancer apparently can develop without intervening steps, but in the vast *majority of endometrial cancers there is a premalignant phase of endometrial hyperplasia.* Common agreement about the terminology of endometrial hyperplasia is awaited, but an attractive thesis is illustrated in Table 22-1. This hypothesis contends that first the endometrium responds to unopposed estrogenic stimulation with

TABLE 22-1
CLASSIFICATION OF ENDOMETRIAL
HYPERPLASIA AND ITS RELATIONSHIP
TO ENDOMETRIAL CARCINOMA

Endometrial Hyperplasia

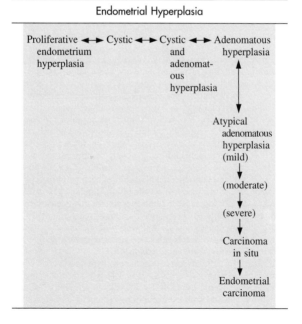

a very florid proliferative endometrium. Continued estrogenic stimulation causes the glands to dilate markedly, and the endometrium assumes a classic Swiss cheese appearance. With still further estrogenic stimulation, the glandular epithelium becomes more prominent. It is postulated that up to this point, with no atypia, the process is spontaneously reversible if estrogenic stimulation ceases or if progesterone is administered.

With continued stimulation, the *adenomatous hyperplasia becomes progressively more atypical.* In some cases, progestin therapy can reconvert the process to normal. Nonetheless, vigilance is required to be sure that the process does not progress to endometrial cancer. The alterations at this stage are based less on the shape, crowding, budding, and glandular branching (architectural atypia) and more on the cytologic atypia—the major determinant of malignant potential. Progressive epithelial cellular atypia includes cellular abnormalities (e.g., piling up of cells), nuclear atypia, and the development of epithelial bridges. This is followed by irregular cell size, prominent nucleoli, occasional nuclear pleomorphism, mitosis, abnormal chromatin configuration, and a high nuclear/cytoplasmic ratio. These alterations are further classified as mild, moderate, and severe. The *incidence of endometrial hyperplasia is age related:* 40–50 years (40%), 50–60 years (25%), <40 years (only 15%). The time required for *conversion to malignancy may be 1–2 years.* If untreated, at least 50% of patients with atypical adenomatous hyperplasia will develop endometrial cancer, whereas only 20%–25% of those with adenomatous hyperplasia will progress to cancer.

Therapy for endometrial hyperplasia is directly related to the degree of hyperplasia, the patient's age, and her desire for retention of reproductive capability. Moderate and severe atypical adenomatous hyperplasia in a woman past the reproductive age or one who does not want more children generally requires hysterectomy. If it is desirable to retain the uterus, and a careful D & C or preferably hysteroscopy with directed biopsies has been performed, therapy may consist of megestrol acetate (40–320 mg/day) for several months to totally suppress the endometrium. The endometrium must be thoroughly sampled at ≤6 month intervals to ascertain the success of therapy. *Regardless of the severity of adenomatous hyperplasia, if abnormal bleeding recurs despite appropriate therapy, the endometrium must be promptly sampled.*

Therapy for mild atypical adenomatous hyperplasia consists of *D & C and perhaps a less potent progestin* (e.g., medroxyprogesterone acetate 10 mg PO daily for 2 weeks to a month). The endometrium must be sampled again in 6–12 months. For continued atypical adenomatous hyperplasia in a woman not desiring reproduction, hysterectomy is justified. For adenomatous hyperplasia, a thorough D & C may be adequate primary therapy if progestin or induction of ovulation is then instituted. The latter is obviously undertaken only in those desiring reproduction. Endometrial sampling should be performed in 1 year to ascertain that the adenomatous hyperplasia has regressed.

The *prevention of endometrial hyperplasia requires recognition of hyperestrogenic states* (e.g., polycystic ovarian syndrome, feminizing tumors, and postmenopausal estrogen replacement). These feature unopposed estrogen, and treatment includes appropriate progestin therapy.

ENDOMETRIAL CARCINOMA IN SITU

Carcinoma in situ of the endometrium is a very *difficult diagnosis to make grossly or on frozen section* at hysterectomy or at D & C. The primary difficulty is that microscopically the endometrial glands are not separated from stroma, myometrium, blood vessels, and lymphatics by a structure analogous to the basement membrane in squamous epithelial lesions. The usual criteria for diagnosis of endometrial carcinoma in situ include histologic staining qualities (endometrial carcinoma often has large, eosinophilic, pale-staining glandular cells whereas lesser lesions are more basophilic), loss of nuclear polarity (enhanced with endometrial carcinoma), and no vascular or lymphatic invasion (both occur with endometrial carcinoma). When the changes of severe atypical adenomatous hyperplasia are at a maximum and these criteria are met, the lesion is termed carcinoma in situ. *Because endometrial carcinoma in situ cannot be distinguished from early invasive carcinoma on biopsy, both should be treated as endometrial carcinoma.*

UTERINE MALIGNANCIES

ENDOMETRIAL CARCINOMA

Carcinoma of the endometrium histologically is usually *adenocarcinoma* (70%–80% in the United States), *adenosquamous carcinoma* (10%–20%), or *adenoacanthoma* (~5%). Other lesions are uncommon to rare. These include clear cell carcinoma, papillary serous carcinoma, secretory carcinoma, mucinous carcinoma, squamous cell carcinoma (from metaplasia or from cellular rests), carcinosarcoma (adenocarcinoma and sarcoma), and sarcoma from endometrial stroma (e.g., chondrosarcoma, leiomyosarcoma, and myxosarcoma).

ETIOLOGY, INCIDENCE, AND IMPORTANCE

Although the etiology of endometrial cancer remains unknown and certainly numerous factors may be operative, *unopposed estrogen is a primary associated factor.* Moreover, the incidence of endometrial carcinoma is directly related to increased estrogen levels (endogenous and exogenous) and the duration of this stimulation. For example, endometrial carcinoma is 4- to 8-fold more common in women using unopposed estrogens for menopausal replacement and is more common in those with feminizing ovarian tumors and polycystic ovarian syndrome. Other known risk factors include *obesity* (20–50 pounds–3 times, >50 pounds–10 times), *nulliparity* (2–3 times), *diabetes mellitus* (2.8 times), and *menopause >52 years* (2.4 times).

Thus, women who have elevated levels of endogenous estrogen, those who are anovulatory, and those requiring estrogen replacement therapy should all receive *close clinical follow-up* (including periodic endometrial sampling) and *consideration for cyclic progestin therapy.*

Endometrial carcinoma is the most common female genital tract malignancy in developed countries. The chance of a woman in the United States developing endometrial carcinoma is ~1%. Overall, endometrial cancer is *most prevalent in women 50–70* years old, and <5% of cases are diagnosed before age 40. When the disease is revealed before age 35, it is almost always in association with a condition of unopposed estrogen; however, a few (27) cases have been reported in conjunction with pregnancy. Just before menopause, about 10% of women with hypermenorrhea will have endometrial carcinoma. The incidence in *nulliparas is 3 times that in multiparas.* The occurrence of endometrial carcinoma is nearly 2 times that of ovarian cancer and >2.5 times that of cervical cancer, and it has a much better prognosis. Table 22-2 details the number of new cases and annual deaths from the most common genital tract cancers.

Pap smears indicating atypical glandular cells of undetermined significance (AGUS) may represent endometrial or endocervical cancer in up to 14% of cases.

PATHOLOGY

Endometrial adenocarcinoma is composed of malignant glands that vary from well differentiated (grade 1) to anaplastic (grade 3). *Endometrial adenosquamous carcinoma consists of malignant glands and malignant squamous epithelium* that are often poorly differentiated. *Adenoacanthoma incorporates malignant glands and benign squamous metaplasia.* It is usually well differentiated.

TABLE 22-2
RELATIVE INCIDENCE AND DEATHS FROM THREE
MOST COMMON GENITAL TRACT TUMORS—1988

Genital Cancers	New Cases	Deaths	Death/New Case Ratio
Endometrial	34,000	3,000	1/11.3
Ovarian	19,000	12,000	1/1.6
Cervical	12,900	7,000	1/1.8

Endometrial carcinoma may *spread* in any of the following ways: within the endometrium as a surface growth (e.g., into the cervical canal), into the myometrium to the peritoneum and parametrium, via the uterine tube to the ovaries, to the uterine and cervical lymphatics, to the uterine arteries and veins, or to the pelvic and abdominal viscera by penetration through the serosa. *Invasion of the myometrium and metastasis occur relatively late* (Fig. 22-2). When invasion of the uterine wall does occur, the lymphatics are involved first and the venous and arterial channels later.

The uterine *lymphatic drainage* includes small lymphatic branches along the round ligament to the femoral nodes, infundibulopelvic ligament drainage to the paraaortic nodes from the tubal and ovarian pedicles, and broad ligament lymphatics to the pelvic nodes. The iliac, obturator, and sacral lymph nodes are commonly involved when there is endocervical involvement by an endometrial cancer. *Reflux of cancer cells through the tubes* results in dependent, lateral and posterior, peritoneal tumor implants. *Vaginal metastases* occur in 10%–15% of patients following hysterectomy. These are most commonly in the *vaginal vault or along the urethra 1–2 cm from the urethral meatus.* Spread may also occur via the uterosacral ligaments and presacral lymphatics to the *iliac and periaortic nodes. Hematogenous metastases to the liver, lungs, and bones are not uncommon.*

CLINICAL FINDINGS

Symptoms and Signs
The *peak incidence of endometrial cancer is at 55–69 years* of age. Endometrial cancer most commonly occurs in a woman who is *infertile, nulliparous, diabetic, obese, and white.* The classic symptom

Massive corpus tumor
and ovarian metastasis

Small fundal lesion   Myometrial invasion

FIGURE 22-2.   Adenocarcinoma of the endometrium.

is *perimenopausal or postmenopausal vaginal bleeding* (in 80% of
cases). In premenopausal women, the usual symptom is abnormal
vaginal bleeding (the most frequent is menorrhagia). About *20% of
postmenopausal bleeding is due to an underlying cancer, with
12%–15% being endometrial.* Hemorrhage is rare, and pain is not
usually a feature of this malignancy unless intrauterine infection or
cervical obstruction occurs or the disease is far advanced. A watery,
serous or sanguineous, malodorous vaginal discharge may occur occasionally.

In early cases, no alterations are detectable by physical examination, but as the cancer progresses, the *uterus usually becomes
larger, more globular, and irregularly softened.* The *cervix may
soften, and the os may appear slightly patulous.* In the older postmenopausal woman, cervical scarring or stenosis may obstruct

external bleeding, and she may experience only *uterine cramping*. With cervical obstruction, *diagnosis often is delayed, and pain, pyometra, or hematometra* may slowly develop. If drainage is not accomplished, the uterus may rupture.

Laboratory Findings

Cytologic examination of cervical and vaginal smears must always be done in these cases, primarily to rule out cervical or vaginal neoplasia. Vaginal cytology reveals endometrial carcinoma cells in only 50% of cases. Indeed, even intrauterine cytologic techniques are less effective than outpatient endometrial tissue sampling (>90%) for diagnosis.

Every suspected case of endometrial carcinoma must have the endocervix evaluated also before therapy is instituted. Hence, it is prudent to obtain endocervical curettage at the same time that the uterus is sounded and the endometrial tissue is sampled. Most frequently, however, a *clinical staging examination with anesthesia* is required, which includes examination under anesthesia, cystoscopy, proctoscopy, and fractional D & C (with accurate uterine measurement).

The histologic differentiation of severe atyptical endometrial hyperplasia, endometrial carcinoma in situ and endometrial carcinoma is often challenging. Thus, it has recently been suggested that cellular proliferation, apoptosis, and Bcl-2 expression may be helpful when distinguishing endometrial carcinoma from non-atypical or atypical endometrial hyperplasia. The histologic finding of lymph vascular space invasion carries a high enough correlation with spread to adjacent lymph nodes that many recommend adjuvant radiation in these cases.

Histopathological grading separates differentiation into three categories: G1 is ≤5% of a nonsquamous or nonmorular solid growth pattern, G2 is 6%–50% of a nonsquamous or nonmorular solid growth pattern, and G3 is >50% of a nonsquamous or nonmorular solid growth pattern. Grading has many other guidelines requiring the expertise of a pathologist.

The *usual laboratory workup* of the endometrial cancer patient includes CBC, UA, liver function tests, BUN, creatinine, 2-h pestprandial blood glucose, stool guaiac, and sigmoidoscopy.

Imaging

Obtain the following radiographs on all endometrial carcinoma patients: *chest x-ray, IVP, and barium enema.* Although hysterosalpingography has been used to detail the site and volume of tumor, it is not recommended because of the possibility of transtubal spread of cancer. *CT scan* is useful in evaluating local invasion as well as the abdomen and retroperitoneal nodes. *MRI improves the accuracy of clinical staging and is very helpful in assessing myometrial invasion and lower uterine segment or cervical involvement.* MRI is more accurate in postmenopausal patients. Thus, the patient's menopausal status needs consideration when using T2-weighted and gadolinium-enhanced T1-weighted MRI to assist in staging of early endometrial carcinoma.

Sonography, particularly endovaginal, is increasingly being utilized to screen women with abnormal uterine bleeding. The imaging should be correlated to other risk factors such as obesity, late menopause, PCOS, use of unopposed estrogens, and use of tamoxifen. As noted previously (see p. 626), women taking tamoxifen have high (~60%) false positivity based on endometrial thickness. In women not on tamoxifen, however, sonography has been demonstrated to have a *high sensitivity for the detection of endometrial cancer, but a low specificity.* There is virtual absence of endometrial malignancy in women with an endometrial thickness ≤5 mm. Further examinations are recommended in the presence of endometrial thickness 6–14 mm. Nearly all patients with an endometrium >15 mm have endometrial carcinoma. In some cases, transvaginal ultrasound may be useful in detecting myometrial invasion.

Sonography is useful to plan the clinical staging examination. Transvaginal sonography is efficient (>75%), specific (78%), sensitive (75%), and inexpensive in the diagnosis of cervical canal involvement in cases of endometrial carcinoma. Preoperative sonography may also assist in predicting lymph node metastasis. The latter prediction is base upon the degree of myometrial invasion and tumor density (both long recognized as indicators for pelvic lymph node metastasis. There are two current methods. The first is direct visualization. The second involves the determination of a Doppler sonographic "resistance index." Patients with tumors having an intratumoral resistance index of <0.4 have a high incidence of lymphatic metastasis. Sonography is also useful in potential cases of hematometra or pyometria.

RECEPTOR ASSAY

Tumor receptor assays for estrogen and progesterone binding should be obtained to assist in planning adjuvant or subsequent hormone therapy. *Generally, the better differentiated the tumor, the higher the estrogen or progesterone receptor binding* (e.g., stage I, grade 1, ~75%; grade 2, ~60%; grade 3, 25%). Recently, VEFG, flt-1, and KDR/flk-1 receptor concentrations were noted to not correlate with the incidence of metastases, recurrence, and survival.

STAGING

Office (ambulatory) hysteroscopy is simple, safe, and also has a high degree of accuracy in diagnosis of endometrial cancer. However, hysteroscopy alone identifies <10% of cervical involvement. Hysteroscopy is *currently recommended by many for the primary evaluation of all postmenopausal uterine bleeding.* Laparoscopic staging may be useful in selected patients.

Staging of endometrial carcinoma is based on the *clinical extent of the disease, the histologic grade* (differentiation of the neoplasm), and the *presence or absence of cancer in the endocervical canal* (Table 22-3). By using this staging at the time of diagnosis, the distribution of endometrial carcinomas is heavily weighted in the lesser categories: stage I 70%–75%, stage II 10%–15%, and the rest are stage III and stage IV. Current staging does not incorporate one other important prognostic indicator, the depth of myometrial invasion (hysterectomy required). This crucial detail, along with degree of anaplasia and cervical involvement, is directly related to nodal metastases, vaginal recurrence, and survival.

Recently, it has been recommended that all patients with endometrial carcinoma undergo complete surgical staging with lymph node dissection. This approach is advocated to maximize the amount of information for treatment planning while having the potential therapeutic advantage of lymph node dissection. *Radiation therapy is reserved for patients with evidence of extrauterine disease.* Alternatively, others have indicated that intraoperative frozen section showing less than one third of myometrial invasion in grade I endometrial carcinoma may not require lymphadenectomy. Future trials will likely resolve these therapeutic disagreements.

DIFFERENTIAL DIAGNOSIS

In the premenopausal female, a pregnancy must be ruled out. Other potentials in the diagnosis include uterine leiomyoma, endometrial hyperplasia, endometrial polyps, cervical polyps, other genital cancers (e.g., cervical, fallopian tube, and ovarian), and metastatic cancers (e.g., bowel, breast, and bladder).

With increasing age, it is more likely that postmenopausal bleeding will be due to endometrial cancer, and by age 80, cancer is responsible in 50%–60% of cases.

TREATMENT

For optimal treatment results in endometrial cancer, therapy should be individualized by gynecologic oncologists in oncology

TABLE 22-3
CLINICAL STAGING OF CARCINOMA
OF THE ENDOMETRIUM[a]

Stage	0	Carcinoma in situ. Histologic findings suggestive of malignant growth. (Cases of stage 0 should not be included in any therapeutic statistics.)
Stage	IA G123	Tumor limited to endometrium
Stage	IB G123	Invasion to less than one half of the endometrium
Stage	IC G123	Invasion to more than one half of the endometrium
Stage	IIA G123	Endocervical glandular involvement only
Stage	IIB G123	Cervical stromal invasion
Stage	IIIA G123	Tumor invades serosa and/or adnexa, and/or positive peritoneal Cytology
Stage	IIIB G123	Vaginal metastases
Stage	IIIC G123	Metastases to pelvic and/or paraaortic lymph nodes
Stage	IVA G123	Tumor invasion of bladder and or bowel mucosa
Stage	IVB	Distant metastases including intrabdominal and/or inguinal lymph nodes

[a]International Federation of Gynecology and Obstetrics, 1989
Note: On occasion, it may be difficult to decide whether the cancer involves the endocervix only or both the corpus and the endocervix. If a clear differentiation is not possible on examination of a specimen obtained by fractional curettage, adenocarcinoma should be classified as carcinoma of the corpus and epidermoid carcinoma as carcinoma of the cervix.

centers. *Surgery and radiation therapy* are the two major therapeutic modalities for endometrial cancer. For stage I, grade 1 endometrial cancer, extrafascial total abdominal hysterectomy and bilateral salpingo-oophorectomy is the primary treatment of choice. In this case, radiation therapy as a primary treatment averages a 20% lower cure rate than extrafascial hysterectomy and bilateral salpino-oophorectomy. The *abdominal approach to surgery* is preferred because it allows the collection of peritoneal washings for cytology, permits evaluation of the peritoneal cavity for cancer spread, and allows survey of the retroperitoneal nodes. The cervix and tubes should be occluded to decrease the chance of cellular dissemination. If the tumor is grade 2 or 3 preoperatively, there is lymph node enlargement, or the surgical specimen (opened in the operating room) reveals deep myometrial penetration, *lymph node dissection* (aortic, iliac, and obturator) should be added if possible. Intraperitoneal radioactive colloids may be added postoperatively if positive washings are reported.

Adjuvant radiation therapy is recommended if there is one-third myometrial penetration by tumor, poor histologic differentiation, papillary serous or clear cell histology, lower uterine segment or cervical involvement, or extrauterine extension and for those at greater risk of metastasis. Adjuvant radiation therapy postoperatively in stage I reduces the rate of vaginal vault recurrence from 3%–8% to 1%–3% and is worthwhile for all other patients with resectable endometrial adenocarcinoma.

For *stage II, the three options include radical hysterectomy and pelvic node dissection, primary radiation (intrauterine and vaginal implants plus external therapy) followed by extrafascial hysterectomy, and radiation without surgery.* For *stage III, therapy is usually total abdominal hysterectomy, bilateral salpingo-oophorectomy, and tumor debulking, followed by external radiation.* However, other variations must be considered (e.g., individualized treatment of patients with vaginal extension). For *stage IV, the uterus, tubes, and ovaries should be removed if possible, and the tumor should be debulked. This should be followed by radiation and hormone chemotherapy.*

Endometrial carcinoma not amenable to surgery or radiation therapy may be treated with long-term (>3 months) progesterone (medroxyprogesterone acetate, 200 mg PO a day, hydroxyprogesterone caproate, or megestrol). The response rate is <35%, with a 20-month average response duration and 13% long-term remission of recurrent disease. Those responding survive 4 times longer than nonresponders, with ~30% of responders alive at 5 years. Indicators of good responsiveness include young patients, high levels of tumor receptors, well-differentiated tumors, positive progesterone receptor status, and localized or late recurrence. Patients with poorly differentiated endometrial carcinoma and/or progesterone receptor levels <50 fmol/mg cytosol protein have only 8%–9% response to medroxyprogesterone acetate.

Response rates of advanced or recurrent endometrial carcinomas are 18%–36% with the following *single chemotherapeutic agents:* doxorubicin, epirubicin, cisplatinum, carboplatin, pacli-taxel, ifosfamide, 5-fluorouracin, and vincristine. Clearly, a single agent does not achieve the 47%–60% response rates of the current standard combined chemotherapy, doxorubicin and cisplatin. A promising current trial is the addition of paclitaxel to doxorubicin and cisplatin, which yields a response rate of 73%.

Pelvic exenteration is the only potentially curative option (~20%) for the minority of patients with central recurrence of en-dometrial cancer after surgical and radiation therapy.

PROGNOSIS

Overall 5-year survival of stage I endometrial carcinoma is 75%–95%. About 90% of recurrences occur <5 years. Those with poorly differentiated tumors or deep myometrial invasion have 5-year survivals of 50%–60%. In the latter group, there are 30%–40% positive pelvic nodes. Other overall 5-year survivals are stage II 50%–60%, stage III ~30%, and stage IV 5%–10%. Black patient's overall survival is lower than other racial or ethnic groups. The reasons for this are not clear.

Currently, the most *important parameters of prognosis are age, tumor stage* (advanced stage has poor prognosis), *histologic type of cancer* (serous carcinoma and clear cell carcinomas have poor prog-nosis), *grade of the tumor, lympho-vascular involvement and ad-nexal involvement.* The poor outcomes associated with adnexal in-volvement likely result from the preponderance of other adverse pathologic factors encountered in these cases. Less significant para-meters include: size of the tumor, tumor location, and peritoneal cytology. Factors currently under investigation include: estrogen and progesterone receptors, p53 status, flow cytometric determina-tions of ploidy and s-phase fraction, and various oncogenes [e.g., HER-2/neu (c erbB-2)].

Tumor ploidy and additional laboratory prognostic indicators may be useful in formulation of treatment policies. For example, patients with diploid, low-risk stage I endometrial cancers have low risk for relapse and have excellent overall survival, whereas those with aneuploid tumors require adjuvant radiotherapy to achieve the same risk of relapse as untreated patients with diploid tumors. How-ever, the expression of p53 in diploid tumors is associated with in-creased relapse.

Trials of successfully treated endometrial cancer patients sub-sequently taking hormonal replacement therapy have been reassur-ing. There is little indication that the estrogen leads to risk of re-currence.

SARCOMAS

Sarcomas of the uterus are heterogeneous, highly malignant tumors derived from mesodermal elements. They are uncommon, constituting *only 2%–3% of all malignant tumors of the uterine corpus.* The etiology of uterine sarcomas is unknown. However, there is a positive correlation between the mixed forms and prior pelvic radiation. Sarcomas usually occur *after age 40* and spread by direct extension, lymphatic, or hematogenous routes. Overall, sarcomas have a *poor prognosis,* but survival of endometrial stromal cell carcinoma is generally linked tumor grade. For example, low grade endometrial stromal sarcomas have a >80% 5-year survival, whereas high grade malignancies usually succumb within 12–30 months.

CLASSIFICATION AND STAGING

Several categories are necessary to classify uterine sarcomas: *homologous* (malignancies that histologically appear native to the uterus), *heterologous* (malignancies appearing foreign to the uterus), *pure* (composed of a single cell line), *mixed* (composed of ≥2 cell lines), and *mesodermal, mullerian, or mesenchymal* (depending on their differentiation). A summary of sarcoma classification is found in Table 22-4. Most clinicians apply the staging for endometrial carcinoma (Table 22-3) to sarcomas.

PATHOLOGY

About 55% of sarcomas (leiomyosarcoma) are derived from smooth muscle by heteroplasia, 40% are mixed mesenchymal or mesodermal tumors (probably related to endometrial stroma cells), <5% are carcinosarcoma, and the rest develop from blood vessels (angiosarcoma) or from connective tissue (reticulum cell sarcoma).

Sarcomas begin as *localized silent tumors,* gradually becoming diffuse and symptomatic on extension into and beyond the myometrium. Pain, obstruction, and inflammation do not occur until the tumor is moderately advanced. Extension into the uterine cavity or the formation of polypoid growths causes leukorrhea and abnormal bleeding. Metastases occur early via the bloodstream or lymphatics.

LEIOMYOSARCOMA

A leiomyosarcoma rarely arises from a leiomyoma. Leiomyosarcomas usually *occur in women in their 50s.* The histologic features

TABLE 22-4
CLASSIFICATION OF UTERINE SARCOMAS[a]

Classification	Sarcoma
I. Pure sarcoma	
A. Homologous	
1. Smooth muscle tumors	Leiomyosarcoma
	Leiomyoblastoma
Metastasizing tumors with benign histology	Intravenous leiomyomatosis
	Metastasizing uterine leiomyoma
	Leiomyomatosis peritonealis disseminata
2. Endometrial stromal sarcoma	
a. Low grade	Endolymphatic stromal myosis
b. High grade	Endometrial stromal sarcoma
B. Heterologous	Rhabdomyosarcoma
	Chondrosarcoma
	Osteosarcoma
	Liposarcoma
C. Other sarcomas	
II. Malignant mullerian mixed tumors	
A. Homologous: Carcinoma and homologous sarcoma	Carcinosarcoma
B. Homologous: Carcinoma and heterologous sarcoma	
III. Mullerian adenosarcoma	Adenosarcoma
IV. Lymphoma	Lymphoma

[a]Modified from P. Clement and R.E. Scully. Pathology of uterine sarcomas. In: *Gynecologic Oncology.* M. Coppleson, ed. Churchill Livingstone, 1981, p 591.

most correlated with outcome include the *number of mitoses* (per 10 hpf), *vascular and lymphatic invasion, serosal extension, and degree of anaplasia.* Mitoses per 10 hpf is closely associated with outcome: <5 usually is benign, ≥5 is diagnostic of leiomyosarcoma, 5–9 is low malignant potential, ≥10 has the worst prognosis. Premenopausal patients have a better prognosis than those who are postmenopausal. The overall 5-year survival is ~20%. However, when stage is considered (I and II), the survival is ~40%.

LEIOMYOBLASTOMA AND METASTASIZING UTERINE SARCOMAS WITH BENIGN HISTOLOGY

Less common or unusual sarcomas, (e.g., leiomyoblastoma, intravenous leiomyomatosis, metastasizing uterine leiomyoma, and leiomyomatosis peritonealis disseminata) must be differentiated from leiomyomas and leiomyosarcomas. Leiomyoblastomas are rare tumors made up of spindle-shaped, epithelial-like cells. They generally have <5 mitoses/hpf and are nearly always benign. Extrauterine intravenous extension of smooth muscle tissue (often described as wormlike) characterizes the rare intravenous leiomyomatosis. Metastasizing leiomyoma is characterized by extrapelvic smooth muscle nodules, found most frequently in the lymph nodes or lungs. Leiomyomatosis peritonealis disseminata is most frequently encountered during pregnancy. It may regress postpartum.

ENDOLYMPHATIC STROMAL MYOSIS

Endolymphatic stromal myosis occurs primarily in younger women (three fourths <50 years) and is frequently mistaken for leiomyomas because the primary clinical findings are abnormal uterine bleeding and an irregularly enlarged uterus. Histologically, these tumors consist of uterine stromal cells with a spindlelike appearance, having <10 mitoses/10 hpf. They are rare, being the least frequent among the uterine sarcomas, and are generally benign.

ENDOMETRIAL STROMAL SARCOMA

These uterine stromal cell sarcomas generally have >10 mitoses/10 hpf and carry a very poor prognosis. Endometrial stromal sarcoma is, like endolymphatic stromal myosis, usually found in women <50 years of age with abnormal bleeding and an irregularly enlarging uterus.

MALIGNANT MULLERIAN MIXED TUMORS (MMMT)

MMMTs occur in older women (generally >62 years) and generally occur clinically as postmenopausal bleeding with a large uterus. Prior pelvic radiation is a known etiologic association. Heterologous and homologous tumors occur with equal (albeit rare) frequency and have similar survival rates (overall 5-year survival ~20%) despite different histologic patterns.

CLINICAL FINDINGS

Symptoms and Signs
A rapidly enlarging uterus or myoma may suggest sarcoma in a young woman or postmenopausal woman. Common complaints relative to sarcoma are abnormal uterine bleeding, abdominal enlargement, leukorrhea, urinary frequency, and pelvic discomfort. Protrusion of polyps through the cervix is ominous. Late manifestations are loss of weight, pain, orthopnea, jaundice, and edema of the legs.

Laboratory Findings
Anemia, increased ESR, and eosinophilia are reported in well-established sarcomas.

Imaging
Chest x-ray films should rule out pulmonary metastases. CT or MRI scans may be useful to detect abdominal or pelvic extension.

Cytologic Diagnosis and Biopsy
Vaginal cytologic examination may disclose malignant cells of endometrial sarcoma and mixed mesenchymal tumors, but they rarely indicate leiomyosarcoma or other sarcomas. Sarcomas arising from the endometrium can be diagnosed by biopsy or D&C, but leiomyosarcomas require more direct sampling.

DIFFERENTIAL DIAGNOSIS

A postmenopausal patient's leiomyoma that is rapidly enlarging, without large doses of estrogen, is a sarcoma until proven otherwise. In the premenopause, rapidly enlarging leiomyomas (particularly submucous) are usually benign. Metastatic carcinoma must also be considered.

TREATMENT

Therapy is largely surgical, with extrafascial total abdominal hysterectomy and bilateral salpingo-oophorectomy (TAH, BSO). In well-differentiated sarcomas, even more radical primary or secondary surgery may be justifiable. Radiation therapy may retard tumor growth and relieve distressing symptoms. However, radiation does not significantly increase life expectancy. Chemotherapy may be palliative and is most commonly used (multiple agent) to treat distant metastases.

Low-grade sarcomas (e.g., stromatosis) have a better prognosis than those of more malignant morphology or extent of growth. Well-encapsulated sarcomas incidentally discovered within leiomyomas metastasize infrequently, and cure is likely. Without treatment, invasive sarcoma of the uterus is fatal <18 months in 75% of patients. After therapy, 20%–30% survive 5 years.

GESTATIONAL TROPHOBLASTIC DISEASES

Gestational trophoblastic disease (GTD) is a general term for five histologically distinct tumors arising from a fertilization event: triploidy (partial mole), *hydatidiform mole* (true or complete mole), *chorioadenoma destruens* (invasive mole), *placental site trophoblastic tumor* (PSTT), and *choriocarcinoma.*

All GTD tumors are the result of a *genetic aberration.* Hydatidiform mole results from fertilization of an empty egg by a single sperm, followed by reduplication of the haploid chromosomes. Thus, hydatidiform molar gestations are diploid (46,XX). Transitional molar gestations are usually trisomic. Partial moles are triploid (69,XXX or 69, XXY), the mechanism being fertilization of a haploid egg with two sperms. Whereas hydatidiform moles carry a 20% risk of malignancy, triploidy pregnancies are rarely malignant.

These tumors all have a characteristic tumor marker, human chorionic gonadotropin (hCG). The GTD tumors are currently the only disseminated solid tumors curable by chemotherapy alone.

HYDATIDIFORM MOLE

Hydatidiform mole occurs in *1/1500 in the United States* and in *1/125 deliveries in Mexico.* It is more commonly associated with *previous molar gestation* (increased over initial risk 20–40 times), *low socioeconomic status, certain geographic locations* (Southeast Asia and

Mexico), *poor diet* (e.g., low protein, low folic acid, low carotene), and <20 years or >40 years. The overall recurrence is <5%.

Common clinical findings include *uterine bleeding in the first trimester* (90%), *expulsion of vesicles* (80%), *rapid enlargement of the uterus* (greater than expected by dates in 50%), *multiple theca lutein cysts* enlarging one or both ovaries (15%–30%), *hyperemesis gravidarum* (10%), onset of *pregnancy-induced hypertension during the first trimester* (10%–12%), *maternal hyperthyroidism* (10%, occurs as a result of thyrotropin secretion by molar tissue), *anemia,* and *absent fetal heart tones.* It is now more frequent to diagnose GTD (particularly hydatidiform mole) in the first trimester as a result of hCG determinations and/or sonography (particularly transvaginal). Indeed, these two tests (beta subunit hCG and sonography) are invaluable in diagnosis, management, and follow-up of GTD tumors. Levels of hCG in urine or serum correspond to the number of viable tumor cells. Standard hCG levels are of value when high, but because most tests will not differentiate between LH and hCG, beta subunit hCG (β-hCG) levels are essential when hCG falls to the normal range of 20–30 mIU (the pituitary level of LH). Normal pregnancy is associated with β-hCG levels, 60,000 mIU/mL, in contrast to levels of >100,000 mIU/mL seen in molar pregnancies.

Sonography of hydatidiform mole demonstrates multiple echoes formed by the interface between the molar villi and surrounding tissue, with no gestational sac or fetus (*"snow storm"* or *"Swiss cheese"* pattern).

Characteristic *gross pathologic findings* are multiple, 1–2 cm diameter, grapelike vesicles filling and distending the uterus. If small, however, hydatidiform moles may grossly resemble an abortus, and the diagnosis will only be made histologically. Edema of the villous stroma, avascular villi, and nests of proliferating syncytiotrophoblastic or cytotrophoblastic elements surrounding villi are characteristic histopathologic findings. Malignant sequelae occur more often if the trophoblastic cells are anaplastic or show proliferation.

Treatment consists of cervical dilatation and uterine evacuation as soon as the diagnosis has been confirmed. Although suction curettage may be safely performed in uteri up to the size of 28 weeks gestation, *each procedure must be undertaken with care.* Patients with larger uteri (>20 weeks size) tend to have a much greater risk of complications and require precautions for emergency hysterectomy, hysterotomy, hypogastric artery ligation, and massive transfusion. However, thoughtful evaluation and preparation for common potential complications is prudent in every case as the complications can be serious, including: *blood loss, anemia, hyperthyroidism to the point of thyroid storm, preeclampsia, hypertension, and respiratory insufficiency.*

Before surgery *blood should be available.* Preoperative preparation for patients with signs of hyperthyroidism includes *beta-blockers* to prevent thyroid storm. A decision should be made as to whether or not *antihypertensives* should be initiated, and an appropriate setting and care made available should pulmonary insufficiency develop.

The *pulmonary insufficiency* associated with evacuation of a molar gestation is multifactorial (trophoblastic embolization, hyperthyroidism, fluid overload, preeclampsia) in origin. Clinically tachypnea, tachycardia, and hypoxia are usually experienced shortly after evacuation. Rales appear in the chest and Po_2 levels are markedly reduced. Chest x-ray is usually marked by diffuse pulmonary infiltrates. The treatment is appropriate cardiovascular and pulmonary support. Generally, symptoms resolve over 72 h.

Intraoperatively, the correct size suction cannula (10–12 mm) and deliberate speed assists in decreasing blood loss. Additionally, oxytocin should be initiated intravenously concurrently with the evacuation and certainly no later than once the uterine contents have been moderately decreased. Sharp curettage should follow suction curettage, and all specimens must be submitted for histopathology. *The Rh negative patient will require Rh immune globulin.*

If no further pregnancies are desired or if there are complicating circumstances, *hysterectomy* may be the therapy of choice in the patient who is a good surgical risk. An example of those with hydatidiform mole who may wish to consider hysterectomy are those >40 y of age. They face both an increased recurrence risk for complete mole and at greater risk for persistent trophoblastic disease.

Ovarian enlargement (due to theca-lutein cysts) is usually directly related to increasing hCG levels. Thus, ovarian enlargement is common, may be present at the time of diagnosis, or develop after evacuation. If expectant management is precluded by pain, shortness of breath, or marked ascites, the cysts may be aspirated under sonographic guidance. Spontaneous resolution usually occurs within 8 weeks and there is little risk of torsion, rupture or bleeding.

CHORIOADENOMA DESTRUENS (INVASIVE MOLE)

Chorioadenoma destruens is simply a hydatidiform mole with myometrial invasion. Grossly, the tumor may penetrate the myometrium to such an extent that uterine rupture and hemoperitoneum occur. In addition to findings typical of a hydatidiform mole, the signs and symptoms in the cases of perforation are those of hemoperitoneum and may be life-threatening. The incidence of malignancy is ~10% in chorioadenoma destruens.

PLACENTAL SITE TROPHOBLASTIC TUMOR (PSTT)

PSTT probably is a rare variant of choriocarcinoma that may arise after pregnancy, abortion, or hydatidiform mole. Only ~100 cases are in the world's literature. Genotypic analysis (PCR allelotyping) has revealed two types, diploid biparental and androgenetic, following monospermic complete hydatidiform moles. PSTT contains intermediate trophoblastic cells with typically positive hPL immunostaining. The clinical presentation may include irregular vaginal bleeding. Sonography or MRI are the most useful imaging methods.

PSTT has four worrisome characteristics. (1) hCG is not as reliable a tumor marker with PSTT as it is in other GTD because it is not secreted in proportion to tumor volume; (2) PSTT is relatively insensitive to chemotherapy; (3) whereas PSTT invades locally and spreads via lymphatics, metastases are often fatal; and (4) there is a hypervascular type in which massive bleeding following D & C may occur. Thus, preoperative sonography is required for detection of this type.

Primary treatment is hysterectomy. Multiagent chemotherapy may produce long term remission, even in recurrent or metastatic PSTT. To date, few cases exist and there appears to be a heterogeneous biologic behavior. A long interval (>2 years) from the antecedent pregnancy to clinical presentation is an adverse prognostic variable. Overall prognosis, however, remains to be determined.

CHORIOCARCINOMA

Choriocarcinoma is an epithelial tumor composed of syncytiotrophoblastic and cytotrophoblastic cells that may accompany or follow any pregnancy, including ectopic. Microscopic examination of the tissue shows trophoblasts in sheets or isolated foci on a hemorrhagic or necrotic background. Choriocarcinomas occur in *1/40,000 normal pregnancies and 3%–5% of molar gestations.*

The predilection for this disorder is *increased 10 times in women of blood group A impregnated by a type O male* (compared to a type A male). Women with *blood type AB have a much poorer*

prognosis than any other blood group when malignancy occurs.
Choriocarcinoma arising primarily has a worse prognosis than if it
occurs after hydatidiform mole.

TRIPLOIDY

More than *90% of cases in this category are secondary to diandric
triploidy.* Triploidy shares vaginal bleeding with hydatidiform mole
as the usual presenting symptom. Although β-Hcg levels are elevated over the expected in ~80% of cases, they rarely achieve the
levels encountered with hydatidiform mole. Sonography reveals a
growth restricted or nonviable fetus with multiple structural anomalies. Oligohydramnios, abnormal placental Doppler indices, and
variable placental size and characteristics are also noted on sonography. The nearly pathognomonic sonographic features of hydatidiform mole are less like to be present in triploidy.

Over 40% of the women with a triploidy pregnancy develop
preeclampsia.

Whereas triploidy is a dominant lethal for the fetus, there is
much less chance of poor prognosis GTD (Table 22-5) in women
having this problem, compared to hydatidiform mole.

TABLE 22-5
FIGO STAGING SYSTEM FOR GTD—1992

Stage	
I	Disease confined to the uterus
II	Disease extending outside the uterus but limited to the genital structures (adnexa, vagina, broad ligament)
III	Disease extending to the lungs, with or without known genital tract involvement
IV	Disease at other metastatic sites
Substage	
A	No risk factor
B	One risk factor
C	Two risk factors
Risk factors	
HCG >100,000 mIU/mL	
Duration from termination of the antecedent pregnancy to diagnosis >6 months	

GENERAL PRINCIPLES OF GTD FOLLOW-UP

It is essential to assure that all cases of GTD are not complicated by malignancy. *Quantitative hCGs* are a sensitive malignancy marker, but must be *obtained serially* in order to determine tumor production as opposed to residual from the primary process. Given the half-life of hCG *it averages 9–11 weeks for the residual to be undetectable.* Thus, in all cases of GTD, *quantitative hCGs are recommended weekly until three consecutive are undetectable.* Following the undetectable series, the quantitative hCGs are obtained *monthly for 6 months.* Pelvic examination should be performed *1 week after evacuation, followed by examination every 4 weeks* to evaluate the change in size of the uterus and the presence of theca lutein cysts. During the observation interval, *pregnancy is contraindicated* and the most effective method of contraception acceptable to the patient is recommended.

Approximately *20% of women with hydatidiform mole treated by evacuation (and 5% treated by hysterectomy) will have persistent GTD as indicated by plateau or rising quantitative hCG levels.* Higher risk of persistent GTD is encountered in: women >40 years of age, those with pretreatment hCG >100,000 mIU/mL, and with uterine size >20 weeks. Triploidy has a persistence risk of 4%.

Choriocarcinoma occurs 1:20,000–40,000 following normal pregnancy. The rate is lower, but the possibility of choriocarcinoma also exists with spontaneous abortion or ectopic gestation. Most cases present with irregular vaginal bleeding and serial hCG levels are elevated. D & C may not reveal choriocarcinoma for it may be metastatic.

GENERAL PRINCIPLES OF GTD MALIGNANCY

Of those GTD patients developing malignancy, hydatidiform mole is responsible for 75% of those with nonmetastatic disease and for 50% of the metastatic disease. The rest occur after abortion, ectopic gestation, or term pregnancy. The presence of an excessively large uterus with multiple lutein cysts is associated with a malignancy risk of 57%. *The most common site of metastases is the lung.*

INITIAL EVALUATION

If malignancy (persistent GTD) is diagnosed, the studies to be performed include: history; physical examination; pelvic examination (including evaluation of the cervix, vagina, urethra, and vulva for metastases); baseline quantitative hCG, CBC, liver function tests, chest x-ray, chest CT scan or MRI; and uterine sonography. Pelvic MRI is obtained if the sonography is abnormal or if there are other suggestions of myometrial invasion. CT or MRI of the brain, liver, and kidneys are obtained if there are signs or symptoms referable to those areas. Establishing the ratio of hCG in CSF to that in serum will be helpful in follow-up of brain metastases. Fortunately, malignancy is most often confined to the uterus.

Recently, it has been reported that the telomerase activity in hydatidiform moles is associate with the development of persistent GTD, invasive moles, and choriocarcinoma.

TREATMENT

For therapy, patients are generally divided into two groups: those with a *natural history suggesting good prognosis* and those with a *likely poor prognosis.* There are several systems for doing this. Table 22-5 is the 1992 revised FIGO staging system for GTD. Probably the most common in clinical usage, it simply classifies GTD as nonmetastic or metastatic, and further classifies the metastatic group as to those with good prognosis and those with poor prognosis. The patients with GTD and a probable *good prognosis* include those who have nonmetastatic disease as well as those with metastatic disease outside the uterus with the following: disease of <4 months duration, metastases confined to lungs or pelvis, serum β-hCG <40,000 mIU/mL, and no prior chemotherapy.

Failure of initial drug therapy occurs in ~6.5% of those with nonmetastatic malignant disease and in ~1% of the good prognosis patients with metastases.

Patients having metastatic disease with *poor prognosis* include the following: quantitative hCG mIU/mL >40,000, disease of >4 months duration, metastases to brain or liver, unsuccessful previous chemotherapy, and those with GTD following a term pregnancy. Even the poor prognosis patients may eventually achieve remission in >85% with proper therapy.

As a general rule, patients with nonmetastatic disease (and other criteria for good prognosis) as well as patients with metastatic disease with good prognosis are treated with a single agent. Methotrexate (usually with leucovorin) is the most common first line agent used in the US, with actinomycin D as an alternative. Following therapy, weekly hCG monitoring is used to ascertain response. Rising or plateau of hCG signals the necessity for retreatment (again, single agent methotrexate or actinomycin D). Patients with nonmetastatic gestational trophoblastic malignancy not desiring fertility are also candidates for hysterectomy.

Patients with poor prognosis may require combinations of chemotherapy, radiation therapy and/or surgery. Such therapy is sufficiently complex to warrant care in an oncology center. A useful chemotherapy (70%–75% remission rates) is etoposide, methotrexate, actinomycin D, cyclophosphamide, and vincristine. In those in whom this regimen is not successful further modifications are necessary. Radiation is most frequently employed for brain metastases. Surgery is used to control acute bleeding from metastases and to treat relapsing or resistant disease.

PROGNOSIS

Three criteria are commonly used to measure prognosis in patients with GTD: *cure rates, risk of subsequent GTD, and ability to subsequently have a normal pregnancy.* The risk of subsequent GTD is somewhat geographically related. For example, in the United States with low risk patients, it is 1%, whereas it is over 4% in Korea. Those with an excellent chance of cure (~100%), being able to subsequently have a normal pregnancy, and a 1% risk (US) of subsequent GTD include: hydatidiform mole, triploidy, and good prognosis persistent GTD successfully treated. However, given the potential for GTD recurrence with subsequent pregnancy, *several precautionary steps are advisable:* institute ultrasound early (<9 wks gestation), in the event of spontaneous abortion the products of conception are histologically examined, at delivery the placenta is histologically examined, and hCG levels are obtained at 6 weeks postpartum.

A *fourth criteria in prognosis is the patient's psychological adjustment to GTD.* Patients with GTD experience clinically significant levels of: anxiety, anger, concerns about future pregnancy, confusion, fatigue, and sexual problems. These symptoms may last for extended intervals and lead to mood disturbances, marital problems and extraordinary concerns about future reproduction. Emotional support and counseling may be necessary.

Patients receiving combination chemotherapy are at increased risk of developing secondary tumors (leukemia, colon cancer, melanoma, and breast cancer) *and require long-term follow up.* This is particularly important to consider if they received etoposide. Prognosis is highly dependent on metastases, sensitivity of the tumor, initial therapy necessary, and other factors. Thus, prognosis (cure) for these complex patients is highly individualized, but in most centers should be 80%–85%.

OVARY

Ovarian tumors are classified as benign (neoplastic and nonneoplastic), *premalignant, or malignant.* Benign nonneoplastic disease of the ovary is usually of an inflammatory or infectious nature and is discussed in Chapter 24 and Chapter 28. Table 23-1 details a classification of nonneoplastic ovarian lesions, Table 23-2 is the WHO classification of ovarian neoplasms, and Table 23-3 gives the characteristics of common ovarian neoplasms.

BENIGN OVARIAN NONNEOPLASTIC CYSTS

The clinical assessment and therapy of benign ovarian masses have been greatly aided by *modern imaging techniques* and the use of *oral contraceptives to decrease pituitary gonadotropin stimulation.* Sonographic scanning is the most frequently applied imaging technique for ovarian masses. Imaging modalities *aid in the differentiation* of ovarian enlargements from other masses or fullness in the pelvis, *determine the structure of a tumor* (solid or cystic, multilocular or unilocular), determine the *size of a tumor* (often difficult by physical examination in obese patients), and *document the change in size of masses over time.* In complex cases (e.g., cancer) more sophisticated imaging techniques (e.g., MRI) may assist in preoperative determinations.

Oral contraceptives administered daily for 4–8 weeks will resolve 80% of functional cystic ovarian masses not requiring surgery. *Surgery for benign lesions in the premenopausal patient is removal of the lesion (cystectomy), not oophorectomy.* The general indications for operative intervention are listed in Table 23-4.

TABLE 23-1
CLASSIFICATION OF OVARIAN TUMORS

Nonneoplastic lesions
  Inflammatory diseases of the ovary
    Adhesive disease due to subacute or chronic
      infections
    Endometriosis
    Peritoneal inclusions
  Nonneoplastic cysts
    Follicle cysts
    Lutein cysts (corpus luteum, theca lutein cysts)
    Polycystic ovarian disease (Stein-Leventhal
      syndrome)
  Focal proliferation
    Thecosis
    Cortical granuloma
    Luteoma of pregnancy
Ovarian neoplasia (mesothelial)
  Mesothelial tumors (primarily epithelial)
    Serous
    Mucinous
    Endometroid
    Mesothelioid tumors
    Mesotheliomas
  Mesothelial tumors (primarily stromal)
    Fibroadenoma
    Cystadenofibroma
    Brenner tumor
    Granulosa-theca cell tumor
    Sertoli-Leydig cell tumor
    Gonadal stromal tumors
  Stromal (mesenchymal) tumors
    Fibroma
    Fibromyoma
    Gonadal stromal tumors
    Sarcoma
  Germ cell tumors
    Dysgerminoma
    Teratoma
      Embryonal
      Extraembryonal
        Endodermal sinus
        Polyvesicular vitelline (yolk sac)
        Choriocarcinoma
  Gonadoblastoma
Metastatic tumors and secondary malignant tumors

TABLE 23-2
WORLD HEALTH ORGANIZATION CLASSIFICATION
OF OVARIAN NEOPLASMS

Common epithelial tumors
Sex cord stromal tumors
Lipid (lipoid) cell tumors
Germ cell tumors
Gonadoblastoma
Soft-tissue tumors (not specific to ovary)
Unclassified tumors
Secondary (metastatic) tumors
Tumorlike conditions (not true neoplasm)

FOLLICLE CYST

Follicle cysts are normal, transient, and often multiple, physiologic structures resulting from faulty resorption of the fluid from incompletely developed follicles. They occur most frequently in *young, menstruating women* and are the most common cysts found in normal ovaries. Their diameter may be *microscopic to 8 cm* (2 cm average). Grossly, they are *translucent, thin walled, and filled with clear to slightly yellow fluid.* Histologically, the wall of the cyst is formed by closely packed, round granulosa cells overlying a deeper layer of spindle-shaped theca cells.

Follicle cysts are usually asymptomatic and disappear spontaneously in <60 days. If symptoms occur, they usually involve an abnormally long or short intermenstrual interval. Intraperitoneal bleeding and torsion are rare complications. Any cyst that continues to enlarge or persist >60 d warrants further investigation. The usual investigation for cysts <4 cm is initial ultrasound examination, reexamination in 6 weeks and again in 8 weeks if the cyst persists. In follicle cysts ≥4 cm or if a small cyst is persistent, oral contraceptives for 4–8 weeks should cause resolution of the cyst.

CORPUS LUTEUM CYST

After ovulation, the granulosa cells become luteinized to form a corpus luteum. If blood leaks into the cavity during this process (which involves marked vascularization), a corpus hemorrhagicum is formed. Resolution involves resorption of the blood, and a corpus luteum cyst remains. A corpus luteum is termed a corpus luteum

TABLE 23-3
SUMMARY OF CHARACTERISTICS OF COMMON OVARIAN NEOPLASMS

	Age[a]	% of all Ovarian Neoplasms	% of Ovarian Cancers	Benign % Bilateral[b]	Malignant %[c] No	Malignant %[c] Yes	Malignant %[c] ±
Epithelial							
Serous	30–50	20–50	35–40	10	70	20–25	5–10
Mucinous	30–60	15–25	6–10	8–10	85	5	10
Brenner tumor	40–50	1–2	<1	6	97	3	
Endometrioid	40–60	5	15–25				
Mesonephroid	>40	<5	5	Rare	70	30	
Germ cell							
Benign cystic teratoma	18–30	20–25	<1	12	>99	<0.5	
Dysgerminoma**	10–30	<1	0.1	5–30			

[a]The age given is for benign tumors, except where ** indicates malignant tumors. In the epithelial tumors, malignancy of each type generally occurs at an older age than the same benign tumor.

[b]Epithelial malignant tumors tend to have a higher incidence of bilaterality (serous cystadenocarcinoma 33%–66%, mucinous cystadenocarcinoma 10%–20%, malignant Brenner tumor up to 15%, endometroid carcinoma 13%–30%). This is not true of the germ cell tumors. Immature teratomas are 2%–5% bilateral, and other germ cell tumors are rarely bilateral, except dysgerminoma.

[c]No, benign tumor %; Yes, malignant tumor %; ±, borderline %.

TABLE 23-4
INDICATIONS FOR SURGICAL EXPLORATION
OF PATIENTS WITH OVARIAN TUMORS

An ovarian cyst ≥5 cm persisting after 8 weeks of
   observation and/or oral contraceptive therapy
Any adnexal mass before menarche
Any adnexal mass after the menopause
A solid mass at any age
A cystic mass >8 cm in diameter

cyst if it is ≥3 cm. Occasionally, these cysts may be as large as 10 cm in diameter (average is 4 cm). Complications of this process may occur as a result of the original hemorrhage or as a result of the corpus luteum cyst.

A hemorrhagic corpus luteum usually causes local pain and tenderness (especially on pelvic examination). If the bleeding is so great that the *ovarian capsule is ruptured, hemoperitoneum* develops. Curiously, rupture is more frequent (two thirds) on the right. Bleeding usually causes a sudden, severe lower abdominal pain (but may have been preceded by aching discomfort). Pain most often occurs 14–60 d after the LMP. Not infrequently ($\sim\frac{1}{4}$th as frequent as bleeding ectopic pregnancy), the blood loss may be so severe that operative intervention (usually laparoscopy) is required to arrest the bleeding. The usual operative intervention is ovarian cystectomy with preservation of the ovary. Although culdocentesis is currently less frequently performed, the necessity for operation was established if the Hct of fluid obtained by culdocentesis was >15%.

If the hemorrhage is less severe, and the pain and tenderness are associated with delayed menstruation or amenorrhea, the corpus luteum cyst must be differentiated from ectopic pregnancy as well as rupture of an endometrioma or adnexal torsion. An *hCG and a sonographic scan usually accomplish this.* In the absence of significant complications (hematoperitoneum or ovarian torsion), symptomatic expectant therapy (analgesia and observation) is advised.

In addition to spontaneously occurring corpus luteum cyst, it is not uncommon for the *corpus luteum of pregnancy to persist after a first trimester pregnancy loss.* All early corpus luteum cysts are purple to brown (depending on how long it has been since bleeding occurred) and smooth. In chronic cases, the wall may be gray-white. On cut surface, the cyst wall is usually yellow-orange, perhaps with a resolving blood clot, but in chronic cases, the cyst remnant may be gray-white to pale yellow. On microscopic examination, both the granulosa and theca cells are luteinized. In chronic cases, the cells may be atrophied due to pressure. The cyst is hormonally active, producing both estrogens and progesterone. Thus, symptomatology consists of menstrual abnormalities, unilateral pelvic pain, and a tender adnexal mass. Once ectopic pregnancy is excluded, conservative therapy (analgesics, observation, and oral contraceptive therapy) may be instituted. Persistent cysts require 4–8 weeks of oral contraceptive therapy to resolve.

THECA LUTEIN CYST

Theca lutein cysts usually are bilateral, small, and much less common than follicle or corpus luteum cysts. Theca lutein cysts are filled with straw-colored fluid. They are *associated with gestational trophoblastic disease* (i.e., hydatidiform mole, choriocarcinoma), *multiple pregnancy or pregnancy complicated by diabetes mellitus or Rh sensitization, polycystic ovaries, and administration of ovulatory agents* (e.g., clomiphene or hCG therapy).

Symptoms are usually minimal (e.g., pelvic fullness or pressure), even though the total ovarian size may be 10–20 cm. *Complications are uncommon* and include rupture (with intraperitoneal bleeding) and ovarian torsion. When theca lutein cysts are discovered, gestational trophoblastic disease must be ruled out. The cysts themselves require no therapy. Gestational trophoblastic disease is discussed elsewhere (p. 643).

Polycystic ovarian disease is seen in women 15–30 years old with bilateral enlarged polycystic ovaries, secondary amenorrhea, oligomenorrhea, and infertility. Obesity is common, and 50% are hirsute. The ovaries have a thick, whitish surface cortex with small fluid-filled follicle cysts below the surface (oyster ovaries).

The diagnosis is suggested from history and physical examination. The FSH is normal, and the LH is tonically elevated (without LH surge). The urinary 17-ketosteroid level may be elevated minimally. Diagnosis is confirmed by ultrasonography and laparoscopy.

Because these patients are anovulatory, the endometrium is stimulated by unopposed estrogen, thus increasing the risk for endometrial carcinoma.

The treatment is induction of ovulation, initially with cyclic clomiphene citrate, but hMG may be necessary (Chapter 29). Wedge resection has been successful in restoring fertility but should be used as a last resort because adhesive disease or ovarian insufficiency may result from surgery.

OVARIAN NEOPLASIA

Ovarian cancer remains the fourth leading cancer death in U.S. women. The lifetime risk of ovarian cancer is 1/70. The *incidence is age related,* with the incidence at <40 years of age being 1.4/100,000, whereas those >60 years have an incidence of ~45/100,000. The median age at diagnosis is 61 years. Family history is the strongest known risk factor and ~10% of cases are thought to have a hereditary basis. Although prophylactic oophorectomy had been advocated for women with two or more affected first degree relatives, identification of those specifically at more risk (BRCA1, BRCA2) allows more precise counseling. Probably the greatest value of this genetic tool is to reassuring those that are negative. Those that are positive currently are reported to have a 15%–30% chance of developing ovarian cancer. Moreover, the value of oophorectomy in mutation carriers has not yet been proven.

Approximately one third of women with borderline ovarian tumors and nearly 20% of those with early stage ovarian cancer have no symptoms. Of those having symptoms, they are similarly nonspecific and occur with roughly the same distribution in women with borderline ovarian tumors and those with early stage ovarian cancer: *abdominal or pelvic pain* (>33%), *bloating* (>30%), *vaginal bleeding* (~20%).

There is considerable public awareness of the nearly symptomlessness of ovarian cancer, the difficulties in diagnosis, and the risks experienced by certain families. This knowledge raises anxieties concerning even the benign processes and mandates thoughtful counseling that anticipates both psychological and medical consequences.

EPITHELIAL TUMORS

Epithelial (mesothelial) tumors comprise 65% of all true ovarian neoplasms and ~85% of ovarian cancers. However considering just epithelial tumors, *over 70% are benign, ~5% are of low malignant potential,* and *less than 25% are malignant.* The maximum number of cases *occurs in the third decade.*

The epithelial tumors arise from the original epithelial lining of the embryonic celomic cavity and are composed of both supporting connective tissue and ovarian stroma. Because ovarian stroma is present, all varieties of this tumor have a potential functional capacity. However, this group of tumors characteristically *does not produce hormones.* The several types of epithelial ovarian tumors include *serous, mucinous, endometrioid, clear cell (mesonephroid), and Brenner tumors.*

As many as *10% of epithelial ovarian tumors may be of low malignant potential.* Collectively, these tumors occur at a *mean age of 40 years.* Pregnancy, breastfeeding, and oral contraceptive use are protective against the development of these tumors. Alternatively, there is serious question relative to ovulation induction agents have a potential causative role in both epithelial ovarian malignancy as well as epithelial tumors of low malignant potential. There has not been an association demonstrated with hereditary ovarian cancer syndromes. *Survival at 7 years is 99% for stage I tumors and 92% for stage II tumors.*

Treatment for low malignant potential tumors is surgical: bilateral salpingo-oophorectomy, pelvic and paraaortic lymph node biopsies, peritoneal washings, and tumor debulking. In younger patients with early stage disease, oophorectomy may be considered. To date, *a role for adjuvant therapy has not been established.*

SEROUS TUMORS

There are *three types of serous tumors: serous cystadenoma, cystadenofibroma, and fibrocystadenoma.* Serous tumors account for *20%–50% of all ovarian neoplasms and 35%–40% of ovarian cancers.* About *70% of serous tumors are benign, 5%–10% have borderline malignant potential, and 20%–25% are malignant.*

Serous Cystadenoma

Serous cystadenomas, which are by far the most frequent of the serous tumors, occur most frequently in *women 30–50 years of age,* and *serous carcinomas occur in women >40 years old.* The tumor may enlarge to fill the abdominal cavity but usually weighs 4.5–9 kg. Few symptoms are reported. Serous tumors are generally discovered on routine pelvic examination. The tumor produces no hormones.

Originally, serous tumors are *unilocular,* contain a thin yellowish fluid, and have a *smooth, fibrous capsule.* Subsequently, they become *multilocular, and papillary excrescences develop on both inner and outer surfaces.* Histologically, serous tumors consist of fallopian tubelike, ciliated epithelial cells (cuboidal or low columnar cells). Small, sandlike, sharp, calcareous concretions (psammoma bodies) often are present within the tumor. In younger women, serous tumors tend to be well differentiated, whereas anaplastic lesions are more common in older patients.

Laboratory findings are not characteristically abnormal. *Imaging is most helpful.* X-ray studies may reveal the small calcifications of psammoma bodies. Sonography or MRI are helpful in detailing the extent and configuration of the tumor. The differential diagnosis includes benign cystic teratomas, dysgerminomas, metastatic malignancy, and retroperitoneal tumors. Complications include malignancy, torsion, rupture, or intestinal obstruction.

Malignancy cannot be predicted by visual inspection. Serous tumors of low malignant potential are bilateral in 35%, with extraovarian extension in 30%. In contrast, *40%–60% of serous carcinomas are bilateral, with extraovarian extension in 85%.* Over half are >15 cm, and malignant tumors may be unilocular or multilocular. Usually the more differentiated the tumor, the more likely it will be benign. Lesser-differentiated serous carcinomas have a poor prognosis.

Malignant changes in cystadenomas are characterized by (1) excessive proliferation and extensive stratification of cells; (2) an intricate pattern with increased glandular elements; (3) spare stroma in proportion to epithelial cells; (4) anaplasia characterized by immature cells, variation in size and shape of cells and nuclei, numerous nucleoli, many undifferentiated cells, and numerous mitotic figures; and (5) invasion of the stroma or the capsule by glandular elements, with intralocular cyst formation.

Treatment of both benign and malignant tumors is *surgical removal individualized according to the operative findings.* Pathology assessment is mandatory.

Cystadenofibroma and Fibrocystadenoma

Cystadenofibroma and fibrocystadenoma are related, usually *benign tumors, most commonly seen in the 40–60 year age group.* There is a predominantly stromal component, with a variety of epithelial elements in the cystic areas. It is thought that cystadenofibroma and fibrocystadenoma are solid variations of serous cystadenomas.

Fibrocystadenomas are *commonly unilateral* (fibrocystadenoma is bilateral in 20%–25%), *<3 cm in diameter* (but up to 30 cm reported), and *asymptomatic.* On rare occasions, a hormone-producing tumor causes feminization. Treatment for cystadenofibroma and fibrocystadenoma is *surgical removal,* usually with hysterectomy and bilateral salpingo-oophorectomy in the postmenopausal woman. In premenopausal women, removal of the tumor (usually salpingo-oophorectomy) and inspection of the contralateral ovary probably is sufficient.

MUCINOUS TUMORS

Mucinous tumors comprise 15%–25% of all ovarian neoplasms and account for *6%–10% of ovarian cancers.* They are *bilateral in 8%–10%.* Mucinous tumors may be huge (>70 kg) but average

16–17 cm in diameter at diagnosis and are seen primarily in two age groups *(10–30 years and >40 years)*. There are usually no symptoms other than fullness from an abdominal mass. Cigarette smoking is a risk factor for mucinous epithelial ovarian cancer.

Mucinous tumors are smooth-walled with a tough parchment like capsule. They usually are *multilocular,* and contain *brownish, thick, viscid liquid.* Histologically, they are lined by endocervical-like or intestinal-like tall columnar epithelial and mucin-producing goblet cells. These tumors often develop a well-defined pedicle.

Mucinous tumors *usually are of low malignant potential,* but mucinous carcinomas account for 10%–20% of epithelial ovarian tumors. Stage I tumors are bilateral in only 10%. Extraovarian extension at diagnosis occurs in ~15% of the low malignant potential and in 40% of mucinous carcinomas.

The mucinous carcinoma has almost entirely intestinal-like cells. The tumor is composed of multiloculated cysts filled with viscous mucin. There may be solid areas of tumor, hemorrhage, or necrosis. However, these findings are not as predictive of malignant potential as in the serous tumors. *The more differentiated the cells, the better the prognosis.*

Peritoneal implantation of mucinous cells after extension or rupture of a mucinous ovarian tumor (usually of low malignant potential) or mucocele of the appendix results in propagation of tall columnar tumor cells and the accumulation of mucin within the abdomen known as *pseudomyxoma peritonei (mucinous peritonitis).* Although benign, this is a very serious complication leading to distention and multiple intestinal obstructions. It has a mortality rate of ~50%.

Treatment is unilateral salpingo-oophorectomy if the tumor is not bilateral and no malignancy is present. If malignancy is present, the primary therapy is surgical. *Chemotherapy is less effective than for other ovarian epithelial cancers.*

Endometrioid Tumors

Benign endometrioid neoplasms grossly resemble the far more common endometriosis (Chapter 28). Some pathologists believe the two must be differentiated from one another because ovarian endometrial neoplasms are composed of cells resembling the endometrial epithelium but do not have endometrial stroma and do not demonstrate the invasive characteristics of disseminated endometriosis. Moreover, it is believed that the endometrioid carcinomas arise from ovarian epithelium, as opposed to originating from endometriosis.

The *importance of endometrioid neoplasms is not their frequency (~5%), but their malignant potential (~20% of all ovarian carcinomas).* Endometrioid carcinoma usually occurs in *women age 40–60 years.* Treatment is similar to that of other ovarian cancers.

As in other ovarian cancers, the better differentiated the endometroid carcinoma, the better the prognosis. Recommended therapy is TAH, BSO, and omentectomy with removal of any affected pelvic tissues. The prognosis is improved if endometriosis is present. *Five-year survival is ~80%.* Adjunctive therapy includes radiation and chemotherapy, including progestational agents if progesterone receptors are present in tumor cells.

Brenner Tumor

The Brenner tumor (2%–3% of all primary ovarian tumors) is probably of epithelial origin. Approximately *1%–2% are malignant, and ~2% occur in association with a mucinous cystadenoma or benign cystic teratoma* in the same or contralateral ovary. Brenner tumors occur in women *40–80 years of age (mean ~60 years).* They are usually *small* (may reach 20 cm) and *unilateral* (5%–15% bilateral). About *10%–15% are associated with endometrial hyperplasia.*

Grossly, Brenner tumors are smooth, gray-white, solid neoplasms. On cut section, the tumor is homogeneous and gray to slightly yellowish with small cystic spaces. Histologically, the tumors have masses or nests of uniform epithelial cells surrounded by fibrous stroma. The epithelial cells have a coffee bean-appearing nucleus from a nuclear membrane indentation. Therapy for benign lesions is simple excision.

CT and MRI imaging of Brenner tumors reveals extensive amorphous calcification in a solid mass or solid component of a multilocular cystic mass. It is rare for the Brenner tumor to undergo malignant transformation, but when this occurs, surgical therapy should be followed by radiation because chemotherapy is ineffective. If the tumor extends beyond the ovary at diagnosis, 5-year survival is extremely rare.

MESONEPHROID TUMORS (CLEAR CELL CARCINOMAS)

Mesonephroid tumors are a small group of ovarian neoplasms composed of scattered glycogen-rich pseudoglomerular cell groupings suggestive of the mesonephros. They commonly are multifocal and may involve the peritoneal surfaces from diaphragm to pelvis. Most ~85% mesonephroid tumors occur in women *>40 years* of age. At least *30% of mesonephroid tumors are malignant.*

Grossly, mesonephroid tumors are unilateral, fairly well encapsulated, grayish brown, smooth, free, semisoft or cystic. Friable tissue and thin serous fluid fill the loculi and tissue spaces. Areas of cystic degeneration and even hemorrhagic extravasation may be seen. Most tumors are 10–20 cm in diameter. Extraovarian extension occurs late and about two thirds are unilateral at presentation. Two main histological types are recognized: a semisolid clear cell variety and a more adenomatous papillary type with groups of prominent protruding hobnail epithelial cells studding the acinous spaces. The tumor cells may be mesothelial, ciliated, secretory, or a combination without mitotic activity. The differential diagnosis includes cystadenomas, metastatic clear cell carcinomas of renal origin, and other poorly differentiated tumors.

Hyperpyrexia and hypercalcemia are associated with mesonephroid carcinoma for obscure reasons. Otherwise, symptoms are similar to those of other ovarian cancers. The tumor must be differentiated from a renal tumor metastatic to the ovary. Treatment requires total abdominal hysterectomy, bilateral salpingo-oophorectomy, and tumor debulking. Radiation or chemotherapy is largely ineffective, and if the tumor has spread, the prognosis is guarded. Five-year survival is ~60% in stage I and almost zero in stage III or IV.

GERM CELL TUMORS

Germ cell tumors are derived from ovarian germ cells and comprise *20%–25% of all ovarian tumors.* Germ cell tumors may occur at any age, but they are *more common in younger women,* constituting *~60% of ovarian neoplasms occurring in infants and children.* Although the vast majority are adnexal, they may be located anywhere from the base of the ovarian mesentery (in which the embryonic germ cells migrate to the gonad) to the ovary. The World Health Organization's classification of germ cell tumors is given in Table 23-5. Nearly all the tumors of this category are *benign cystic teratomas.*

TERATOMAS

Generally, *teratomas are tumors with one or more of the three embryologic layers, ectoderm, mesoderm, and endoderm.* They may be *benign* (mature) or *malignant* (immature). Teratomas are also categorized by the *predominant tissue type* and their *gross configuration (solid or cystic).* Mature tissues (teeth, hair, skin, muscle, bone, cartilage) are easily recognized in the neoplasm. The extraembryonic tissues are of trophoblast or endodermal sinus origin. Teratomas are *usually asymptomatic* unless complications, such as rupture, torsion, fistula formation, or peritonitis, occur. *Malignant*

TABLE 23-5
WORLD HEALTH ORGANIZATION CLASSIFICATION
OF GERM CELL TUMORS

Dysgerminoma
Endodermal sinus tumor
Embryonal carcinoma
Polyembryoma
Choriocarcinoma
Teratomas
  Immature
  Mature
    Solid
    Cystic
      Dermoid cyst (mature cystic teratoma)
      Dermoid cyst with malignant transformation
Monodermal and highly specialized
  Struma ovarii
  Carcinoid
  Struma ovarii and carcinoid
  Others
Mixed forms

---

teratomas are uncommon. If there is a thyroid preponderance (struma ovarii) or carcinoid preponderance in the teratoma, clinical symptoms (hyperthyroidism, carcinoid syndrome) may become evident.

Benign Cystic Teratomas (Dermoid Tumors)
Benign cystic teratomas are the most common ovarian tumors during the early reproductive years (18–30 years). Benign cystic teratomas are *parthogenic in origin.* Overall, they comprise *20%–25% of primary ovarian tumors, and about 10%–15% are bilateral.* Benign cystic teratomas contain ectodermal (and often mesodermal) tissue in the form of macerated skin, hair, bone, and teeth. The cyst is filled with a heavy, greasy sebaceous material. A long pedicle is often present.

    Benign cystic teratomas may be minute, but most weigh <0.5 kg, and they may be much larger. The tumor wall is smooth and tough. The neoplasm generally has a yellowish cast from sebaceous material within the tumor. On opening the tumor, striking amounts of *grumous sebaceous material* and hair are revealed. The various structures noted above may be apparent on gross or histologic examination. Most commonly, the cysts are lined by epidermal-like stratified squamous epithelium with sudoriparous and sebaceous glands as well as numerous hair follicles. Solid tumors are rare (<0.1% of all ovarian tumors).

Clinically, benign cystic teratomas *float upward in the abdomen,* elongating the ovarian pedicle and causing them to lie anterior and superior to the uterus (Kustner's sign). This is in contrast to other ovarian tumors, which are generally found posterior to the uterus. Few symptoms are related to this freely shifting, lower abdominal tumor unless it exceeds 10 cm (when it may exert nonspecific pressure symptoms). Thus, benign cystic teratomas are usually asymptomatic, although three major complications may cause striking symptoms. *Torsion* may occur with the usual abdominal pain. *Rupture* leads to peritonitis, and *impaction* in the pelvis during pregnancy can cause nonengagement of the fetus.

Imaging is very useful for diagnosis because calcified bone or teeth may be seen on ultrasonic scans or by radiography. Laboratory studies may reveal functional thyroid tissue (*struma ovarii*) in ~5% or the presence of *carcinoid* or *choriocarcinoma* revealed by their respective metabolites [T_4, 5-hydroxyindoleacetic acid (5-HIAA), and hCG]. Teratomas are only one of the reasons that cystic tumors are not aspirated for diagnostic or therapeutic purposes. *Teratoma leakage causes chemical peritonitis with subsequent adhesion formation* and the long term possibility of bowel obstruction. Of course, should the tumor contain malignancy then aspiration may lead to spread of cancer.

Treatment is surgical removal of the tumor (*cystectomy*), leaving as much ovarian tissue as is identifiable to preserve fertility. Occasionally, it may be necessary to perform *unilateral oophorectomy,* but that is unusual. Care should be taken not to spill tumor contents into the pelvic cavity. At the time of surgery, the contralateral ovary should be inspected carefully. However, surgical incision (bivalving the ovary) for inspection is not only unnecessary, it is so inimical to future reproduction that it has been largely abandoned.

Malignant changes in mature teratomas occur very infrequently (<0.5%). Of these, squamous epithelial malignancies are the most common. When the tumor is confined to the ovary it is usually treated by excision. However, if the tumor has broken through the ovarian capsule, the prognosis is poor even with radiation or chemotherapy or both. Malignant struma ovarii may be treated effectively with [131]I.

Carcinoid elements in a teratoma may cause a carcinoid syndrome in ~30% of patients. Carcinoids occur in older women and tend to be unilateral and slow growing. If the patient is young and childbearing is desired, stage IA tumors may be treated by unilateral salpingo-oophorectomy. More advanced cases and all of those who do not desire childbearing should be treated by bilateral salpingo-oophorectomy. Postoperatively, 5-HIAA may be used to monitor the success of treatment.

Malignant Teratomas

Overall, immature (malignant) teratomas account for <1% of all ovarian tumors, but they are the *second most common germ cell malignancy (after dysgerminoma)*. Moreover, since ~75% occur at <20 years of age, malignant teratomas comprise ~20% of malignant ovarian tumors in women under 20. Malignant teratomas are *rarely bilateral*, but ~5% of cases have a contralateral benign teratoma. Characteristically, these tumors *grow rapidly and pain* as an early feature. However, they do not produce hCG or AFP. At diagnosis, *two thirds are confined to the ovary*.

Malignant teratomas may be of three varieties: *choriocarcinoma* (tumor marker hCG), *endodermal sinus tumor* (tumor marker AFP), or *polyvesicular vitelline. Dysgerminoma will be associated in ~30%.*

Therapeutic decisions must incorporate tumor grade and the preservation of childbearing. Because the tumor is nearly always unilateral, removal of the affected ovary is the only surgery required, but this must be immediately followed by combined chemotherapy. Preservation of the unaffected ovary maintains fertility in these young patients. If the tumor is confined to one ovary, there is no convincing evidence that bilateral salpingo-oophorectomy and hysterectomy will improve the outcome over unilateral salpingo-oophorectomy. For all ovarian tumors over grade 1 and those with metastasis, however, *adjunctive chemotherapy* is required. Additionally, if metastases exist, efforts should be made to sample as much of the tumor as possible. Following surgery, prolonged chemotherapy [e.g., VAC (vincristine, dactinomycin, and cyclophosphamide)] has demonstrated effectiveness. Second-look surgery has documented the ability to convert immature to mature elements (which require no more therapy).

In the adult experiencing malignant degeneration of a benign teratoma, the tumor most often found is a squamous cell carcinoma. Nonetheless, mucinous cancers, malignant melanoma, mixed tumors, thyroid cancer, and others have been reported. The prognosis depends on the tumor type, grade, and extent of disease at diagnosis. The most common adjunctive therapy after surgery is total pelvic radiation, but this is not usually successful.

DYSGERMINOMAS

Dysgerminomas are the most frequent malignant germ cell tumors and the most frequent ovarian malignancy in young women.

Dysgerminomas account for *0.1% of ovarian malignancies and represent only 1% of germ cell tumors.* Dysgerminomas are not hormonally active, being analogous to male seminomas. Dysgerminomas occur most commonly *10–30 years of age (80% <30 years, 50% <20 years).* They tend to grow rapidly and are *bilateral in 10%–30% of cases.* Clinically, dysgerminomas are most frequently identified because of abdominal enlargement (tumor growth and ascites). Acute pain may accompany capsular rupture.

These typically *unilateral tumors are 3–5 cm in diameter* in most cases. Dysgerminomas are grayish brown, smooth, rounded, thinly encapsulated, nonadherent, and semisolid (rubbery). On cut surface, the appearance is edematous and brainlike. Histologically, dysgerminomas are composed of primitive germ cell nests separated by lymphocytic infiltrated fibrous trabeculae. It is the tumor type occurring in dysgenetic gonads. Hemorrhage and cystic degeneration are common. Histologic grading cannot be applied to dysgerminomas.

Giant cells representing trophoblastic elements may secrete *hCG,* which may cause a weakly positive pregnancy test in a rare patient. *Lactate dehydrogenase* can be a tumor marker for dysgerminomas. As in most tumor markers, if it is initially elevated it us useful to follow serially after therapy. *A teratoma may be associated with the dysgerminoma,* but because of the high incidence of dysgenetic gonads in such patients, *a karyotype should be performed. If any portion of a Y chromosome is present, bilateral oophorectomy is indicated,* because of the high incidence of gonadoblastoma in the contralateral ovary.

If confined to one ovary, treatment by *unilateral salpingo-oophorectomy is as effective (5-year survival >90%) as more extensive surgery. A 20% recurrence rate (particularly in tumors >15 cm) is likely,* but since the *tumors are radiosensitive* (some cured after <3000 rad), radiotherapy is effective in elimination of recurrences. Close follow-up (CT scans, MRI) of patients is mandatory. Sampling the contralateral ovary at surgery is necessary because of the incidence of bilaterality. More advanced tumors should be treated with a combination of surgery and radiotherapy. Chemotherapy is useful in cases where radiotherapy fails or is not feasible, and given the effectiveness of platinum-based agents, may become the primary adjuvant therapy. For example, there are beneficial reports for even metastatic dysgerminoma treated with conservative surgery (reproductive function preservation) and bleomycin, etoposide, and cisplatin.

Prognosis is related to tumor type (pure dysgerminomas have a better prognosis than mixed germ cell tumors), unilateral occurrence (better than bilateral), tumor size (better if <15 cm), encapsulation (better than spread beyond the capsule), lack of nodal metastasis, and absence of ascites. If the tumor is bilateral or if extraovarian extension has occurred, surgery should consist of TAH and BSO followed by chemotherapy (platinum-based adjuvant therapy is particularly effective) or radiotherapy or both. The 5-year survival rate for unilateral disease (stage IA) is ~95%. In more advanced disease, the 5-year survival rate is <70%.

OTHER GERM CELL TUMORS

Endodermal sinus (yolk sac) tumors are *rare (<1% of ovarian) malignancies.* They occur primarily in young women (*median 19 years*) and may even affect small children. Endodermal sinus tumors produce *AFP,* which may be used for both identification and follow-up. Treatment for stage IA is unilateral salpingo-oophorectomy. More advanced cases should receive chemotherapy (e.g., VAC). The prognosis must be guarded.

Embryonal carcinomas are rare malignant germ cell tumors that produce hCG and AFP. They occur primarily in young women and are treated similarly to endodermal sinus tumors.

Nongestational choriocarcinoma is a rare but highly malignant germ cell tumor occurring in young women (<20 years). Like gestational choriocarcinoma, these tumors produce hCG. Nongestational choriocarcinoma must be treated with multiple-agent chemotherapy after surgical excision.

Combinations of the various germ cell tumors are called *mixed germ cell tumors.* Therapy must be individualized with consideration of the germ cell elements present.

SEX CORD STROMAL TUMORS

These tumors are derived from the *sex cords and specialized stroma* of the developing ovary. Cumulatively, sex cord stromal tumors represent ~6% of ovarian neoplasms. Although this tumor classification contains the majority of hormonally active ovarian tumors, some have no or *low potential for hormone production* (e.g., fibroadenoma, cystadenofibroma). Others have a *high functional potential* (e.g., granulosa-theca cell, Sertoli-Leydig, gonadal stromal tumors).

Tumors in this category may have a male or female differentiation based on their sex cord component (*female* is granulosa cell sex cord and theca cell or fibroblast stromal elements; *male* is Sertoli cell sex cord and Leydig cell stromal component).

GRANULOSA-THECA
CELL TUMORS

Granulosa-theca cell tumors may develop in *any age group*. They account for ~5% *of patients with precocious puberty* (<9 years). If granulosa-theca tumors occur during the menstrual years, ~5% *will cause amenorrhea and signs of estrogen excess*. Because of tonically elevated and unopposed estrogen levels, ovulation is inhibited, and the proliferative endometrium may become hyperplastic. Other symptomatology in the postmenopausal years is related to estrogen stimulation (breast soreness, fluid retention, nausea). In addition to endometrial hyperplasia, endometrial carcinoma may occur.

Granulosa-theca cell tumors are usually yellow-orange and <15 cm in diameter. Some may be microscopic. They usually are usually *unilateral* (3%–8% bilateral). Granulosa cell tumors are constituted primarily of granulosa cells with lesser thecal or fibrous elements. Characteristically, the granulosa cells surround Call-Exner bodies (eosinophilic areas) set in a follicular pattern. Luteinization may occur, and the primary hormone production is estrogen. Mitoses are normal in the proliferating granulosa of the normal developing follicle. Hence, mitotic figures are not abnormal in these tumors. The histologic pattern is not directly correlated with clinical malignant potential. The very well differentiated tumors tend to be benign, but these tumors *overall tend to be low-grade malignancies,* often with late (>5 years) recurrences (some after 10–15 years).

Treatment is *surgical excision of the ovary* containing the tumor unless both ovaries are involved or no further children are desired, in which case, total hysterectomy and bilateral salpingo-oophorectomy are advised. Both chemotherapy and radiation therapy are useful adjuncts. Prognosis is adversely affected by tumors >15 cm in diameter, advanced clinical stage, tumor rupture, or high incidence of mitoses in the tumor. The 10-year survival rate is ~90%.

The luteoma of pregnancy is discussed elsewhere.

SERTOLI-LEYDIG CELL TUMORS

The Sertoli-Leydig cell tumor classically is a gonadostromal lesion with tubular differentiation. These *tumors are rare* (<500 cases reported) and occur in women in the reproductive age. Sertoli-Leydig cell tumors cause hirsutism and masculinization in one third of patients. Rarely, they produce estrogens.

Grossly, Sertoli-Leydig cell tumors are unilateral, small, solid tumors with a smooth capsule. The color varies, but most are yellowish brown. They have histologic components that resemble the testis (tubules of Sertoli cell surrounded by Leydig cells). A karyotype should be performed to rule out the Y chromosome.

Therapy has generally been surgical, but insufficient data exist to detail adjunctive therapy. Since the tumors behave as low-grade malignancies, the *5-year survival is high* (70%–90%). Prognosis is adversely affected when tumors are poorly differentiated or are in an advanced stage.

FIBROMAS AND THECOMAS

These tumors represent up to *4% of ovarian tumors* and include the *fibroma, fibrothecoma, and thecoma*. Fibroma is by far the most frequently seen in this category, and fibroma tends to become larger than the others. Fibromas are not usually hormonally active and are usually found on routine pelvic examination as a firm adnexal mass. Tumors in this category arise from the undifferentiated mesenchymal component. They are most commonly seen in patients aged *40–60 years*. When functioning components are present (thecal cells), expect signs of estrogen stimulation.

Grossly, tumors of this group are typically *unilateral, grayish white, encapsulated, round, lobulated tumors, which rarely are >10 cm* diameter. Thecomas consist entirely of stromal (theca) cells, and fibromas are composed of fibrous (spindle-shaped) cells. Combinations of the two components occur.

Meigs-Demons syndrome (transudative hydrothorax and ascites associated with a benign ovarian tumor) may be present. Oophorectomy results in resolution of Meigs-Demons syndrome in <2 weeks.

In premenopausal patients, these usually benign tumors should be treated by unilateral salpingo-oophorectomy. If the patient is postmenopausal, hysterectomy and bilateral salpingo-oophorectomy are advised. The prognosis is good.

GYNANDROBLASTOMAS

These rare sex cord stromal tumors consist of both *female and male cell types*.

GONADAL STROMAL TUMORS (WITH OR WITHOUT TUBULAR STRUCTURES)

These tumors may be *well-differentiated* (Pick's adenoma), *intermediate* (poorly defined tubules with gonadal stromal cells with interstitial cell foci), or *sarcomatoid (stromal) tumors* (no tubular structures). Gonadal stromal tumors are *usually feminizing*. They are *unilateral* (bilateral in <5%) and *infrequently progress to malignancy* (<10%). The patient is usually a younger woman, although all ages have been reported. Treatment is aimed at preserving the uterus and one ovary unless the karyotype reveals a Y chromosome.

HILUS CELL TUMOR

The hilus cell tumor is a *virilizing ovarian neoplasm* (hirsutism, alopecia, enlarged clitoris, and sometimes, deepening of voice) in perimenopausal or early postmenopausal women. Endometrial hyperplasia may develop in some patients, suggesting simultaneous androgenic and estrogenic effect. The tumor is brown to yellowish brown, typically unilateral, and *<4–5 cm in diameter.* An adrenal tumor and familial hirsutism must be ruled out. Treatment is surgical removal of the tumor. The prognosis is good.

GONADOBLASTOMA

Gonadoblastomas are *rare tumors with germ cell* (often dysgerminoma-like) *and sex cord-stromal* (often immature granulosa and Sertoli cell-like) elements. In pure form, these tumors do not metastasize. There is a *higher occurrence of gonadoblastoma in phenotypic females with a Y chromosome.* Such patients should be advised to have the gonads removed.

Like the germinoma, the *gonadoblastoma is also common in dysgenetic gonads.* Most patients will be phenotypic and genetic females, but a karyotype should be performed to rule out a Y component. The pathologic features of this tumor are the unencapsulated germ cell, an attempt at tubule formation, folliculoid pattern with nests of granulosa cells surrounding large eosinophilic bodies, and focal calcification. Therapy consists of *bilateral salpingo-oophorectomy.*

LIPOID TUMORS

These very rare tumors (<100 cases) may cause virilization or excess cortisol production and are composed of cells that resemble cells of the adrenal cortex, Leydig cells, or luteinized ovarian cells. Occasionally, metastases have occurred. Treatment requires removal of the involved ovary, but data are insufficient to detail total therapy.

UNCLASSIFIED TUMORS

Multifocai neoplasia and ovarian neoplasia associated with other types of genital cancer are difficult to classify. Because the ovarian mesothelium and the endometrium have a common embryonic origin, tumors may arise in separate foci in the ovary and endometrium without representing metastatic disease. If the lesions are truly multifocal, the prognosis is much improved (80% 5-year survival) compared to metastatic disease (30%–35%).Treatment of multifocal ovarian cancer is the same as for endometrial carcinoma, (i.e., TAH and BSO). Because 25% of the ovarian tumors are not palpable at surgery, they may be an incidental finding during therapy for primary uterine cancer.

SECONDARY (METASTATIC) TUMORS

METASTATIC TUMORS FROM GENITAL PRIMARY MALIGNANCY

Metastatic disease to the ovary from the lower genital tract is *rare* (1%–2%) but may represent direct extension through the broad ligament rather than true metastatic disease.

METASTATIC OVARIAN TUMORS FROM EXTRAGENITAL PRIMARY MALIGNANCY

Metastases to the ovary are common, especially if the *primary cancer is in the breast or gastrointestinal tract.* These represent *1% of all ovarian neoplasia.* They are commonly *bilateral (75%)* and may reach massive proportions. The cell pattern will vary depending on the primary malignancy. One recognizable tumor, *Krukenberg tumor,* is characterized by coarse, abundant, occasionally edematous stroma with islands of moderately large epithelial cells with mucin-laden or vacuolated cytoplasm and eccentrically placed, small hyperchromatic nuclei resembling signet rings. The primary tumor is usually stomach but may be intestinal, breast, or thyroid in origin. Slight estrogen production is not unusual. Treatment is surgical, with removal of as much tumor as possible, followed by adjunctive chemotherapy. The overall prognosis is discouraging.

MALIGNANT AND PREMALIGNANT OVARIAN NEOPLASIA

Approximately *15% of ovarian tumors are malignant.* Over *80% of deaths from ovarian cancer occur between ages 35 and 75 years.* The lifetime risk of developing ovarian cancer in the United States (*unchanged in 30 years*) *is 1.4%.* Because these tumors are difficult to diagnose and treat early, the *5-year survival rate is only 35%–38%,* despite improved chemotherapy and radiotherapy.

STAGING

The most widely used staging for ovarian neoplasia is that of the International Federation of Gynecology and Obstetrics (FIGO) (Table 23-6). Recall that *ovarian cancer staging includes all of the operative findings,* in contrast to cancer of the cervix and vulva, where staging is based on the nonoperative clinical findings.

PATHOPHYSIOLOGY

Although ovarian cancer accounts for 15%–20% of female reproductive tract cancer, it causes more deaths than the others combined. Ovarian cancer is usually silent until palpable or widely disseminated.

Ovarian cancer is *more frequent in infertile women* or in those who have had *repeated spontaneous abortion, delayed childbearing, or breast cancer.* In the United States, the incidence is *6–7/100,000,* with about *equal rates in blacks and whites.*

Malignant ovarian tumors in children are most often of germ cell origin, whereas those of adult women are malignant epithelial tumors (>90%), of which 70% have metastasized outside the pelvis at the time of diagnosis. The site of metastatic disease is as follows: peritoneum (85%), pelvic and aortic lymph nodes (80%), omentum (70%), contralateral ovary (70%), mediastinal or supraclavicular lymph nodes (50%), liver (35%), pleura (33%), lung (25%), uterus (20%), vagina (15%), bone (15%), spleen (5%–10%), kidney (5%–10%), adrenal (5%–10%), skin (5%–10%), vulva (1%), and brain (1%).

The ovaries may become the site of *metastases of other primary tumors or may be involved by simple extension.*

DIAGNOSIS

There is *no routine screening test available for ovarian cancer,* although *clinical trials employing sonograph are underway.* Symptoms of pain may occur with significant distention, inflammation, torsion, or traction. Pelvic pressure may be reported if the tumor is large. Enlarging abdominal girth, weight gain or loss, and gastrointestinal symptoms ranging from indigestion to intestinal obstruction may occur with ovarian cancer. Diagnosis depends on appropriate clinical, laboratory, and surgical evaluation.

TABLE 23-6
INTERNATIONAL FEDERATION OF GYNECOLOGY
AND OBSTETRICS (FIGO) STAGING OF OVARIAN
NEOPLASMS (MODIFIED, 1994)

Stage	Characteristics
Stage I	Growth limited to the ovaries.
IA	Growth limited to one ovary; no ascites present containing malignant cells; no tumor on the external surface; capsule intact.
IB	Growth is limited to both ovaries; no ascites present containing malignant cells; no tumor on the external surface; capsule intact.
IC	Tumor is classified as either stage IA or IB but with tumor on surface of one or both ovaries; or with ruptured capsule(s); or with ascites containing malignant cells present or with positive peritoneal washings.
Stage II	Growth involving one or both ovaries with pelvic extension.
IIA	Extension and/or metastases to the uterus and/or tubes.
IIB	Extension to other pelvic tissues.
IIC	Tumor is either stage IIA or IIB, but with tumor on surface of one or both ovaries; or with capsule(s) ruptured; or with ascites present containing malignant cells present or with positive peritoneal washings.
Stage III	Tumor involves one or both ovaries with peritoneal implants outside the pelvis and/or positive retroperitoneal or inguinal nodes; superficial liver metastasis equals stage III; tumor is limited to the true pelvis but with histologically proven malignant extension to small bowel or omentum.

(Continued)

TABLE 23-6
(Continued)

Stage		Characteristics
	IIIA	Tumor grossly limited to the true pelvis with negative nodes but with histologically confirmed microscopic seeding of abdominal peritoneal surfaces.
	IIIB	Tumor of one or both ovaries with histologically confirmed implants of abdominal peritoneal surfaces, none exceeding 2 cm in diameter; nodes are negative.
	IIIC	Abdominal implants >2 cm in diameter and/or positive retroperitoneal or inguinal nodes.
Stage	IV	Growth involving one or both ovaries with distant metastases; if pleural effusion is present, there must be positive cytology to assign a case to stage IV; parenchymal liver metastasis equals stage IV.

CLINICAL EVALUATION

A careful history and complete physical examination are most important in the evaluation of potential ovarian malignancy. The most common physical findings are *adnexal masses, an abdominal mass, ascites, or nodulation.* Any fixed mass in the posterior cul-de-sac must be considered as possibly malignant, as is any large, fixed mass.

LABORATORY EVALUATION

Preoperative evaluation for suspected ovarian cancer includes complete blood count and typing, blood chemistry, urinalysis, cervical and vaginal cytology, liver function tests, coagulation profile, and proctosigmoidoscopy.

Sustained elevation of CA 125 occurs in >80% of patients with nonmucinous epithelial ovarian carcinomas, but is insufficiently specific to be diagnostic. For example, CA 125 elevations occur in

~1% of the general population and is most commonly associated with the following benign conditions: endometriosis, leiomyoma, PID, hepatitis, congestive heart failure, cirrhosis and nonovarian malignancies. Other serum tumor markers useful in the management of epithelial ovarian malignancies are CA 15-3, CA 19-9, carcinoembryonic antigen (CEA), lipid-associated sialic acid, and NB/70K. While alpha-fetoprotein, hCG, and lactate dehydrogenase may be of some usefulness in follow up of ovarian gem cell tumors, they (like CA125) are not sufficiently specific or sensitive to be diagnostic. Finally, the management of stromal tumors may be assisted by measurements of: inhibin, estrogens, androgens and alpha-fetoprotein.

IMAGING

Transvaginal sonography is now accepted as a portion of the initial evaluation for potential ovarian cancer. The sonographic criteria suggesting malignancy include: *bilaterality, solid and cystic component, excrescences, thick septations and the presence of free peritoneal fluid. Chest X-ray* rules out parenchymal involvement or pleural effusion. If screening *mammography* has not been performed within 6–12 months, it should be performed. Other imaging evaluations are dictated by the patient's signs or symptoms and may include: barium enema, upper gastrointestinal series, intravenous pyelography, and CT or MRI imaging. Liver and bone scans are currently less frequently indicated.

SURGICAL EVALUATION

Surgical exploration is necessary to obtain tissue for histologic study, to stage the tumor, and, hopefully, to effect cure. A *midline incision of sufficient size to allow intact tumor removal and complete exploration is necessary. Peritoneal washing* is performed if there is no peritoneal fluid available for cytologic sampling in unilateral disease. Lavage with 100 mL saline should be performed in four areas.

- Undersurface of the diaphragm (a cytological preparation similar to a Pap smear may be substituted)
- Lateral to the ascending colon
- Lateral to the descending colon
- The pelvic peritoneal surfaces

Washings are less helpful if malignant extension to the peritoneal surfaces or omentum has occurred or if the entire tumor cannot be removed. Both visualization and palpation of all peritoneal surfaces and abdominal organs are mandatory to search for metastatic disease. Any suspicious area(s) should be biopsied. Recall that staging is based on integration of clinical, surgical, histological, cytological, and pathological findings. Frozen sections may be helpful, but permanent histologic sections must be reviewed carefully before prognosis is given. *Under-staging is common in presumed early stage malignancies because of occult metastases in the: retroperitoneal nodes (10%), omentum (15%), and diaphragm (15%).*

TREATMENT

Standard therapy consists of total abdominal hysterectomy (TAH), bilateral salpingo-oophorectomy (BSO), and omentectomy. Retroperitoneal nodes should be palpated and biopsied if suspicious. In some cases, the disease is too extensive for total hysterectomy, adnexectomy, and omentectomy. In such cases, as much tumor as possible should be removed to improve the results of adjunctive therapy (chemotherapy and radiation therapy). However, more radical surgery has not been proven to be of added benefit in these advanced cases.

In the woman with an epithelial or germ cell neoplasm, stage IA that is well to moderately differentiated or of low malignant potential who understands the risks for late recurrence (10-year survival ~95%) and who wishes to preserve childbearing potential, surgery may be more conservative (i.e., unilateral salpino-oophorectomy).

Chemotherapy has not proven to further benefit (over surgery) those with stage IA or IB ovarian malignancies that are borderline, well or moderately-differentiated. Cisplatin and paclitaxel chemotherapy is the currently preferred initial adjunctive therapy for more advanced stages, and may be administered intravenously or directly intraperitoneally. Radiation therapy rarely has a role in primary treatment because of the disease's wide spread and proximity to regions likely to be quite radio-sensitive (e.g., liver, kidneys, bone marrow).

Reexploration (second-look surgery) may be of benefit if remarkable response to adjunctive therapy is documented in previously inoperable cases. Response rates of 40%–45% can be anticipated.

Follow-up of those with Ca_{125} elevations prior to surgery is facilitated by serial measurement of this tumor antigen. Indeed, in most cases this may be the most sensitive indication of tumor cell mass and may be used to suggest treatment failure as well as to indicate if second-look surgery is necessary. The *therapy of recurrent ovarian malignancies must be highly individualized.*

THE OVIDUCT

BENIGN TUMORS

These neoplasms are usually *asymptomatic and are not palpable.* They usually are discovered incidentally during surgery or investigative procedures.

Cysts of the uterine tube are fairly common, most often occurring near the fimbriated end as the result of occlusion of the accessory lumina of the tube during embryogenesis. On rare occasion, pregnancy may develop in the cyst or torsion may occur. Otherwise, they are asymptomatic.

Epithelial polyps may be located in the cornual portion of the tube. More distal tubal polyps are rare. Mesotheliomas are <1.5 cm in diameter. They are asymptomatic and found incidentally. Leiomyomas occur primarily in the cornual portion of the tube. Tubal teratomas have the same elements as ovarian teratomas but are located on the uterine tube.

MALIGNANT TUMORS

PRIMARY OVIDUCT CARCINOMA

Primary tubal carcinoma is the *least common cancer of the female reproductive tract.* It is associated with nulliparity in ~50% of the cases and usually becomes symptomatic in the early 50s. Like ovarian cancer, there are few complaints other than an intermittent serosanguineous discharge in ~30%. Occasionally, vaginal cytologic studies will be positive and lead to further investigation. Ascites is rare. Early in the disease, a slightly tender adnexal mass may be palpated during pelvic examination. Interestingly, the frequency and pattern of chromosomal changes detected in tubal carcinoma are very similar to those observed in serous ovarian and uterine carcinomas, suggesting common pathogenesis.

Ultrasonography may demonstrate a partially cystic, partially solid mass separate from the ovary and uterus. Hysterosalpingography should be avoided because dispersal of malignant cells into the peritoneal cavity may occur. *Laparoscopy is of little value, since treatment is surgical excision.* Barium enema and chest x-ray should be part of the workup, but liver and bone scans are rarely necessary. Late manifestations are lower abdominal discomfort or enlargement and intestinal obstruction.

The vast majority *(95%) of primary tubal cancer is papillary adenocarcinoma. In 40%–50%, bilateral tumors are found,* which may represent bilateral primary disease rather than metastases. With time, the papillary tumor progresses to papillary-alveolar, then to alveolar carcinoma. Extratubal extension does not necessarily portend poor prognosis.

Treatment is hysterectomy and bilateral salpingo-oophorectomy. Surgery is followed by chemotherapy or radiation therapy.

OTHER MALIGNANT TUMORS OF THE OVIDUCT

Other tumors of the oviduct include mixed mesodermal tumors, choriocarcinoma, and mesonephroma. Therapy is essentially the same as for the same tumor type located in the ovary or uterus.

ADNEXAL TORSION

Most commonly, *torsion of the ovary and tube occur together,* although the ovary alone may occasionally be twisted on its pedicle. *Adnexal torsion accounts for ~3% of gynecologic operative emergencies.* Adnexal torsion *occurs more often in children.* In adults (the average patient is in her mid-20s), *50%–60% of torsions occur with an ovarian mass* (most common at ~8–12 cm), and the most common ovarian tumor involved is *benign cystic teratoma.* However, solid benign tumors, serous cysts, and even paraovarian cysts may have a predilection to cause torsion. Pregnancy is also a predisposition. The *right ovary is involved more frequently* than the left. Interestingly, if a woman has one episode, she has a *10% chance of contralateral involvement.*

The usual symptom of adnexal torsion is *abdominal pain.* This pain is *acute and unilateral.* Associated *nausea and vomiting* occur in two thirds of patients. Intermittent pain may have preceded the final event, and a sudden change in position may be the precipitating factor. Expect *tenderness to palpation, but rebound tenderness is uncommon.* As the infarction progresses, there may be low-grade fever and leukocytosis.

Until recently, imaging studies (sonography and MRI) were limited and usually employed to rule out other processes. However, color Doppler sonography has proven valuable in both confirmation of the process as well as ascertaining the presence or absence of arterial and venous blood flow to the adnexa. If no blood flow is observed, it is nearly certain that hemorrhagic necrosis has occurred.

This is an important advance in diagnosis for it *discriminates which adnexa are viable and may be treated conservatively.*

Grossly, the involved adnexa is cyanotic to nearly black in color and edematous. On cut section and histology, hemorrhagic infarction is found. A twisted pedicle with vascular compromise must not be untwisted because *untwisting may discharge an embolus.* An *oophorocystectomy* should be performed by doubly ligating the pedicle slightly below the area of the twisting, taking care not to include adjacent structures (e.g., the ureter).

With foreknowledge of the vascular status of the adnexa, it may be possible to salvage the ovary or tube with incomplete torsion (i.e., without vascular compromise) by carefully releasing the torsion, performing a cystectomy if there is an associated ovarian cyst, and stabilizing the ovary by *shortening the ovarian ligament* with sutures. In many cases, this may be accomplished by laparoscopy. Although risk of emboli must be recognized, that has been infrequent when there is not vascular compromise. Additionally, consideration should be given to *shortening the contralateral ovarian ligament* because of the enhanced risk of torsion.

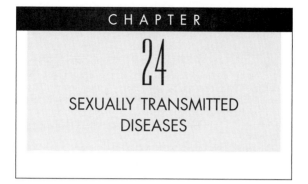

A *sexually transmitted disease (STD) is any infection acquired primarily through sexual contact.* STD is a *general term,* and the causative organisms, which are harbored in the blood or body secretions, include viruses, mycoplasmas, bacteria, fungi, spirochetes, and minute parasites (e.g., crab lice, scabies). Some of the organisms involved are found exclusively in the genital (reproductive) tract, but others exist simultaneously in other systems. Additionally, various STDs often coexist, and *when one is found, others should be suspected.* There is a range of intimate bodily contact that may transmit STDs, including kissing, sexual intercourse, anal intercourse, cunnilingus, anilingus, fellatio, and mouth or genital to breast contact. Physicians are required to *report most STDs* to local public health departments.

The *vast majority of female genital tract infections are acquired sexually.* Female genital tract infections are divided into *lower genital tract and upper genital tract (or pelvic) infections.* The lower genital tract infections (including a number of STDs and their sequelae) are discussed in Chapters 20 and 21, and they include viral infections (herpes simplex, human papillomavirus, and molluscum contagiosum) and vulvar infestations (pedicularis pubis and scabies). Common types of vulvovaginitis (e.g., *Trichomonas,* bacterial vaginosis, and *Candida*) and some of the sequelae of STDs (e.g., infections of Bartholin glands and cervicitis) also are discussed in Chapter 20. This chapter deals with upper genital tract infections, the most serious, most directly sexually transmitted diseases and their sequelae.

HUMAN IMMUNODEFICIENCY VIRUS (HIV) INFECTIONS

The human immunodeficiency virus (HIV) was first reported to cause disease in 1981. In the United States, *AIDS is now the fifth leading cause of death among women of childbearing age.* More-over, it is the leading cause of death in this age group in New York City. This is now a *worldwide crisis,* with millions affected, especially in developing countries. One of the problems in recognition of HIV infection is a *long, asymptomatic latency of 2 months to 5 years.* The mean age at diagnosis of HIV infection is *35 years.*

The virus is present in blood and all body fluids and is *transmitted by sexual contact (>70%),* by parenteral exposure to infected blood or body fluids, or by transplacental passage of the virus from mother to fetus. The highest-risk groups for HIV infection are *homosexuals, bisexual men, intravenous drug abusers, and hemophiliacs receiving blood transfusions.* Others at high risk are *prostitutes* and *heterosexual partners of men in the high-risk groups.* All blood must be screened for HIV before transfusion to minimize transfusion risk. *Women acquire the virus more easily from men* rather than the reverse because the concentration of HIV in semen is high and mucosal breaks at the introitus or vagina with intercourse occur more commonly than do breaks in penile skin.

Although anti-HIV antibodies develop within 12 weeks of exposure, *45%–90% of persons infected with HIV will develop symptoms of an acute infection similar to mononucleosis within a few months.* They experience weight loss, fever, night sweats, pharyngitis, lymphadenopathy, and an erythematous maculopapular rash. Most of these symptoms resolve within a few weeks, although the patients remain infectious despite being asymptomatic. Some will progress to develop symptoms of *AIDS-related complex* (ARC), with *early immunosuppression* (decreased CD4+ lymphocytes). ARC is usually marked by generalized lymphadenopathy, weight loss, diarrhea, malabsorption, and wasting. Some patients experience *further immunosuppression and develop AIDS* (any of the symptoms of acute sepsis, opportunistic infections, Kaposi's sarcoma, cognitive difficulties, or depression). Once AIDS has been diagnosed, mortality is >90%. Immunologic abnormalities associated with AIDS include (but are not limited to) lymphopenia, decreased T helper cells, decreased T lymphocytes, hypergammaglobulinemia, and an inverted T4/T8 ratio.

Because there is *no cure for HIV,* current therapy only slows the progression of the disease. Hence, there is *every reason to stress prevention.* Other than abstinence or having a monogamous relationship with a known noninfected partner, using latex condoms lubricated with nonoxynol 9 is the most effective method of limiting the risk of infection. If a woman is HIV positive, she should be counseled (1) not to donate blood, plasma, tissue, or organs; (2) to avoid pregnancy; (3) to maintain a monogamous relationship;

and (4) to assiduously use condoms lubricated with nonoxynol 9 during any sexual contact.

HIV antibody testing begins with the *enzyme-linked immunosorbent assay (ELISA)*, which has a >95% sensitivity and a >99% specificity if repeatedly positive. *If the ELISA is positive, a Western blot assay* must be performed to confirm the diagnosis. False-negative results are rare unless the patient is too early in the disease to have formed antibodies. *HIV screening* (after informed consent has been obtained and assurances of confidentiality provided) should be encouraged for women in the following categories: *intravenous drug users, prostitutes, sex partner(s) of men who are HIV positive or at risk for HIV, those with other sexually transmitted disease, those who received blood transfusions between 1978 and 1985, those with clinical signs and symptoms of HIV infection, inhabitants of a country with high endemic heterosexual HIV infection, prison inmates, and one who considers herself at risk.*

Pregnancy does not appear to alter the progression of HIV infection, but the *chance of the fetus acquiring the virus is 20%–50%.* The neonate may be infected during labor and delivery by maternal blood or body fluids or may be infected during breastfeeding. The mode of delivery does not influence the development of pediatric AIDS. The acute illness associated with HIV in pregnancy may be misdiagnosed if HIV serologic testing is not performed. When HIV infection is diagnosed during pregnancy, treatment should be delayed because of the teratogenic potential of the medications used. The pregnant HIV-infected woman should be screened for other STDs, along with evaluation for opportunistic infection. A baseline serologic study for CMV and toxoplasmosis, TB skin testing, and chest radiograph are recommended. Recently AZT and other chemotherapeutic agents have been found to decrease maternal–fetal and neonatal transmission of HIV. When caring for HIV positive mothers, health care providers should obtain the very latest information in this important and rapidly evolving area.

Care of the HIV-positive woman and her infant in the peripartum and postpartum interval includes protection of health care workers by using universal infection control guidelines (e.g., water-repellent gowns, gloves, masks, goggles for potential splash situations, wall or bulb suctioning). Scalp electrodes and fetal scalp blood samples should be avoided (potential entry site for HIV if fetus is not already infected). Circumcision should not be done if the neonate is HIV positive. Because anti-HIV IgG antibody passes through the placenta, the infant may be seropositive without being infected. Abnormal facial features have been described in some HIV-positive newborns, but this is not common.

If neonatal/pediatric AIDS develops, the course of the disease is much more rapid than in adults, with death in months rather than years.

GONORRHEA

Neisseria gonorrhoeae (one of the most common causes of STD) is a *gram-negative diplococcus* that usually resides in the female in the urethra, cervix, pharynx, or anal canal. The infection primary involves the columnar and transitional epithelium of the genitourinary tract. The organism is very fastidious and sensitive to drying, sunlight, heat, and most disinfectants. Special media (e.g., Thayer-Martin) are required to achieve optimal recovery. Culture of the lower genital tract is usually obtained by rotating a cotton swab for 15–20 sec deep in the *endocervical canal.* If a *rectal swab* is taken, the incidence of recovery increases from 85% to >90%. In upper genital tract infections (salpingitis, peritonitis) proven by laparoscopically obtained culture, only ~50% of the lower genital tract cultures will reveal *N. gonorrhoeae.*

After exposure to an infected partner, 60%–90% of women and 20%–50% of men will become infected. *Untreated, 10%–17% of women will develop pelvic inflammatory disease (PID).* If a woman is positive for *N. gonorrhoeae,* she has a *20%–40% chance of also having chlamydial infection, syphilis, or hepatitis.*

Early symptoms typically include *vaginal discharge, urinary frequency, and rectal irritation.* Some report burning, itching, or inflammation of the vulva, vagina, cervix, or urethra, *although most women are asymptomatic.* Bartholin duct(s) and gland(s) may be involved, as evidenced by swelling or abscess formation (Chapter 20). Acute pharyngitis and tonsillitis may occur, but this is uncommon. Rarely, the asymptomatic carrier will develop a disseminated infection with *polyarthralgia,* tenosynovitis, and dermatitis or meningitis or endocarditis. Although *ophthalmic infection* most commonly occurs in neonates born to an infected mother, adult ophthalmitis may result from autoinoculation.

The diagnosis may be presumed when a stained smear from the involved sites reveals *intracellular gram-negative diplococci.* However, confirmation after growth on selective medium is essential. The culture for gonorrhea must include penicillin resistance testing because 2%–3% of strains in the United States are penicillin resistant. Gonorrhea must be reported to the state public health authorities.

The patient and all sexual partners must be treated. Other concomitant diseases must be ruled out and treated if present. The preferred adult regimen for uncomplicated disease is ceftriaxone 125 mg IM (single dose), cefixime 400 mg PO (single dose), or spectinomycin 2 g IM (single dose for patients with cephalosporin intolerance). Although spectinomycin is not reliable therapy for pharyngeal infection, ceftriaxone and cefixime are effective in all sites. Given the high rate of coinfection, treatment for chlamydial infection (see the following section) is necessary. Because of the emergence of resistant organisms, repeat cultures should be performed within 7 d of completion of therapy to ensure cure.

Disseminated disease requires hospitalization. Meningitis and endocarditis must be confirmed or ruled out. Recommended therapy is ceftriaxone 1 g IM or IV qd or cefotaxime or ceftrizoxime 1 g IV q8h. Patients with allergy to beta-lactamase drugs may be treated with spectromycin 2 g IM q12h. If sensitivity testing confirms that the organism is penicillin-sensitive, ampicillin 1 g q6h may be given. Whichever regimen is chosen, therapy should be continued for 7 days. The prognosis for properly treated gonorrhea is good, but future fertility may be compromised.

CHLAMYDIAL INFECTIONS

Chlamydia trachomatis is an obligate intracellular microorganism with a cell wall similar to that of gram-negative bacteria. Although they are classified as bacteria, contain both DNA and RNA, and divide by binary fission. *Chlamydia* grow only intracellularly, as do viruses. Since most of the *C. trachomatis* serotypes attack only columnar epithelial cells (except the aggressive L serotypes), signs and symptoms tend to be localized to the infected area (e.g., eye or genital tract) without deep tissue invasion.

CERVICITIS

C. trachomatis cervical and tubal infections occur in women of young age (2–3 times higher in women <20 years), *with numerous sexual partners, of low socioeconomic status, with other STDs, and with oral contraceptive use.* Barrier contraception tends to decrease the infection rate. *Pregnant women have an incidence of 8%–12%.*

SIGNS AND SYMPTOMS

Typically, a mucopurulent discharge develops with cervical chlamydial infection, and the cervix shows hypertrophic inflammation (mucopurulent cervicitis). The infection may be *asymptomatic in 15%* of nonpregnant, sexually active women.

LABORATORY FINDINGS

The most frequently used method of detection is a *direct fluorescein-conjugated monoclonal antibody test* (available in kit form). This is rapid, sensitive (85%–93%), and specific (~99%). Specimens are generally obtained as described for gonorrhea (p. 684). Tissue culture is required for culture of *C. trachomatis,* and because of the high cost, limited availability, and 2–6 day delay, it is used infrequently. Although Giemsa staining of conjunctival specimens in neonates is fairly successful in identifying chlamydial inclusions, this technique is only 40% accurate in genital infections.

DIFFERENTIAL DIAGNOSIS

N. gonorrhoeae is the only other predominant organism causing a mucopurulent cervicitis. Thus, fluorescent antibody tests or cultures on selective medium are mandatory for differentiation. Both organisms may be present simultaneously.

TREATMENT

Cure rates of >95% can be achieved with the use of one of several regimens. The preferred regimen is tetracycline 500 mg PO qid for 7 days or doxycycline 100 mg bid for 7 days. If tetracyclines cannot be taken or are contraindicated, erythromycin base 500 mg qid for 7 days or erythromycin ethylsuccinate 800 mg qid for 7 days may be prescribed.

COMPLICATIONS

The primary complication of *C. trachomatis* cervical infection is *salpingitis.* Unfortunately, if the patient is *pregnant and untreated,* the vaginally delivered neonate will develop *chlamydial conjunctivitis in 50% of cases and late onset pneumonitis in 10%.* Premature delivery and early postpartum endometritis are also associated problems.

SALPINGITIS

C. trachomatis salpingitis may be as prevalent as that caused by *N. gonorrhoeae.* However, there are marked differences in the pathophysiology and symptomatology. *C. trachomatis* salpingitis (which is also an ascending infection) has an *insidious onset,* it usually causes *minimal symptoms,* and the organism remains in the tube (primarily in the epithelium) for months. In contrast,

N. gonorrhoeae infections have an *acute onset,* cause more *acute symptoms,* and remain in the tubes only 24–48 h. Gonorrheal infections appear to have a much greater cytotoxic effect on the tubal epithelium.

Although *C. trachomatis* salpingitis usually causes fewer symptoms, the gross appearance of the tubes suggests even more severe involvement. Salpingitis is a consequence of *C. trachomatis* cervicitis. Treatment of *C. trachomatis* salpingitis may be accomplished with tetracyclines or erythromycin. The sequelae of *C. trachomatis* salpingitis include ectopic pregnancy and infertility, although the exact incidence of these complications is unknown.

LYMPHOGRANULOMA VENEREUM

The L serotypes of *C. trachomatis* cause lymphogranuloma venereum, which usually occurs in tropical or subtropical areas (including the southern United States). The *incubation period is 7–21 days,* and *men are affected 6 times more often than women.* In the United States, <500 cases/year are reported, and most occur in men.

Lymphogranuloma venereum begins with a vesicopustular eruption that progresses to very painful inguinal and vulvar ulceration, lymphedema, and secondary bacterial invasion. Clinically, a depression between the groups of inguinal nodes and the genitocrural fold produces the appearance of a *double genital crural fold* (the groove sign). There is a reddish to purplish blue, hard induration that occurs *10–30 days after exposure.* Anorectal lymphedema causes painful defecation and blood-streaked stools. Later in the disease, *progressive rectal strictures* form, which may even prevent defecation. *Vaginal strictures* may cause distortion and narrowing, with resultant dyspareunia. Headache, arthralgia, chills, and abdominal cramps may occur late in this disease. Late complications include *vulvar elephantiasis.*

The *diagnosis* is confirmed by tissue culture and serotype determination, but complement fixation for *Chlamydia* with titer ≥1:16 is presumptive, as is a rising titer (>1:64 is diagnostic). Immunofluorescent testing is available. The differential diagnosis for the cutaneous lesions includes granuloma inguinale, tuberculosis, syphilis, chancroid, vulvar cancer, genital herpes, and Hodgkin's disease. With systemic symptoms, meningitis, arthritis, peritonitis, and pleurisy must be considered.

Treatment for lymphogranuloma venereum includes doxycycline 100 mg PO bid for 21 days. Persistent disease requires a second course. Alternative drugs include tetracycline, erythromycin, or sulfisoxizole, each at 500 mg PO qid for 21 days. After the disease is under control, surgery may be necessary (e.g., partial vulvectomy). Abscesses should not be excised but treated by aspiration. Anal strictures should be dilated weekly. A diversionary colostomy may be required for severe anal stricture.

SYPHILIS

Syphilis is a disease caused by the spirochete *Treponema pallidum,* which is transmitted by direct contact with an infectious moist lesion. These organisms can pass through intact mucous membranes or abraded skin or may be acquired transplacentally. A single sexual encounter with an infected partner carries ~*10% chance of acquiring syphilis.* Untreated, the disease progresses from *primary to secondary to latent and, finally, to tertiary syphilis.* Congenital syphilis has its own course and symptoms. *There are >280,000 new cases of syphilis in the United States each year.*

The primary lesion of syphilis is the *hard chancre,* an indurated, firm, painless papule or ulcer with raised borders, which appears *10 days to 3 months* (average is 3 weeks) after the treponemes have entered the body. The chancre may be located on the external genitalia, cervix, or vagina or any area of skin or mucous membrane of the body but is often not noted in women. The *primary lesion persists for 1–5 weeks* and is followed in most by spontaneous healing. Any lesion suspected of being a chancre should be subjected to *darkfield examination,* seeking treponemes, because culture is not available. Serologic tests for syphilis should be performed weekly for 6 weeks or until positive (usually reactive 1–4 weeks after the chancre appears).

The *generalized cutaneous eruption (macular, maculopapular, papular, or pustular) of secondary syphilis appears 2 weeks to 6 months after the primary lesion.* The rash is a diffuse, bilateral, symmetric papulosquamous eruption that may *involve the palms and soles.* Perineal lesions (moist papules, *condyloma latum*) are present and positive for treponemes on darkfield examination or immunofluorescent studies. Other mucous patches may be present, as well as patchy alopecia, hepatitis, or nephritis. Generalized lymphadenopathy is typical. The secondary lesions *last 2–6 weeks and heal spontaneously.* Serologic tests are almost always positive at this stage.

Latent syphilis is untreated syphilis after secondary symptoms have subsided. These patients remain *infectious for 1–2 years* and may have relapses resembling the secondary stage. Latency may be lifelong or end with the development of *tertiary syphilis, which occurs in one third of patients.*

Tertiary syphilis is marked by the presence of *destructive lesions of skin, bone (gummas), cardiovascular system (e.g., aortic aneurysm or insufficiency), or nervous system disorders* (e.g., meningitis, tabes dorsalis, paresis). Tertiary syphilis is *fatal in 25%* of those affected.

Although the maternal course of syphilis is unaltered by pregnancy, it is *frequently not recognized unless detected by serologic screening.* The treponemes may pass transplacentally throughout pregnancy, but if the disease is discovered and treated <18 weeks gestation, the fetus appears to suffer few sequelae. *After 18 weeks, the classic signs of congenital syphilis occur in the fetus.* The risk of fetal infection is greater during the secondary stage than during the primary or latent stages. The incidence of stillbirth and premature delivery is increased with syphilis. Hydramnios may be present. The placenta is involved; it has a waxy, hydropic appearance. Infection late in pregnancy results in fetal or neonatal infection in 40%–50%.

Congenital syphilis occurs in the fetus or newborn whose mother has untreated syphilis. Depending on time of acquisition of infection, there may be *signs of intrauterine infection* (e.g., hepatosplenomegaly, radiographic changes in bone, anemia, jaundice, lymphadenitis, and meningitis) *or the baby may appear unaffected,* only to develop signs and symptoms equivalent to secondary syphilis sometime after birth.

Classically, the *newborn with congenital syphilis may be undergrown, with wrinkled facies* because of reduced subcutaneous fat. The skin may have a *brownish (café-au-lait) tint.* The most common lesion of early congenital syphilis in the newborn is a *bullous rash,* so-called syphilitic pemphigus. Large blebs may appear over the palms and soles and, occasionally, in all other areas. Seropurulent fluid from the lesions swarms with treponemes. Mucositis identical with that of secondary syphilis in older patients may be noted in the mouth and upper respiratory passages of the newborn. The nasal discharge (*syphilitic snuffles*) is very infectious because it contains large numbers of *T. pallidum.*

The bones usually show signs of *osteochrondritis,* and on x-ray, an *irregular epiphyseal juncture* (Guerin's line) is characteristic. Abnormalities of the eyes and other organs or the central nervous system may be apparent at birth, or defects may develop later in untreated cases. Any infant with the stigmata of syphilis should be placed in isolation until a definitive diagnosis can be made and appropriate treatment given.

Because serologic testing evaluates IgG antibodies that are transplacentally acquired, the baby will be positive if the mother is positive. Effective neonatal treatment is shown by progressively falling titers over weeks to months.

LABORATORY FINDINGS

Visualization of the treponemal organisms requires the presence of a moist cutaneous lesion for *darkfield examination* (fresh smear), immunofluorescent staining (dried smear), or silver staining for the treponemes in a biopsy specimen. Because the organisms are demonstrable for only a short time, *diagnosis usually relies on history and serologic testing.*

Screening for syphilis is accomplished primarily by *nonspecific nontreponemal antibody testing* (e.g., VDRL, RPR). All pregnant women should be tested at the first visit. High-risk patients should be screened at 28–32 weeks gestation and at delivery. These tests become *positive 3–6 weeks after infection.* The titers are high in secondary syphilis and fall to low titers or even become negative in late syphilis. *Titers that have a 4-fold drop or are falling in early syphilis indicate adequate treatment.*

False-positive tests may be associated with collagen disease, infectious mononucleosis, malaria, leprosy, febrile illnesses, vaccination, drug addiction, old age, and pregnancy itself. The titer seen with false-positive tests usually is low. However, any positive test should be investigated by an antitreponemal antibody test. The most widely performed antitreponemal antibody test is the fluorescent treponemal antibody absorption (FTA-ABS) test. The test remains positive regardless of therapy. Thus, titers are not determined.

DIFFERENTIAL DIAGNOSIS

The *differential diagnosis for primary syphilis* includes chancroid, granuloma inguinale, lymphogranuloma venereum, herpes, carcinoma, scabies, trauma, lichen planus, psoriasis, drug eruption, aphthosis, mycotic infection, Reiter's syndrome, and Bowen's disease.

The *differential diagnosis for secondary syphilis* includes pityriasis rosea, psoriasis, lichen planus, tinea versicolor, drug eruption, "id" eruptions, perleche, parasitic infection, iritis, neuroretinitis, condylomata accuminata, acute exanthems, infectious mononucleosis, alopecia, and sarcoidosis.

TREATMENT

Treatment should be initiated if exposure has occurred even if evidence of disease is not present. During pregnancy, it is better to treat any suspicion of disease rather than risk congenital syphilis.

Contacts and patients with early syphilis (primary, secondary, and latent <1 year) should be treated with one of the following regimens: (1) benzathine penicillin G 2.4 million units IM, (2) tetracycline hydrochloride 500 mg PO qid or doxycycline 100 mg bid for 14 days (for penicillin allergy but not during pregnancy), or (3) erythromycin (stearate, ethylsuccinate, or base) 500 mg PO qid for 15 days (30 g total) for penicillin allergy and if unable to take tetracycline. A short-lived (<24 h) febrile reaction occurs in 50%–75% of those receiving penicillin therapy, presumably due to a release of toxic treponemal products. The fever, which occurs 4–12 h after injection, is a *Jarisch-Herxheimer reaction.*

Congenital syphilis is treated with benzathine penicillin G 50,000 units/kg IM if the infant is asymptomatic and there is no evidence of neurosyphilis. Symptomatic congenital syphilis or neurosyphilis is treated with aqueous crystalline penicillin G 50,000 units/kg/day IV, divided in two doses for 10 days or aqueous procaine penicillin G 50,000 units/kg daily for 10 days.

CHANCROID

Chancroid (soft chancre) is caused by the gram-negative rod *Haemophilus ducreyi* and is uncommon in the United States (<1500 cases/year). This infection begins in females as a papule or vesicopustular lesion on the perineum, cervix, or vagina *3–5 days* after exposure. The lesion *progresses over 48–72 h to a very tender saucer-shaped ragged ulcer.* Several ulcers may develop in a cluster. The heavy discharge produced by the ulcer(s) is foul-smelling and infectious. Over 50% of patients develop *painful inguinal lymphadenitis* that may become necrotic and drain spontaneously. Aspiration of pus from a bubo may yield the organism. Syphilis must be ruled out, although the differential diagnosis also includes herpes simplex, lymphogranuloma venereum, and granuloma inguinale.

Treatment includes sitz baths, soap and water plus antibiotics. The *therapeutic regimen will vary depending on sensitivity of the pathogen.* Ceftriaxone 250 mg IM qd, erythromycin 500 mg PO qid, and trimethoprim (160 mg)/sulfamethoxazole (800 mg) PO bid have been effective. Treatment should continue for a minimum of 10 days until the ulcer(s) and lymph nodes are healed. Abscessed nodes should be aspirated rather than incised and drained.

GRANULOMA INGUINALE

Granuloma inguinale is caused by *Calymmatobacterium granulomatis.* A characteristic finding in the lesions is the *Donovan body* (bacteria encapsulated in mononuclear leukocytes). It is almost never seen in the United States (~100 cases/year) but is common in India, Brazil, and the West Indies. The incubation period is *1–12 weeks.* Granuloma inguinale may be spread by repeated sexual or nonsexual contact.

The disease usually is localized to the vulva and inguinal area but may involve the cervix, uterus, ovary, or mouth. It begins as an asymptomatic papule or nodule that ulcerates to form a red, granular area with sharp borders. The ulcer drains a foul-smelling discharge. *Healing is extremely slow,* but there are few local or systemic manifestations. Satellite ulcers may coalesce into one large ulcer. Buboes may occur late in the disease. Pain may be present if the urethra or anus is involved.

Late complications include *dyspareunia* if the introitus constricts from chronic disease. The differential diagnosis includes carcinoma, chancroid, lymphogranuloma venereum, and syphilis. The diagnosis is confirmed by finding Donovan bodies in a biopsy specimen or smear using Wright, Giemsa, or a silver stain.

The drug of choice for *treatment* of granuloma inguinale is tetracycline 500 mg qid for a minimum 21 days. Other choices include erythromycin 500 mg qid for 14–21 days, doxycycline 100 mg bid for 21 days, or sulfamethoxazole 1 g bid for 21 days.

PELVIC INFECTIONS

Infections may occur in any or all portions of the upper genital tract: endometrium (endometritis), uterine wall (myositis), oviducts (salpingitis), ovary (oophoritis), uterine serosa and broad ligaments (parametritis), and pelvic peritoneum (peritonitis). Although the exact incidence of upper genital tract infection is unclear, *over 10%* of U.S. women of reproductive age have received treatment for an upper genital tract infection. A functional classification of pelvic infections is shown in Table 24-1.

Organisms may disseminate to and throughout the pelvis in any of five ways.

- *Intraluminal.* Nonpuerperal acute pelvic inflammatory disease nearly always (~99%) follows a progression of entrance of pathogens through the cervix into the uterine cavity. Infection then spreads to the uterine tubes, with pus eventually entering the peritoneal cavity from the ostia. Organisms known to spread by this mechanism include *N. gonorrhoeae, C. trachomatis, Streptococcus agalactiae, cytomegalovirus,* and herpes simplex virus. Three fourths of

TABLE 24-1
FUNCTIONAL CLASSIFICATION OF
PELVIC INFECTIONS

Pelvic inflammatory disease (PID)
  Limited (salpingitis)
  Pelvic abscess (cul-de-sac or tuboovarian)
Puerperal infections
  Cesarean section (common)
  Vaginal (less common)
Postgynecologic procedure infection
  Acute PID after diagnostic instrumentation
  Abortion-related infections
    Postabortal cellulitis
    Incomplete septic abortion
  Cuff cellulitis and parametritis
  Vaginal cuff abscess
  Tuboovarian abscess
Pelvic infection secondary to other infections or
  intraabdominal accidents
  Appendicitis
  Diverticulitis
  Tuberculosis
  Traumatic viscus rupture

women with acute PID have concomitant endometritis, whereas ~40% of those with mucopurulent cervicitis and 50% of those with positive *C. trachomatis* or *N. gonorrhoeae* endocervical cultures have concomitant endometritis. The *endometritis phase is generally asymptomatic, often brief, and occurs at the end of a menses.*

- *Lymphatic.* Puerperal infections (including abortion) and IUD-related infections are disseminated through the lymphatic system, as are nonpuerperal *Mycoplasma* infections.
- *Hematogenous.* Hematogenous dissemination of pelvic disease is limited to certain diseases (e.g., tuberculosis) and is uncommon in the United States.
- *Intraperitoneal.* Intraabdominal infections (e.g., appendicitis, diverticulitis) as well as intraabdominal accidents (e.g., perforated viscus or ulcer) may lead to an infectious process involving the internal genital system.

- *Contiguous.* The postgynecologic surgical infections are the result of local spread of infection from areas of tissue necrosis and infection.

PELVIC INFLAMMATORY DISEASE (PID)

Given the anatomic intimacy and functional proximity of the reproductive system, it is *infrequent that infection is confined to just a single anatomic site.* Thus, *PID is a general clinical term for upper genital tract infections.* PID is an extraordinary health problem. There are about *1 million cases of acute PID a year in the United States,* and the total cost is estimated to exceed $7 billion per year. Over a quarter of PID cases require hospitalization. PID affects 1%–2% of sexually active females yearly and is more frequent in young women (75% of those affected are <25 years). In the United States, PID annually results in 2.5 million physician visits, nearly 270,000 inpatient admissions, about 120,000 operative procedures, and 0.29 deaths/100,000 women age 15–44.

There are a number of *risk factors* for PID, but the greatest risk centers about *sexual activity.* PID, which usually arises after a menstrual period, in sexually active females accounts for 85% of cases, but 15% occur after procedures in which the mucosal surface is injured (e.g., IUD insertion, endometrial biopsy, curettage, hysterosalpingogram). In <1% of PID, transperitoneal spread to the upper genital tract occurs from appendicitis, diverticulitis, or traumatic rupture of a viscus.

The risk of acquiring any STD is directly related to the number of sex partners. A woman with ≥10 lifetime sexual partners is >3 times more likely to have PID than a woman with one partner. Young age (*adolescence*) is a risk factor because of the less stable sexual relationships marking this time of life and possibly because of less immunity. *Other risk factors for PID include:* contraceptive practice (barrier methods markedly reduce the risk), ethnicity (in United States, African-American women report 17%, Caucasians 10%), postmarital status (3 times that of never married), bacterial vaginosis, vaginal douching and cigarette smoking.

Approximately two thirds of acute pelvic infections are polymicrobial. N. gonorrhoeae is responsible for one third of acute PID, *N. gonorrhoeae* with a mixed endogenous anaerobic and aerobic flora is responsible for another one third, and mixed anaerobes and aerobes are responsible for the remaining third. In combination with other organisms, *C. trachomatis* is found in up to 30% of cases. The aerobes and anaerobes found in PID usually are normal vaginal and gastrointestinal flora. The anaerobes (e.g., *Bacteroides, Peptostreptococcus,*

Peptococcus) predominate in abscesses. Common aerobes include *Escherichia coli,* group B *Streptococcus, Streptococcus faecalis,* and coagulase-negative *Staphlococcus. Mycoplasma hominis* and *Ureaplasma urealyticum* do not appear to be pathogenic in PID.

The *signs and symptoms of acute PID are generally nonspecific but are related to both the extent of the infection and the organisms* involved. *Lower abdominal pain* of <7 days duration occurs in >90% of patients with acute PID. The pain is usually characterized as constant and dull (but may be aching, burning, cramping, or stabbing) and is enhanced by movement or sexual activity. Endocervical infection is present in 75% of patients with PID. Abnormal vaginal bleeding, increased discharge or abnormal vaginal odor occurs in 40% of patients. Other symptoms are nonspecific, including fever (30%), malaise, gastrointestinal (vomiting, diarrhea, constipation, and tenesmus), urinary (dysuria, frequency, and urgency), and headache.

The *white blood cell count* may be normal, increased, or decreased and *should not be relied on to rule out PID.* Abdominal x-ray films (KUB and upright) may demonstrate adynamic ileus or free peritoneal gas or both. *Transvaginal sonography may be the most useful imaging and will reveal peritoneal fluid, thickne` ed edematous structures, hydrosalpingx,* and so forth. Sonography may also be useful for monitoring therapy. Culdocentesis is simple, relatively painless, and may be diagnostic, but is not currently used a great deal because of sonography and laparoscopy.

Laparoscopy is the "gold standard" for definitive diagnosis. Evaluating the *fluid* within the abdomen is of assistance in interpreting the visualized alterations. *Pus* suggests a ruptured tuboovarian abscess, ruptured appendix, ruptured viscus, ruptured diverticular abscess, or a uterine abscess involving a myoma. *Cloudy fluid* suggests pelvic peritonitis (as seen with acute gonococcal salpingitis), adnexal torsion, or other causes of peritonitis (e.g., appendicitis, pancreatitis, cholecystitis, perforated ulcer, carcinomatosis, or echinococcosis). *Blood* may be found with ruptured ectopic pregnancy, hemorrhage from corpus luteum cyst, retrograde menstruation, ruptured spleen or liver, gastrointestinal bleeding, or acute salpingitis.

If laparoscopy is performed the *sterile collection of specimens is mandatory.* Acute PID may be polymicrobial, but in two thirds *N. gonorrhoeae, C. trachomatis,* or both, are recovered. The other one third have mixed anaerobic organisms (*Prevotella* species and peptostreptococci) and facultative bacteria (*Gardnerella vaginalis,* streptococci, *Escherichia coli,* and *Haemophilus influenzae*). Reports are beginning to accumulate linking bacterial vaginosis and PID.

The infection may be so widespread that in *5%–10% of acute PID, perihepatic inflammation* develops. Here, the symptoms are right upper quadrant distress, pleuritic pain, and right upper quadrant tenderness. This condition is called the *Curtis-Fitzhugh syndrome and often results in perihepatic adhesions.*

Early diagnosis and prompt effective treatment may decrease the sequelae (e.g., pelvic adhesions, tissue necrosis, abscess formation, intestinal obstruction, infertility, and tubal pregnancy), but *25% of women with acute PID develop significant complications.* There is a *6–10 times increase in ectopic pregnancy and a 4 times increase in chronic pelvic pain, dyspareunia, and pelvic adhesions. Infertility is enhanced (20% of patients with just one attack—a 7 times increase),* depending on the number and severity of attacks. *Tuboovarian abscess occurs in 5%–10% of hospitalized acute PID patients.*

PID may be *decreased or prevented* by limiting the number of sexual contacts; determining if sexual contacts have STDs; using condoms, spermicides, diaphragms and spermicides; and employing postcoital toilet (urination, washing, or douching with antiseptic solution).

ACUTE SALPINGITIS

As noted previously, *the most common organisms* initiating acute salpingitis-peritonitis is *Neisseria gonorrhoeae* and *Chlamydia trachomatis.* Approximately 15% of asymptomatic infections will result in acute salpingitis.

Symptoms and Signs

Typically, salpingitis occurs in *young* (often teenage) women who have *multiple sexual partners* and are not using vaginal contraception. *Symptoms typically begin shortly after cessation of menses* or following instrumentation. The onset of *lower abdominal and pelvic pain* (frequently bilateral) is usually *acute* but may be insidious. Pain may radiate from the back down the leg(s). There may be a purulent vaginal discharge. Systemic symptoms include *fever (30%),* headache, malaise, nausea, and vomiting.

Physical examination reveals *abdominal tenderness,* usually of the lower quadrants. *Rebound tenderness is noted in the presence of peritonitis.* Bowel sounds may be decreased or absent. The paraurethral and Bartholin glands may be inflamed and discharging purulent material. The cervix often exudes a purulent discharge. *Movement of the cervix or uterus is exquisitely painful.* The adnexa are tender to palpation. The criteria for diagnosis of salpingitis are summarized in Table 24-2.

TABLE 24-2
CRITERIA FOR DIAGNOSIS OF SALPINGITIS

Criteria	
Abdominal direct tenderness, with or without rebound tenderness	
Tenderness with motion of cervix and uterus	All 3 necessary for diagnosis
Adnexal tenderness	
	plus
Gram stain of endocervix positive for gram-negative, intracellular diplococci	
Fever (>38°C)	
Leukocytosis (>10,000)	One or more necessary for diagnosis
Purulent material (WBCs present) from peritoneal cavity by culdocentesis or laparoscopy	
Pelvic abscess or inflammatory complex on bimanual examination or on sonography	

Modified from W.E. Hager, D.A. Eschenbach, M.R. Spence, et al. Criteria for diagnosis and grading of salpingitis. *Obstet Gynecol* 61:114, 1983.

Laboratory Findings

A smear of the cervical discharge nearly always reveals infection and may suggest the etiology (e.g., gram-negative diplococci of *N. gonorrhoeae*), but confirmation is essential, using selective media for *N. gonorrhoeae* and LCR or PCR for *C. trachomatis*. The WBC may be elevated or normal. *Women with suspected PID should have a quantitative hCG test because 3%–4% of them will have ectopic gestation.* Culdocentesis usually produces cloudy fluid, which should be sent for cell count, (>30,000 WBC/mL is associated with PID), gram stain, culture, and sensitivity.

If abdominal x-ray films show evidence of free air under the diaphragm, laparotomy is mandatory. Ultrasonic scanning is useful in the patient who is too tender to examine properly to rule out ectopic gestation or to reveal abscesses.

Differential Diagnosis

Included in the *differential diagnosis* are appendicitis, ectopic pregnancy, ruptured corpus luteum cyst with hemorrhage, diverticulitis, infected septic abortion, degeneration of a uterine leiomyoma, torsion of an adnexal mass, endometriosis, acute urinary tract infection, ulcerative colitis, and regional enteritis.

Treatment

Free peritoneal air is a surgical emergency, but the decision to *hospitalize for treatment is most frequently based on the following findings:* peritonitis in upper quadrants (nonpelvic peritonitis), gastrointestinal symptoms (including ileus), tuboovarian abscess, pregnancy, uncertain diagnosis, presence of an intrauterine device, history of instrumentation, inadequate response to outpatient therapy, or nulliparity.

Patients requiring hospitalization should be put at bedrest, initially kept NPO, given IV fluids, and placed on nasogastric suction for abdominal distention or ileus. Antibiotic therapy should be IV until the patient has shown clinical improvement for 48 h. Recommended[*] drug regimens include: cefotetan 2 g IV every 12 h, or cefeoxitin 2 g IV every 6 h, plus doxycycline 100 mg IV or PO every 12 h. An alternative[*] regimen is clindamycin 900 mg IV every 8 h, plus gentamicin, IV loading of 2 mg/kg followed by maintenance of 1.5 mg/kg every 8 h. For both regimens, 24 h after clinical improvement, parenteral therapy may be discontinued; however oral doxycycline 100 mg bid should be administered for 14 d. Alternative parenteral regimens recommended by various authorities include: ofloxacin 400 mg IV every 12 h plus metronidazole 500 mg IV every 8 h, ampicillin-sulbactam 3 g IV every 6 h, plus doxycycline 100 mg IV or PO every 12 h, Ciprofloxacin 200 mg IV every 12 h plus doxycycline 100 mg IV or PO every 12 h plus metronidazole 500 mg IV or PO every 8 h.

An *IUD should be removed* once therapy has been begun. Analgesics with or without codeine may provide relief.

Surgical exploration is reserved for those in whom life is threatened, the condition deteriorates, a tuboovarian abscess ruptures, a pelvic abscess is pointing into the cul-de-sac, the abdominal symptoms persist despite intensive therapy, and there are persistent masses. In women not desiring future childbearing, the tuboovarian masses may be removed. In the majority, however, every effort should be made to preserve ovarian function, especially in those who may want in vitro fertilization, when the uterus should remain.

---

[*]Centers for Disease Control and Prevention: 1998 guidelines for treatment of sexually transmitted diseases. *MMWR* 1998;47(RR-1):82–84.

Treatment is reasonable on an *outpatient basis for the majority of mild PID* (~75% of cases). The patient must not be pregnant and must not appear acutely ill, and the diagnosis must be certain. The recommended* outpatient oral regimens is ofloxacin, 400 mg PO bid for 14 d, plus metronidazole 500 mg PO bid for 14 d. The recommended* outpatient parenteral regimens include: ceftriaxone 250 mg IM once, or cefoxitin 2 g IM plus probenecid 1 g PO. Other possibilities* include other parenteral third-generation cephalosporins (e.g., ceftizoxime or cefotaxime) plus doxycycline 100 mg PO bid for 14 d. Additionally, many authorities advocate adding metronidazole 500 mg bid PO to the previously noted IM regimens to cover the anaerobes associated with bacterial vaginosis. Alternatively amoxicillin-clavulanic acid plus doxycycline 100 mg PO ever 12 h for 14 d may be used. The patient should be reevaluated in 48–72 h after starting therapy. If she fails to improve, she should be hospitalized for treatment. Other indications for hospitalization include: inability to follow or tolerate an oral regimen, severe illness (high fever, nausea, vomiting), tuboovarian abscess, and an immunodeficiency state. Follow-up examination, including cervical cultures, should be performed 2 weeks after therapy to assure a cure.

Prognosis

The prognosis depends on *prompt therapy with broad-spectrum antibiotics and rest*. *Complications* include hydrosalpinx, pyosalpinx, tuboovarian abscess, infertility, ectopic pregnancy (at least 2 times increased), and chronic pelvic pain (20% after just one episode). Probably between 1%–2% of U.S. women are *infertile* as a result of PID. Approximately 6% of aggressively treated gonococcal salpingitis will result in infertility, whereas 17% of nongonoccal case will suffer infertility. *Laparoscopy is useful in relating the extent of the disease to future infertility.* About 10% with observable mild disease will be infertile, compared to >40% of those with severe disease. *The prognosis for fertility decreases substantially with each infection.* Infertility is present in 12%–18% with the first (or only) episode of acute salpingitis, 25% with two episodes, and 60% with three episodes of salpingitis.

Recurrent infections are so common (25%) that in the past a designation of chronic infection was given to cases in which therapy was appropriate but the patient returned with another infection. Thus, *effective treatment of sexual partners is mandatory.* The partners of women with *N. gonorrhoeae* and *C. trachomatis* are usually teated with ceftriaxone 125 mg IM plus 100 mg of doxycycline PO bid for 7 d. An alternative is azithromycin 1 g PO (a single dose).

PELVIC ABSCESS

Cul-De-Sac Abscess

Pelvic abscesses may be tuboovarian or in the cul-de-sac. Most often, pelvic abscesses follow acute pelvic infection or septic abortion, although they may follow appendicitis, perforated viscus, or recurrent pelvic infection. *Bacteroides* (either *fragilis* or *bovis*) is the most commonly cultured organism. The symptoms may be those of *acute pelvic infection plus a fluctuant mass in the adnexa or cul-de-sac.* Pain usually is more severe than with acute PID or salpingitis, especially to the rectum and back and during defecation.

The *differential diagnosis* includes tuboovarian abscess, periappendiceal abscess, ectopic pregnancy, retroflexed and incarcerated uterus, endometriosis, diverticulitis with perforation, and carcinomatosis.

Antibiotic treatment must be effective against both aerobic and anaerobic bacteria. Recommended regimens include (1) penicillin G 20–30 million units IV per day, plus chloramphenicol 4–6 g IV per day (monitor for idiosyncratic aplastic anemia); (2) penicillin G 20–30 million units IV per day, clindamycin 600–1200 mg IV qid, and gentamicin 5 mg/kg per day; (3) cefoxitin 8–12 g IV per day and gentamicin or tobramycin 5 mg/kg/day; and (4) cefotaxime 6–8 g IV per day.

The patient should be *reevaluated frequently* (and gently) for *signs of peritoneal involvement or dissection into the rectovaginal septum with fixation.* If any of these occur, *surgical intervention is necessary.* If extension downward occurs, vaginal drainage with a large Pezar-type catheter should be accomplished. This should be followed by low-pressure irrigation with sterile saline q6h until the space is obliterated. If fever persists despite antibiotic therapy, percutaneous drainage and irrigation of the cul-de-sac may be performed.

If peritoneal signs develop or if the patient's condition deteriorates despite therapy, an exploratory laparotomy is indicated. When the patient has no further desire for children, total abdominal hysterectomy (TAH), bilateral salpingo-oophorectomy (BSO), and lysis of adhesions should be performed. More conservative surgery may be dictated by age, parity, condition of the tubes and ovaries, and desire for childbearing. In some cases, salvage of even an ovary may be desirable.

Although the *prognosis for fertility is guarded, the overall prognosis is good* if the abscess is localized and is treated early. If rupture into the peritoneum occurs, the prognosis is serious.

Tuboovarian Abscess (TOA)

Although tuboovarian abscess may occur after an initial episode of acute salpingitis, it *most often is associated with recurrent adnexal infections* (Fig. 24-1). The ovarian site of ovulation is thought to be a portal of infection for abscess formation. *TOA is bilateral in 60%–80%.*

Fulminant peritonitis with a 5%–10% mortality rate results from sudden rupture of an abscess, whereas a slow leak may result in signs and symptoms of a cul-de-sac abscess. Granulomatous disease (e.g., tuberculosis, actinomycosis) and use of IUDs are associated with TOA.

Patients may be asymptomatic or clearly be in septic shock. The *typical patient has a history of previous pelvic infection, is young, with low parity, and has had symptoms for <1 week.* The onset is usually 2 weeks after menses, with pelvic and abdominal pain (of varying degrees), nausea, vomiting, fever, and tachycardia. The entire abdomen is tender, and guarding may be present. Because of extreme tenderness of the adnexa, pelvic examination may be difficult. Culdocentesis may rupture the abscess, thus ultrasonography is preferred for diagnosis. The WBC count may be low, normal, or greatly elevated. The abdominal x-ray may show adynamic ileus or free air under the diaphragm if rupture has occurred.

The *differential diagnosis in the asymptomatic patient* may be ovarian cyst, ovarian neoplasm, unruptured ectopic pregnancy,

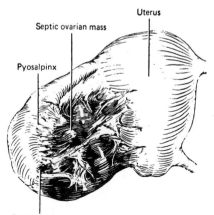

FIGURE 24-1. Tuboovarian abscess.

uterine leiomyoma, hydrosalpinx, or periappendiceal abscess. In the *symptomatic patient* whose tuboovarian abscess remains unruptured, the differential diagnosis includes appendiceal abscess, appendiceal rupture, diverticular abscess, perforated diverticulum, perforated peptic ulcer, porphyria, and diabetes mellitus. Complications include septic shock, septic emboli, peritonitis, bowel obstruction, recurrent infection, ectopic pregnancy, and infertility.

Treatment depends on whether or not the abscess is symptomatic and whether or not it has ruptured. If the tuboovarian abscess is *unruptured and asymptomatic, it* may be treated by antibiotics (see below). If the *mass does not shrink within 2–3 weeks* of antibiotic therapy or increases in size, surgery is indicated. Usually TAH and BSO are performed, although a more conservative approach (unilateral adnexectomy) is reasonable in select patients. If the abscess is *unruptured but symptomatic,* the patient should be hospitalized, placed at bedrest in semi-Fowler position, and maintained NPO with nasogastric suction applied, and she should receive IV fluids with close monitoring of electrolytes. Antibiotics should be administered IV in one of the following combinations.

Penicillin G (or ampicillin) and chloramphenicol
Penicillin G (or ampicillin) plus metronidazole
Clindamycin plus an aminoglycoside (gentamicin, amikacin, tobramycin)
Cefoxitin or cefamandole plus either clindamycin, metronidazole, or choramphenicol
Moxalactam or cefotaxime with or without clindamycin, metronidazole, chloramphenicol, or an aminoglycoside

If the initial therapy results in improvement, continue oral antibiotics (tetracycline, doxycycline) for 10–14 days. If rupture or leakage is suspected or if the patient does not respond to antibiotic therapy, perform an exploratory laparotomy. About 50% of patients with unruptured symptomatic tuboovarian abscess will require surgery.

A ruptured tuboovarian abscess is a life-threatening emergency and must be treated as such. Admit the patient to an intensive care unit (or its equivalent) in preparation for surgery. Monitor urine output hourly, and monitor the central venous pressure, administer oxygen, and correct hypovolemia. Corticosteroids (e.g., methylprednisolone succinate 15–30 mg/kg IV q4–6h for 4 doses) may be advisable. Surgery must be performed as soon as the patient has stabilized sufficiently to tolerate a major operation.

The abdomen should be entered through a midline incision. The pus encountered should be sent for aerobic and anaerobic culture. The entire abdomen should be explored, and all abscesses should be drained. Thorough irrigation with suction is necessary. Normally, TAH and BSO are performed, but therapy must be individualized. Supracervical hysterectomy may be necessary to shorten operative time in the unstable patient. Drains should be inserted through the open vaginal cuff or cul-de-sac. Leave drains in place as long as there is purulent discharge. Close the fascia but leave the subcutaneous space open.

The *prognosis for survival with an unruptured tuboovarian abscess is excellent, although fertility is markedly diminished. Mortality from ruptured tuboovarian abscess is 5%–10%, with sterility a consequence of hysterectomy and oophorectomy.*

POSTOPERATIVE PELVIC INFECTIONS

Hysterectomy carries a high rate of infection presumably because the vaginal flora cannot be eliminated from the operative site. The common infectious sequelae of hysterectomy includes *cuff induration* (cellulitis), *infected cuff hematoma* (cuff abscess), *salpingitis, pelvic cellulitis, suppurative pelvic thrombophlebitis,* and *tuboovarian abscess.* These infections are usually *polymicrobial.* The incidence of posthysterectomy infection may be lowered to 5% by a single dose of prophylactic antibiotic therapy.

Postoperative infection usually begins as cuff cellulitis that spreads from the vaginal apex to the parametrial tissues. If there is a hematoma present, an abscess forms. Antibiotic therapy and adequate drainage may halt further progression to salpingitis, diffuse pelvic cellulitis, and tuboovarian abscess. If the pelvic veins become involved (as is common with anaerobic infection), suppurative pelvic thrombophlebitis results, and septic emboli may occur to lungs, brain, spleen, and other sites.

CLINICAL FINDINGS

Postoperative pelvic infection causes *fever* (>38°C or >100°F) within 24–36 h in 50% of patients. Alternatively, temperature elevation may be due to atelectasis, urinary tract infection, or phlebitis. Early onset of fever without symptoms may resolve spontaneously, whereas fever by 72 h may require antibiotic therapy.

Examination of the *vaginal cuff* after hysterectomy may disclose hyperemia, edema, and purulent or seropurulent exudate whether the wound is infected or not. If the host immune system cannot control the inoculum of vaginal flora, the *parametrium* will usually become indurated, causing pain and tenderness. Infection may then spread to the tubes *and ovaries, followed by paralytic ileus.*

Spiking *diurnal fever* after the sixth postoperative day is suggestive of suppurative pelvic thrombophlebitis. The patient may not appear toxic (despite a high temperature) unless septic embolization has occurred.

Palpation is difficult, but *ultrasonography may detect an infected pelvic hematoma.* Typically, there may be no abnormality other than fever. An unexpectedly low HCT and fever are suggestive of an infected hematoma.

Because laboratory and x-ray findings are not often helpful in making the diagnosis of postoperative pelvic infection, the *diagnosis must be made clinically.* If the next step is a workup for postoperative fever, it is useful to recall the clinical mnemonic *3 Ws (wind, water and wound).* Include in the differential diagnosis atelectasis, which causes fever within 12–36 h and is suggested by auscultation and demonstrated by chest x-ray films. Dehydration may cause mild fever within 24–48 h of surgery and usually can be suspected by the patient's clinical appearance, fluid losses, urine output, and HCT. The abdominal incision may become infected and should be probed carefully if the pelvic examination is unremarkable. Except for extremely virulent infections (e.g., clostridia), it is uncommon for the abdominal wound to cause marked fever before the third postoperative day.

Other causes of postoperative fever to be ruled out include *phlebitis and urinary tract infection.* Phlebitis of a superficial vein at an IV site may cause fever, especially if antibiotics are being infused. Urinary tract infection is common after gynecologic surgery because of the use of indwelling catheters. However, fever usually occurs principally when pyelonephritis is present.

COMPLICATIONS

Complications of postoperative infections include wound abscess, tuboovarian abscess, pelvic or intraabdominal abscess, metastatic septic emboli, and septicemia.

PREVENTION

Conscientious attempts should be made to prevent or decrease sepsis because of the severity of postoperative pelvic infection. Helpful measures reportedly include:

- Preoperative vaginal douches with topical antibacterial agents (e.g., povidone-iodine, hexochlorophene) for several days
- Preoperative insertion of antibacterial vaginal creams or suppositories (especially if vaginitis or cervicitis is present)

- Meticulous operative hemostasis without strangulation of tissues
- Use of nonreactive suture material
- Suction drainage at sites of suboptimal hemostasis (with vaginal surgical margin left open or closed)
- Prophylactic antibiotics preoperatively with two optional additional doses 6 and 12 h postoperatively (note: usual drugs for single-dose prophylaxis are cefonicid, ceforanide, cefotaxime, cefotetan, ceftriaxone, and cefuroxime)
- Treatment of a mild infection before it becomes severe

TREATMENT

Treatment depends on diagnosis. A cuff hematoma or abscess must be adequately drained and antibiotics must be initiated. Single-agent therapy with one of the newer cephalosporins usually eliminates fever within 48–72 h. Large hematomas will require suction drainage and more prolonged antibiotic therapy. Tuboovarian abscess therapy has been described previously. Diagnosis of suppurative pelvic thrombophlebitis is made by exclusion when fever persists after 7–10 days of antibiotic administration. Heparin to a therapeutic dose, e.g., 5000 units q6h IV should be administered. If fever persists despite heparin and antibiotic therapy, addition of another antibiotic effective against anaerobic organisms (e.g., clindamycin, chloramphenicol, metronidazole) is recommended. Surgical intervention is usually necessary only if heparin therapy is contraindicated, if embolization continues despite adequate therapy, or if the patient fails to respond to therapy.

PELVIC TUBERCULOSIS

Pelvic tuberculosis (TB), often resulting from lymphatic spread of pulmonary TB, is rare in the United States and complicates pulmonary tuberculosis in about 5%. Direct extension to other abdominal organs from the pelvic organs is common. The pelvic organs primarily involved are oviducts and the endometrium.

Clinical findings may be minimal. Presentation may be for infertility, although pelvic pain, dysmenorrhea, or signs of tuberculous peritonitis may be present. Patients with abdominal symptoms may complain of low-grade fever and weight loss. Tuberculous peritonitis is usually accompanied by ascites. If the pelvic TB is found incidentally during pelvic surgery, it may be mistaken for chronic pelvic inflammation. However, the adhesions are much more dense, with loss of cleavage planes, the tubes are segmentally dilated, and the tubal ostia are usually not occluded with TB.

The *diagnosis may be suspected* given a history of TB, positive TB skin test, or chest x-ray consistent with TB. Hysterosalpingography during infertility workup may be suggestive when films reveal an irregular tubal lining, segmental areas of tubal dilatation, and saccular diverticula extending from the ampulla (characteristic of granulomatous disease). Abdominal x-ray may show calcified inguinal and periaortic lymph nodes. The diagnosis is confirmed when acid-fast bacteria are found on Ziehl-Neelsen stain and mycobacteria are cultured on Lowenstein-Jensen medium from samples obtained from menstrual discharge, curettage, or peritoneal biopsy.

The *differential diagnosis* includes schistosomiasis, enterobiasis, lipoid salpingitis, carcinoma, chronic pelvic inflammation, and mycotic infections. Complications are sterility and TB peritonitis.

Treatment consists of a 24–36 month course of standard TB drugs using a combination of several of the following drugs: isoniazid (INH), streptomycin, ethambutol, cycloserine, and rifampin. The reader is referred to medical texts describing specific TB therapeutic regimens.

The prognosis is good if diagnosis is made early and treatment is instituted, but the incidence of fertility remains low.

ABNORMAL UTERINE BLEEDING

Abnormal uterine bleeding may be caused by: hormonal factors, complications of pregnancy, systemic diseases, endometrial abnormalities (polyps), uterine or cervical problems (leiomyomas), or cancer. The pattern of abnormal bleeding is often very helpful in determining the etiology; thus, a number of terms differentiate the various types of abnormal uterine bleeding.

Menorrhagia (hypermenorrhea) is prolonged or heavy menstrual flow that may be further complicated by clots. Menorrhagia may be caused by leiomyomas (often submucous), pregnancy complications, endometrial hyperplasia, adenomyosis, malignancy, or coagulopathies.

Metrorrhagia (intermenstrual bleeding) is defined as bleeding at any time between menstrual periods. The causes of metrorrhagia include midcycle (ovulatory) bleeding, endometrial polyps, endometrial or cervical cancer, endogenous estrogen production, and exogenous estrogen administration.

Menometrorrhagia is bleeding occurring at irregular intervals. Generally, the amount and duration of bleeding vary. The causes of menometrorrhagia are the same as those of metrorrhagia.

Polymenorrhea is menstrual-like bleeding that occurs too frequently. The usual cause of polymenorrhea is anovulation, but occasionally a shortened luteal phase may be the fault.

Postcoital bleeding must be investigated to rule out cervical cancer, although the most common causes are benign and include cervical eversion, cervical polyps, and cervical or vaginal infections.

Hypomenorrhea (cryptomenorrhea or spotting) is unusually light menstrual bleeding. Possible causes are obstructions (e.g., hymenal or cervical), uterine synechiae (Asherman's syndrome), and inappropriate oral contraceptive dosage (correctable).

Oligomenorrhea is defined as menstruation occurring at an interval >35 days.

The differential diagnosis of abnormal uterine bleeding must include the possibility of *gynecologic but nonuterine bleeding*. The most common causes of *vulvar and vaginal bleeding* are: atrophic vulvovaginitis, infectious vulvovaginitis, local trauma, and genital cancer. *Cervical* causes of bleeding include eversion, erosion, cervical polyps, pedunculated leiomyomas, and cancer. With the exception of *tubal* ectopic gestation, other causes of bleeding from the uterine tube are unusual (e.g., fallopian tube cancer). The *ovarian* causes of vaginal bleeding include functional ovarian cysts, estrogen-producing tumors, polycystic ovaries (PCO), and ovarian neoplasms.

Uterine causes of abnormal bleeding are endometritis, endometrial hyperplasia, endometrial cancer, endometrial polyps, adenomyosis, submucous leiomyomas, IUD abnormalities, or reaction to oral contraceptives or exogenous steroids. *Systemic conditions* that may cause abnormal uterine bleeding include hypothyroidism, hepatic dysfunction (abnormal estrogen metabolism), coagulopathies, blood dyscrasias, and extreme weight loss (e.g., eating disorders or excessive exercise leading to anovulation). The use of *anticoagulants or adrenal steroids* may also lead to abnormal uterine bleeding.

Nongynecologic causes of bleeding that may be confused with abnormal uterine bleeding include anorectal or urological problems.

The *history of abnormal uterine bleeding* must detail the intervals between bleeding, the duration and amount of the bleeding, the character of the blood loss (e.g., color, consistency, and clots), and when the abnormal pattern began. Additional information useful to evaluate the bleeding, includes: obstetric history, contraceptive history, postcoital bleeding, LMP, LNMP, menarche (or menopause), and alteration(s) in general health. A patient-generated contemporaneous menstrual record is useful.

Evaluation of abnormal uterine bleeding requires a general physical examination, noting systemic health. In addition to the pelvic examination, a cytologic smear assists to screen for cervical (and in some cases uterine) malignancy. An enlarged or irregular uterus suggests leiomyomas, and a symmetrically enlarged uterus is more commonly noted with endometrial cancer or adenomyosis. Pelvic examination should reveal vulvar, vaginal, and cervical lesions (e.g., atrophic, inflammatory, neoplastic), and bimanual examination should reveal uterine, tubal, or ovarian masses.

If pregnancy is not a factor (a *pregnancy test* may be required), and the patient is in satisfactory hemodynamic status, the *endometrium may be sampled* by endometrial aspiration, endometrial biopsy, or ambulatory hysteroscopy. Currently, hysteroscopy with directed biopsies as well as endocervical curettage is favored because of the more comprehensive results. Whereas D & C is used less frequently, it remains the method of choice in patients with continuing heavy blood loss. The exact modality for diagnosis depends on the patient's age, parity, anatomy, and amount of blood loss.

Treatment of abnormal uterine bleeding must be individualized depending on the diagnosis.

DYSFUNCTIONAL UTERINE BLEEDING (DUB)

DUB is abnormal uterine bleeding occurring without anatomic abnormalities of the uterus or endometrium. Dysfunctional uterine bleeding is most common at the extremes of reproductive age (20% of cases are in adolescents, 40% are in patients >40 years). A *persistent corpus luteum cyst* or a *short luteal phase* may cause dysfunctional uterine bleeding, but most patients are *anovulatory;* thus, the term "anovulatory bleeding" is most appropriate once *uterine* or *endometrial* causes are excluded. Anovulation results in continuous estrogen stimulation of the endometrium, with resultant hyperplasia, periodic partial endometrial breakdown, and irregular bleeding. Anovulatory cycles are characterized by irregularity of cycle length (longer), duration (variable), and amount of flow (heavier). Additionally, anovulation does not usually have midcycle pain and vaginal discharge, premenstrual breast engorgement and tenderness, or dysmenorrhea.

Anovulation may result from *primary ovarian dysfunction* (e.g., functioning ovarian tumors), from *secondary ovarian dysfunction* (e.g., polycystic ovaries), or, most commonly, from a cumulative group of influences on the hypothalamus (e.g., emotional stress, vigorous exercise, obesity, pituitary disorders, changes, rapid changes in body weight). *Aberrations of interacting hormonal systems* may primarily or secondarily lead to anovulation, examples include: adrenal hyperfunction (e.g., congenital or acquired adrenal hyperplasia), adrenal insufficiency, obesity, hyperthyroidism, and hypothyroidism. Additionally, a variety of *drugs and medications* may create anovulation (e.g., anticholinergics, gonadal steroids, monamine oxidase inhibitors, morphine, phenothiazines, and reserpine).

At menarche, anovulation with subsequent irregular menses is common. Usually, only pelvic examination and exclusion of pregnancy are necessary before therapy is begun. The *therapeutic goals* are control of bleeding, stabilization of the endometrium, and induction of controlled menstruation. The endometrium may be stabilized and the bleeding checked (usually in 12–14 h) by the administration of estrogen-progestin oral contraceptives. After the oral contraceptives are withdrawn, 5–7 d of heavy bleeding followed by renewal of more normal endometrium may be expected. An alternative is administration of *progesterone* (e.g., medroxyprogesterone acetate 10 mg/d for 10 d). Occasionally, it may be necessary to give high doses of conjugated estrogens first to control very heavy bleeding. Finally, prescribe *cyclic therapy* (either oral contraceptives or estrogen and estrogen-progesterone, e.g., conjugated equine estrogens 1.25 mg/d for 1–25 d, medroxyprogesterone acetate 10 mg/d for 10–25 d) for three to six cycles. Often after 2–3 months of cyclic therapy, spontaneous ovulation and normal menstruation may occur.

Endometrial sampling, exclusion of organic lesions, and exclusion of systemic or coagulation disorders before initiating therapy (as above) is increasingly important with increasing age. In the premenopausal woman endometrial sampling is crucial. Hysteroscopically guided biopsies and endocervical curettage are especially revealing. The work up must exclude: benign endometrial neoplasia (most commonly polyps, leiomyoma), chronic endometritis, intrauterine syneciae, intrauterine device, benign cervical lesions (polyps, erosion, cancer), vaginal lesions, malignancy (cervical or endometrial carcinoma), pregnancy bleeding (abortion, ectopic, hydatidiform mole, retained products of conception, subinvolution, placental polyp), and coagulopathies (ITP, von Willebrand disease, platelet abnormalities).

Although a *Hct or Hgb is necessary in nearly all patients, further laboratory work-up is guided by the history and physical examination.* Some patients will need coagulation studies, others will require thyroid studies and/or serum prolactin levels, or other indicated studies. Cerebral imaging studies need be obtained only on patients evidencing hyperprolactinemia or hypopituitarism. Serum androgen levels (testosterone, dehydroepiandrosterone sulfate) are indicated for patients with signs of hyperandrogenism.

Therapy must be individualized. Factors to consider include: age, amount and duration of blood loss, health status, intercurrent diseases, and reproductive desires. Nearly all patients will require oral or parenteral iron therapy. Endometrial sampling is ideally obtained prior to hormonal therapy (see a previous discussion) in all save the adolescent patient. Hormone therapy, unless contraindicated, will resolve irregular bleeding in the majority of hemodynamically stable patients. The most common agents used (see above) are: oral or parenteral progestagens, combination oral contraception (generally starting with ≤35 mcg of estrogens and increasing as necessary), or estrogenic/progestagen combinations. After initial control most patients are continued on cyclic estrogen-progesterone therapy.

Acute hemorrhage, often in a patient already anemic from chronic blood loss, *mandates more aggressive therapy.* In patients who have risk of cancer (e.g., long-term anovulation, perimenopausal) or who are experiencing extraordinary bleeding, the first step may be a fractional D&C and/or hysteroscopy. The D&C will control the hemorrhage in well over 50% of cases. In less acute patients, sonography may assist in the exclusion of polyps or leiomyoma. The most common medical approach to arrest hemorrhage is the use of high dose estrogen (conjugated estrogens, 20 mg IV q 2–4 h). Generally, this approach will stop the bleeding over a 12–24 hour interval. After the bleeding has materially slowed or stopped, daily oral estrogens are administered for three weeks (equivalent to 2.5–3.75 mg conjugated estrogens). At that time, a progestagen (e.g., medroxyprogesterone acetate 10–20 mg) is added to the estrogen therapy for 7–10 days.

If fertility is not desired and the various medical and surgical therapies are unsuccessful (or if hormones are contraindicated), hysterectomy may be considered. Alternatively, endometrial ablation may be utilized.

POSTMENOPAUSAL BLEEDING (PMB)

PMB is defined as bleeding occurring after >12 months of amenorrhea in a woman of menopausal age (>45 years). Postmenopausal bleeding is far more likely to be of pathologic origin than is abnormal uterine bleeding during the reproductive years. Therefore, it is *mandatory that postmenopausal bleeding be thoroughly investigated.* Although pelvic sonography is useful in detection of thickened endometrium as well as endometrial polyps and leiomyoma, the endometrium must be selectively sampled for histology. In the past, as well as many cases today, this evaluation is accomplished by fractional D&C. However, hysteroscopy with selected biopsies and endocervical curettage are increasingly being employed.

Although nongynecologic bleeding is more common in this age group, it is always wise to exclude gynecologic causes. The differential diagnosis of pathologic causes of PMB includes atrophic endometrial bleeding, endometrial hyperplasias (cystic, adenomatous, and atypical), endometrial polyps, submucous leiomyomas, sarcoma, endometrial carcinoma, cervical carcinoma, endocervical carcinoma, fallopian tube carcinoma, estrogen-producing ovarian tumors, and ovarian carcinoma.

AMENORRHEA

Amenorrhea, the absence of menstruation for 3 or more months during the reproductive years, is a symptom not a diagnosis. The most common causes of amenorrhea are physiologic (i.e., pregnancy, nursing, or the puerperium). When pathologic, amenorrhea may be caused by genetic, anatomic, ovarian failure, or endocrine disorders. Amenorrhea may be further classified as primary or secondary.

PRIMARY AMENORRHEA

Primary amenorrhea is failure of menses to occur by age 16 years or within 2 years of full secondary sexual characteristic development. It is infrequent (0.1%–2.5%), and the etiologies causing primary amenorrhea may be pathophysiologically classified by physical examination, with emphasis on breast development (secondary sexual characteristics), the external genitalia, and whether or not a uterus is present. Most commonly, the external genitalia are normal.

AMBIGUOUS GENITALIA

Those patients with ambiguous genitalia usually have been exposed to excessive androgens in utero. Ambiguous genitalia usually are encountered at a much earlier age and are discussed on page 598.

BREAST DEVELOPMENT
AND UTERUS PRESENT

Primary amenorrhea with normal breast development and a uterus *occurs in one third of cases.* Of these, one quarter are caused by hyperprolactinemia. Others are due to exogenous estrogens. The rest of these patients have diagnoses similar to those with secondary amenorrhea (Table 25-1, Group A). Thus, testing and therapy should proceed as is discussed for secondary amenorrhea.

BREAST DEVELOPMENT ABSENT
AND UTERUS PRESENT

This category is the *most commonly encountered situation (one half) in patients with primary amenorrhea* (Table 25-1, Group B).

Gonadal Failure
The causes of gonadal failure are *mainly chromosomal or genetic:* partial or total absence of an X chromosome (e.g., 45,X; 46,XX;

TABLE 25-1
DIFFERENTIAL DIAGNOSIS OF PRIMARY
AMENORRHEA WITH NORMAL EXTERNAL GENITALIA
BASED ON BREAST DEVELOPMENT AND UTERINE
PRESENCE OR ABSENCE

	Uterus Present	Uterus Absent
Breast development present	**Group A** Hypothalamic Pituitary Ovarian Uterine	**Group C** Congenital uterovaginal agenesis Androgen insensitivity (testicular feminization)
Breast development absent	**Group B** Gonadal failure CNS–hypothalamic–pituitary disorders	**Group D** 17,20-Desmolase deficiency Agonadism 17α-Hydroxylase deficiency (46,XY)

p-; or q-), mosaicism (e.g., X/XX), pure XX and XY gonadal dysgenesis, and 17 α-hydroxylase deficiency (with 46,XX karyotype). Two or more normal X chromosomes are necessary for normal ovarian development. Without them, fibrous bands (gonadal streaks) often replace normal ovarian development, and there is no ovarian hormonal production and no secondary sexual characteristics. Gonadotropin levels in such cases are high, as with ovarian failure. Other stigmata of X chromosome abnormality include short stature (<63 inches) and major cardiovascular or renal anomalies in one third of these patients.

The most common X chromosome abnormality is *Turner's syndrome* (45,X), which occurs in 1 in 2000 live births. Individuals with Turner's syndrome or Turner's mosaicism (45,X/XX) have normal migration of the oogonia to the genital ridge. Although some fetal ovarian development may occur, it soon undergoes accelerated degeneration, resulting in streak ovaries. Individuals with mosaicism have been reported to menstruate briefly, but conception is very rare. Females with deletion of the short arm of an X chromosome phenotypically resemble those with 45,X.

Gonadal dysgenesis is considered *pure if the primitive oogonia do not migrate to the genital ridge,* resulting in streak gonads that cannot produce hormones. This probable genetic disorder includes normal stature and phenotype in both 46,XX and 46,XY. If this maldevelopment occurs with 46,XX, there will be no ovarian hormones produced. However, development of both internal and external genitalia is not dependent on estrogen. Primary amenorrhea is the usual result. When the syndrome is incomplete, a few such individuals may have some follicles and occasional menstruation. In 46,XY karyotypes, failure of primitive germ cells to migrate to the genital ridge results in a streak gonad that produces neither testosterone nor mullerian-inhibiting hormone (MIH). The resulting internal and external genitalia are female. Because estrogen is not produced, breast development does not occur, and the doctor usually is consulted because of delayed onset of puberty rather than primary amenorrhea.

Patients with *17 α-hydroxylase deficiency are very rare.* They lack the enzyme necessary to convert progesterone to cortisol and, thus, have high progesterone levels and low cortisol levels. They also may have hypernatremia (with hypertension) and hypokalemia, as well as elevated ACTH and mineralocorticoid levels. These patients require sex steroids and cortisol replacement.

CNS–Hypothalamic–Pituitary Abnormalities
Patients with these lesions have *low gonadotropin and estrogen levels.*

Hypothalamic Disorders
Normal hypothalamic function requires pulsed release of GnRH from the arcuate nucleus into the hypophyseal portal system about every hour. GnRH causes release of LH and FSH from the pituitary, which stimulate ovarian follicular growth and ovulation. Absence of GnRH, abnormal transport of GnRH, or abnormal pulsation of GnRH will result in *hypogonadotropic hypogonadism.*

Defective GnRH Transport
Conditions that will interfere with GnRH transport include those that destroy the arcuate nucleus or compress or disrupt the pituitary stalk. These problems include trauma, tumors (e.g., craniopharyngioma, germinoma, glioma, teratoma, or endodermal sinus tumor), Hand-Schuller-Christian disease, sarcoidosis, tuberculosis, and radiation.

Defective GnRH Pulse Production

If the GnRH pulse frequency or amplitude is severely reduced, little or no FSH and LH will be released, no ovarian follicles will develop, and estradiol will not be secreted. Although this may be idiopathic, it is seen also in prepubertal girls and in those with anorexia nervosa, severe stress, starvation, prolonged vigorous exercise, and hyperprolactinemia. If GnRH pulsation amplitude or frequency is less severely reduced, there may be diminished LH and FSH production that may result in follicular stimulation insufficient for full development and ovulation, but estradiol will be secreted. This too may be idiopathic, or the condition may occur as the result of stress, hyperprolactinemia, marked athletic activity, or early eating disorders.

Congenital Absence of GnRH

Congenital absence of GnRH (Kallmann's syndrome) is associated with anosmia (see p. 532). LH and FSH are not released from the pituitary so that follicular development and ovulation cannot occur.

Pituitary Disorders

Pituitary lesions (excluding chromophobe adenomas) are rarely the primary cause of amenorrhea. Congenital absence of the pituitary is exceptional and lethal. On rare occasions, isolated congenital abnormalities of LH or FSH occur, resulting in anovulation and amenorrhea. Acquired pituitary dysfunction may occur as the result of Sheehan's syndrome (postpartum necrosis of the pituitary secondary to severe hypotension from hemorrhage), hemosiderosis (destruction of the cells producing FSH and LH by iron deposits), and pituitary hyperplasia or pituitary adenomas (both cause high prolactin levels).

BREAST DEVELOPMENT PRESENT AND UTERUS ABSENT

Congenital Uterovaginal Agenesis (Rokitansky-Kusnter-Hauser Syndrome)

Congenital absence of the uterus is usually an *isolated developmental defect occurring in 1 in 4000–5000 female births* (Table 25-1, Group C). This contributes about 15% of individuals with primary amenorrhea. The ovaries function normally. Therefore, these individuals generally have normal secondary sexual development and no endocrinopathies. However, the uterus and upper (or total) vagina are absent. Associated abnormalities include renal (one third), skeletal (one eighth), and an enhanced rate of cardiac and other abnormalities (also see p. 532).

Androgen Insensitivity

Primary amenorrhea is often the reason individuals that have 46,XY karyotype but are phenotypically female seek medical assistance. The fetus does not develop male genitalia unless testosterone and its active metabolite dihydrotestosterone (DHT) are present. Thus, any disorder of fetal testosterone production, metabolism, or its receptors will result in a phenotypic female. In addition, the fetal testis produces mullerian-inhibiting factor (MIF), which is responsible for regression of the mullerian structures (i.e., uterus, uterine tubes, and upper two thirds of the vagina).

Androgen insensitivity (*testicular feminization*) occurs with normal fetal testosterone production as the result of either absent or defective androgen receptors in the genital anlagen and mesonephric ducts. Because MIF production is normal, the mullerian structures regress, and there are no uterine tubes, uterus, or upper vagina. Physical examination reveals a blind ending or absent vagina. Since these patients produce some estrogen, breast development may be normal, but there is minimal or no pubic and axillary hair. The abnormality may not be diagnosed until they are investigated for primary amenorrhea. The diagnosis is confirmed by karyotype and measurement of testosterones (which will be in the normal adult male range).

BREAST DEVELOPMENT ABSENT AND UTERUS ABSENT

Any enzymatic defect in the biosynthesis of testosterone that occurs before the production of androstenedione will result in an individual with female external genitalia but no mullerian structures (i.e., MIF is produced). If the enzymatic defect occurs after androstenedione is formed but there is no testosterone production, the patient will have ambiguous external genitalia and no mullerian structures (Table 25-1, Group D).

This group includes <1% of all primary amenorrhea patients and comprises *17,20-desmolase deficiency, agonadism, and 17 α-hydroxylase deficiency.* Generally, they are male in karyotype, have elevated gonadotropin levels, and have testosterone in the normal or below-normal female range. With both 17,20-desmolase deficiency and 17 α-hydroxylase deficiency, individuals have an enzymatic defect in the path of testosterone synthesization. As a result, they develop female, not male, external genitalia. The testes produce MIF, causing female internal genitalia regression.

Regression of the fetal testis at <7 weeks results in a clinical picture indistinguishable from pure gonadal dysgenesis. If regression of the testis occurs between 7 and 13 weeks, MIF and testosterone production have had time to affect genital differentiation sufficiently to result in ambiguous genitalia.

SECONDARY AMENORRHEA

Secondary amenorrhea is the lack of menses for ≥ 3 months in a woman who has previously had normal menstruation or lack of menses for three typical intervals in the oligomenorrheic woman. Secondary amenorrhea occurs in 0.7%–3% of women. It is predisposed by age (<25 years), by previously having menstrual irregularities, by extraordinary emotional stress, or by marked physical stress.

OVARIAN DYSFUNCTION

The most common cause of ovarian dysfunction is *polycystic ovaries* (*Stein-Leventhal syndrome*). Pathologic findings consist of ovaries with multiple small antral follicles, well-developed stromal tissue, and a thick pseudocapsule. The abnormality is believed to be the result of increased androgen (from either the ovary or adrenal gland), with subsequent conversion to estrogen ovary or adrenal gland), with subsequent conversion to estrogen in the adipose tissue. Because levels of sex steroid-binding globulin are low, free estrogen levels are increased. Elevated estrogen stimulates the pituitary to increase the LH/FSH ratio, which results in aberrant follicular development, anovulation, and increased ovarian androgen production. That androgen is, in turn, converted to more estrogen: a vicious cycle. Amenorrhea may be primary or secondary.

OVARIAN FAILURE

Primary ovarian failure is demonstrated by the presence of elevated gonadotropins and low estradiol (*hypergonadotropic hypogonadism*). Secondary ovarian failure is demonstrated by normal or low gonadotropins and low estradiol (*hypogonadotropic hypogonadism*) and usually is secondary to hypothalamic dysfunction. If ova are depleted <35 years, ovarian failure is considered premature, and premature menopause is the result.

Cause of primary gonadal failure include idiopathic premature ovarian failure, steroidogenic enzyme defects, true hermaphroditism, gonadal dysgenesis, ovarian resistance syndrome, post operative injury (after wedge resection or bivalved operations), autoimmune oophoritis, postinfection, post-radiation, and postchemotherapy. Many of these become evident by careful history and examination.

Ovarian resistance (Savage's syndrome) is characterized by ovaries containing primordial germ cells and elevated levels of circulating FSH and LH. Receptor resistance is postulated.

SYSTEMIC CAUSES

In addition to previously listed processes, obesity may result in amenorrhea, presumably by the same hormone imbalance mechanism as that found in polycystic ovarian syndrome. Other endocrinopathies causative of obesity include hypothyroidism, Addison's disease, Cushing's syndrome, and chronic renal failure.

DIAGNOSIS OF AMENORRHEA

The diagnostic goal is to determine which organ is primarily responsible for amenorrhea so that appropriate therapy, if any, can be initiated. *A careful history and physical examination are mandatory. The history should establish:* pubertal events, symptoms of decreased estrogen (hot flashes, night sweats, and dyspareunia), family history, anatomic or genetic anomalies, medications or drugs (including psychotrophics, herbs, and dietary additives), galactorrhea, previous surgical or medical therapies, endocrinopathies, intercurrent diseases, dietary habits, employment, exercise routines, and stress. *Increased androgens may be confirmed by both history and physical examination:* acne, decreased breast size, hirsutism, voice deepening, temporal balding, increased muscle mass. The *general physical examination* specifically evaluates: height and weight, habitus, distribution of body and head hair, and breast development (see p. 539 for Tanner staging). The pelvic examination evaluates the development of the external and internal genitalia. During the history and physical examination it is useful to consider several circumstances.

ANATOMIC ABNORMALITIES

There are five common anatomic disorders in 46,XX individuals that may lead to amenorrhea.

- *Mullerian dysgenesis* (congenital absence of the uterus and upper vagina)
- *Vaginal agenesis* (congenital absence of the vagina)
- *Transverse vaginal septum* (from the failure of fusion of the mullerian and urogenital sinus-derived portions of the vagina)
- *Imperforate hymen* (does not allow menstrual blood egress from the vagina)

- *Asherman's syndrome amenorrhea* secondary to intrauterine synechiae. Asherman's syndrome may occur as the result of such procedures as myomectomy and cesarean section but most often follows complicated D&C (e.g., vigorous elimination of endometrium, infected products of conception) or it may result from tuberculous endometritis.

Imperforate hymen, transverse vaginal septum, and vaginal agenesis can be identified or ruled out by examination.

Of prime importance in evaluating primary amenorrhea is to determine whether or not the patient has a uterus (by examination or sonography). If the uterus is absent, a karyotype and testosterone level should be obtained.

Hyperandrogenism

The *clinical stigmata of hyperandrogenism* include: excessive hair growth (facial, midline body), temporal hairline recession, deepening of the voice, altered body habitus (toward a male type), male type pubic hair distribution and clitoral enlargement. When the evaluation of amenorrhea detects any of these changes the workup involves evaluation for androgen dysfunction (see p. 786).

Galactorrhea-Hyperprolactinemia

Consideration of the *differential diagnoses* of galactorrhea-hyperprolactinemia should begin when galactorrhea is noted on history or physical examination in a patient with elevated prolactin levels. The differential diagnosis includes pituitary tumor, hypothyroidism, idiopathic hyperprolactinemia, drug-induced hyperprolactinemia (dopamine antagonists, e.g., phenothiazines, thioxanthines, butyrophenone, diphenylbutylpiperidine, dibenzoxazepine, dihydroindolone, and procainamide derivatives; catecholamine-depleting agents; and false transmitters, e.g., alpha-methyldopa), interruption of the normal hypothalamic–pituitary relationship, and peripheral neuronal stimulation varying from chest wall stimulation (e.g., thoracotomy, mastectomy, thoracoplasty, burns, herpes zoster, bronchogenic tumors, bronchiectasis, chronic bronchitis), nipple stimulation, spinal cord lesions (e.g., tabes dorsalis, syringomyelia) to CNS disease (e.g., encephalitis, craniopharyngioma, pineal tumors, hypothalamic tumors, pseudotumor cerebri).

The *workup* for amenorrhea associated with galactorrhea-hyperprolactinemia begins (assuming a recent prolactin level) with obtaining serum level of TSH. If the TSH is elevated, treat the hypothyroidism. If TSH is normal, obtain a CT or MRI scan of the sella turcica. If the sella appears normal and prolactin levels are <50–100 ng/mL, repeat the prolactin level every 6 months and sella

turcica scans every 1–2 years. If the sella is abnormal or the prolactin level is >50–100 ng/mL or if visual fields are restricted, an
adenoma or hyperplasia may be present.

EVALUATION OF AMENORRHEA

Pregnancy

If a uterus and patent vagina are present, *pregnancy should be ruled
out* before extensive testing is begun, whether amenorrhea is primary or secondary. In the absence of pregnancy and demonstrable
endocrinopathies, progestin challenge testing may prove useful.

Progestin Challenge Test

The diagnostic workup for the patient who has secondary amenorrhea with normal prolactin levels and absence of galactorrhea often begins with a progestin challenge test to determine whether or
not the ovary is producing estrogen. Although the test is not definitive, it is often helpful if utilized as one component of the complete evaluation. Medroxyprogesterone acetate 5–10 mg PO daily
for 5–10 d is the progestin most often used. The exogenous progestin
administered will produce menses if the endometrium has been
normally primed with estrogen If the progestin challenge is positive (menses occurred) and the patient has evidence of hirsutism,
polycystic ovary syndrome, ovarian tumor, or adrenal tumor should
be suspected. If the patient with a positive challenge test, but has
no other stigmata (e.g., hirsuitism), *mild hypothalamic dysfunction*
is likely, possibly the result of such factors as emotional or physical stress, weight loss, obesity, or psychologic disorder, or the problem may be idiopathic.

   If bleeding does not follow, either there is no (or inadequate)
estrogen or the patient has Asherman's syndrome. *Asherman's
syndrome* can be diagnosed by hysterosalpingography, but is best
ascertained by hysteroscopy. Inadequate estrogen may be tested
by administration of estradiol 2.5 mg PO for 25 days with
medroxyprogesterone acetate 10 mg PO on days 16–25.

Laboratory Studies

Once pregnancy, anatomic abnormalities, hyperandrogenism, and Asherman's syndrome have been ruled out, LH, FSH, prolactin, thyroid-
stimulating hormone (TSH), and estradiol are usually obtained. Next,
a karyotype should be considered if there is potential for chromosomal abnormality.

   An LH of >20 mIU/mL or an LH/FSH ratio of >2.5 may aid
in the diagnosis of *polycystic ovarian syndrome*. Increased FSH

levels generally indicate *ovarian failure*. If FSH is >40 mIU/mL, *gonadal failure* is the diagnosis. If the FSH level is <40 mIU/mL, severe *hypothalamic dysfunction* is present (hypogonadotropic hypogonadism). If the estradiol concentration is >50 pg/mL or if the LH is significantly greater than FSH, viable oocytes may exist.

If initial prolactin levels exceed 20 ng/mL, the test may bear repeating because it may be elevated by stress, exercise, anxiety, sleep, and food ingestion. With elevated prolactin levels and normal thyroid function, *a pituitary adenoma* (or empty sella) is suspected. Thus, imaging studies (CT or MRI) to evaluate the pituitary are necessary. If a pituitary neoplasm is ≥10 mm visual fields and complete pituitary testing are recommended.

When TSH is elevated, the prolactin may or may not also be elevated (increased secretion of TRH). In borderline cases of hypothyroidism, an abnormal increase in TSH levels will occur in response to exogenous thyrotropin-releasing hormone (200–500 picograms IV).

If prolactin, TSH, and FSH levels are normal or low, thoughtful correlation of the clinical picture and determination of testosterone and DHEA-S may be useful, for not all hyperandrogenic women display classic symptomatology. When testosterone is >200 ng/mL, *an ovarian androgen secreting neoplasm* should be considered. If DHEA-S is >7.0 picograms/dL, an *adrenal androgen* secreting neoplasm may be present.

The investigation of *autoimmune* causes includes: CBC, sedimentation rate, total serum protein (with albumin/globulin ratio), thyroid antibodies (to rule out thyroiditis), antinuclear antibodies, and rheumatoid factor. Screening for other endocrinepathies includes: calcium and phosphorus (hyperparathyroidism), cortisol (hypoadrenalism), and a glucose tolerance test (diabetes mellitus).

TREATMENT OF AMENORRHEA

Management of the amenorrheic patient depends on the individual's desire to *ovulate* (menstruation, pregnancy) and the *etiology of the amenorrhea*. If amenorrhea is secondary to hypothyroidism, thyroid hormone replacement may be the only therapy required. If the patient has *amenorrhea-galactorrhea with pituitary macroadenoma (>10 mm)*, surgical removal of the adenoma should be considered. However, the cure rate is only 5%–10% and postoperatively, ~50% will require bromocriptine to induce ovulation. Thus, many authorities recommend initial bromocriptine therapy (~6 months) with close follow up. If the patient has *amenorrhea-galactorrhea without adenoma or with microadenoma (<10 mm),* therapy with bromocriptine alone (2.5 mg PO bid) will induce ovulation in 80%–90%. The dosage can be titrated until the serum prolactin level falls to normal. The drug may be discontinued once an ovulatory pattern is established or continued until pregnancy occurs.

If the patient has *primary ovarian failure* (hypergonadotrophic amenorrhea), the likelihood for ovulation is practically nonexistent unless the cause is autoimmune oophoritis, which may respond to treatment of the underlying disease and/or corticosteroid therapy. Hormonal replacement therapy is indicated. Because the condition may not be permanent and intermittent failure occurs, pregnancy occurs in up to 10% of patients with *hypergonadotrophic amenorrhea;* thus, contraception is necessary for those not wishing to reproduce. Ovulation induction (usually with hMG) has a low probability of success and oocyte donation with embryo transfer currently offers the greatest chance of reproduction for these patients. If the *karyotype reveals a Y chromosome and the patient is <30 y old,* the ovaries should be removed to decrease the risk of tumor formation.

Progestin challenge-negative patients (hypoestrogenic hypothalamic amenorrhea) desiring pregnancy may be treated with clomiphene citrate (50-100 mg PO q d for 5 d) to induce ovulation. Care must be taken to avoid overstimulation of the ovaries. If clomiphene is ineffective hMG or hMG-hCG may be added. Because the primary problem is a deficiency or abnormal pulse frequency of GnRH, pulsatile GnRH can be administered SC or IV to induce ovulation, although GnRH therapy is expensive. In those not desiring pregnancy hormonal replacement therapy and monitoring for osteoporosis is indicated.

Progestin challenge-positive patients almost always respond to clomiphene citrate. The initial dosage is 50 mg PO daily for 5 days. Ovulation usually occurs 5–10 days after the fifth dose. If the starting daily dose is insufficient, increase it gradually to a maximum of 250 mg/day. If there is still no response and androgens are elevated, adding corticosteroids may be effective. If combination therapy is ineffective, hMG may be added to the regimen.

If *polycystic ovaries* are present, and pregnancy is desired, the drug of choice is clomiphene citrate, followed by hMG if unsuccessful. Although surgical wedge resection may lead to ovulation, it may also lead to adhesions and mechanical infertility and, thus, should be reserved until other therapy has been tried and proven to be unsuccessful. Intermittent progestins or oral contraceptives are used for those women with PCO not desiring pregnancy (see p. 787).

Progestin challenge-negative patients who desire menses without ovulation are best treated with oral contraceptives combining estrogen 0.625–1.25 mg on days 1–25 plus 5–10 mg medroxyprogesterone on days 16–25 to maintain bone density and prevent genital atrophy. Adequate daily calcium intake should be assured.

Progestin challenge-positive patients should be given progestins to avoid endometrial hyperplasia and the increased risk of endometrial carcinoma. This can be accomplished easily using oral contraceptives in patients <35 years. Otherwise, give medroxyprogesterone acetate 10 mg PO daily for 10–13 days every 1–2 months.

Anatomic abnormalities obstructing outflow are corrected and the potential damage of retrograde menstruation assessed. An absent vagina may be treated surgically or by the use of increasing size dilators. With hysteroscopic lysis of *intrauterine synechiae,* ~80% of women will subsequently successfully deliver.

PROGNOSIS OF AMENORRHEA

Because amenorrhea is amenable to therapy in almost all cases, the *prognosis is good. The exceptions are premature ovarian failure and reproductive organ absence.* With the use of either one or a combination of hormones (e.g., hMG, GnRH, and corticosteroids) and medications (e.g., bromocriptine, clomiphene citrate), almost all other amenorrheic patients with ovaries may be induced to ovulate.

COMPLICATIONS OF MENSTRUATION

DYSMENORRHEA

The definition of *dysmenorrhea is severe, painful cramping in the lower abdomen just before or during the menses.* Other symptoms may include sweating, tachycardia, headaches, nausea, vomiting, diarrhea, and tremulousness. Dysmenorrhea is probably *the most common complaint* of gynecologic patients, affecting 75% of all women. Of those affected, 50% report mild symptoms (i.e., no systemic symptoms, medications not often required, and work rarely affected), 30% have moderate symptoms (i.e., few systemic symptoms, medication required, and work moderately affected), and 20% have severe symptoms (i.e., multiple symptoms, poor medication response, and work inhibited). Dysmenorrhea is more likely to occur in women who have first-degree relatives with dysmenorrhea and is less likely to occur in those who have delivered a child or take birth control pills. Additionally, dysmenorrhea is more commonly seen in women with heavy exercise regimes.

Primary dysmenorrhea denotes women without pathologic indications or conditions potentially causative of the symptomatology. Primary dysmenorrhea begins near menarche (<20 years). It is likely that elevated prostaglandim $F_{2\alpha}$ in the secretory endometrium leads to painful uterine contractions and other symptoms of primary dysmenorrhea. Indeed, prostaglandin-synthetase inhibitors (PGSIs) alleviate symptoms in nearly three fourths of sufferers. A special rare form of dysmenorrhea is *membranous dysmenorrhea*. It is the painful passage of the intact endometrial lining through the cervix.

Relief of mild primary dysmenorrhea is usually possible with aspirin or acetaminophen. For some mild cases, nearly all moderate cases, and some severe cases, PGSIs (ibuprofen 400–800 mg q6h, naproxen 250–500 mg q6h, naproxen sodium 275–550 mg q6h, and mefenamic acid 250–500 mg q6h) generally afford relief of acute pain. *Cyclic administration of oral contraceptives, usually low dose but with a higher estrogen content, will prevent dysmenorrhea.* Cervical dilation rarely helps. Very occasionally, medication will not help, and surgical therapy becomes necessary. Procedures that have been used include uterosacral ligament division, presacral neurectomy, and hysterectomy. Obviously, such choices must be weighed carefully, and all options must be discussed with the patient.

Secondary dysmenorrhea includes conditions or pelvic pathology that cause the pain. Secondary dysmenorrhea is usually acquired later in life (>30 years). Conditions capable of causing dysmenorrhea include endometriosis (p. 755), adenomyosis (p. 766), pelvic infection and adhesions (p. 755), pelvic congestion, cervical stenosis, endometrial polyps causing acervical outflow obstruction, conditioned behavior, stress, and tension.

Pelvic congestion syndrome is caused by engorgement of the pelvic vessels and is characterized by burning or throbbing pelvic pain, worse on standing and at night. The vagina and cervix may reveal vasocongestion, and there may be uterine enlargement, with tenderness. Laparoscopy reveals uterine congestion as well as engorgement or varicosities of the broad ligament and pelvic veins. The pathophysiology is not understood, and the condition appears to be related to tension and psychosomatic problems. Therapy (usually counseling) is directed toward relief of tension and psychosomatic problems, but occasionally even medical pain management fails, and presacral neurectomy or hysterectomy becomes a last resort.

During menses, cervical stenosis (either external or internal os) may impede menstrual flow. This increases intrauterine pressure and leads to retrograde menstrual flow through the fallopian tubes. Cervical stenosis may be congenital, secondary to cervical injury (e.g., childbirth), caused by infections, or due to operative injury (e.g., electrocoagulation, conization). Clues to diagnosis include scant menstrual flow with severe cramping throughout menses, scarring of the cervix, and difficulty passing a uterine sound. The diagnosis may be confirmed by hysterosalpingogram. Therapy consists of progressive cervical dilation using laminaria or dilators of progressive size. Pregnancy and delivery (cervical dilation) are usually curative.

Very occasionally, an endometrial polyp or polypoid leiomyoma will act as a ball-valve during menses. This may be confirmed by sonography, hysteroscopy, or hysterosalpingography. Treatment consists of hysteroscopic resection of the lesion.

Conditioned behavior as an etiology for dysmenorrhea requires that a reward or control results from the symptoms and that no other cause can be found. Confirmation of this as an etiology may be accomplished by use of a personality profile test (e.g., Minnesota Multiphasic Personality Index). Treatment involves sensitive reeducation or reconditioning. Stress and tension as a cause for dysmenorrhea are usually characterized by a history of gradual onset, with the symptoms worsening at times of stress. Therapy is directed to stress reduction.

PREMENSTRUAL SYNDROME (PMS)

PMS is variably defined and the etiology remains unknown. Moreover, there is disagreement concerning symptoms and criteria for diagnosis. More than 150 symptoms have been related to PMS. The more common behavioral symptoms include: fatigue (92%), irritability (91%), labile mood (sadness, anger, 81%), depression (80%), oversensitivity (69%), crying spells (65%), social withdrawal (65%), forgetfulness (56%), and difficulty concentrating (47%). The more common physical complaints are: abdominal bloating (90%), mastodynia (85%), acne (71%), appetite changes and food cravings (70%), extremity edema (67%), headache (60%), and gastrointestinal upset (48%).

Dalton has indicated that to be defined as PMS, *sufferers must exhibit* (at the minimum) edema, weight gain, restlessness, irritability, and increased tension. *Symptomatology must occur in the second half of three consecutive menstrual cycles*, and there must be a *symptom-free interval of at least 7 days in the first half of the cycle* (although this may not occur in up to 25% of patients). PMS must be *severe enough to require medical intervention.* PMS occurs to some degree in up to 90% of women; 20%–40% are mentally or physically limited, and 2%–3% have severe distress with true incapacitation. PMS rarely occurs in adolescents, and the peak incidence is in the late 20s to early 30s. Severe PMS is often a symptom of other problems. Indeed, 50%–60% of women with severe PMS have bipolar disorder, anxiety, or personality disturbances. Additionally, PMS increases in marital or familial stress. One of the useful diagnostic tools is a *daily symptom diary* with relation to the menstrual cycle.

Treatment of PMS is emperic and directed toward the symptomatology. Therapy is extremely controversial and has included (all of undocumented efficacy) progesterone (400 mg/day vaginal suppositories in the second half of the menstrual cycle), oral contraceptives, vitamins (B_6 50–200 mg/day), diuretics (spironolactone is the only diuretic found effective in clinical trials), PGSIs, bromocriptine (only for those with hyperprolactinemia, mastodynia, and breast engorgement and certainly the elimination of caffeine and chocolate should be the first step), minerals, natural substances for sedation, and laxatives. Other therapeutic suggestions include high-protein well-balanced diet, more regimented daily life (especially exercise and rest), and restriction of salt, sugar, caffeine, alcohol, and smoking.

The use of relaxation techniques (including biofeedback), and behavioral techniques appear at least as effective as most medications. Group support, empathy, and a special interest in the problem are essential to successful management. Medical therapy of PMS, unless an underlying cause is identified, remains unscientific. Currently, spironolactone and fluoxetine (Prozac) are probably the most commonly used medications. Alprazolam is also used, but only in patients who can be reliably monitored.

CHAPTER

26

CONTRACEPTION

DEFINITION, USAGE, EFFECTIVENESS

Contraception (pregnancy avoidance) is practiced for many reasons, such as pregnancy planning, limiting the number of children, avoiding medical risks of pregnancy (especially with heart disease, diabetes mellitus, or tuberculosis), and controlling the world population. The use of contraception is increasing in developed countries, but some forms are economically out of reach for those in developing countries.

Of the U.S. female population age 15–44 years, it is estimated that 30% are not sexually active, 5% are not using contraception, 5% have surgical sterilization, and 60% are using a contraceptive. Table 26-1 shows an approximate distribution of the different contraceptives used in the United States and their relative effectiveness. Contraceptives *usually fail when they are unacceptable* (and therefore not often used) or when pregnancy inadvertently occurs. This is difficult to quantify, but the latter is termed the *failure rate and is expressed as pregnancies per 100 women at 1 year, or per 100 woman-years. Pearl's index is another way of expressing the pregnancy rate.*

$$\text{Pregnancy rate} = \frac{\text{Pregnancies} \times 1200}{\text{Woman-months of use}}$$

The *life table method* is an actuarial expression of pregnancy (or discontinuation) at various intervals and may be a superior method for quantifying contraceptive information. Whatever type of assessment is used, it is important to differentiate between method effectiveness and use effectiveness. *Method effectiveness is the rate of contraceptive effectiveness when always used correctly, whereas*

TABLE 26-1
TYPES OF CONTRACEPTIVES USED IN THE
UNITED STATES AND FAILURE RATES

	% Using Method[a]	First Year Failure[b]	Theoretical Effectiveness[b]
Sterilization			
Female	20	0.4	0.4
Male	15	0.15	0.1
Norplant® System	<1	0.1	0.1
Oral contraceptive[c]	>30		
Combination		1–3	0.1
Progestin only		5	0.5
Depoprovera®	Unknown	0.3	0.3
IUD	<6		
Copper		0.8	0.6
Progesterone		2	1.5
Condom (without spermacide)			
Male	13	12	3
Female	<1	21	5
Diaphragm (with spermacide)	6	18	6
Cervical cap	<1		
Nulliparous		18	9
Parous		36	26
Spermicide	4	18–21	6
Rhythm	Unknown	4–20	1–9
Withdrawal	3	4–19	4
Douche	<0.5	4–20	Unknown
No contraception	Unknown	85	85

[a]% of women using contraception.

[b]Pregnancy per woman years.

[c]The majority of women are on combined oral contraceptives but exact distribution unknown.

use effectiveness is the overall effectiveness in actual use. Effectiveness is materially enhanced by: women wishing to prevent (as opposed to delay) pregnancy, those >30 years, those having higher education, and women of higher socioeconomic status.

TABLE 26-2
THE ORAL CONTRACEPTIVES AVAILABLE IN THE
UNITED STATES

Brand Name®	Estrogenic Component (mg)	Progestagenic Component (mg)
Alesse[1]	Ethinyl estradiol 0.02	Levonorgestrel 0.1
Brevicon[1]	Ethinyl estradiol 0.035	Norethindrone 0.5
Demulen 1/35[1]	Ethinyl estradiol 0.035	Ethynodiol diacetate 1.0
Demulen 1/50[1]	Ethinyl estradiol 0.050	Ethynodiol diacetate 1.0
Desogen	Ethinyl estradiol 0.03	Desogestrel 0.15
Estrostep[1,2]	Ethinyl estradiol 0.02/0.03/0.035	Norethindrone 1.0/1.0/1.0
Levelin[1]	Ethinyl estradiol 0.03	Levonorgestrel 0.15
Lo/Ovral[1]	Ethinyl estradiol 0.03	Norgestrel 0.3
Micronor[3]		Norethindrone 0.35
Modicon[1]	Ethinyl estradiol 0.035	Norethindrone 0.5
Nor-Q D[3]		Norethindrone 0.35
Nordette[1]	Ethinyl estradiol 0.03	Levonorgestrel 0.15
Norinyl 1/35[1]	Ethinyl estradiol 0.035	Norethindrone 1.0
Norinyl 1/50[1]	Mestranol 0.05	Norethindrone 1.0
Ortho-Cept[1]	Ethinyl estradiol 0.03	Desogestrel 0.15
Ortho-Cyclen[1]	Ethinyl estradiol 0.035	Norgestimate 0.250
Ortho-Novum 1/35[1]	Mestranol 0.035	Norethindrone 1.0

(Continued)

TABLE 26-2
(Continued)

Brand Name®	Estrogenic Component (mg)	Progestagenic Component (mg)
Ortho-Novum 1/50[1]	Mestranol 0.050	Norethindrone 1.0
Ortho-Novum 777[1,2]	Ethinyl estradiol 0.035/0.035/0.035	Norethindrone 0.5/0.75/1.0
Ortho-Novum 10/11[1,4]	Ethinyl estradiol 0.035/0.035	Norethindrone 0.5/1.0
Ortho Tri-Cyclen[1,2]	Ethinyl estradiol 0.035/0.035/0.035	Norgestimate 0.18/0.215/0.25
Ovral[1]	Ethinyl estradiol 0.05	Norgestrel 0.5
Ovrette[3]		Norgestrel 0.075
Tri-Norinyl[1,4]	Ethinlyl estradiol 0.035/0.035	Norethindrone 0.5/1.0
Tri-Levelen[1,2]	Ethinyl estradiol 0.03/0.04/0.03	Levonorgestrel 0.05/0.075/0.125
Triphasil[1,2]	Ethinyl estradiol 0.03/0.04/0.03	Levonorgestrel 0.05/0.075/0.125

[1]Available in both 21- and 28-day, [2]three-phase administration, [3]progestagen only, and [4]two-phase administration.

Laws regarding the prescription and sale of contraceptives vary from state to state and country to country. In the United States, regulations may vary also with regard to the prescription of contraceptives to patients <18 years.

There is *no perfect contraceptive* when one considers both side effects and effectiveness. All contraceptives have advantages and disadvantages, which must be integrated carefully with the patient's status. Therefore, *careful individualization* is necessary to avoid undesirable side effects and to optimize patient acceptance. Informed consent regarding the benefits, risks, and alternatives of contraceptives should be documented. At the time of this writing, there are 52 prescription regulated means of contraception available in the United States: two devices (diaphragms, IUD), one implant, one injectable, and forty-eight different formulations of oral contraceptive (Table 26-2).

METHODS OF CONTRACEPTION

BEHAVIORAL ALTERNATIVES

COITUS INTERRUPTUS

Withdrawing the penis before ejaculation is moderately effective in preventing pregnancy. It has the disadvantages of requiring male self-control and the occurrence of pregnancy from semen escaping before ejaculation or semen deposition at the vaginal introitus.

PERIODIC ABSTINENCE

Because women are *fertile for only* ~24 h after ovulation, conscientious avoidance of intercourse for the 2 days before ovulation and 2–3 days after ovulation should provide effective contraception. The difficulty is to determine prospectively, with reasonable certainty, when ovulation will occur. Thus, *several adjuncts* may be used to increase precision in identifying the time of ovulation. Three methods are commonly available to predict the day of ovulation. The *calendar method* predicts ovulation 14 d before the next menstrual period as determined by months of careful documentation of the length of the woman's menstrual cycles. *Basal body temperature* (BBT) is recorded immediately on awakening, before any activity is performed. The BBT rises abruptly 0.3–0.4°C (0.5–0.7°F) with ovulation (Fig. 26-1).

Checking the cervical mucus for consistency may assist in determination of ovulation. This has been used as an aid to the rhythm method. The *laboratory determination* of the abrupt surge of LH and progesterone with ovulation is the most reliable method of determining ovulation. However, one must obtain serial serum LH or progesterone levels, which is expensive and impractical for the avoidance of pregnancy. All in all, the BBT determination and cervical mucus assessment are the most reliable, practical methods to determine the infertile periods of the cycle. Nevertheless, ~20% of fertile women have such menstrual cycle variability that accurate prediction of ovulation is difficult, if not impossible. As a consequence, the failure rate of the rhythm method is high.

PROLONGATION OF LACTATION

Prolonged nursing (1–2 years, without supplementation) provides some contraceptive benefit (i.e., pregnancy is delayed 5–10 months

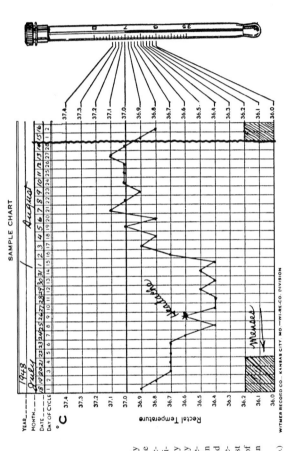

FIGURE 26-1. Basal body temperature recording. The temperature (vaginal or rectal) must be taken immediately on awakening every morning, before any activity whatsoever. The thermometer is allowed to remain in place for at least 5 min, and the recording is made immediately. This procedure must be continued over a period of at least 3 cycles to obtain an accurate chart.

(Courtesy of Witmer Record Co.)

732

on average compared with those who do not nurse). However, since about *6% of women will ovulate before the first postpartum menstrual period,* relying on lactation alone for contraception is questionable.

PERICOITAL INTERVENTIONS

DOUCHING AFTER COITUS

The intent of this method is to wash semen out of the vagina before sperm can enter the cervix. Because *sperm are found in the cervical mucus within 90 sec of ejaculation,* the effectiveness of this method of contraception is marginal.

CONTRACEPTIVE SPONGE

A polyurethane sponge containing the *spermicide* nonoxynol 9 is available without prescription for insertion before intercourse. It is *effective for 24 h after wetting,* and a loop to the sponge facilitates removal. It is less effective than diaphragm and spermicide. Occasional cases of *toxic shock syndrome* (TSS) have been reported in association with the use of the sponge.

SPERMICIDAL PREPARATIONS

A variety of *spermicidal creams, jellies, foams, gels, and suppositories are available* without prescription and are effective as spermicides as well as barriers to contraception. All of these agents require insertion into the vagina before each coitus. Failure may occur with improper insertion or if inadequate time is allowed for vaginal dispersal of the agent. Some women or men will experience chemical irritation requiring discontinuance or change to a different product or method. Some of the available preparations also provide a good prophylactic effect against sexually transmitted diseases (STD) caused by *Neisseria gonorrhoeae, Treponema pallidum, Candida albicans,* and *Trichomonas vaginalis,* for example.

BARRIER METHODS

VAGINAL DIAPHRAGM

This simple rubber device acts as a mechanical barrier between the cervix and penis, and it holds contraceptive cream or jelly to the cervix and upper vagina. The diaphragm must be fitted properly during a pelvic examination using fitting rings.

The disadvantages of this method are the need for fitting, the need for insertion in anticipation of intercourse, and the possibility of the diaphragm becoming dislodged during coitus. Diaphragms are less effective in the first few months of use (presumably because the patient is less familiar with usage).

CERVICAL CAP

The cervical cap is a barrier device covering the cervical portio. The latest cap has a one-way valve allowing uterine and cervical fluids to escape while preventing entrance of sperm. Cervical caps probably should not be left in place for >72 h to avoid infection. The disadvantage of this method is that each cap must be individually molded for every patient because cervical anatomy varies greatly.

CONDOM

The condom is a penile sheath made of latex, rubber, plastic, or animal membrane that serves as a barrier. The addition of a vaginal spermicide makes this method very effective if used properly. The additional advantage of protection against STD is lost if the animal membrane variety is used or if petroleum jelly is used with the latex product. Among the disadvantages, manufacturing defects occur in ~3/1000. Moreover, if withdrawal of the penis occurs after detumescence, semen may leak into the vagina. Both partners may complain of decreased sensation during intercourse. The widespread availability, low cost, and effectiveness in prevention of STDs, however, make it the most commonly used barrier contraceptive in the world. The "female condom" is a latex or rubber membrane that can be inserted into the vagina. It has a higher rate of pregnancy than the male condom.

ORAL CONTRACEPTIVES (OCs)

There are 26 different oral contraceptives available in the United States, and nearly all offer 21 or 28 (7 placebo or iron) day regimens. The various compounds share many similarities (Table 26-2). In the various formulations there are only *two compounds with predominant estrogenic activity,* whereas *seven have progestagenic effect(s). The estrogens are ethinyl estradiol* (contained in all the ≤0.035 mg preparations) *and mestranol,* its 3-methyl ether derivative (contained in only three of the formulations). *The progestins are: desogestrel, ethynodiol diacetate, levonorgestrel, norethindrone, norethindrone acetate, norgestimate, and norgestrel* (Table 26-2). Desogestrel and Norgestimate are advocated to have less androgenic side effects than the other progestagenic agents. There are *five three-phase dosage regimens, two two-phase dosage regimens, and three progestin only formulations.*

Synthetic estrogens and progestin combinations given to prevent ovulation also create a cervical mucous inimical to sperm passage and are almost 100% effective in preventing pregnancy when taken as directed (*pregnancy rate of ~0.2%/year*). Combination pills containing both estrogen and progestin (often in different combinations) are taken daily for 20–21 days, with no pill or inert pills taken for 7–8 days to maintain a 28-day cycle. Withdrawal bleeding usually occurs 3–5 days after completing a 20–21 day regimen of two hormones. Low doses of progestin daily is a reasonably reliable method of contraception (2–7 pregnancies per 100 woman years); however, ovulation is not prevented. The exact mechanism of action is unknown, but may well be simply the cervical mucous alterations. The *advantages* of progestin only oral contraceptives include no estrogen side effects and no sequencing of pills, with the daily administration. The *disadvantages* are irregularity of the ovulatory cycle, occasional abnormal bleeding patterns, and an increased incidence of ectopic pregnancy. There is probably no enhancement of thromboembolism, hypertension, nausea, and breast tenderness. Ideal patients for this method may be those with estrogen intolerance or lactating women (although long-term effects on the offspring from the small amount of progestin in the milk are unknown).

Method of Action

With the combined contraceptive regimen, FSH and LH levels remain constantly low. Thus, the follicle is not stimulated to develop, and ovulation does not occur. They also cause scant, viscid cervical mucus, alter the endometrium, and reduce ovarian responsiveness to gonadotropin stimulation. With lower dose and progestin only formulations the cervical mucus changes may be responsible for contraceptive activity.

BENEFITS AND RISKS

In addition to extremely effective contraception, the *advantages* of combination oral contraceptives are improvements in menstruation, prevention of benign conditions, prevention of gynecologic malignancies, and possible general health benefits. Specific menstrual improvements include: decreased incidence of heavy menstrual bleeding, fewer menstrual irregularities, less dysmenorrhea, and regulation of menses in anovulatory women. Benign conditions beneficially influenced by oral contraception are: functional ovarian cysts (fewer), iron deficiency anemia (less blood loss), benign breast disease (fibroadenoma and cystic changes), ectopic pregnancy (virtually eliminated), and pelvic inflammatory disease (50% decreased). Gynecologic malignancies, which are decreased with oral contraceptives, include endometrial adenocarcinoma (<50%) and epithelial ovarian cancers (~50% decrease). The general health benefits include increased bone mineral density (less osteoporosis) and prevention of rheumatoid arthritis. Additionally, combination oral contraceptives may help to prevent or arrest endometriosis.

There are two major *disadvantages* of oral contraceptives. The first is an increased incidence of thromboembolic disease, especially in smokers (4–5 times nonusers). The death rate from thromboembolic disease in users is 3/100,000. Although certainly less than the death rate from pregnancy and delivery (9/100,000, excluding illegal abortions), it is a risk. The second is the increased incidence of coronary artery disease (2.7 times nonusers age 30–39 and 5.7 times nonusers age 40–44) in women who smoke. This association is so strong that oral contraceptives are contraindicated in women >35 who smoke.

All *side effects* are reduced with lower-dose products. Even so, the estrogenic components occasionally cause depression, mood changes, sleepiness, nausea, breast tenderness, fluid retention (usually <3–4 lbs), hypercoagulability (ethinyl estradiol), and hypertension (transient). Indeed, the occurrence of hypertension warrants checking (~4–6 weeks, then annually) the blood pressure after initiation of therapy. Progestagens may cause weight gain, acne, nervousness, or failure of withdrawal bleeding. Both act to cause chloasma. There is lowered effectiveness if oral contraceptives are taken with rifampicin (often used to treat tuberculosis). Additionally, barbiturates, sulfonamides, cyclophosphamide, ampicillin, and penicillin may exert a similar effect. Thus, the use of barrier contraceptives is recommended when oral contraceptive users must take these medications.

Oral contraceptive use *does not cause atherosclerosis and is not associated with increased incidence of breast, endometrial, or cervical cancer.* The occurrence of liver cancer (rare) may be slightly increased. Oral contraceptive use does not, overall, appear to impede future pregnancies.

CONTRAINDICATIONS

Oral contraceptives are *contraindicated* in pregnancy (virilization of female fetus), but OC use during early pregnancy does not increase the risk of fetal malformation. Other contraindications include: nursing mothers (decreased milk production), those with vascular disease (thrombophlebitis, thromboembolism, atherosclerosis, stroke), lupus, diabetes mellitus, severe heart disease, SS hemoglobinopathies, hypertension, hyperlipidemia, smoking habit and age >35 years, and cancer of the breast or endometrium. *Relative contraindications* include migraine headaches, depression, and heavy smoking at age <35 years. Women with oligomenorrhea, amenorrhea (except for polycystic ovarian syndrome), or galactorrhea should have a definitive diagnosis before starting oral contraceptives.

PRESCRIBING ORAL CONTRACEPTIVES

The specific prescribing information should be consulted prior to initiating any oral contraceptive. A complete history and physical examination should identify contraindications to oral contraception. A CBC, UA, and cervical cytology are obtained. Also documented (written) informed consent is obtained. In patients ≥35 years old or those with a family history of diabetes, vascular diseases, or liver disease, the following should be determined: a 2 h postprandial blood glucose, HDL and LDL cholesterol, total cholesterol, triglycerides, and liver function studies. Follow-up of any abnormality is mandatory.

Products containing 30–35 μg of ethinyl estradiol are often used as a trial oral contraceptive. Oral contraceptives may be given to sexually active adolescents who have had a minimum of three regular (ovulatory) menses without fear of causing epiphyseal closure. After a first trimester abortion, oral contraceptives may be started immediately. In contrast, they should be started 1 week after second trimester abortions. In nonnursing mothers, oral contraceptives may be started 2–3 weeks after delivery.

The patient should be seen after 3 months for a nondirected history and blood pressure recording. Thereafter, the patient should be seen annually for history, blood pressure, weight, physical examination, and cervical cytology.

POSTCOITAL PILL

The postcoital pill is an *emergency method of contraception taken within 72 h of unprotected intercourse.* If coitus occurs 2–6 days before ovulation, ovulation usually will be suppressed and pregnancy avoided by the use of oral contraceptives. The failure rate is 0%–2.4%. The prevention of pregnancy after coitus is often used in women who have been raped, but any reproductive age woman having unprotected intercourse within 72 h may desire this emergency contraception. If menses does not occur within 21 d of the treatment, appropriate pregnancy testing should be initiated.

Two tablets of ethinyl estradiol 0.05 mg and dl-norgestrel 0.5 mg q12h for two doses (a total of 4 pills), or the equivalent, is effective (1.6% pregnancy rate). The greatest side effect is nausea and vomiting (15%–66%), which usually responds to antiemetics. Mifepristone (RU 486) has also been used postcoitally. Compared to oral contraceptives it has a lower rate of pregnancy as well as fewer side effects.

PARENTERAL HORMONAL CONTRACEPTION

INJECTABLE PROGESTAGENS

Hormones injected in depot form may effectively prevent pregnancy for up to 1 year. This method prevents ovulation by suppressing anterior pituitary function (subsequently blocking gonadotropin production). The only agent available in the United States is a 21-carbon progesterone, depomedroxyprogesterone acetate (DMPA-Depo-Provera®) of which 150 mg is given every 90 days. It is initiated within 5 d of menstrual onset. With this agent, the resultant hormonal imbalance may cause atrophy of the endometrium and irregular or absent menstrual bleeding for months. Indeed, *menstrual irregularities* (unpredictable irregular bleeding and spotting lasting ≥7 d) *are so common* with this agent that women should be counseled that it will occur.

Advantages of DMPA include less iron deficiency anemia, less bleeding in those with menorrhagia, less dysmenorrhea, and the privacy of use. It also assists in menstrual hygiene problems associated with severe mental retardation. Other benefits include a decrease in PID, hematological improvement in women with sickle cell disease, and fewer seizures in those with seizure disorders. A frequent *disadvantage* is delay in reestablishing ovulation after discontinuation of the injections (6–12 months). Another disadvantage is a light reduction in bone mineral density (compared to nonusers).

IMPLANTABLE PROGESTIN CAPSULES

In this method, implantation capsules of progestin (levonorgestrel) are inserted through a 2 mm skin incision beneath the skin of the nondominant upper inner arm in a fan-shaped pattern under local anesthesia. The skin, about four fingerbreadths from the medial epicondyle, is cleansed with three applications of an antiseptic solution (e.g., providone-iodine), a sterile fenestrated drape is applied, and an intradermal wheal is created with a local anesthetic through a 25 gauge needle. Using an 18- to 22-gauge 1.5-inch needle, 1 mL of local anesthetic (e.g., 1% lidocaine with 1:4000 epinephrine) is injected along each anticipated site for the capsule. The proximal ends of the capsules are 15 degrees apart (and close enough to be removed by a single small incision) in a splayed pattern extending over 75–90 degrees. Using a sharp trocar or a #11 scalpel blade, an incision is made and the capsules are inserted from the most medial to the most lateral. The incision, which does not require suturing, is covered with a compression dressing (to prevent bruising) for 24 h. Implants must be replaced after 5 years.

The circulating levonorgestrel appears to prevent pregnancy by impaired oocyte maturation, luteal insufficiency, and progestin mediated hostile cervical mucous. Irregular bleeding is the most common side effect, but 5%–10% of women will have amenorrhea. Of nonmenstrual abnormalities leading to cessation, the most frequent is headache.

INTRAUTERINE CONTRACEPTIVE DEVICES (IUD)

Of the many intrauterine contraceptive devices that have been on the market over the years, only one type is currently available in the United States, Copper TCu 380A. IUDs are inserted into the endometrial cavity and prevent implantation through a variety of local mechanisms.

The device usually is inserted during the menses to ensure the avoidance of pregnancy and better patency of the cervical canal. The device can be inserted at any time during the menstrual cycle, however (Fig. 26-2).

The cervix is cleansed using a topical antiseptic, the anterior lip is grasped with a single-toothed tenaculum, and with gentle traction, the uterine cavity length and direction are determined using a sound. This is followed by insertion of the IUD using its accompanying insertion tube. The monofilament plastic tail is allowed to protrude from the cervix to aid later removal and to allow periodic digital palpation by the patient as a check (usually after each menses) for its presence. Complications of insertion include pain and, occasionally, syncope (especially in nulligravidas). Care and appropriate insertion technique should avoid perforation of the uterus (rare).

FIGURE 26-2.   Insertion of the Copper T.
(From H.J. Tatum. In: R.C. Benson, ed., *Current Obstetric & Gynecologic Diagnosis & Treatment,* 4th ed. Lange, 1982.)

The advantages of the IUD include long-term protection without active participation by the patient except for occasional digital checking for expulsion. Fertility returns promptly after the device is removed. The disadvantages of the IUD include continued cramping in some, expulsion during menses (especially in the first few months after insertion), abnormal bleeding (less frequent if the device is the proper size), and ectopic pregnancy (3.8%). If the patient cannot feel the IUD string and did not notice expulsion, she should be examined and radiographs should be taken to locate the device. The string may have separated, but the device may also have perforated the uterus (<1/1000 insertions). If the patient becomes pregnant with a device in place, she must be warned of the enhanced rate of septic abortion, and pregnancy termination should be offered.

Contraindications to IUD include pregnancy, severe cervicitis, malignancy of the genital tract, recent class III or IV cytologic (Pap) smear without definitive diagnosis and treatment, uterine bleeding of unknown etiology, abnormal uterine cavity, acute or subacute salpingitis, cervical canal stenosis, and previous ectopic pregnancy.

An IUD should be removed when uterine cramps are severe, when bleeding is excessive or prolonged (increased bleeding during the first three or four menses after insertion are to be expected), when perforation has occurred (IUD removal by laparoscopy or colpotomy may be possible), if the device is displaced into the cervix, if pregnancy occurs (spontaneous abortion risk is 50% if not removed), and if bacterial salpingitis occurs (most frequently <4 weeks after insertion).

THE NONREPRODUCTIVE YEARS

CLIMACTERIC

The climacteric, or *perimenopause,* is that phase of the aging process in which a *woman passes from reproductive to nonreproductive capability (generally age 45–55 years).* The perimenopause normally lasts ~4 years and is marked by altered ovarian function (e.g., cycle length increases or decreases and anovulation is more common). *Menopause is defined as permanent cessation of menstruation* following the characteristic altered ovarian function.

The physiology of the climacteric requires a brief review of ovarian physiology. Primordial germ cells migrate to the genital ridge by 5 weeks of gestation. Successive mitotic cellular divisions form oogonia, which in turn give rise to oocytes. Although there are approximately 7 million oogonia present in the fetus at 20 weeks of gestation, their numbers gradually decline, leaving 2 million at birth and only 300,000 at puberty. This reduction continues until menopause. The oogonia are reduced by atresia (the primary cause of loss) and ovulation (400–500 per lifetime). As the menopause approaches, ovulation is more erratic, the ovary becomes less responsive to the gonadotrophic hormones, estrogen production is more erratic and often lower, and the level of FSH increases. *Menopause occurs when the ovaries and oocytes response to gonadotropins markedly diminishes or disappears.* The average age of menopause in the United States is *49–50 years,* and it relates to health and genetic background. The age of menopause is not correlated with age at menarche, height, weight, parity, or prolonged use of oral contraceptives.

Early menopause has been associated with smoking, infection, chemotherapy (especially alkylating agents), radiation, surgical procedures that impair ovarian blood supply, tumors, or surgical removal of the ovaries. Early menopause has even been related to left-handedness, although menopause is not classified as being premature unless menses cease at <35 y of age.

PREMENOPAUSE

The length of the *menstrual cycle shortens* from 35 d at age 15 years, to 30 d at age 25 years, to 28 d at age 35 years. This is due to shortening of the follicular phase of the cycle; the luteal phase is unaffected by aging. The transition from premenopause to menopause may be marked by *wide variations in menstrual cycle* length. This transition period tends to be shorter when menopause occurs at an early age. Because the maturation of follicles in the premenopausal period is irregular, ovulation may or may not occur. Although the likelihood of conception occurring during this transition period is less, *precautions should be taken* until 1 year after menopause. Hormone secretion by these follicles is variable but diminished.

Progesterone levels remain similar to those in younger women, but premenopausal women have lower *estradiol* levels. Although LH levels are similar to those in younger women, FSH levels are elevated, especially during the early follicular phase. The elevated FSH levels may stimulate the release of bursts of estradiol from the residual follicles, causing estrogen stimulation of the endometrium, which in the absence of regular progesterone secretion results in irregular bleeding.

HORMONAL CHANGES WITH MENOPAUSE

With the cessation of follicular activity, major changes in estrogen, progesterone, androgen, and gonadotropin secretion occur within 6 months (Table 27-1). In sum, estrogen and progesterone materially decreases at, or before, the time of menopause as well as when the ovaries are removed or sufficiently altered to cease physiologic functioning. Growth hormone (GH) and dehydroepiandrosterone sulfate (DHEA) also decrease at menopause. Whereas the latter hormones undoubtedly have importance, investigation of the impact of hormonal replacement of GH and DHEAS is just beginning.

ESTROGEN

With menopause, *estrogen production, especially estradiol, declines even further from the levels in the premenopause.* The residual estradiol is produced indirectly by the adrenal glands. Both estrone (the major contributor) and testosterone are converted to estradiol in peripheral tissues. Estrone has a diurnal variation with a peak level in the morning and a nadir in early evening. Peripheral aromatization

TABLE 27-1
MEAN SERUM CONCENTRATIONS OF HORMONES
IN PREMENOPAUSAL AND
POSTMENOPAUSAL WOMEN

Hormone	Premenopausal (ng/mL)	Postmenopausal (ng/mL)
Androstenedione	1.5	0.6
Dehydroepiandrosterone	4.2	1.8
Dehydroepiandrosterone-S	1600	300
Estradiol	0.05	0.013
Estrone	0.08	0.029
Progesterone	0.47	0.17
Testosterone	0.32	0.25

of adrenal androstenedione to estrone accounts for most of the estrone production.

PROGESTERONE

Because progesterone is produced by the corpus luteum, postmenopausal progesterone *levels are only 30%* of those seen in ovulating women during the follicular phase. The adrenal gland is presumed to be the source of the small amount of progesterone in postmenopausal women.

ANDROGENS

Androstenedione is the predominant androgen secreted by developing follicles. With cessation of follicular development in postmenopausal women, androstenedione levels *fall by 50%*. Diurnal variation of androstenedione can be shown to follow adrenal gland activity after menopause. The ovary secretes only 20% of androstenedione after menopause. *Overall, postmenopausal testosterone production is decreased by less than a third.* Diurnal variation is notable. The postmenopausal ovary secretes a relatively large portion of testosterone. This continued testosterone production combined with relatively low estrogen levels may result in slight virilism. Dehydroepiandrosterone (DHEA) and dehydroepiandrosterone sulfate (DHEAS) are produced primarily by the adrenal gland (<25% by the ovary). With aging, *DHEA production falls by 60%*

and DHEAS falls by 80%. In the relative absence of estrogen and progesterone, however, there may be a slight expression of the androgenicity (e.g., facial hair).

GONADOTROPINS

After menopause, *LH and FSH increase substantially.* FSH and LH levels are both 4–30 mIU/mL during reproductive life, except briefly during the preovulatory surge, when they increase to >50 mIU/mL and >100 mIU/mL, respectively. After menopause, the levels of both are >100 mIU/mL. FSH rises sooner and at a more rapid rate than does LH. Both FSH and LH show pulsatile bursts every 1–2 h, thought to be secondary to pituitary response to hypothalamic release of gonadotropin-releasing hormone (GnRH). Low estrogen levels increase pituitary sensitivity to GnRH.

CLINICAL FINDINGS

REPRODUCTIVE TRACT

Both the *duration and flow of menstrual blood gradually diminish* prior to the menopause until only spotting is followed by cessation. On rare occasion, abrupt cessation occurs. In some women, vaginal bleeding will be heavier or more frequent, occasionally with intermenstrual bleeding. Menopause cannot be diagnosed until cessation of menses has exceeded 6–12 months.

Decreased estrogen levels are responsible for *atrophic changes* in the entire reproductive tract. The vaginal epithelium thins, and the capillary bed is closer to the surface, making the vagina appear hyperemic. Minimal trauma may result in mild vaginal bleeding. Bacterial invasion may occur. The vaginal rugae gradually disappear. As time passes, and the capillary bed further decreases, the vagina becomes pale, shiny, and smooth.

Vaginal cytological smears may be obtained to assess estrogenic activity. Either the maturation index (a differential count of the parabasal, intermediate, and superficial squamous cells) or the cornification count (the percentage of precornified vs. cornified cells) may be used. Because there can be great variation in the findings, the vaginal smear should be used only as a gross estimate of estrogenic status of the woman. It cannot diagnose the climacteric state, although cytology may be helpful in determining the dosage of replacement estrogen required to reverse vaginal atrophy and may help to diagnose genital tract malignancy or infection.

The *cervix contracts in size, and cervical mucus production decreases.* The *uterus and tubes atrophy* as the myometrium and endometrium shrink. This change is of benefit to women with leiomyomas or adenomyomas because these lesions tend to atrophy as well. Endometrial biopsy may show tissue changes ranging from a scanty basal atrophic pattern to a moderately proliferative pattern. When glandular hyperplasia is present, excessive estrogenic stimulation is occuring and further investigation is necessary.

Because the decrease in ovarian size is substantial after menopause, *a palpable ovary* in a postmenopausal woman (the palpable ovary syndrome) should be considered neoplastic until otherwise explained. *Progressive loss of pelvic tissue tone* accompanies estrogen deficiency and contributes to the increased incidence of enterocele, rectocele, cystourethrocele, and uterine prolapse often seen in postmenopausal women.

URINARY TRACT

Estrogen maintains the epithelium of the bladder and urethra. Hence, estrogen deficiency causes *atrophic cystitis and urethritis,* characterized by urgency and frequency without dysuria or pyuria. Urethral tone decreases, occasionally allowing the meatus to protrude (a reddened caruncle).

BREASTS

Breast size *decreases progressively* during the climacteric and the breasts become *less dense.*

HOT FLUSHES

Hot flushes, or flashes, will *occur in 75% of women* who lose ovarian function, either through menopause or by bilateral oophorectomy. The episodic sudden flushing causes perspiration even in a cool environment. The vasomotor episodes are described as starting with a sensation of pressure in the chest or head that increases until a feeling of heat or burning is experienced in the face, neck, and chest, immediately followed by sweating, especially involving the head, neck, chest, and back. Some report palpitations, vertigo, weakness, fatigue, or a feeling of faintness. The frequency may be from 1–2 per h to 1–2 per week. The durations of the episodes vary from momentary to 10 min, with an average duration of 4 min. If flushes occur, 80% can expect them to recur for 1 year, and at least 25% will experience flushes for 5 years.

Only slight changes in blood pressure or heart rhythm have been demonstrated, but *cutaneous vasodilatation, decreased core temperature, sweating, and increased pulse rate* are documented. The symptoms may relate to a malfunction of the central thermoregulatory system. Despite a falling core temperature, the patient feels hot and attempts cooling by fanning or moving to an open door or window. Apparently at climacteric, the set point for temperature in the hypothalamus is reset temporarily at a lower point. Withdrawal of estrogen rather than lack of estrogen appears to be responsible because young girls or those with gonadal dysgenesis do not have hot flushes (unless estrogen is given, then withdrawn). There appears to be a correlation of hot flushes with the pulsatile release of gonadotropins. If the flushes occur at night, frequent awakening may lead to sleep deprivation (with subsequent fatigue, irritability, anxiety, and memory loss). The most effective treatment is estrogens. Progestins also have been shown to be effective in treatment of hot flushes.

CARDIOVASCULAR SYSTEM

Heart disease in women <55 years of age is less common and less severe than in men of the same age. For each decade >55, however, the death rate from heart attack increases 2 times in men and 3 times in women. Smoking increases the risk in both groups. The risk of heart disease increases the younger the age at menopause.

Estrogen replacement therapy decreases the risk of heart disease and decreases the death rate as well. Cholesterol levels increase about 16 mg/dL with menopause, but replacement estrogens do not lower this increase. Estrogens increase the high-density lipoproteins by 10% and decrease the low-density fraction. Replacement estrogens increase triglyceride levels. This effect on lipid metabolism may be profound in cases of familial hyperlipidemia.

Although menopause has no consistent effect on blood pressure, replacement estrogens increase both systolic and diastolic blood pressure. The change in blood pressure associated with estrogen therapy occurs via the renin–angiotensin–aldosterone system, thus resulting in vasoconstriction and fluid retention. The *increase is usually mild,* and no increased incidence of stroke has been documented because of this shift. Menopause does not affect carbohydrate metabolism. Replacement estrogen either has no effect on carbohydrate metabolism or may decrease glucose tolerance slightly without increasing insulin secretion.

In the United States, the *decrease in the female death rate from heart disease has coincided with the increased use of replacement estrogen therapy.* The female death rate has declined by >30%, whereas male deaths from heart disease declined only 20% during the same time.

OSTEOPOROSIS

Osteoporosis is a systemic skeletal disease characterized by low bone mass and microarchitectural deterioration of bone tissue, with a consequent increase in bone fragility and susceptibility to fracture. Quantification of the process has not been universally adopted, but all standards relate loss to the young adult mean bone mass: *osteopenia is 1–2 or 2.5 SD below, whereas osteoporosis is 2–2.5 SD below the young adult mean bone mass.* A decrease of 1 SD is associated with ~2 times fracture risk. Bone mass loss occurs with aging in both sexes, but is worse and occurs earlier in women than in men (beginning as early as age 30 and 45–50, respectively). Menopause dramatically accelerates bone mass density (BMD) loss. A useful generalization is that *after menopause 3% of BMD is lost per year for the first 5 years and 1% per year thereafter.* Patients at risk for osteoporosis may lose as much as 5% of BMD per year.

It may be that *osteoporosis is the most significant health hazard associated with the climacteric* because of the resulting fractures (1.3–1.5 million annually in the United States), disability, and invalidism. Although hip fractures account for only 15% of total fractures the morbidity and mortality is remarkable. Death within 12 months of hip fracture occurs in 20%, with 25% of survivors confined to long-term care facilities, and 50% suffering loss of mobility.

There are *racial differences* in the incidence of osteoporosis: the highest incidence in Caucasians, although Asians are not far behind. Hispanics are intermediate in risk and African Americans at the lowest risk. A *family history* of osteoporosis is predisposing. Estrogen deficiency appears to be the most common risk factor. *Thin* women and those who *do not exercise* are more susceptible. *Smoking* increases osteoporosis. *Excessive use of alcohol and high caffeine intake* are also risk factors.

The bone loss is the result of bone resorption exceeding bone formation, with a calcium loss of approximately 15 mg/d between 50 and 70 years of age (net loss 100 g). Trabecular bone loss is greater than cortical bone loss (50% and 5%, respectively). The exact mechanism is unclear, but *estrogen replacement therapy results in decreased bone resorption and decreased bone calcium loss.* However, new bone formation does not occur with this therapy. Effects of estrogen on parathyroid hormone receptors and calcitonin are being studied. Osteoporosis in itself is not painful, but fractures are. Vertebral body fractures are most common, leading to a hunched posture (dowager's hump). Hip and arm fractures are increased substantially, as well as rib fracture, often after seemingly trivial accidents.

Early diagnosis is important, and therapy must be initiated early enough to decrease the risk of pathologic fractures. Bone mass measurements are an excellent means of measuring trabecular bone mass.

If the presentation of osteopenia or ostoporosis is atypical, other influences or bone diseases must be considered. *Medications adversely influencing bone mass* include: glucocorticoids, thyroxine, and heparin. *Diseases associated with decreased bone mass include:* osteomalacia, multiple myeloma, osteitis deformans (Paget's disease of bone), metastatic cancer, or hyperparathyroidism. These may be differentiated by serum calcium, phosphorus, and alkaline phosphatase levels. Occasionally, 24-h urinary calcium, parathyroid hormone, or serum protein electrophoresis will also be useful. In rare cases, *evaluation of bone formation* (serum bone alkaline phosphatase, serum osteocalcin, and serum procollagen I extension peptides) or bone resorption (urinary *N*-telopeptide collagen cross links, collage cross links, urinary deoxypyridinoline, and urinary hydroxyproline) may be necessary.

SKIN

Estrogen receptors are present in skin, especially of the face, thigh, and breasts. With aging, the *skin becomes thinner, with a loss of elasticity leading to wrinkling.* These changes are most pronounced in areas exposed to sunlight (e.g., face, neck, hands). In animal studies, estrogen increases skin cell growth, changes dermal collagen content, alters skin vascularization, and enhances dermal water. However, estrogen in skin creams or lotions may cause systemic problems and should only be used under physician direction, if at all.

HAIR

Changes in hair (thinning) may be in part the result of low estrogen with sustained testosterone levels. The fine hair decreases on the face with the growth of coarse hair, especially on the upper lip (moustache) and chin. Pubic and axillary hair decrease, and slight baldness may appear. Body and extremity hair may increase or decrease.

PSYCHOLOGIC ASPECTS

Psychologic disturbances increase during the climacteric. Hot flushes, sleep disturbance, and vaginal atrophy may play a significant role. Many family changes may be occurring concomitantly, with slight alterations in the woman's appearance. The incidence of severe psychiatric illness is not increased by menopause, but estrogen therapy may improve the emotional state by relieving hot flushes, insomnia, or vaginal atrophy.

EXCESS ENDOGENOUS ESTROGENS

Occasionally, women will show signs of estrogen excess, with uterine bleeding, mastodynia, edema, leiomyoma growth, and increased endometriosis. When such symptomatology of estrogen excess develop in postmenopausal women, one of three mechanisms is likely: (1) increased androgen production, (2) increased aromatization of androgens, or (3) excess estrogen production. Increased androgen production is usually associated with an ovarian or adrenal neoplasm. Increased aromatization of androgen is associated with hyperthyroidism, obesity, or liver disease. Increased androgenic estrogen may be associated with obesity likely due to the increased conversion of androstenedione to estrone in adipose tissue.

TREATMENT

ESTROGENS

Hormonal replacement therapy (HRT), casually used synonymously with estrogen replacement, today also includes certain uses of progesterone, as well as the use of certain estrogen analogs (selective estrogen receptor modulators). When a woman seeks relief of symptoms of the climacteric, a discussion of the physiologic changes she is experiencing may be helpful to *understand the therapeutic goals.* She should be made aware of the benefits of and alternatives to estrogen replacement therapy. Although often an essential component, *HRT is only a portion of total therapy. Other components include: lifestyle alterations to reduce factors causing osteoporosis, diet, calcium, vitamin D, and exercise.*

Absolute contraindications to estrogen replacement are undiagnosed vaginal bleeding, acute liver disease, chronic hepatic dysfunction, acute vascular thrombosis, neuroophthalmologic vascular disease, and endometrial or breast carcinoma (estrogen may stimulate the growth of malignant cells). Estrogens are not contraindicated in treated cervical carcinoma. Undesirable *side effects* may be seen in patients given estrogens with hypertension, seizure disorder, uterine leiomyomas, fibrocystic disease of the breast, familial hyperlipidemia, some collagen diseases, chronic thrombophlebitis, diabetes mellitus, migraine headaches, or gallbladder disease.

The use of replacement *estrogen without progestins in the postmenopausal woman increases her risk of developing endometrial carcinoma.* Although the incidence of endometrial cancer is increased, the risk of death from this is not increased if careful observation of these patients allows diagnosis of cancer in the early stages.

There may be a *slightly increased risk of breast carcinoma* with the use of replacement estrogens. However, studies have not shown consistent results relative to those at greatest risk. Nonetheless, high estrogen doses have been implicated in breast cancer development.

Thromboembolic disease may be worsened due to the estrogen effect on the clotting mechanism. Estrogen increases the coagulability of blood via platelet changes, the coagulation system itself, and the fibrinolytic sequence. Estrogen also increases vascular endothelial proliferation and decreases venous blood flow slightly. The low doses of estrogen used in replacement therapy, however, usually do not significantly increase the risk of thromboembolic disease. This must be considered, however, in certain women.

Gallbladder disease increases with estrogen replacement, presumably due to the increase in cholesterol and triglycerides. *Heart disease is decreased with the use of low-dose estrogens.* Because the age-adjusted mortality rate of death from heart disease is 4 times that of death from breast cancer or endometrial cancer combined, this benefit should be stressed.

PROGESTIN-ESTROGEN THERAPY

Long-term study and usage provides clear evidence that estrogen replacement therapy significantly reduces the incidences of osteoporosis, vasomotor symptoms (hot flushes), central nervous system symptoms (i.e., insomnia, irritability, poor memory, anxiety, and headaches), and improves genital atrophy. Estrogen replacement therapy may even reverse cognitive changes and improve cognitive function. Additionally, there is observational evidence that estrogen is associated with reduced cardiovascular morbidity and may retard the progression of senile-associated dementia, especially Alzheimer's disease. The mechanisms by which estrogen accomplishes the various beneficial effects remains unclear, but a portion of the cardiovascular effect may be the demonstrated improvement in the lipoprotein profile (decrease LDL, increase HDL). The improvement of genital atrophy may assist some patients, but there is no evidence that estrogen enhances libido. The addition of androgens to estrogen introduces additional risks, but may assist in increasing libido.

Current recommendations include *progestin therapy with estrogen therapy* because studies have shown that the *risk of endometrial carcinoma is decreased* if endometrial tissue exposed to estrogen is periodically opposed by progestin. The duration of progestin therapy is critical for this effect, since 7 d/month is ineffective, whereas 13 d is protective. Long-term estrogen replacement is necessary to prevent osteoporosis (e.g., 4 years is insufficient). The effects of long-term progestin therapy are unknown but seem to be limited to periodic vaginal bleeding. If the patient has no uterus, progestins are not indicated.

Although the hormones may be replaced orally or by injection, certainly the *oral method is more convenient.* The starting dosage of estrogen is 0.625 mg/d of oral conjugated equine estrogens or estropinate for 25 d, with no therapy for the rest of the month. If the lower dose does not prevent hot flushes, a higher dose may be given and tapered as soon as possible. Norethindrone (Norlutate) should be avoided, because this preparation blocks the beneficial effects of estrogen on lipid metabolism. If the uterus is present, *medroxyprogesterone acetate 10 mg/d should be given during the last 13–15 d of estrogen replacement each month.*

If estrogen replacement is contraindicated or refused, hot flushes may be reduced in 90% by medroxyprogesterone 150 mg/m IM or 10–40 mg/d PO. Less effective than estrogen is norgestrel 250 Mg/d PO. Conjugated estrogen vaginal cream 1 g every other day may relieve symptoms of vaginal atrophy.

Although progesterone replacement therapy (usually megestrol acetate, norethindrone, or medroxyprogesterone acetate) is effective in *reducing vasomotor symptoms it is not as effective as estrogens.* To be efficient, large doses are required and there may be undesirable side effects. Additionally, when used in combination with estrogens MPA reduces the increased HDL levels. Micronized progesterone does not reduce the beneficial lipid effects of estrogens.

SELECTIVE ESTROGEN RECEPTOR MODULATORS

Raloxifene, a nonsteroidal benzothiophene, acts as an estrogen agonist in both bone (inhibits osteoclast function) and liver (decreases

LDL). It is administered PO at 60 mg q d and after 24 months has been demonstrated to increase bone density by 1%–2%.

ADDITIONAL THERAPY (OSTEOPOROSIS)

Elemental *calcium supplementation* (1000–1500 mg PO q d) benefits treatment of osteoporosis. Indeed, there is evidence that childhood calcium intake influences adult hip bone mass. Daily phosphorus intake of >2000 mg may adversely influence bone mass and the postmenopausal recommended daily intake is <*700 mg*. Although vitamin D deficiency is uncommon, *vitamin D supplementation* is recommended for the treatment of osteoporosis.

Alendronate, a bisphosphonate, inhibits the function of osteoclasts, thereby reducing bone resorption. Alendronate 10 mg PO q d is recommended to be taken with 8 oz of water in the morning 30 mins before anything else by mouth. Treatment for 3 years has been demonstrated to increase (6%–9%) bone mass and decrease fractures. Alendronate has a half-life of >10 years, but may cause abdominal pain, musculoskeletal pain, and upper GI bleeding.

Low-dose calcitonin plus calcium has been shown to increase body calcium stores for up to 2 years. Calcitonin is administered as a nasal spray containing 200 IU once a day. While a potential side effect is rhinitis, calcitonin does increase bone density and decrease fractures.

High-dose *sodium fluoride* will increase trabecular bone by stimulation of osteoblasts. It is administered at 75 mg q d PO. There is question about the new bone's integrity, but it has been demonstrated to decrease fractures. Flouride may cause both gastric irritation and lower extremity pain.

PREVENTION (OSTEOPOROSIS)

Prevention of osteoporosis is life long. Adequate calcium in childhood and adolescence is necessary. Life-long exercise (avoidance of a sedentary life style) assists in building a stronger skeleton. Lifestyle risks fostering osteoporosis (smoking, alcohol) can be avoided. Alternatives to the medications influencing bone loss should be sought. The use of hormonal replacement therapy is an essential component of prevention. Finally, the risks of falling in the elder years may be minimized.

CHAPTER

28

ENDOMETRIOSIS AND ADENOMYOSIS

ENDOMETRIOSIS

Endometriosis is the *extrauterine occurrence of endometrial glands and stroma,* most often involving the ovaries or dependent visceral peritoneal surfaces. Although benign, *endometriosis is progressive, tends to recur, may be locally invasive, may have widespread disseminated foci (rare), and may exist in pelvic lymph nodes* (30%). The etiology is unknown, but several mechanisms may be important in pathogenesis. Endometriosis is a significant gynecological problem, occurring in *7%–10% of the general population* and up to 50% of premenopausal women. Endometriosis is found in 20%–50% (mean *38%) of infertile women,* and in *71%–87% of those with chronic pelvic pain.* Endometriosis is responsible for *20% of all gynecologic operations* and is the *single leading nonobstetric cause (>5%) of hospitalization for women age 15–44 years.*

PATHOLOGY

Although some contend that it may be entirely a microscopic diagnosis, with no grossly visible alterations, most authorities maintain that grossly visible changes are necessary for a clinical diagnosis. Early lesions appear as red petechiae on the pelvic peritoneal surfaces. With accumulation of menstrual-like detritus, these multifocal lesions develop into small (1–10 mm), flat to cystic, dark (blue, brown, or black) lesions with hemorrhage into adjacent tissues. Collectively, these changes are often described as a powder-burn appearance. They also cause thickening and scarring of the contiguous peritoneal surfaces. As the disease progresses, the size and number of these lesions increase, and extensive adhesions form. The largest cysts occur in the ovary, where they are termed *endometriomas* and are filled with thick, chocolate-colored blood breakdown products.

755

Pelvic endometriosis is characteristically *multifocal,* involving (in order of decreasing frequency) the ovary (50%), cul-de-sac, uterosacral ligaments, posterior uterine surface and broad ligaments, and the remaining pelvic peritoneum. The bladder (10%–15%), ureters (<1%), and bowel (rectosigmoid 10%–15%, appendix 14%–30%) may be affected by implants leading to scarring, obstruction, or blood in the urine or stool. Distant sites of endometriosis are rare but have been reported in the lung, brain, and kidney.

The most characteristic histology (endometrial glands, stroma, and hemorrhage into adjacent tissues) is found in early lesions. With progression, the wall of the implant may be lined by a monolayer of connective tissue cells, or no lining may be identifiable. Indeed, *viable endometrial glands and stroma may not be found in about 25% of cases.* Characteristically, the fibrotic cyst wall contains *hemosiderin-laden macrophages.* In part, these progressive alterations may explain the *8% incidence of disagreement* between the operative and pathologic diagnoses, for pathologists characteristically diagnose endometriosis if two or more of the following histological features are present: endometrial epithelium, endometrial glands, endometrial stroma, and hemosiderin-laden macrophages.

Ca_{125} levels are elevated in endometriosis and have specificity of >85% and sensitivity of 20%–50% for moderate to severe disease. However, Ca_{125} lacks correlation to both minimal disease and recurrences; thus, Ca_{125} is of limited use.

PATHOLOGIC PHYSIOLOGY

Although a *single etiology for endometriosis has not emerged,* several observations and potential mechanisms seem to generally explain pathogenesis. Endometriosis has a *multifactorial inherited predisposition.* The risk of endometriosis in first-degree female relatives of an afflicted woman is increased 7 times. Women with a family history of endometriosis develop the disease earlier in life, and it is more likely to be advanced when compared to those without first-degree relatives with endometriosis.

Retrograde menstruation (which probably occurs in the majority of women) with direct implantation of fragments of viable endometrium was a cause of endometriosis advocated by Sampson. This readily explains the usual distribution of lesions. However, retrograde menstruation does not explain why distant metastases occur or why the majority of women do not develop endometriosis. Another theory is that *multipotential cells of the celomic epithelium may undergo metaplasia.* This induction phenomenon as a cause for endometriosis was advocated by Meyers and subsequently modified by others as either a spontaneous or induced alteration (perhaps by factors within the menstrual discharge). The metaplasia theory assists in answering some (e.g., deep rectovaginal septal) cases but fails to provide a complete answer. Women with endometriosis may have a *defect in local cell-mediated immunity.* Finally, *lymphatic and vascular metastasis* may explain the rare remote endometrial implants, to the lung, for example.

Any *outflow obstruction* leading to a greater incidence and amount of retrograde menstruation predisposes to endometriosis. Other clinical predispositions include: *early menarche, regular cycles, and a longer and heavier than normal flow.* The only factors thought to decrease the incidence of endometriosis are those that lower estrogen levels.

How endometriosis causes pelvic pain and infertility is only partially understood; however, pain and infertility may be related mechanically by direct extension of the process. Alternatively, patients with endometriosis have an increased number of anovulatory cycles, luteal phase defects, luteinized but unruptured follicles, and galactorrhea. These problems all seem related to a relative hyperprolactinemia. In addition, there are increased amounts of prostaglandin precursors, prostaglandins (Pg), and prostaglandin metabolites in the peritoneal fluid and peritoneal washings from infertile patients with endometriosis. Notably increased are thromboxane B_2, 6-ketoprostacycline $F_{1\alpha}$, $PgF_{2\alpha}$, and PgE. Enhanced amounts of peritoneal fluid also roughly parallel the severity of endometriosis.

Endometriosis may enhance spontaneous abortion. In support, several studies have detailed a decrease in the rate of spontaneous abortion (44%–82%) after therapy eliminating endometriosis.

DIAGNOSIS

Typical patients with endometriosis are in their mid-30s, nulliparous, involuntarily infertile, and have secondary dysmenorrhea and pelvic pain. The diagnosis of endometriosis may be difficult because one third of endometriosis cases are asymptomatic, there is no correlation between extent of the disease and symptomatology (i.e., minimal disease may cause severe pain, whereas large endometriomas may be asymptomatic), endometriosis frequently appears in atypical fashions (e.g., teenagers, multigravidas, and asymptomatic ovarian tumors), and the symptomatology varies with the anatomic site of endometriosis.

SYMPTOMS AND SIGNS

The *usual symptomatology* includes pelvic pain, dysmenorrhea, infertility, abnormal bleeding, and dyspareunia. The most common *signs on physical examination* include: uterosacral ligament nodularity, adnexal mass, nodularity in the rectovaginal septum, and cervical (external) endometriosis.

Pelvic Pain

Pelvic pain is the cardinal symptom of endometriosis. Characteristically, the pain is chronic and recurrent and presents as acquired or secondary dysmenorrhea. The pain *usually occurs 24–48 h premenstrually and subsides sometime after the onset of menstruation;* however, discomfort may include the entire menstrual interval. The pain is characterized as *constant,* usually in the *pelvis or low back* (sacral); however, pain may be unilateral or bilateral and may radiate to the legs or groin. When compared to primary dysmenorrhea, the pain is more constant and less often in the midline. Other pelvic symptoms include severe cramping, pelvic heaviness, and pelvic pressure.

Gastrointestinal symptoms may occur, whether or not the bowel is actually involved (e.g., cyclic abdominal pain, intermittent constipation, diarrhea, dyschezia, and blood in the stool). Urinary symptoms include urinary frequency, dysuria, perimenstrual hematuria, or hydronephrosis. Deep penetration with intercourse may evoke severe pain (dyspareunia), which may last for 1–2 h. Unusual symptoms about the time of menses have been reported: seizures (central nervous system implants) and hemothorax or hematemesis (pulmonary implants).

Infertility

Endometriosis is diagnosed nearly *twice as often in infertile women* as in those who are fertile. Thus, it must be suspected in every case of infertility (Chapter 29).

Abnormal Bleeding

Abnormal bleeding, not associated with anovulation, occurs in 15%–20% of women with endometriosis. The characteristic patterns are premenstrual spotting or menorrhagia or both.

PHYSICAL EXAMINATION

External endometriosis usually occurs *on the cervix* and is associated with an enhanced frequency of internal endometriosis. Other external endometriosis is usually *iatrogenic,* occurring in surgical incisions. On physical examination, endometriosis classically causes *tender nodularity of the uterosacral ligaments*. With progression, the uterus becomes retroverted and fixed, usually with posterior cul-de-sac scarring and tenderness. The *ovaries* may be enlarged (rarely symmetrically), tender, and fixed to adjacent structures (e.g., broad ligament or lateral pelvic sidewall). In advanced cases, the pelvic structures become rigid and unyielding.

Laparoscopy

Laparoscopy is *generally used to confirm the diagnosis* of endometriosis. Biopsy of selected implants may reveal the characteristic pathology. Although this is not necessary to complete the diagnosis, it is useful for subsequent therapy and overall prognosis. The American Fertility Society's classification (Table 28-1) quantifies severity based on the characteristic of the lesions, resultant adhesions, ovarian cysts, scarring and retraction, fixation of pelvic structures, and obliteration of the cul-de-sac. The *classification does not correlate well* with: pain, dyspareunia, or pregnancy following treatment. It does, however, *allow a uniform recording of findings* and may be useful in following individual patients as well as comparing results of various therapies. Occasionally, confirmation of the diagnosis and staging are accomplished during a laparotomy (e.g., for ruptured ectopic pregnancy).

Most recently, laparoscopic analysis of pain ("pain mapping") has been performed in selected awake patients by methodically stimulating the pelvis under direct visualization. This reveals that the pain arises from normal peritoneal surfaces adjacent to lesions and extends well beyond visible lesions. Thus, pain most likely comes from lesions involving peritoneal surfaces innervated by peripheral spinal nerves (vs. autonomic nervous system innervation).

ENDOMETRIOSIS DURING ADOLESCENCE AND AFTER MENOPAUSE

Endometriosis is present in *two thirds of adolescents who have significant morbidity associated with their menses*. Adolescents account for 8% of women with endometriosis. Of the teenagers with endometriosis, 10% have congenital obstruction to menstrual outflow. The *symptoms* in this age group most indicative of endometriosis are increasing acquired dysmenorrhea, chronic pelvic pain, bowel changes with menses, and abnormal vaginal bleeding. Thus, *diagnostic laparoscopy should be considered* in truly symptomatic adolescents. Rarely, postmenopausal endometriosis is due to the use of unopposed exogenous estrogens.

TABLE 28-1

AMERICAN SOCIETY FOR REPRODUCTIVE MEDICINE, REVISED CLASSIFICATION OF ENDOMETRIOSIS, 1996.

THE AMERICAN FERTILITY SOCIETY
REVISED CLASSIFICATION OF ENDOMETRIOSIS

Patient's Name_____ Date_____

Stage I (Minimal) — 1–5   Laparoscopy_____ Laparotomy_____ Photography_____
Stage II (Mild) — 6–15   Recommended Treatment_____
Stage III (Moderate) — 16–40
Stage IV (Severe) — > 40
Total_____   Prognosis_____

PERITONEUM	ENDOMETRIOSIS	< 1cm	1–3cm	> 3cm
	Superficial	1	2	4
	Deep	2	4	6
OVARY	R Superficial	1	2	4
	Deep	4	16	20
	L Superficial	1	2	4
	Deep	4	16	20

	POSTERIOR CULDESAC OBLITERATION	Partial		Complete
		4		40

OVARY	ADHESIONS	< 1/3 Enclosure	1/3-2/3 Enclosure	> 2/3 Enclosure
	R Filmy	1	2	4
	Dense	4	8	16
	L Filmy	1	2	4
	Dense	4	8	16
TUBE	R Filmy	1	2	4
	Dense	4*	8*	16
	L Filmy	1	2	4
	Dense	4*	8*	16

*If the fimbriated end of the fallopian tube is completely enclosed, change the point assignment to 16.

Additional Endometriosis:_____ | Associated Pathology:_____

To Be Used with Normal Tubes and Ovaries	To Be Used with Abnormal Tubes and / or Ovaries
L R	L R

DIFFERENTIAL DIAGNOSIS

The *differential diagnosis of endometriosis* includes primary dysmenorrhea, chronic pelvic inflammatory disease, leiomyoma with degeneration, pelvic adhesions, adenomyosis, ovarian malignancy, and functional bowel disease. Less commonly, the following conditions should be considered in the differential diagnosis: salpingitis isthmica nodosa, chronic ectopic gestation, carcinoma of the colon or rectum, and diverticulitis. *Rupture of an endometrioma* appears as an acute abdomen and must be differentiated from bleeding corpus luteum, ectopic gestation, appendicitis, and diverticulitis.

MINIMAL DIAGNOSTIC CRITERIA

In some cases, the symptomatology and physical examination are so classic that the diagnosis seems obvious, and it is tempting to base the diagnosis entirely on the history and physical examination. However, the diagnosis must exclude other conditions because of the serious life-long implications for the patient. Thus, it is recommended that *laparoscopy with documented visualization of gross lesions and pathologic demonstration of characteristic criteria be utilized for diagnosis.* Additionally, laparoscopic visualization allows *staging of the disease.*

THERAPY

One must *individualize therapy* for endometriosis to include the patient's desire for fertility, her age, severity of symptoms, location of the lesions, stage of the disease, and other concurrent significant abnormalities. Various therapeutic options are outlined in Table 28-2.

Empiric medical therapy (based purely on clinical symptoms without definitive surgical diagnosis) is currently being studied, but at the minimum includes pretreatment exclusion of other conditions, and initial treatment with oral contraceptives and nonsteroidal antiinflammatory drugs. Before this approach could be recommended, further studies are necessary to detail the full efficacy, safety and cost effectiveness.

OBSERVATION AND PALLIATION

Observation is warranted in some patients (e.g., those with minimal disease or near the menopause) but should be undertaken with the knowledge that physical examination alone is not likely to detect

TABLE 28-2
THERAPY OPTIONS FOR ENDOMETRIOSIS

A. Observation
B. Palliation
   1. Analgesics
   2. Nonsteroidal anti-inflammatory agents
   3. Prostaglandin synthetase inhibitors
   4. Pregnancy
   5. Infertility studies
C. Endocrine therapy
   1. Progestogens
   2. Estrogen-progestogens
   3. Danazol
   4. GnRH agonists
D. Surgical therapy
   1. Conservative surgery
   2. Procedures for pain relief
   3. Definitive surgery

any very gross disease. *Analgesic therapy is purely palliative,* regardless of the agent used, but may be useful in combination with other therapy.

Pregnancy was once described as curative for endometriosis, but this is untrue. Indeed, endometriomas may increase rapidly in size during the first trimester of pregnancy but generally decrease in size during the third trimester. Rupture of endometriomas has been reported at any time during pregnancy. Once menses return after the puerperium, endometriosis will continue to progress.

ENDOCRINE THERAPY

Progestogens and
Estrogen-Progestogen Combinations

Both *progestogens* (oral or IM) and *estrogen-progestogen combinations* (oral contraception) have demonstrated usefulness in controlling pain associated with endometriosis. This is true both in comparison to placebo as well as danazol. Thus, some authorities recommend this as a first therapeutic step, particularly in patients with minimal disease. Additionally, the safety of this approach is well established.

Whereas cyclic hormones may induce endometrial growth, continuous estrogen-progestogen or progestogen alone suppresses the growth pattern. Thus, constant (daily) regimens of estrogen and progestin, oral contraceptives, or progestogen all cause endometrial atrophy. *Low estrogen combination oral contraceptives with high progestin activity* are most commonly used in the treatment of endometriosis as 1 tablet per d starting on the third d of menses until breakthrough bleeding occurs. When this develops, doubling the dosage generally will relieve the breakthrough bleeding, and after 5 d of elevated amounts, the dosage may be returned to 1–2 pills per d. This may be continued for 6–9 months.

There may be an initial (first 6 weeks) slight exacerbation of clinical symptoms and even a slight risk of endometrioma rupture. Side effects include nausea, breast tenderness, weight gain, chloasma, depression, irritability, edema, and rarely hypertension. Alternatively, medroxyprogesterone may be used (100 mg IM every 2 weeks for four doses, then 200 mg per month for four doses). Medroxyprogesterone may be associated with a long or extremely variable interval before ovulation resumes (1 year is not uncommon). Thus, the patient's desire for pregnancy and their ability to tolerate an interval of anovulation or irregular bleeding after therapy should be considered when medroxyprogesterone is used. Breakthrough bleeding is the most frequent side effect, but unpleasant mood alterations may cause patient discontinuance. These therapies currently are reserved for those with mild endometriosis who do not desire immediate fertility and are not candidates for other treatments. These regimens are less effective (both objectively and subjectively) than danazol and have a greater patient discontinuance (one third) because of side effects. Uncorrected pregnancy rates are 30%.

Danazol

Danazol (17 α-ethinyltestosterone) remains useful in medical treatment of endometriosis. Danazol is mildly androgenic and anabolic, but it also binds to androgen receptors, progesterone receptors, and sex hormone-binding globulin. This results in a threefold increase of free testosterone. The result is marked *endometrial atrophy* (both within the uterus and within the lesions). Amenorrhea and inhibition of ovulation occur with 4–6 weeks of therapy. Unfortunately, because of these clinical alterations, the overall effect was erroneously termed pseudomenopause. The clinical state induced by danazol, although it is hypoestrogenic and hypoprogestational, more *closely resembles that induced by androgens*. It lacks most of the physiologic alterations of the menopause.

The dosage of danazol for suppression of endometriosis is 400–800 mg/d PO for 6–9 months. For therapy >6 months, serum liver enzymes should be determined. Danazol may be started on the fifth day after menses. For the first month, barrier contraceptives should be used because danazol may masculinize a female fetus should pregnancy occur. Success is most marked when treating endometriomas <2 cm in diameter. After a full course of therapy, 90% of patients will be objectively improved and 75% will report symptomatic improvement; however, 15%–30% will have recurrence of symptoms in <2 years. The fertility rate is improved to 40% (uncorrected).

Danazol is *expensive, and 80% of patients have side effects* (10%–20% severe enough to discontinue the medication). The most common side effects in a representative series include acne (>15%), hot flashes (15%), uterine spotting (10%), gastrointestinal disturbances (8%), weakness and dizziness (8%), hirsutism (6%), edema (6%), decreased breast size (5%), weight gain (8–10 lb in 5%), and change in libido (3%–5%). Less common side effects include muscle cramps (4%), voice changes (3%), atrophic vaginitis (3%), and migraine headaches (2%). Although more difficult to quantify, emotional lability and depression also may occur.

Gonadotropin-Releasing Hormone (GnRH) Agonists

By relatively long-term binding to LHRH receptors, the GnRH analogs suppress the pituitary–ovarian axis, creating low levels of FSH and LH as well as estrogen and progesterone levels in the menopause range. This causes endometrial atrophy. Administration of GnRH agonists is usually subcutaneous or intranasal. This is *effective (85%) in objectively decreasing endometriosis*. Ovulation resumes relatively quickly (~45 days) after discontinuation of the medication. GnRH agonists have demonstrated efficacy and safety for treatment of the pelvic pain related to endometriosis.

GnRH agonists create estrogen deficiency, which is clinically manifest by vasomotor symptoms and loss of bone mineral density. Thus, GnRH agonists have been generally *limited to 6-month courses*. When therapy is to exceed 6 months (long-term) an "add back" regimen is advocated. Indeed, progestins, progestins and organic bisphosphonates, low-dose progestins and estrogens have all been demonstrated to have value for both vasomotor symptoms and to retard loss of bone mineral density. However, the safety and efficacy of long-term GnRH use has not been firmly established.

SURGICAL THERAPY

The *indications for surgery for endometriosis* are summarized in Table 28-3. Increasingly, endocrine therapy is being applied before and after surgery, but comprehensive studies of combined therapy

TABLE 28-3
INDICATIONS FOR SURGICAL THERAPY IN ENDOMETRIOSIS

Rupture of endometrioma (a surgical emergency)
Ureteral or bowel obstruction
Tuboovarian masses (>5 cm)
Endometriomas (>8 cm)
Severe, incapacitating symptoms
Pain worsening with medical therapy
Infertility for >1 year despite conventional therapy

remain to be reported. *Conservative surgery* is performed to retain and enhance the patient's reproductive capability. The *goals* are removal of all macroscopic endometriosis, division of adhesions (especially ovarian and tubal), preservation of reproductive function, and restoration of normal anatomy. All this may be accomplished by *laparoscopy* using the argon laser for photocoagulation and the Nd:YAG or CO_2 laser for vaporization of endometriotic foci. Although some controversy remains as to whether or not surgical excision or laser vaporization affords better long term outcomes. With conservative surgery, a D&C may be a wise addition to ascertain that no obstruction exists to menstrual outflow, as the latter may enhance retrograde bleeding, a predisposition of endometriosis.

At *laparotomy,* microsurgical techniques should be used (e.g., operative site magnification, minimal tissue trauma, fine polyglycolic suture, possibly corticosteroids, and prophylactic antibiotics). With laparotomy, it is good practice to do a round ligament uterine suspension to prevent the uterus and adnexa from adhering in the cul-de-sac. Elective appendectomy remains controversial because of the slightly enhanced risk of infection.

Pregnancy rates following conservative surgery are inversely related to the stage of the disease, (i.e., 75% with mild endometriosis, 50%–60% for moderate disease, and 30%–40% for severe disease). Recurrence necessitating further surgery occurs in >10% of patients within 3 years and in 35% of patients within 5 years. The *initial severity of endometriosis does not predict recurrence.* Pregnancy delays, but otherwise does not influence recurrence rates.

Indications for surgery to relieve pain are severe midline dysmenorrhea or dyspareunia or both. For the former, a presacral neurectomy is most often accomplished, whereas uterosacral ligament resection is the most common operation for treatment of the latter. These procedures often are performed through the laparoscope.

In patients who do not desire future reproduction or who have debilitating disease despite medical and conservative surgical therapy, *ablative surgery* may be the best alternative. In the younger woman (generally to the mid-30s), ovarian preservation with total abdominal hysterectomy may be indicated. Only 10% of patients thus treated will suffer progression of their endometriosis.

Definitive surgical therapy involves removal of all sites of *endometriosis, abdominal hysterectomy, bilateral salpingo-oophorectomy, lysis of adhesions, and appendectomy.* The last is recommended because of a 14%–30% finding of microscopic endometriosis in the appendix. It is prudent to place the patient who has had definitive surgical therapy on medroxyprogesterone or continuous oral contraceptive therapy for 1 year even though the risk of *recurrence after definitive surgical therapy is 3%.*

Endometriosis of the *bowel most commonly involves the appendix or rectosigmoid* and is usually only a small serosal involvement. Occasionally, large bowel cramping, lower abdominal pain, dyschezia, perimenstrual blood in the stool, palpation of a rectal shelf, or palpation of a pelvic mass may clinically signal more extensive involvement. Endocrine therapy is not effective in advanced cases. Surgical therapy must be individualized and may vary from superficial excision to bowel resection.

Most *urinary tract endometriosis* is an incidental finding of peritoneal involvement over the bladder and responds well to medical or surgical therapy. Ureteral obstruction, however, may occur without the usual symptoms (hematuria, flank pain) in one third of patients. The obstruction is nearly always in the *distal third of the ureter* and responds poorly to medical therapy. The usual surgical therapy is ureterolysis or ureteroneocystostomy.

PREVENTION

The only currently effective preventive measure for endometriosis is to *ensure adequate menstrual outflow.* Other suggestions remain unproven, including early marriage, early pregnancy, avoidance of partial salpingectomy, irrigation or isolation of operative sites, and annual pelvic examinations.

Hormonal replacement after definitive surgical therapy is not contraindicated.

ADENOMYOSIS

Adenomyosis is the presence of endometrial glands and stroma within the myometrium. It may be a diffuse process, with many areas demonstrating continuity between the endometrium and the glands and stroma within the myometrium, or the adenomyotic foci may be isolated in the myometrium. Expect hypertrophy of the smooth muscle adjacent to the ectopic endometrial glands and fibrosis. In large isolated areas of adenomyosis, the process resembles a leiomyoma and is termed *adenomyoma*. Adenomyosis regresses after menopause. It is a pathologic diagnosis of unknown etiology.

The usual *symptoms* of adenomyosis include hypermenorrhea (50%) and often severe acquired premenstrual and menstrual dysmenorrhea (30%). However, *30% of patients are asymptomatic*. Classically, physical examination reveals the uterine fundus to be diffusely enlarged. Occasionally, softened areas of adenomyosis may be noted just before or during early menstruation. The condition is *more likely to occur* in parous women >30, and it is uncommon in nulliparas. Adenomyosis is found in 20% of hysterectomy specimens, but the correct diagnosis is made preoperatively in less than one third of cases. MRI is useful in the detection of adenomyosis but is seldom used for this purpose. Adenomyosis frequently is complicated by chronic anemia (common), primary adenocarcinoma (rare), and endolymphatic stromal myosis (stromatosis) (also rare).

The *differential diagnosis* includes pregnancy, submucous leiomyoma (leiomyomas are associated in 50%–60% of cases of adenomyosis), pelvic endometriosis (complicates 15% of adenomyosis), pelvic congestion syndrome, idiopathic uterine hypertrophy, and endometrial cancer.

Treatment of adenomyosis is symptomatic if childbearing potential is retained. Hormone therapy is not beneficial. Occasionally, an isolated adenomyoma can be removed surgically, but the usual curative therapy is hysterectomy.

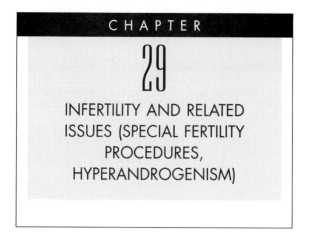

INFERTILITY AND RELATED
ISSUES (SPECIAL FERTILITY
PROCEDURES,
HYPERANDROGENISM)

INFERTILITY

Infertility is defined as the *failure to conceive after one year of attempting pregnancy. Primary infertility* denotes those patients who have never conceived. *Secondary infertility* applies to patients who have conceived previously. Approximately *15% of couples* experience infertility, which may result from subfertility or sterility (the innate inability to conceive) in either partner or both. The female is responsible in 40%–50% of cases. The male is responsible in 30% and is contributory in another 20%–30% of couples. However, it is crucial to recall that *multiple etiologies are found in 40% of infertile couples.*

The *incidence of infertility has increased* (perhaps 100% over the past 20 years) in developed countries because of increasing sexually transmitted disease (especially gonorrhea and *Chlamydia,* causing subsequent tubal damage), an increased number of sexual partners (increasing the potential for acquiring STDs), intentionally delaying pregnancy, the contraceptive(s) used, and smoking (>1 pack/day decreases the chance of pregnancy by >20%). Infertility accounts for 10%–20% of all gynecologic office visits.

Fertility rates are established using *fecundibility* (the chance of pregnancy per month of exposure). Only 25% of young healthy couples having frequent intercourse will conceive per month (60% by 6 months, 75% by 9 months, and 90% by 18 months). *Fecundibility declines with age*, and the effect is more pronounced in women than in men. By 36–37 years of age, the chance of pregnancy is less than half that at 25–27 years of age.

Careful evaluation should detect probable cause(s) for infertility in 85%–90%. Happily, even without therapy, 15%–20% of infertile couples may be expected to achieve pregnancy over time. Therapy, excluding in vitro fertilization, will result in pregnancy in 50%–60%.

ETIOLOGY

The *causes of infertility* may be classified as male-coital factors (40%), cervical (5%–10%), uterine-tubal (30%), ovulatory factors (15%–20%), and peritoneal or pelvic factors (40%). A few genetic causes (e.g., primary amenorrhea) are recognized.

MALE-COITAL FACTORS

Male factors include *abnormal spermatogenesis, abnormal motility, anatomic disorders, endocrine disorders, and sexual dysfunction.* The anatomic abnormalities possibly responsible are congenital absence of the vas deferens, obstruction of the vas deferens, and congenital abnormalities of the ejaculatory system.

Abnormal spermatogenesis may occur as the result of mumps orchitis, chromosomal abnormalities, cryptorchidism, chemical or radiation exposure, or varicocele. Abnormal motility is seen with absent cilia (Kartagener's syndrome), varicocele, and antibody formation.

The male factor endocrine disorders include thyroid disorders, adrenal hyperplasia, exogenous androgens, hypothalamic dysfunction (Kallmann's syndrome), pituitary failure (tumor, radiation, surgery), and hyperprolactinemia (tumor, drug-induced). An elevated FSH commonly indicates parenchymal testicular damage, since inhibin, produced by the Sertoli cells, is the primary feedback control of FSH secretion.

CERVICAL FACTORS

Cervical factors of female infertility may be *congenital* (DES exposure, mullerian duct abnormality) or *acquired* (infection, surgical treatment).

UTERINE-TUBAL FACTORS

Uterine-tubal factors are most *commonly structural abnormalities* (e.g., DES exposure, myoma, failure of normal fusion of the reproductive tract, infections, previous ectopic pregnancy).

OVULATORY FACTORS

Ovulatory factors involve *CNS function, metabolic disease, or peripheral defects*. CNS defects include chronic hyperandrogenemic anovulation, hyperprolactinemia (empty sella, tumor, or drug-induced), hypothalamic insufficiency (including Kallmann's syndrome), and pituitary insufficiency (trauma, tumor, or congenital). Metabolic diseases causing ovulatory factor defects are thyroid disease, liver disease, renal disease, obesity, and androgen excess (adrenal or neoplastic). Peripheral defects may be gonadal dysgenesis, premature ovarian failure, ovarian tumor, or ovarian resistance.

PERITONEAL OR PELVIC FACTORS

The two most common pelvic or peritoneal factors are *endometriosis and sequelae or infection* (e.g., appendicitis, pelvic inflammatory disease). Laparoscopy in women with unexplained infertility will reveal previously unsuspected pathology in at least 30% of patients. Endometriosis exerts a greater pejorative effect on fertility than can be explained on the basis of physical alterations (p. 755).

DIAGNOSIS

Infertility evaluations should follow a progression of testing and procedures that takes into account *probability* (including individualization for the couple), *invasiveness, risks, and expense*. The basic evaluation usually requires 6–8 weeks to complete. Even if the history suggests a probable cause of infertility, completion of the evaluation of all major factors should be accomplished to avoid overlooking a secondary or contributory factor.

The *initial assessment* should include medical history for female infertility factors, including pubertal development, present menstrual cycle characteristics, contraceptive history, prior pregnancy and outcome, previous surgery (especially pelvic), prior infection, abnormal Pap smears and therapy, drugs and therapy, diet, weight stability, exercise, and history of in utero DES exposure (now rare).

EVALUATION OF MALE FACTORS

The *initial test for male infertility is the semen analysis* because a normal semen analysis usually excludes a significant male factor (Table 29-1). The specimen should be obtained after 2–3 days abstinence and evaluated in the laboratory within 30–60 min of ejaculation.

TABLE 29-1
NORMAL SEMEN ANALYSIS VALUES

Parameter	Normal Value
Volume	2–5 ml
Viscosity	Full liquefication <60 min
Count	40–250 M/ml (previously, down to 20 M/ml)
Motility	1st h ≥60%; 2–3 h ≥50%
Normal morphology	>60%
Dead sperm	<35%
White blood cells	<10/hpf

The frequency of male factors (as well as risk and cost effectiveness) *mandates male diagnosis in the initial phase of infertility investigation.* The medical history for male factor infertility should include frequency of intercourse, difficulty with erection or ejaculation, prior paternity, past history of genital tract infections (e.g., mumps orchitis or chronic prostatitis), congenital anomalies, surgery or trauma (e.g., hernia repair, direct testicular trauma), exposure to toxins (medications, lead, cadmium, or radiation), diet, exercise, alcohol consumption, smoking >1 pack/d), illicit drug use, in utero exposure to DES, and unusual exposure to high environmental heat.

The *physical examination* should consider habitus and hair distribution (e.g., testosterone effect). The urethral meatus should be in the normal location. Testicular size may be compared to standard ovoids. Eliciting a Valsalva maneuver in the standing position should aid in the detection of a varicocele. Transrectal prostatic massage generally will produce sufficient secretions for microscopic examination. Excessive leukocytes in this or the semen analysis indicate infection.

If the semen analysis is abnormal or borderline, the man's medical history over the past 2–3 months should be reviewed, recalling that *spermogenesis requires 74 d.* A repeat semen analysis should be performed 1–2 weeks later for comparison. Consider referral to a urologist specializing in infertility if a significant abnormality persists.

Because sperm must reach the ovum before fertilization can occur, infertility in the presence of normal semen values suggests that there may be an abnormally high attrition of sperm. *Cervical mucus studies* may clarify this problem.

In vitro fertilization is the ultimate test for male factor infertility. *A sperm penetration test may be useful.* This uses a hamster egg to demonstrate the ability of the sperm to penetrate a zona-free oocyte using a known fertile donor as control. Abnormality is indicated by <10% penetration. Negative penetration of healthy appearing, mature ova by partner sperm with simultaneous positive penetration by donor sperm may provide the diagnosis.

EVALUATION OF CERVICAL FACTORS

Cervical factors are evaluated by *physical examination* and an appropriately *timed postcoital mucus test*. History of in utero DES exposure, abnormal Pap smears, cryotherapy, postcoital bleeding, or conization is suggestive of persistent cervical problems.

Normal cervical mucus in the preovulatory phase is thin, watery and acellular and dries in a *ferning pattern*. Mucus in this state acts as a facilitative reservoir for sperm. Cervical mucus is best evaluated on *days 12–14 of a 28 d cycle*. The amount and clarity of the mucus are recorded, and the pH should be ≥6.5. Spinnbarkeit (the stretchability of a strand of mucus) is ascertained by drawing out the mucus vertically (it should stretch to ≥6 cm).

The *Sims-Huhner test* evaluates the initial interaction of the sperm with cervical mucus. The test should be conducted in the periovular interval. Timing of the test may be *enhanced using vaginal ultrasound* to determine the presence or absence of a dominant follicle. Mucus is collected 2–4 h after intercourse. The mucus is placed on a clean glass slide under a coverslip and observed.

There should be *>20 sperm/hpf*, and large numbers of active sperm will be seen in the thin, acellular mucus. Lower numbers (<20/hpf) of motile sperm in favorable mucus may be present in normally fertile couples due to the stress of coitus at a prescribed time. The *absence of sperm suggests aspermia or improper coital technique or specimen collection*. Finding an adequate number of *immobile sperm* in favorable mucus requires an investigation for autoantibodies in the male or serum antibodies in the female. If a sufficient number of sperm are present but *poorly motile*, further assessment of the mucus and timing of the test is indicated. If the mucus tests are repeatedly abnormal despite apparently favorable mucus, a crosscheck using donor mucus and donor sperm is reasonable. *Antibody studies* may determine the antigenic site (sperm head, midpiece, or tail) and are more likely to be positive in men who have a history of trauma, infection, or previous surgery.

DIAGNOSIS OF UTERINE-TUBAL FACTORS

Both history and careful pelvic examination are essential initial steps in detection of uterine-tubal factors. *Key details of the history* include menstrual problems, pelvic infections (pelvic pain), STD, appendicitis, and abdominal trauma or surgery. *Suggestive findings on pelvic examination* include uterine irregularities, pelvic masses, and uterine deviation or fixation.

It is uncommon for submucous myomata, endometrial polyps, or bicornuate uterus to cause infertility, although each of these is associated with an enhanced rate of abortion. *Tubal fimbrial occlusion is the most common* of the three usual locations, followed by midsegment and isthmus-cornual occlusion. Midsegment occlusion is nearly always due to tubal sterilization but may be secondary to tuberculosis. The major causes of *isthmic-cornual occlusions* are infection, maldevelopment, endometriosis, adenomyosis, or salpingitis isthmica nodosum.

Hysterosalpingography (HSG) (Fig. 29-1), hysteroscopy, laparoscopy, or a combination of these is required to determine *patency of the tubes*. HSG is performed as an outpatient procedure using a radiopaque dye (first water-soluble and, after patency is assured, an oil-based contrast medium) instilled into the uterine cavity via a small transcervical catheter. Radiographs should document

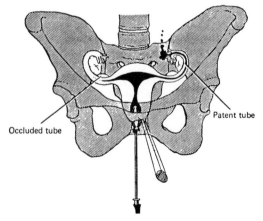

Patent tube

Occluded tube

FIGURE 29-1. Hysterosalpingography.

the fluoroscopically observed findings. Uterine contour, tubal patency, and ability of the dye to freely transit the tubes to enter the pelvis are evaluated. The oil-based dye provides a better image but has a greater risk of retention and granuloma formation. The water-based dye causes less cramping and allows better definition of the rugae. *Abnormal findings* include intrauterine synechiae (Asherman's syndrome), congenital malformations of the uterus, polyps, submucous leiomyomas, proximal or distal tubal occlusion, and salpingitis isthmica nodosa.

The *major risk of HSG is infection.* Thus, HSG should not be performed during even suspected active inflammation or when there is an adnexal mass. Broad-spectrum antibiotic therapy (e.g., doxycyline) may be prudent if recent STD screening has not been performed. The test is also *contraindicated* if there is allergy to the dye.

Laparoscopy may demonstrate tubal abnormalities (e.g., agglutinated fimbria, endometriosis) that probably would not be seen on HSG. *Hysteroscopy performed concomitantly with laparoscopy* may give further information regarding uterine contour or polyps. Endometriosis (Chapter 28) is an important cause of infertility and is suggested by a history of worsening dysmenorrhea or dyspareunia but usually cannot be diagnosed short of visual inspection. Some endometriosis may be eliminated during laparoscopic diagnosis if informed consent has been obtained and preparations have been made for laser surgery or operative pelviscopy.

Laparoscopy may be indicated relatively early in the investigation of infertility if pelvic factors are suggestive or in older patients, whereas it may be the last test performed in a young woman when all other studies are negative. It may be considered together with ovarian stimulation and ovum collection in longstanding infertility using in vitro fertilization or by placing sperm and ovum directly into the tube to allow a trial of normal transport to the uterus.

EVALUATION OF OVULATORY FACTORS

Ovulating women usually have regular cycles (22–35 d). Substantiating symptoms may be useful, especially premenstrual (breast changes, bloating, and mood change). The physical examination and proper timing, coupled with cervical mucus evaluation, may determine ovulation. Some affirmation of ovulation may be obtained by basal body temperatures (BBTs, see Fig. 26-1) and endometrial biopsy. Currently, measurements of the midluteal serum progesterone (attempting to detect the surge), as well as serial

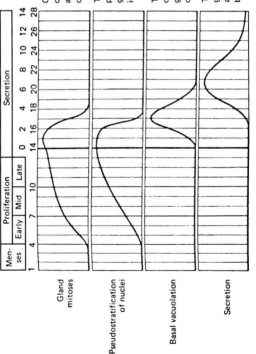

Gland mitoses indicate proliferation. They occur during menstruation because repair and breakdown are progressing simultaneously at that time.

This is characteristic of the proliferative phase but persists until active secretion begins. It is not resumed until the glands have involuted during menstruation.

This is the earliest morphologic evidence of ovulation found in the endometrium. It begins approximately 36–48 hours following ovulation.

This curve represents visible secretion in the gland lumen; active secretion falls off more abruptly. In the later stages, the secretion becomes inspissated.

FIGURE 29-2. Dating the endometrium. Approximate relationship of useful morphologic factors. (Modified after J.P.A. Latour. From Noyes, Hertig, and Rock, Dating the endometrial biopsy. *Fertil Steril* 1:3, 1950.)

Men-	Proliferation			Secretion											
ses	Early	Mid	Late												

Stromal edema — This factor varies with the individual—particularly the rise during proliferation, which may be almost absent. The edema that accompanies secretion is more constant.

Pseudodecidual reaction — This is evident first around the arterioles and progresses until just before menstruation, when a superficial compact layer is formed.

Stromal mitoses — These are most abundant during the proliferative phase, absent during active secretion, and reappear during the stage of predecidual formation.

Leukocytic infiltration — Throughout the cycle there are always a few lymphocytes. Polymorphonuclear infiltration begins about 2 days before the onset of flow.

FIGURE 29-2. (*Continued*)

777

gonadatropin (FSH and LH) evaluations are more commonly used to evaluate ovulation.

BBT is taken on awakening before any other activity. After ovulation, a temperature elevation of 0.4°F occurs due to the thermogenic effect of progesterone. Progesterone levels as low as 5 ng/mL may indicate ovulation, but midluteal levels usually are >10 ng/mL.

Irregular menses, absence of premenstrual molimina, continued ferning of dried cervical mucus, low midluteal progesterone levels, and absence of midcycle BBT elevation all indicate *probable failure of ovulation*. Treatment of ovulation failure is discussed under therapy. Abnormal BBTs, spontaneous abortion(s), endometriosis, and poor cervical mucus may indicate a *luteal phase defect*. Confirmation of this diagnosis is accomplished by endometrial histologic study, including dating of endometrial biopsies (best taken from the superior, anterior uterine fundus) in relation to menses. Dating of the endometrium is accomplished by the criteria illustrated in Figure 29-2. Should the histologic date of the biopsy lag by more than 2 d in two cycles, this diagnosis is confirmed.

An additional ovulatory abnormality is the *luteinized unruptured follicle (LUF) syndrome*. In LUF, the oocyte is trapped or not released from the follicle (as determined by laparoscopy) despite indirect signs of ovulation.

When investigating endrocrine associations of infertility, determination of diabetic status as well as any androgen abnormalities will reveal a significant number of patients with these causes of reproductive dysfunction.

EVALUATION OF PERITONEAL AND PELVIC FACTORS

In women with unexplained infertility, *laparoscopy can identify previously unsuspected pathology in 30%–50% of patients*. The most common condition diagnosed is endometriosis. Other conditions (e.g., unexpected adhesions) also may be encountered.

TREATMENT

MALE AND COITAL FACTORS

Smoking, alcohol, and drug use should be stopped. Eliminate sources of increased scrotal temperature (e.g., saunas, hot tubs, or jockey shorts underwear) with their adverse effect on spermatogenesis. *Lubricants and douching should be eliminated.* The woman should *lie on her back for at least 15 min following coitus* (to facilitate semen retention and progression). Infrequent or poorly timed intercourse is a common cause of infertility. Hence, *coitus every 2 d during the periovulatory interval* (e.g., days 12–16 of a 28 d cycle) should be advised.

Azoospermia because of chromosomal abnormalities, congenital abnormalities (other than congenital absence of the vas deferens), and elevated FSH *cannot be reversed*. Therefore, artificial insemination with donor sperm or adoption are the only alternatives. There have been occasional reports of successful pregnancy in congenital absence of the vas deferens by using sperm aspirated from the epididymis and in vitro fertilization. *Hypothalamic or pituitary hormone insufficiency*-induced azoospermia may be treated by *replacement hormone therapy*, with varying results. Successful reversal of azoospermia secondary to vasectomy by performance of a *vasovasostomy* is influenced by the duration of occlusion and whether or not autoantibodies have formed. Patency can be achieved in 75%–90%, with resultant pregnancy rates of 33%–70%.

Varicoceles are present in approximately one third of men evaluated for infertility, and varicocelectomy has been shown to improve sperm parameters in up to two thirds. However, postoperative pregnancy rates in controlled studies reveal no statistical difference between the treated and untreated.

Low semen volume is a problem notoriously difficult to treat. This is usually treated by artificial insemination with the man's semen *(AIH)*. Here, 0.1 mL of liquefied semen is placed in the endocervical canal and the rest in a cervical cup. When *high semen volume is accompanied by low sperm count, a split ejaculate technique* may be useful. In this technique, the first portion of the ejaculate, which has a much higher sperm count, is collected and used for AIH. If necessary, several first ejaculates may be pooled and saved by freezing, to be used later for AIH.

Oligospermia (low sperm count) or *asthenospermia* (low sperm motility) if *due to an endocrinopathy* may respond to specific hormonal therapy (e.g., human menopausal gonadotropin—hMG)—for hypothalamic–pituitary failure, bromocriptine for hyperprolactinemia, or thyroid replacement for hypothyroidism). In idiopathic oligoasthenospermia, *clomiphene* (not FDA approved for this purpose) may be useful. When specimen quality cannot be improved by other means, the semen may be *washed and the sperm concentrated into a smaller volume by slow centrifugation.* The resultant semen then is only used for intrauterine insemination accurately timed by daily LH levels or ovulatory stimulation.

If sperm autoantibodies are present, suppression of the immune response by *steroids* may be initiated. However, in vitro fertilization may be necessary in some of these cases to achieve pregnancy.

Intrauterine insemination with washed semen (to eliminate prostaglandins) has been shown to be effective in cases where the sperm parameters are normal and the postcoital examinations are abnormal. This is not true in the reverse instance. If postcoital tests are normal but the sperm characteristics are not, intrauterine insemination of the abnormal sperm offers little benefit.

In vitro fertilization and gamete intrafallopian transfer (GIFT) offer therapy most likely to be successful in male factor infertility with abnormal sperm factors. Both are invasive and expensive procedures. Moreover, several attempts may be necessary to achieve pregnancy (reported pregnancy rate per cycle is 15%–20%).

CERVICAL FACTORS

If the *cervix is abnormal* as a result of treatment (e.g., coagulation, cryotherapy) or congenital malformation, intrauterine insemination with washed sperm over three cycles should achieve pregnancy in 30%–40%. If *cervical mucus is not adequate at midcycle*, low-dose estrogen administered during the mid- to late follicular phase of the cycle may be effective. Human menopausal gonadotropins may be necessary to improve the cervical mucus when low-dose estrogen is ineffective. Nonetheless, close monitoring is recommended to avoid multiple gestation or hyperstimulation syndrome. If these are ineffective, intrauterine insemination may be performed. When the cervical mucus is *altered by inflammation or infection*, empiric tetracycline therapy (doxycycline 100 mg bid for both partners) is advocated.

UTERINE-TUBAL FACTORS

Microsurgical tuboplasty is 60%–80% effective in achieving pregnancy with tubal occlusion. However, correction of isthmic occlusions and neosalpingostomy are significantly less successful. *Ectopic gestation occurs in 10% of conceptions after surgical tubal repair.* Fibroids significantly distorting the endometrial cavity or submucous myomas may warrant removal in the treatment of infertility. Periadnexal adhesions may be lysed by operative laparoscopy.

OVULATORY FACTORS

When anovulation is the etiology of female factor infertility, successful *induction of ovulation will result in pregnancy <1 y in 80%.* If pregnancy does not occur despite documented ovulation, other factors must be investigated. *Ovulation can be induced in 90%–95%*

of anovulatory patients, except those with an elevated FSH. An elevated FSH is pathognomonic of ovarian failure or ovarian resistance, and no further testing is warranted. The only hope for pregnancy is embryo or ovum donation. A *pregnancy rate of up to 20% per transfer is likely,* but the ethical, psychologic, and legal issues of this procedure must be considered.

The initial drug used to induce ovulation is *clomiphene citrate.* Of anovulatory women whose ovaries are producing estrogen, 70% will ovulate with this drug. Ideally, it is given for 5 d in the early follicular phase because it acts as an antiestrogen. Ultrasound and hormonal testing may be required to evaluate patient response. Dosage or timing adjustment or additional hormone therapy (e.g., steroids, estrogen, or midcycle hCG) may be necessary to achieve success.

Stimulation with *human menopausal gonadotropins* (hMG) generally is reserved for those who do not respond to clomiphene, those who respond but no pregnancy results, in cases of hypothalamic insufficiency, or in unexplained infertility. Monitoring of estrogen levels and ultrasonic determination of the number of follicles stimulated as well as the degree of maturity of ova are requisites. Most often, administration of hCG is necessary to trigger ovulation. Although *ovulation can be achieved in 85%–90%* using hMG, the risk of *multiple births is 20%.*

If investigation reveals an *elevated prolactin level,* a TSH determination is necessary to rule out hypothyroidism. If present, hypothyroidism should be treated. Many drugs can elevate prolactin levels, and these should be terminated. After pituitary adenoma and hypothyroidism have been eliminated in the etiology of elevated prolactin, bromocriptine therapy may be initiated and continued until pregnancy is confirmed. Despite its use in early pregnancy, there is no documented increase in the incidence of malformation or spontaneous abortion over that seen in the general population.

If the infertility is secondary to an *inadequate luteal phase,* clomiphene may be used successfully in the early follicular phase to recruit additional follicles (thus enhancing progesterone levels in the luteal phase). Other methods of therapy to be considered for an inadequate luteal phase are progesterone supplementation during the luteal phase and hCG injections.

PERITONEAL AND PELVIC FACTORS

Endometriosis and the residual of salpingitis are two of the most common causes of infertility. If medication or conservative surgery is ineffective in treating endometriosis or adhesive problems (regardless of cause), IVF or GIFT may be offered.

COMBINED FACTORS

When combined factors are documented, therapy can be performed sequentially or simultaneously depending on individual circumstances.

UNEXPLAINED INFERTILITY

When no etiology for infertility can be found, no specific therapy is likely to be successful. *Even without therapy, the couple can be given the statistical chance of pregnancy of 60% within 3–5 years.* If age is a factor or infertility has been long-standing, advanced reproductive technologies warrant discussion with the involved couple. The option of giving hMG (Pergonal) combined with timed inseminations offers some hope short of IVF. If the former is unsuccessful, IVF should be offered.

PSYCHOLOGIC ASPECTS OF INFERTILITY

Infertile couples need *considerable psychologic support*. Infertility may engender feelings of inadequacy, loss of self-image, or fears regarding their own sexuality. This is particularly true of the one found to be infertile. Anger, accusations, or depression may predominate as frustration and disappointment recur on a monthly basis when pregnancy is not achieved. Some may become so obsessed with basal body temperatures, timed intercourse, and other aspects of therapy that the couple's interpersonal relationship suffers. An additional burden or stress may be the expense of investigation and therapy. Many insurance carriers pay little or nothing toward the expense involved.

Infertility can engender the progression through all of the phases of the *grief reaction:* denial, anger, bargaining, depression, and acceptance. Many couples become willing to try any technique that they may read or hear about, especially from well-meaning friends or relatives. Support groups may be of help—the national organization RESOLVE can provide informal support and referral for professional counseling.

Emphasize the fact that unlike many disorders (e.g., appendicitis), infertility can rarely be reversed overnight and that the couple should accept a process that may take months rather than days or weeks to diagnose and treat. Pregnancy usually occurs in 6–9 cycles if a true cause can be found. A time limit must be set for the expected resolution of the problem to avoid endless procedures or regimens delaying acceptance of failure and initiation of alternatives (e.g., acceptance of childlessness or adoption).

ASSISTED REPRODUCTIVE
TECHNOLOGY (ART)

IN VITRO FERTILIZATION

In vitro fertilization-embryo transfer (IVF-ET) is the technique of removing the ovum (egg) from the ovary, fertilizing it in the laboratory, then placing the resulting embryo into the uterus. Since the first IVF-ET success in 1978, it has become invaluable in the treatment of otherwise untreatable infertility. Success in achieving pregnancy after ovum retrieval is *15%–20% per cycle*, and 70%–80% of those carry the pregnancy to term. The usual indications for IVF-ET are bilateral tubal abnormality (e.g., postsalpingectomy, post severe salpingitis), antisperm antibodies, extensive endometriosis, oligospermia, and long-standing unexplained infertility.

TECHNIQUE

Superovulation
Several methods may be used, including (alone or in combination) luprolide acetate, clomiphene citrate, hMG, hFSH, and GnRH.

Ultrasound Scans
Determining the number and growth of ovarian follicles is necessary, since at least 2–3 follicles should be developing simultaneously to enhance the possibility of successful ovum retrieval.

Hormonal Monitoring
Serum *estradiol* levels are useful in predicting which cycle is most likely to result in pregnancy. *LH levels* are closely followed because an unexpected LH peak may result in ovulation before a scheduled ovum aspiration.

Ova Retrieval
Ova are aspirated *24–36 h after injection of hCG or the onset of a spontaneous LH surge*. Aspiration may be accomplished via laparoscopy or under indirect visualization using ultrasound and a percutaneous-transvesical or transvaginal approach. The advantage of the ultrasonographic technique is that this program may be outpatient oriented and there is no need for anesthesia. After the ovary is identified, each preovulatory follicle is punctured, and the contents are aspirated. The aspirate is immediately transferred to the laboratory.

Ova Identification and Classification

The ova are *identified microscopically and classified as mature* (expanded cumulus oophorus) *or immature* (compact cumulus). Mature ova have undergone the first meiotic division and are fertilized 5 h after aspiration. Immature ova may be incubated for up to 36 h before fertilization.

Sperm Capacitation

Because freshly ejaculated sperm cannot fertilize an ovum, the *sperm must be capacitated* by a short incubation in culture medium.

Fertilization

With each ovum are mixed 10,000–50,000 motile sperm, and incubation is initiated.

Incubation

An atmosphere of 5%–20% O_2 and 5% CO_2 and culture medium supplemented by maternal serum or human cord serum are used for incubation. During incubation, the preparation is examined for the presence of *pronuclei* (fertilization has occurred) *or blastomeres* (cleavage has occurred).

Embryo Transfer

The fertilized ova are *placed in the uterus after 48–72 h* incubation, usually at the 2-cell to 8-cell stage, although more recently many are awaiting blastocyst stage for embryo transfer. This is accomplished by aspiration of the ova into a small catheter, which is then passed transcervically. The ova are injected into the uterine cavity to complete the process.

Potential complications of the procedure are those associated with anesthesia and laparoscopy and those of any pregnancy. For example, *ectopic pregnancy* may occur. Because of the increased risk of *multiple gestation* with subsequent fetal wastage, most centers implant only three to four embryos a cycle. If there are excess fertilized ova, the options include freezing (for later use or donation to another infertility patient), discarding them (unwise), or experimentation (controversial).

OVUM TRANSFER

Ovum transfer is removal of an ovum from a fertile woman after insemination (usually by an infertile woman's husband) at the time of ovulation (LH peak). The ovum donor and the recipient must ovulate within 2 days of each other. Three to 4 days after insemination, the uterus of the donor is lavaged to attempt ovum retrieval (hopefully fertilized). Because the process is patented, the technique may be performed only in clinics licensed to do so. The major complication is failure to lavage a fertilized ovum from the donor, resulting in undesired pregnancy.

GAMETE AND ZYGOTE INTRAFALLOPIAN TUBE TRANSFER (GIFT, ZIFT)

Both GIFT and ZIFT are used only in patients with patent uterine tubes. GIFT is usually accomplished with superovulation. The ova are collected, ova and sperm are mixed, and then immediately placed into the uterine tube, where natural fertilization can occur. In ZIFT the process is similar to IVF-ET, except the zygote is transferred into the fallopian tube as opposed to the uterus.

OUTCOMES OF ASSISTED REPRODUCTIVE TECHNOLOGY

Annually, the United States Assisted Reproductive Technology results are reported from the American Society for Reproductive Medicine and the Society for Assisted Reproductive Technology's Registry in the journal *Fertility and Sterility*. The interested reader is referred to this source for timely information. *Recent trends* indicate: an increasing number of programs reporting assisted reproductive technology treatment, an increase in reported cycles, and increasing overall success rates (as measured by deliveries per retrieval). In 1996 (at the time of writing the latest data available), 300 assisted reproductive technology programs (likely all of the U.S. centers) contributed data to the registry, revealing the following:

- 65,863 total assisted reproductive technology cycles (average of 219.5 cycles per program) were performed.
- 44,647 cycles were IVF (with and without micromanipulation—ICSI) with 26.0% deliveries per retrieval.
- 2879 cycles of gamete intrafallopian transfer (GIFT) resulted in 29.0% deliveries per retrieval.
- 1200 cycles of zygote intrafallopian transfer (ZIFT) were performed with 30.9% deliveries per retrieval.
- 9610 frozen embryo transfers (FET) resulted in 16.8% deliveries per transfer.
- 3768 donor oocyte cycles had an overall success of 39.1% deliveries per transfer.
- 1076 cryopreserved embryo transfers from donated oocytes resulted in 20.8% deliveries per transfer.

- 688 assisted reproductive technology cycles using a host uterus resulted in 31.3% deliveries per embryo transfer.
- 1341 cycles were reported as combinations of more than one treatment type.
- Overall 14,702 deliveries were reported resulting in 21,196 neonates.

These pooled data do not define variation in the patient characteristics known to affect prognosis, including (but not limited to): maternal age, the duration of infertility, the presumed cause(s) of infertility, the patient's prior history of treatment of infertility, and diethylstilbestrol exposure. As such, the pooled data should be used with caution in counseling individual patients for their characteristics may alter prognosis more than the particular assisted reproductive technology employed.

The complex process of assisted reproductive technology is costly, involving: history, physical examination, endocrine testing with rapid turn around times, ultrasonic monitoring of follicle ripening, surgical fees, gamete and embryo laboratory fees, anesthesia, facility use fees, and medications. The expenses vary per condition and per technique as well as not being comparably reported. Therefore, only a gross estimate of cost per cycle is possible, probably being between $7,000–12,000. Infertility diagnostic and therapeutic techniques are generally not covered by traditional payers; therefore, most patients usually pay directly. Undoubtedly this decreases utilization by those without sufficient economic resources. Thus, it is difficult to assess utilization strictly on a population base. In countries where there is payer coverage for infertility (e.g., Denmark), IVF has been utilized up to 6500 cycles per 1 million women in the reproductive age.

HYPERANDROGENISM

The primary androgen produced by the ovaries is androstenedione, and the primary androgen from adrenal glands is dehydroepiandrostene sulfate (DHEAS). Androgen production in the ovary is stimulated by pituitary LH and in the adrenal is stimulated by pituitary ACTH. Most androgens are bound to specific proteins in the circulation and, while bound, are largely biologically inactive. On reaching the target tissue, androgens are further metabolized, often regaining biologic activity. For example, testosterone is 99% bound while in the circulation but, on reaching the skin, is converted to dihydrotestosterone (by 5 α-reductase), an even more potent androgen than testosterone. The sebaceous glands are very sensitive to androgens, and oily skin and acne are early signs of hyperandrogenism. The hair follicle is moderately responsive to androgens, and hirsutism is a further response to increasing androgenicity. Finally, with marked androgenicity, signs of masculinization appear in the woman (virilization). These include temporal balding, deepening of the voice, breast atrophy, increased muscle mass with loss of female body contour, male type pubic hair pattern, and cliteromegaly.

The total testosterone produced by a mature female is 0.35 mg/day. Ovarian secretion accounts for 0.1 mg, 0.2 mg comes from peripheral conversion of androstenedione, and 0.05 mg is from peripheral conversion of DHEAS. The ovary and adrenal gland secrete about equal amounts of androstenedione and DHEA. Thus, about two thirds of a woman's daily testosterone comes from the ovaries. Therefore, increased levels of testosterone suggest an ovarian origin. Hyperandrogenism may be associated with several disorders.

POLYCYSTIC OVARIES
(PCO, POLYCYSTIC SYNDROME [PCOS], STEIN-LEVINTHAL SYNDROME)

Polycystic ovaries are the most common cause of female hyperandrogenism. The etiology of PCO is unknown, but heredity, central catecholamine abnormalities, obesity, and stress are associated factors. The most common symptom is *infertility*, which occurs in 75% of patients. Other manifestations of PCO include *hirsutism* (70%), *menstrual irregularities* (amenorrhea 50%, functional bleeding 30%, and dysmenorrhea 25%), *obesity* (40%), *insulin resistance, and virilization* (20%). Only 15% of those with PCO will have biphasic body temperature, and even less will have cyclic menses. A feature of PCO is enlarged ovaries (often 5 cm) that have a smooth, white, thickened pseudocapsule, immediately beneath which are numerous follicular cysts surrounded by hyperplastic luteinized theca interna cells.

PCO is marked by *increased gonadotropin-releasing hormone* (GnRH) pulse frequency and tonically elevated levels of LH (generally >20 mIU/mL). Estradiol not bound to sex hormone-binding globulin (SHBG) is increased (total estradiol is not) because of a decreased SHBG (due to increased androgen levels and obesity), which stimulates GnRH pulsatility. This results in *androgen excess* (from both ovaries and adrenals) and anovulation. However, the *hyperandrogenism is mild* (if elevated, testosterone 70–120 ng/dL and androstenedione 3–5 ng/dL); about *one half have elevated DHEAS* levels.

Because the FSH levels are usually low, *an LH/FSH ratio >3 may be useful in diagnosis of PCO* (when LH is >8 mIU/dL).

TABLE 29-2
PROBABLE INTERRELATIONSHIPS IN PCOS[a]

Hypothalamus	Pituitary	Ovaries/ Adrenals	Circulation	Result
GnRH pulsatility	↑LH	↓E$_2$ ↑T	↓ Unbound E$_2$ ↓ SHBG	Excess androgen Anovulation LH/FSH ratio >2–3
		↑A$_2$	↑Unbound T + A$_2$	

[a]GnRH, gonadotropin-releasing hormone; LH, luteinizing hormone; FSH, follicle-stimulating hormone; E$_2$, estradiol; T, testosterone; A$_2$, androstenediol; SHBG, sex hormone-binding globulin.

Ovaries of PCO patients do not produce more estradiol from androstenedione (in fact, because of less FSH, the ovaries have lower aromatase levels). The increased circulating androstenedione is peripherally converted to estrone, resulting in elevated estrone levels. The important interrelationships in PCO are graphically demonstrated in Table 29-2.

Mild hyperprolactinemia is found in 20% of women with PCO.

Transvaginal sonography is of increasing importance in women with PCO to detect the characteristic ovarian image as well as to measure the endometrial thickness (a gross measure of hyperplasia). Prior to therapy, endometrial sampling is nearly always indicated to rule out endometrial hyperplasia and endometrial carcinoma.

Therapeutic goals in women with PCO must be highly individualized and may include: pregnancy, control of hirsutism, and prevention of endometrial hyperplasia (from unopposed estrogen). Patients should be made aware that therapy for this condition is long-term and that although short-term treatment may achieve a desired goal, the underlying condition persists, placing them at risk.

When the PCO patient is *anovulatory, not hirsute, and does not desire pregnancy*, therapy with intermittent progestin or oral contraceptive agents (if not contraindicated) is recommended to prevent the risk of endometrial hyperplasia and carcinoma. When the PCO patient is *mildly hirsuite and does not desire pregnancy*, oral contraceptives will: arrest the hirsuitism, lower gonadatropin levels, and decrease the risk of endometrial hyperplasia. Continuous progestin therapy is a less attractive alternative because of the side effects (mastodynia, bloating, depression). For greater amounts of hirsutism there are no effective pharmacological agents; thus, physical adjuncts (bleaching, electrolysis, depilation, etc.) are usually recommended. If *pregnancy is desired,* medical therapy is the therapeutic choice. Clomiphene citrate is the ovulatory agent customarily used first and should achieve ovulation in ~75% and pregnancy in 35%–40%. Other ovulation methods used (largely if clomiphene citrate fails) include: hMG-hCG, purified human FSH and hCG, and pulsatile GnRH. Ovarian wedge resection was commonly used in the past, but today is indicated when: all other therapies fail, there is a question of ovarian tumor (ovarian size or high androgen levels), and fertility is not an issue.

STROMAL HYPERTHECOSIS

The *peak age of women with stromal hyperthecosis is 50–70 years,* in keeping with the gradual onset of this uncommon disorder. Like

PCO, stromal hyperplasia is associated with enlarged ovaries (5–7 cm in diameter). Stromal hyperthecosis is usually bilateral and is characterized by stromal proliferation with foci of luteinization. There are no subcapsular cysts like those found in PCO. The theca cells produce gradual but ever increasing amounts of androstenedione, leading to elevated testosterone (usually >2 ng/dL). Again, in contrast to PCO, stromal hyperthecosis patients tend to have advancing virilization over a course of years.

ANDROGEN-PRODUCING OVARIAN NEOPLASMS

Neoplastic androgen-secreting ovarian disorders typically have a *rapid onset of hirsutism, amenorrhea, and virilization.* These neoplasms are usually *unilateral and palpable* on *pelvic examination.* Testosterone is the most commonly secreted androgen (usually >200 ng/dL) in these disorders. The most common of the tumors causing hyperandrogenism are the *Sertoli-Leydig cell* and *hilus cell tumors.* The neoplasms produce testosterone and almost always lead to virilization. The less common ovarian neoplasms leading to hyperandrogenism include *lipoid cell* (adrenal rest) *tumors* (produce testosterone or DHEAS or both), *granulosa-theca cell* tumors (can produce testosterone in addition to increased estradiol), *Brenner tumors,* and *Krukenberg tumors* (unusual, rarely produce testosterone). Also to be considered are *ovarian tumors,* whether benign or malignant, primary or metastatic in origin. They do not secrete androgens but stimulate the ovarian stroma to do so.

Sertoli-Leydig cell tumors are uncommon (<1% of solid ovarian tumors). They are most often diagnosed in menstruating women (20–40 years) and are associated with hirsutism, virilization, and a palpable ovarian mass (85%). *Hilar (Leydig) cell tumors* are most frequent after the menopause. They are not usually palpable but cause rapid development of virilization. Testosterone levels are high, but DHEAS levels are normal. *Gonadoblastomas* are a very rare cause of hyperandrogenism, most often occurring in phenotypic females with gonadal dysgenesis and a Y chromosome.

Hyperandrogenism during pregnancy may be caused by a luteoma of pregnancy or by hyperreactio luteinalis. Hyperreactio leuteinalis is defined as bilateral cystic ovarian enlargement. The ovaries may be 20–30 cm in diameter and consist of innumerable thin-walled cysts. These give the mass a bluish to gray ovarian color and a honeycombed appearance. The cysts are lined by luteinized thecal lutein cells from the ovarian connective tissue.

A luteoma of pregnancy is a unilateral or occasionally bilateral (30%) benign solid ovarian tumor (50%) caused by a hyperplastic reaction of ovarian theca lutein cells. They are discrete and brown to reddish brown and may have a cystic component. Luteomas are more common in black multiparas.

Both luteoma and hyperreactio luteinalis are benign and hCG-dependent. They regress after pregnancy and should not be removed unless other problems intervene (e.g., torsion). The majority of cases are asymptomatic and are found incidentally. Should symptoms occur, they are usually nonspecific (i.e., a sense of pressure, ascites, or increasing abdominal girth). Although the majority are not hyperandrogenic, some produce high levels of testosterone and androstenedione. Thus, the mother is virilized in 30%, and a female fetus is at risk of virilization.

HYPERANDROGENISM OF ADRENAL ORIGIN

Excess androgens from the adrenal glands *may be the result of* neoplasia, inborn errors of biosynthesis of adrenal hormones, or inappropriate stimulation of the adrenal gland. Adrenal neoplasias typically produce DHEA with blood levels >7000 ng/mL. On rare occasions, testosterone will be secreted (blood levels >200 ng/mL). Androgens are intermediates in the biosynthetic pathway for cortisol. Consequently, a disorder that causes an increase in cortisol production (e.g., Cushing's syndrome) may concomitantly increase androgen levels.

CUSHING'S SYNDROME

Cushing's syndrome may have three etiologies: adrenal tumors, ectopic production of adrenocorticotropic hormone (ACTH) by a non-pituitary tumor, or excess production of ACTH by the pituitary (Cushing's disease). All result in *excessive production of glucocorticoids*. The *classic findings* include centripetal obesity, dorsal neck fat pads, abdominal striae, muscle wasting, weakness, hirsutism, and menstrual irregularity. Cushing's syndrome is diagnosed by the *dexamethasone suppression test*. The test involves administering dexamethasone 1 mg PO at 11 PM followed by an 8 AM blood cortisol (normal is <5 nanog/mL).

Androgen-producing adrenal tumors are usually adenomas or carcinomas. Characteristically, symptoms have a rapid onset. The tumors produce DHEA, DHEAS (>8 μ/mL), and androstenedione. CT or MRI scan of the adrenals facilitates diagnosis.

CONGENITAL ADRENAL HYPERPLASIA (CAH)

CAH results from *enzymatic deficiencies (21-hydroxylase or 11B-hydroxylase) inherited as autosomal recessive traits*. The 21-hydroxylase deficiency is the most common form. Because both conditions result in diminished cortisol biosynthesis, ACTH is increased. ACTH leads to enhanced intermediate compounds before the enzymatic defect. Thus, elevations of 17-hydroxypregnenolone and 17-hydroxyprogesterone (17-OHP) occur and are subsequently converted to DHEA and androstenedione. The latter compounds are in turn peripherally converted into testosterone. Female infants with this disorder are often diagnosed shortly after birth due to ambiguous genitalia. CAH is the most common cause of ambiguous genitalia in the newborn.

Milder deficiencies also occur and may not be diagnosed until puberty or later. *CAH may account for 5% of women with hirsutism*. Characteristically, these women have a history of prepubertal accelerated growth but overall reveal short ultimate height and postpubertal hirsutism. They may exhibit mild virilization and DHEAS levels >5 mg/mL. Measurement of 17-OHP >8 ng/mL facilitates diagnosis. However, when 17-OHP is 3–8 ng/mL, an ACTH stimulation test may be diagnostic.

DIAGNOSIS

A complete medical history is essential. This must include the menstrual and family history. Onset of symptoms should be noted as well as drug ingestion, whether current or in the recent past. Use of body building programs and food supplements should not be overlooked. Physical examination should include vital signs, body habitus, hair pattern, and presence or absence of skin and fat changes consistent with Cushing's syndrome, as well as signs of virilization in addition to hirsutism. The pelvic examination should consider ovarian size or masses.

Initial laboratory testing should include serum testosterone and DHEAS levels. Serum testosterone <200 ng/mL rules out testosterone-secreting neoplasms, whereas serum DHEAS <7000 ng/mL eliminates significant adrenal pathology. A testosterone level >200 ng/mL is indicative of ovarian tumor until proven otherwise (i.e., study of the adrenals is essential only if no ovarian mass is present). If the patient is anovulatory or oligoovulatory, FSH, LH, and prolactin levels may be helpful. Elevated LH levels (especially LH/FSH ratio >3) suggest PCO. Prolactinoma may cause elevated prolactin levels.

Screening for hypercortisolemia requires a 24-h urine for urinary-free cortisol or 17-hydroxycorticosteroids (17-OHCS). More definitive testing includes an overnight dexamethasone suppression test. Obtain an outpatient baseline plasma cortisol determination. Administer dexamethasone 1 mg PO at 11 PM the same day. Obtain a plasma cortisol level again at 8 AM the next day. The cortisol level will be suppressed (<5 ng/mL) in normal patients but not in Cushing's syndrome. False positives may occur in obesity, chronic illness, or with phenytoin use.

If cortisol suppression does not occur, a 2-day low-dose dexamethasone test is in order. This is performed after two baseline 24-h urine collections for free cortisol and 17-OHCS levels have been obtained. Dexamethasone 0.5 mg is given q6h PO for 2 d. A 24-h urine is collected during the second day for free cortisol and 17-OHCS. Normal patients' 17-OHCS will be suppressed to <2 mg/g of creatinine. Moreover, free cortisol levels will be below normal values. In contrast, in Cushing's syndrome, the 17-OHCS will be >2.5 mg/g of creatinine.

Cushing's disease may be distinguished from Cushing's syndrome by using higher doses of dexamethasone over a 2-day test (disease shows suppression from baseline levels). Then, ACTH levels should be elevated.

Late-onset congenital adrenal hyperplasia is uncommon in adult women. It may be diagnosed by documenting increased serum 17-OHP. Mild deficiency may be detected only by ACTH stimulation to demonstrate the partial block of 21-hydroxylase activity.

DIFFERENTIAL DIAGNOSIS

The *differential diagnosis of hyperandrogenism* must include idiopathic hirsutism, polycystic ovary syndrome, stromal hyperthecosis, androgen-producing ovarian tumors, Cushing's syndrome or disease, congenital adrenal hyperplasia (adult manifestations), androgen-producing adrenal tumors, androgen excess in pregnancy (luteoma or hyperreactio luteinalis), exogenous or iatrogenic androgen administration (testosterone, danazol, anabolic steroids, or synthetic progestins), and abnormal gonadal or sexual development (idiopathic hirsutism, polycystic ovarian syndrome, and stromal thecosis are the most frequent).

TREATMENT

Therapy *depends on the etiology of the hyperandrogenism* as well as the desire for childbearing. Ovarian and adrenal tumors must be treated surgically. Congenital or acquired adrenal hyperplasia should be treated with hydrocortisone. Cushing's disease (tumor) is treated by transsphenoidal pituitary surgery. If unsuccessful, pituitary radiation or bilateral adrenalectomy is indicated. Acromegaly is treated by transsphenoidal hypophysectomy.

After serious disease and neoplasm are ruled out and a decision is made regarding further childbearing, *medical therapy is indicated.* This entails ovarian or adrenal suppression or the blocking of peripheral androgen effects. If infertility is a problem, ovulation induction is advisable after complete evaluation using appropriate drugs (clomiphene, bromocriptine, hMG, GnRH).

GnRH inhibits the secretion of gonadotropins from the pituitary to inhibit the secretion of androgens and estrogens from the ovary. Although reported to be effective in >60%, long-term effects are unknown. Further studies are warranted before general use of GnRH is advocated. Wedge resection of the ovary is not recommended as treatment for hyperandrogenism. Although it may induce ovulation, androgen levels decrease only transiently, and its success rate to decrease hirsutism is only 15%.

PROGNOSIS

Although the underlying cause may be corrected, the signs of hyperandrogenism may be difficult or impossible to reverse. Therefore, therapeutic efforts focus primarily on hirsutism.

HIRSUTISM

ANDROGEN-DEPENDENT HIRSUTISM

Hirsutism, the excessive growth of terminal hair, is the *most common sign of female hyperandrogenism.* Terminal hair is one of the two types of body hair. It is longer, coarser, pigmented, and in some areas of the body hormonally responsive. The other type of body hair is vellus hairs (short, fine, nonpigmented, and not responsive to hormones). Whereas the amount of terminal hair is hereditarily determined, endocrine factors influencing the sebaceous gland and hair follicle include: androgen secretion (amount and duration), concentration of sex hormone-binding globulin, peripheral conversion of weaker to stronger androgens, and sensitivity to androgens. Hirsutism is but one manifestation of hyperandrogenism. Hirsutism generally has a gradual onset and, in milder forms, occurs primarily on the upper lip and chin.

With increasing severity, hair growth progresses to the cheeks, intermammary chest, abdomen, inner thighs, lower back, and intergluteal areas. Whereas the testosterone levels in virilization are usually >2 ng/mL, with hirsutism, the levels are <1.5 ng/mL.

The disorders to be differentiated from hirsutism are *virilism* (as noted earlier and characterized by more extensive androgen-stimulated changes, (see p. 786), idiopathic hirsutism, and hypertrichosis. Hypertrichosis denotes excessive growth of the vellus hair (e.g., forehead, distal extremities). *Hypertrichosis* may result from starvation, traumatic skin irritation, drugs (e.g., phenytoin, diazoxide, minoxidil), and such disorders as acromegaly, porphyria, dermatomyositis, hypothyroidism, Hurler's syndrome, trisomy E, and Cornelia de Lange syndrome.

Most women with hirsutism will have no specific cause identified. These cases are probably the result of *altered androgen metabolism* (increased conversion of testosterone to dihydrotestosterone (see the discussion that follows). *Increased androgen production* may occur from the ovaries and adrenal glands by hypersecretion of testosterone precursors that are converted to testosterone at other sites or by direct secretion of testosterone or conversion to dihydrotestosterone (by 5 α-reductase). *Adrenal causes of excessive androgen production include:* dysfunctional excesses, congenital adrenal hyperplasia, Cushing syndrome and androgen secreting neoplasms. *Ovarian causes of excess androgen production include:* PCO, sertoli-Leydig cell tumors, granulose cell tumors, and gynandroblastomas. Only free androgen is biologically active and almost all androgens in the circulation are bound to sex hormone-binding globulin or albumin. Thus, *decreased androgen binding* may lead to may cause relative hyperandrogenicity. Hirsutism from *exogenous androgen administration* must be considered in every case.

The evaluation of hirsutism includes thoughtful documentation of the physical extent. Androgen producing tumors are ruled out by total testosterone and DHEAS. If the testosterone is >200 ng/mL a transvaginal sonography should be performed to rule out ovarian neoplasms. If the testosterone is ≤200 ng/mL, the DHEAS assists in sorting different therapeutic classes. When the DHEAS <500 nanog/mL, the patients may be treated symptomatically. If the DHEAS is 500–700 nanog/mL, cosyntropin stimulation is necessary to rule out congenital adrenal hyperplasia. If the DHEAS is >700 nanog/mL, an MRI is necessary to rule out adrenal tumors. Exceptions to this schema includes Cushing syndrome, hyperprolactinemia, and adult onset congenital adrenal hyperplasia (see previous discussion).

The *most common drugs used to treat hirsutism* are oral contraceptives, medroxyprogesterone, dexamethasone, and spironolactone. Dexamethasone is effective in many whose hirsutism is of adrenal origin. The dose is 0.5–1 mg orally at night. Morning cortisol levels must be monitored to prevent oversuppression of the adrenals, however.

Combination oral contraceptives (estrogen and progestins) are effective in decreasing hair growth in 50%–60%, although achieving normalized testosterone levels may require 3 months. The effect of therapy is the inhibition of LH secretion by progestins and increased testosterone binding by SHBG (estrogen elevates SHBG). SHBG-bound testosterone will not be bound by receptors. In addition, combination oral contraceptives decrease DHEAS levels, possibly by suppressing ACTH release. This, in turn, decreases adrenal androgens. Progestins alone may be given in regular form (Provera, 30–40 mg/d) or in depot form (Depo-Provera, 150–400 mg IM every 3 months). Because the depot form may cause long-term suppression of the ovary, it should not be used if pregnancy is desired in the near future. In addition to the LH suppression, medroxyprogesterone acetate acts by increasing metabolic clearance of testosterone.

The *growth cycle of terminal hair is long* (6–24 months), and once stimulated, much lower levels of androgen are necessary to sustain that growth. Therefore, patients should be *cautioned not to expect a therapeutic response for 6–12 months*. However, some decrease in hair diameter and lightening of hair color may be noted during that time. If adequate suppression of testosterone and DHEAS for 6–12 months has been documented without a decrease in hirsutism, the dose may be increased and another medication may be added or substituted. If the androgen levels do not decrease as expected with therapy or if hirsutism is progressive despite therapy, further evaluation for a slow-growing neoplasm should be initiated.

IDIOPATHIC HIRSUTISM (FAMILIAL OR CONSTITUTIONAL HIRSUTISM)

When hirsutism is present without ovarian or adrenal dysfunction and exogenous sources of androgens are absent, it is termed *idiopathic*. Idiopathic hirsutism is particularly common in those of Mediterranean or Near East descent. This condition is caused by abnormal peripheral androgen metabolism, (i.e., increased 5α-reductase activity converting normal levels of testosterone into higher than normal levels of DHT and adiol-G). *Spironolactone, cimetidine, and cyproterone acetate afford effective therapy by blocking peripheral testosterone activity or interfering with 5a-reductase activity.*

Spironolactone lowers testosterone levels by inhibiting the biosynthesis of androgens and by competing for androgenic receptors in the hair follicle itself. The dosage is 50–200 mg/d. Cimetidine reduces hirsutism by peripheral inhibition of binding of dihydrotestosterone to androgen receptors. The dose is 300 mg PO 5 times per d.

Cosmetic therapy consists of bleaching, waxing, or depilatory use. Shaving and plucking may cause infection or scarring and are not recommended. Because permanent hair removal via electrolysis is expensive and painful, its use should be recommended only after 6–12 months of medical therapy.

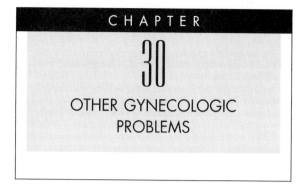

CHAPTER

30

OTHER GYNECOLOGIC PROBLEMS

UTERINE POSITION AND MALPOSITION

UTERINE POSITION

Uterine position and axis are described by both the relationship to an imaginary line, equidistant from all bony structures through the true pelvis, and the relationship of the uterine axis to the cervical axis. The term *version, with the appropriate prefix,* ante- or retro-*designates the uterine axis vis-à-vis the central pelvis. Flexion is the angulation of the axis of the uterus in relation to the axis of the cervix* (Figs. 30-1 and 30-2).

The uterine axis usually deviates from that of the cervix by being anterior or posterior, and this is termed anteflexion or retroflexion. The corpus of the uterus is *anteflexed in nearly 80%* of women, and in the remaining 20% the corpus is retroflexed. Thus, retroversion implies that the axis of the body of the uterus is directed toward the hollow of the sacrum, but the cervix remains in its normal axis (Fig. 30-3). *Retrocession* implies that both uterus and cervix (to a lesser degree) are displaced backward toward the sacrum—away from the midpoint of the pelvis (Fig. 30-4).

Normally, because of the flexibility of the uterine supports, the position of the uterus may vary transiently as a result of pelvic inclination during sitting, standing, or lying down. In nulliparas and multiparas with good pelvic support, the cervical axis is usually directed posteriorly in the vaginal vault, *almost at a right angle to the vaginal axis.* Enlargement of the uterus by pregnancy or tumor may alter the relative fundal position. The uterus and cervix are often aligned with the vaginal axis following parturition or with relaxation of the pelvic floor because of laxity of the transverse cervical and round ligaments.

FIGURE 30-1. Anteflexion of uterus.

FIGURE 30-2. Retroflexion in an anteverted uterus.

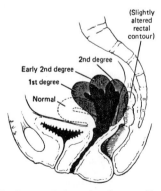

FIGURE 30-3. Degrees of retroversion of uterus without retroflexion.

FIGURE 30-4. Retrocession of uterus.

UTERINE MALPOSITION

Uterine prolapse (even moderate) is nearly always associated with uterine retroversion or retrocession. *Nonfixed lateral uterine displacement* generally indicates displacement by tumors or shortening of the supports. *Fixed (adherent) lateral uterine* displacement may indicate endometriosis, adhesions, a tuboovarian mass, or tumor. Pelvic infections or endometriosis may obliterate the cul-de-sac and result in fixed uterine retroversion. A pyosalpinx or hydrosalpinx may draw the corpus backward and downward by its weight, whereupon adhesions add restriction to cause immobility. Speculum examination of the patient with retroflexion and retroversion of the uterus will reveal the cervix to be anterior, higher in the vagina than normally encountered, and pointing toward the symphysis pubis (as opposed to its normal posterior vaginal inclination). Bimanual examination ordinarily confirms this finding.

Differential diagnosis of unusual uterine positions includes a fundal fibroid, an ovarian tumor resting in the cul-de-sac, adherent retroposition of the uterus, salpingitis, or endometriosis. The diagnosis is most frequently clarified by a pelvic ultrasound examination.

Of *women with retroposed uteri, <5% will have a complaint* referable to posterior flexion or version of the uterus. When symptoms occur, they are most frequently backache, dysmenorrhea, or dyspareunia. These symptoms usually respond to correction of the retroposition of the uterus, which may be accomplished by manual replacement (rectovaginal manipulation of the corpus) (Fig. 30-5) and support using a vaginal pessary (Hodge type) (Fig. 30-6).

Uterine anteversion
encouraged

Uterine anteversion
accomplished

FIGURE 30-5. Bimanual replacement of uterus.

During early *pregnancy, a retroflexed uterus may become incarcerated,* often because of adhesions, and lead to acute urinary retention. In addition, because adherence interferes with normal fetal growth and development, abortion may result. This has been simply treated by catheterizing the bladder and using a vaginal mercury-filled balloon to gently displace the uterus anteriorly.

Adherent uterine fixations rarely cause uterine symptomatology. However, evaluation and appropriate therapy may be indicated for

Pessary inserted
with patient in
lithotomy position

Patient in
knee-chest position.
Uterus anteverted
and pessary seated.

Final seating of
pessary and
support of uterus

FIGURE 30-6. Insertion of Hodge pessary if bimanual replacement of uterus is not successful.

the underlying process creating the deviation. There are few indications for uterine suspension as a primary surgical therapy, although uterine suspension may assist in preventing uterine adherence to other pelvic structures in cases of pelvic endometriosis (p. 755).

RELAXATION OF PELVIC SUPPORT

NORMAL SUPPORT OF PELVIC STRUCTURES

The cervix is normally relatively fixed in place by the dense fibrous and smooth muscle *cardinal ligaments,* which extend laterally to the pelvic sidewalls. At or just above the cervicouterine juncture, the relatively strong, primarily fibrous *uterosacral ligaments* attach posterior-lateral and extend to the sacrum to further support the uterus and cervix. The *broad ligaments,* a far weaker superior extension of the cardinal ligaments, are composed primarily of peritoneum and blood vessels.

The broad ligaments support the uterus laterally, and the *round ligaments* attach to the superior-lateral aspects of the corpus. Thus, the ligamentous support to the uterus is movable, in contrast to that of the cervix, which is not. The vagina is supported in part by the strong *lower extension of the cardinal ligaments* but pierces and is partly elevated by the muscles of the *pelvic diaphragm* (levator ani) and the perineum (perineal body, bulbocavernous muscle). *Support of the lower vagina is intimately involved with that of the bladder and rectum.*

With failure of support, the uterus, vagina, bladder, or rectum may first prolapse into, and finally protrude from, the vagina. It is so common for multiple problems to occur as a result of the basic defect that many authorities prefer the term *symptomatic pelvic relaxation* as the primary diagnosis, with a secondary description of the specific defects (e.g., cystocele) and their extent.

VAGINAL HERNIAS

At least half of all parous women develop some degree of *vaginal hernia* (the most common are cystocele and rectocele), usually after the menopause. Approximately 10% of these are symptomatic and require treatment.

Vaginal herniations are caused by defects of the endopelvic connective tissue, fascia, or pelvic floor musculature. Such defects may *occur as a result* of congenital weaknesses, childbirth trauma, excessive strain on normal structures (e.g., straining with constipation), or musculofascial lacerations. Vaginal herniations rarely occur early in life, even after a traumatic delivery. The defects usually become evident only months or years later. The long delay in childbirth trauma becoming manifest is thought to be related to both intrinsic damage at the time and conversion of fibroelastic supports to fibrous (scar) tissue. The latter is much more prone to attenuation later. Thus, the climacteric and persistent stress of increased intraabdominal pressure cause gradual stretching of the damaged supports of the pelvic floor, bladder, or rectum.

Other contributing factors to prolapse are those that increase intraabdominal pressure and enhance strain on the pelvic structures. The following processes are associated with enhanced rates of vaginal herniation: congenitally deficient or relaxed pelvic support, obesity, chronic respiratory problems (asthma, chronic bronchitis, and bronchiectasis), ascites, and sacral nerve disorders (injury to S1–4, the most common is diabetic neuropathy).

UTERINE (AND CERVICAL) PROLAPSE

Prolapse of the uterus occurs most commonly in postmenopausal multiparous Caucasians. When the uterus prolapses, it carries the upper vagina with it. Figure 30-7 illustrates this condition.

Clinically, patients complain of a *pelvic heaviness or dragging sensation.* Other complaints may include low back pain, a sense of "something falling out," or a mass coming from the vagina. On physical examination, the *descensus is apparent when the patient strains* (i.e., increases intraabdominal pressure) or is demonstrated by gentle traction on the cervix (by grasping it with an Allis clamp or tenaculum).

The *extent of uterine prolapse parallels the seriousness of separation or attenuation of its supporting structures.* The degree of prolapse is *graded by the extent of the cervical prolapse.* A first-degree prolapse occurs when the cervix remains within the vagina, a second-degree prolapse exists when the cervix protrudes beyond the introitus, and a third-degree prolapse (complete procidentia) implies that the entire uterus is outside the vulva. Often, the same grading is applied to other vaginal hernias to detail their extent.

The *differential diagnosis* of cervical or uterine prolapse includes only a nonprolapsed, hypertrophied, elongated, and often engorged, cervix. Rarely do cervical or uterine tumors have similar symptomatology.

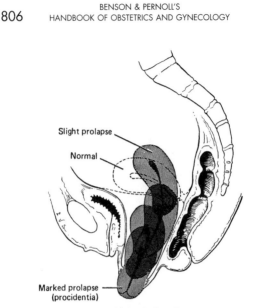

Slight prolapse

Normal

Marked prolapse
(procidentia)

FIGURE 30-7.   Prolapsed uterus.

CYSTOCELE AND URETHROCELE

A *cystocele* is the prolapse of the bladder from its normal position into the vagina (Fig. 30-8). This hernia represents loss or a weakness of the pubocervical fascia. A *urethrocele* is defined as protrusion (a sagging) of the urethra into the vagina and is caused by loss of urethral attachments beneath the symphysis pubis. The urethra may assume a funnel-like configuration. Frequently, *the two defects occur together (cystourethrocele).* The usual *symptomatology* of a cystocele includes a sensation of vaginal fullness, pressure, or falling out. On examination, a *cystocele* is marked by a soft, reducible mass bulging into the anterior vagina. With perineal depression and straining, the *mass descends.* Frequently, with a cystocele there is *increased residual urine,* enhancing the possibility of urinary tract infection.

If there is an associated urethrocele, a *downward and forward rotation of the urethra may be noted.* Damage to the pubococcygeus portion of the levator musculature and the endopelvic fascia, often associated with a large cystocele, weakens and displaces the bladder neck and urethra. With a urethrocele, if the bladder is even partially

FIGURE 30-8. Cystocele.

filled and the patient strains (e.g., cough), there may be *stress incontinence of urine.*

RECTOCELE

Loss of the rectovaginal septum and posterior vaginal wall support results in hernial protrusion of the rectum into the vagina, a rectocele (Fig. 30-9). The *symptomatology* of a rectocele includes a bearing-down sensation and vaginal fullness or heaviness. Additionally, patients with a rectocele may complain of constipation or the feeling of incomplete emptying of the rectum with bowel movement. In the most severe cases, the patient must *place one or two fingers in the vagina (reducing the rectocele) to have a bowel movement.*

On physical examination, a rectocele is revealed by retracting the anterior vaginal wall upward while having the patient perform

FIGURE 30-9. Rectocele.

a Valsalva maneuver. The *rectum bulges into or through the vagina.*
Confirmation of the defect is afforded by placing one finger in the
rectum and one in the vagina to detail the hernia and confirm loss
of the rectovaginal septum. Most patients with rectocele also have
hemorrhoids. In extreme forms, rectocele may lead to obstipation
or fecal impaction.

ENTEROCELE

*Herniation of the cul-de-sac (pouch of Douglas) is defined as an
enterocele.* This hernia often contains loops of small bowel or omentum (Fig. 30-10). The bowel and omentum may be adherent to the
peritoneum or freely movable. *Enterocele may occur between the
uterosacral ligaments into the rectovaginal septum with the uterus
in place but is much more common following vaginal or abdominal hysterectomy.*

Enteroceles are difficult to diagnose. *Symptomatology is usually
minimal* (heaviness or internal weakness) or the same as with a rectocele. It is occasionally possible to differentiate the enterocele from
a rectocele on physical examination by defining two hernias. This
may be accomplished by seeking the bulge of the enterocele just
above that of a rectocele as a bivalve speculum is slowly withdrawn
from the vagina of the supine patient. The diagnosis can be confirmed by performing rectovaginal examination and asking the patient to cough. An impulse is felt against the fingertip opposing an
enterocele (upper bulge) but not a rectocele (lower bulge). Also, if
the enterocele is large enough to prolapse through the vaginal vault,
transillumination may reveal bowel shadows; however, rectocele

FIGURE 30-10. Enterocele and prolapsed uterus.

and enterocele are often only differentiated at the time of surgery. Enterocele is rarely a cause of intestinal obstruction.

DIFFERENTIAL DIAGNOSIS

Cysts of vestigial (*wolffian*) origin, *semisolid tumors of the vaginal septa, and large inclusion cysts* may be mistaken for cystocele or rectocele. A sizable cystocele may conceal a *urethrocele. A bladder or urethral diverticulum* may be mistaken for a cystocele or urethrocele. The fullness of a high rectocele, prolapsed and adherent adnexa, a markedly retroflexed uterus, a soft cervical or uterine myoma, or retained fecal material may be confused with enterocele.

DIAGNOSIS

There are *no specific tests of value for detailing or diagnosing vaginal hernias.* The workup generally is related to ascertaining fitness for surgery and excluding malignancy and other defects of the genital system. The diagnosis of urinary stress incontinence is reviewed on page 811. With complete procidentia any ulceration must be shown to be benign and resolved preoperatively.

TREATMENT

Treatment of vaginal hernias in postmenopausal patients usually involves the *local or systemic administration of estrogen* to enhance the vaginal mucosa, increase the blood supply to the region, and promote muscular tone. *Kegel exercises* (isometric contraction of the pubococcygeus muscles) may strengthen the musculature of the pelvic floor. In young women (who desire more children), it is common to defer surgical repair until after childbearing is complete or, when repair must be performed, to deliver subsequent pregnancies by cesarean section. In the woman who wishes to preserve her childbearing capability or in the medically compromised, *pessary support* (p. 854) is palliative.

Therapy of uterine/cervical descensus most commonly is *vaginal hysterectomy and resupport of the vagina using the uterosacral and cardinal ligaments. It is uncommon for cystocele to occur without some degree of rectocele, and vice versa.* Until recently, the usual primary procedure for a cystocele and urethrocele was an anterior colporrhaphy. However, recurrence of stress urinary incontinence was high. Currently, *urodynamic testing is performed before surgery* so that the procedure most likely to effect cure may be determined. Many authorities recommend that even minor rectoceles be corrected at the time of urinary surgery to obviate the need for additional surgery at a later date.

Patients with *recurrent cystourethroceles,* those with severe stress incontinence of urine, and those in whom an abdominal procedure is necessary for other reasons may be treated with a pubovaginal sling, Marshall-Marchetti-Krantz, Burch, or similar cystourethropexy (suspension) procedure (p. 819). Posterior colporrhaphy is used to treat rectoceles. Repair of enteroceles is challenging (p. 875), and the recurrence rate is >15% in all types of vaginal hernias after surgical repair.

GYNECOLOGIC UROLOGY

Because the female reproductive tract and lower urinary tract are so intimately related, consideration must be given to the lower urinary tract in evaluation of many gynecologic diseases.

ANATOMY AND PHYSIOLOGY

The urinary bladder is composed of *three tightly woven muscle layers. Two of these layers extend into the urethra,* forming longitudinal and circular muscle layers. Controversy exists as to whether or not a genuine striated muscle sphincter of the urethra exists because the pubococcygeus muscle acts as the sphincter of the urethra.

Innervation of the bladder is complex, with both autonomic and somatic nerves controlling the storage and expulsion of urine. Parasympathetic nerves from S2–4 stimulate bladder contractions. Beta-adrenergic fibers predominate in the bladder, and alpha-adrenergic fibers are dominant in the urethra. The smooth muscle of the urethra is contracted by the alpha-adrenergic system, and relaxation of the bladder and urethra are stimulated by the beta-adrenergic component. The pudenal nerve innervates the striated muscle present in the urethra.

The detrusor muscle relaxes as the bladder fills, thus allowing the intraluminal pressure to remain low. Although a smooth muscle, normally there is voluntary control, allowing micturition only when desired. When injury or disease is present, the intrinsic function of this muscle may be lost, resulting in incontinence.

Control of micturition involves the *complex interplay of several systems.* The urethra has two muscular layers (circular and longitudinal). Functionally, the pubococcygeus muscle acts as a striated muscle sphincter of the urethra. Urination is controlled by parasympathetic nerves from S2–4 (cholinergic nerve fibers), which stimulate bladder contractions, preganglionic sympathetic fibers from T10–L2, which are also cholinergic, postganglionic fibers from T10–L2 (adrenergic nerves) with beta fibers terminating mainly in the bladder and alpha fibers in the urethra.

Alpha-adrenergic stimulation contracts the ureteral smooth muscle. Beta-adrenergic stimulation relaxes both bladder and urethra. The detrusor muscle is composed of three muscular layers. It relaxes (within normal limits of volume) in response to increasing bladder volume, thus maintaining the same pressure.

BASIC EVALUATION OF URINARY PROBLEMS

COMMON SYMPTOMS OF URINARY DISORDERS

Dysuria

Dysuria is painful urination, often described as a burning sensation as urine flows through the urethra. Dysuria is a *symptom of cystitis or urethritis* but may result from chemical irritation, trauma, or atrophy (from estrogen deficiency). Dysuria must be differentiated from the burning associated with urine flowing over inflamed vulvar or vaginal tissues.

Frequency

Urinary frequency is *a relative term,* being defined as an increase in the number of voidings per 24 h for a given individual. Normal frequency varies from 2–7 times per waking day; thus, "frequency" is defined as more than 7 micturitions per 24 h. Urinary tract infection *(UTI)* is most often responsible for frequency, although interstitial cystitis, diabetes mellitus, emotional problems, or diuretics must be considered.

Urgency

Urgency is a *sudden sensation of a need to void* (often described as overwhelming). It is common in urinary tract disorders, especially with infection and interstitial cystitis.

Nocturia

Women who awaken *more than once per night* to void have nocturia. It may be the result of infection, a sleep disorder, or a neurologic problem. Voiding more than once per night is common for the elderly. Recall that pregnancy, peripheral edema, and congestive heart failure cause diuresis in the recumbent position.

Enuresis
Enuresis is bedwetting. Although common in younger children, in an adult enuresis may be associated with: detrusor instability, a neurologic condition, or a psychogenic disorder.

Hesitancy
Hesitancy is the *inability to start readily or maintain a stream of urine.* This may be the result of poor urethral relaxation, inadequate detrusor contraction, partial urethral obstruction (from severe relaxation of pelvic supports), or overcorrection by cystourethropexy.

Postvoiding Fullness
A feeling of *bladder fullness immediately after voiding* is rarely a result of elevated residual urine volumes. Instead, it is often due to irritation (e.g., infection, trauma, inflammation, or foreign body), vaginal atrophy, or relaxation of pelvic supports. Residual urine volumes are generally low in postvoiding fullness.

Urinary Incontinence
Urinary incontinence affects up to a third of women >60 years old, but is not entirely confined to the elderly (15%–20% of women <60 years old have incontinence). *Urinary incontinence occurs in >50% of nursing home residents and may be the largest contributor to nursing home admission.* Probably less than half of the women with urinary incontinence seek medical assistance, relying on absorbent pads or life-style changes to cope with the problem.

The *physical consequences* of urinary incontinence (e.g., perineal irritation, vaginal discharge, dyspareunia, and unpleasant odors) provide a constant reminder of the condition. The *emotional distress* accompanying these changes is difficult to quantify, but includes fears about "having an accident" in public, insecurity concerning their appearance or odor, embarrassment, and depression. Incontinence often leads to social distress including isolation and alteration of sexual relationships. Thus, the *impact on the individual is profound.*

The *societal problems posed by urinary incontinence are also profound.* The care issues in the elderly incontinent often necessitate nursing home placement are only a reflection of the total problem. The direct costs in the United States probably approach $20 billion per year.

All too frequently, urinary incontinence in the elderly *may be a symptom or sign of other problems.* Indeed, *spontaneous resolution occurs in up to one third of cases.* In these cases the most common *causative factors include:* urinary tract infections, drugs, delirium, depression, excess urine production due to excess intake, fluid mobilization, endocrinological problems, restricted mobility, or fecal impaction. Whereas such problems may be detailed by a thoughtful history, physical examination, or minimal testing, more than two thirds of cases will have the condition "urinary incontinence" that must be further differentiated into stress incontinence and urge incontinence.

Leakage of urine associated with the desire to void is termed *urge incontinence,* whether the urge is sudden or gradual in onset. In normal micturition the detrusor muscle contracts reflexly after voluntary relaxation of the pelvic floor. Urge incontinence occurs when there is sufficient detrusor hyperactivity to initiate micturition without the voluntary relaxation of the pelvic floor. Thus, the condition is also known as *detrusor instability and motor urge incontinence. Two variants of detrusor instability are described.* Detrusor hyperreflexia refers to detrusor hyperactivity with concomittent neurologic disease (e.g., Parkinson disease, stroke). Detrusor hyperreflexia with impaired contractility usually occurs in the elderly. The involuntary detrusor contraction is usually sufficient to initiate the flow of urine, but too weak to complete voiding. Thus, these individuals have urge incontinence and urinary retention. Urge incontinence and stress incontinence may be concomitant.

Stress incontinence of urine is the involuntary loss of urine associated with increased intraabdominal pressure. Examples of activities that increase intraabdominal pressure include sneezing, coughing, laughing, stepping up or down, and lifting. It is useful to ascertain the frequency of occurrence of stress incontinence and the amount of urine lost. The condition of stress incontinence is extensively discussed in the next section.

HISTORY

Detailed obstetric, medical, and surgical histories are necessary to *clarify the patient's symptoms.* The *obstetric details* of each delivery should be pursued, including: gravidity, parity, mode of delivery, instrumentation (if used) for delivery, size of the fetus, position of the fetus, and postpartum complications (including urinary incontinence). Examples of the *medical problems* of importance to incontinence are diabetes mellitus, thyroid disease, back pain, back injuries, and any neurologic disorders (e.g., cerebrovascular accidents, multiple sclerosis, Parkinson's disease). *Surgical issues* to be pursued in the history include any prior pelvic, gynecological, urological, or anorectal procedures.

A *drug history* is important to screen for the commonly prescribed medications which may influence micturition (e.g., alpha methyldopa, anticholinergic, antihistamines, diazepam, diuretics, phenothiazines, and prazosin).

A *voiding diary,* recording the time and volume of spontaneous voiding for a 24–72 h interval, is a useful historical tool in evaluating incontinence. Although the historical information is invaluable in the total evaluation, even the best of histories will reveal the correct diagnosis in only 50%–70% of cases. Thus, further evaluation is essential.

PHYSICAL EXAMINATION

In the evaluation of urinary problems, a *general physical examination* (including neurological evaluation of the lower thoracic, lumbar, and sacral nerves) and a *complete pelvic examination* should be performed. Evaluation for the *relaxation of pelvic support(s)* is important. The vagina should be inspected for evidence of inflammation, discharge, atrophy, scarring, stricture, abscess, or neoplasia. Urethral epithelial atrophy resulting from lack of estrogen stimulation is commonly associated with lower urinary tract symptoms in postmenopausal women.

The bladder and urethra should be *palpated for tenderness or mass. Milking the urethra* (stripping from proximal to distal) may disclose a discharge indicative of infection or diverticulum. To evaluate perineal neurologic integrity, assess the sensation of the perineum, the reflexes evaluated, and muscle strength. Evaluate the ability to contract and relax the pubococcygeus muscles and anal sphincter voluntarily.

Descent of the bladder or urethra is assessed during straining, with the patient in the dorsal lithotomy position. A lubricated cotton applicator is placed in the urethra to the urethrovesical junction The angle formed by the applicator stick and a line parallel to the floor is measured at rest and during a Valsalva (straining) maneuver. If the angle is <15 degrees both during rest and straining, good pelvic support is likely. If the angle is >30 degrees during straining, there is poor pelvic support. An angle of 15–30 degrees is inconclusive.

A *urinary stress test* should be performed to evaluate incontinence. The bladder is filled with a known volume of fluid (e.g., 300 mL) until it feels full but not uncomfortable. The patient is asked to stand with the feet a shoulder-width apart and to either cough eight or ten times or perform the Valsalva maneuver. The perineum is observed for leakage of urine. If incontinence occurs during the stress maneuver and ends shortly after straining is discontinued, the most likely cause is poor anatomic support. If the leakage is continuous or delayed, inadequate detrusor muscle control is likely. If the test is negative, mild incontinence may still be present, and further testing is necessary. Stress tests that include elevation of the vaginal wall during the test are not valid for predicting the effectiveness of surgery because they only show the effect of mechanical obstruction of the urethra. The full evaluation of urinary incontinence requires more complex evaluations. Increasingly, sonographic evaluations are playing a role in the evaluation of incontinence.

EVALUATION AND THERAPY OF COMMON URINARY PROBLEMS

URINARY TRACT INFECTION (UTI)

Because of the shorter urethra in females, *UTI is more prevalent in women than in men,* with an increasing incidence from adolescence to old age of 2%–20%. Pregnancy increases the incidence of UTI 2–3 times and the incidence after uretheral catheterization is 3%. The *organisms causing UTI are usually from the vagina or rectum* and may ascend from the urethra (urethritis) to the bladder (cystitis) to the kidney (pyelonephritis). If urine contains >100,000 bacteria/mL in two clean-catch or one catheterized specimen, it is considered infected. Persons with poor hygiene, who void infrequently, or who have chronic urinary residual volume are *most likely to develop UTI,* as are those with renal stones, urinary tract anomalies, urinary reflux, or prolonged bladder catheterization.

The *signs and symptoms of UTI may be minimal to severe,* with dysuria, frequency, and urgency common in urethritis. Cystitis may be accompanied by suprapubic discomfort as well as urgency incontinence. Fever is usually present only with pyelonephritis. Back pain and anorexia are often associated findings in pyelonephritis, but asymptomatic renal infection does occur.

The *laboratory findings* suggesting UTI include pyuria (>6–8 WBC/hpf) in centrifuged urine sediment. Epithelial cells are usually of vaginal origin. A positive urine culture is diagnostic for many bacteria but will be negative in chlamydial infection. Cystitis is often accompanied by hematuria. If WBC casts are present, pyelonephritis is likely. The WBC count on CBC may be elevated with pyelonephritis but may be normal in urethritis or cystitis.

The *differential diagnosis* includes vaginitis, especially from *Trichomonas* and herpes simplex. Pressure on the bladder from a pelvic mass may suggest cystitis.

Treatment for UTI is usually directed toward *Escherichia coli,* the most common offending organism. If it is the first episode of UTI and is uncomplicated, the drugs of choice are trimethoprim-sulfamethoxazole, and nitrofurantoin. Once *culture and sensitivity* patterns are known, the drug dose or choice may be changed. Chronic or recurrent infections frequently are associated with resistant organisms requiring cephalosporins or aminoglycosides.

Dysuria may be relieved by urinary anesthetics (e.g., phenazopyridine hydrochloride). Administration of a single dose of antibiotic may cure simple cystitis. Pyelonephritis may require prolonged, even IV antibiotics. If bacteriuria persists after appropriate therapy, cystoscopy and intravenous pyelography (IVP) are indicated to rule out structural defects, stone, or tumor. Some recurrent UTIs result from contamination of the urethra during sexual intercourse and may be prevented by voiding immediately after intercourse, urinary antibiotics after intercourse, or nightly antibiotic prophylaxis.

Patients experiencing the symptoms of *recurrent urethritis with negative bacterial cultures have urethral syndrome.* Their symptomatology may be caused by organisms such as herpes simplex, *Chlamydia,* anaerobic bacteria, *Ureaplasma,* or *Mycoplasma.* Patients with urethral syndrome should be investigated for evidence of *chemical or mechanical irritation of the urethra,* as well as *diverticula, stenosis, or a meatus opening into the vagina.*

GENUINE STRESS URINARY INCONTINENCE (GSUI, ALSO TERMED TRUE STRESS INCONTINENCE AND ANATOMIC URINARY STRESS INCONTINENCE)

GSUI is *the involuntary loss of urine through the urethra simultaneously with an increase in intraabdominal pressure in the absence of detrusor muscle contraction.* Because intraabdominal pressure is also transmitted (incompletely) to the proximal urethra, such activities as exercise or coughing may result in the loss of the pressure gradient and allow urine to escape.

Several mechanisms may be responsible for GSUI: (1) anatomic descent of the proximal urethra below its normal intraabdominal position during stress-causing activities; (2) altered anatomic relationships between the urethra and bladder, resulting in vector forces directed from the bladder along the axis of the urethra; and (3) failure of the neuromuscular components that reflexly increase intraurethral pressure in response to increased intraabdominal pressure.

The etiology of urinary incontinence is complex and the onset of symptoms often long delayed after the causative factor(s). Contributors to urinary incontinence include: vaginal birth, aging, familial or genetic, smoking, gynecological surgery, underlying disease states (especially asthma, neurological conditions), occupational and recreational factors.

The *diagnosis of GSUI does not hinge on one test.* The criteria include normal urinalysis, negative urine culture, poor anatomic support (as evidenced by the cotton-tipped applicator test, x-ray, cystourethroscopy), demonstrable leakage with stress, and normal cystometrogram or urethrocystometry. *Complex cases (~10%) will require multichannel urodynamics or other technologically advanced techniques.* Figure 30-11 details the common normal and abnormal bladder and urethral configurations.

The signs and symptoms of GSUI are predominantly *stress incontinence,* although frequency, urgency, urge incontinence, and

Normal support. (Continent.)

Type II stress incontinence. (Loss of posterior urethrovesical angle, downward and backward rotational descent of urethra and bladder neck.)

Note: This is not a cystocele but may simulate one. Often called urethrocele, but this is a poor descriptive term.

Type I stress incontinence. (Loss of posterior urethrovesical angle, slight or no displacement of normal urethral axis, minimal findings on pelvic examination.)

Cystocele. (Continent.)

FIGURE 30-11. Anatomic configuration of the bladder in normal (continent) women and women with stress incontinence. Drawn from cystourethrograms.

(From T.H. Green, Jr, *Gynecology: Essentials of Clinical Practice,* 3rd ed. Little, Brown, 1977.)

postvoiding fullness are common complaints. Dysuria and hematuria are uncommon unless there is a concomitant UTI. Approximately 75% of patients will have cystocele, urethrocele, or both.

Because treatment is based on correction of the anatomic abnormality, *studies demonstrating poor support of the urethra are necessary before surgical correction.* In 95%, the cotton-tipped applicator test will be abnormal. In the 5% with normal results, incontinence is the result of funneling of proximal urethra, severe scarring of the urethra, or atony of the urethral sphincteric mechanism. Urethral scarring will prevent movement of the applicator despite poor pelvic support. Therefore, a normal test should be followed by a *straining cystogram or voiding cystourethrogram.*

If a urinary stress test is negative, a *pad test* may be performed to document incontinence. A preweighed sanitary napkin is used to measure the volume of urine lost during exercise or whatever activity that precipitates stress incontinence in that woman. Colored fluid may be instilled into the bladder to visually demonstrate loss of urine.

A *cystometrogram* must be performed to rule out unstable bladder, overflow incontinence, reduced bladder capacity, or abnormal bladder sensation. If the bladder capacity is <300 mL or >800 mL, surgery is contraindicated.

Urethroscopy and cystoscopy may show diverticula, fistulas, neoplasia, calculi, or inflammation. Dynamic urethroscopy observes the urethrovesical junction during bladder filling and straining. If pelvic support is adequate during increased intraabdominal pressure maneuvers, the urethrovesical junction will close proximal to the tip located in the proximal urethra. If anatomic support is poor, the urethrovesical junction closes over the tip of the urethroscope.

Obtaining a *urethral pressure profile* can show weakness of the urethral sphincteric mechanism at rest, although this may not be exclusive to patients with GSUI. It is most helpful in determining which patients with GSUI will not benefit from surgical correction (i.e., when urethral closing pressures are very low at rest).

Treatment

Treatment may be either surgical, medical, behavorial, or a combination. GUSI is rarely cured by medical management. Surgical techniques that are successful initially may be followed by recurrence over the years due to the effects of aging and other disease processes that affect the continence mechanisms.

Medical Measures

Kegel isotonic exercises consist of repeated contractions of the pubococcygeus muscles to strengthen a weak pelvic floor musculature.

The patient is instructed to squeeze the muscles used to stop urination 150–200 times per day. Good improvement is seen in 15%–30% with GSUI, with some improvement in another 30%–40%. If the exercises are repeated less frequently or if the pubococcygeus muscles are separated in the midline, improvement may be marginal.

If the cause of incontinence is atrophic change from estrogen deficiency, *estrogen replacement will result in resolution of stress incontinence in 10%–30% of postmenopausal women.* Vaginal estrogen provides the most rapid response, but oral preparations maintain the patient's status as well as do vaginal preparations.

If the patient is taking *medications* that stimulate ganglionic or alpha-adrenergic blocking activity (e.g., guanethidine, methyldopa, or prazosin), discontinuing their use may result in improved urethral tone and improved continence. Alpha-adrenergic agonists (e.g., phenylpropanolamine, pseudoephedrine) also may improve stress incontinence.

Other methods, such as electrical stimulation of the pelvic floor to increase urethral closure pressure and Teflon or collagen injected periurethrally to compress the urethral mucosa and cause a mild obstruction to urinary flow, have been performed with some success.

Surgical Measures

The *goal of surgical procedures for incontinence is to elevate and support the urethrovesical junction to improve pressure transmission to the urethra during stress maneuvers.* The best results are obtained if the operative procedure for GSUI is *combined with correction of pelvic support defects.* The procedures may be accomplished vaginally or abdominally. The cure rate depends on patient selection, accuracy of preoperative diagnosis, skill of the surgeon, and length of follow-up. Cure rates for the abdominal procedures are 85%–90% and for vaginal procedures 75%–85%.

The predominant abdominal procedures are the *pubovaginal sling, Marshall-Marchetti-Krantz (MMK) procedure, the Burch procedure, the paravaginal procedure,* or various modifications. With the exception of the pubovaginal sling, these procedures consist of placing sutures in the periurethral, vaginal, or perivaginal tissue to elevate the urethrovesical junction and attaching these sutures to relatively strong and permanent structures. The MMK uses the periosteum of the pubic symphysis for suture fixation, whereas the Burch procedure uses Cooper's ligaments. The obturator fascia, arcus tendineus of the pelvic fascia, insertion of the rectus fascia, and the periosteum of the pubic ramus have all been employed in various modifications.

A *pubovaginal sling* using autologous fascia (e.g., rectus fascia, fascia lata, or round ligaments) or synthetic material is accomplished through a combined vaginal and abdominal approach. The sling is submucosally passed under the urethra at the urethrovesical juncture and then both ends (or polygycolic sutures attached to the ends) carried through the endopelvic fascia, space of Retizus, abdominal musculature (just lateral to the Rectus muscles), and rectus fascia. The sling or sutures is then loosely tied and/or sutured superficial to the rectus fascia. This provides excellent support, without undue restriction, of urethrovesical junction motion. For many authorities, the pubovaginal sling has become the technique of choice for difficult cases and most surgical failures. An interval of bladder reaccomodation is usually managed by intermittent self-catheterization or use of a suprapubic catheter.

Vaginal procedures for stress incontinence are based on the assumption that weakening of or damage to the endopelvic fascia between the vagina and bladder is responsible for the poor support. The initial procedure (Kelly plication) involves an anterior colporrhaphy with plication at the urethrovesical angle through a midline vaginal incision. Because long-term success is limited using the endopelvic fascia, employing stronger structures (e.g., autologous fascia, pubourethral ligaments, periosteum of the pubic ramus, and pubococcygeus muscles) has met with better results.

Patients with urethral scarring or atony not amenable to standard surgical therapy may benefit from placement of an *artificial urethral sphincter* that obstructs the urethra until the patient desires to void, at which time the artificial sphincter is emptied by an internal pumping system to relieve the urethral obstruction and allow the urine to flow.

Surgical complications include UTI, delayed postoperative voiding, dyspareunia, frequency-urgency syndrome, and surgically induced unstable bladder, in addition to iatrogenic damage to the urinary tract, postoperative fistula, and bladder calculi from sutures perforating the bladder mucosa.

The prognosis for medical management is usually an improvement in symptoms but not cure. *Surgical management is the only definitive cure for GSUI.* A poorer prognosis is likely for patients who have had a previous surgical failure, low urethral closing pressure at rest, concomitant local disease, combined urinary incontinence (GSUI plus motor urge incontinence), or systemic diseases that make healing or technical performance of surgery difficult (e.g., diabetes mellitus, obesity).

DETRUSOR INSTABILITY

Detrusor instability incontinence results *from involuntary uninhibited detrusor muscle contractions.* If the cause is neurologic, it is termed *hyperreflexic bladder.* Most cases are idiopathic, although infection and obstruction may contribute.

Because the urine loss is unpredictable and large volumes may be lost, this condition may cause even more distress than does GSUI. About 1%–2% of adult females suffer from motor urge incontinence, with the highest incidence occurring in the geriatric population.

Normal micturition sequence is relaxation of the urethral sphincteric mechanism, followed by contraction of the detrusor muscle 1–3 sec later. The sequence is unchanged in motor urge incontinence, but the patient cannot voluntarily inhibit the action. It may occur at any bladder volume and may be spontaneous or provoked by physical, psychologic, tactile, or auditory stimuli. Approximately 25%–50% of patients with motor urge incontinence are incontinent only with provocation. About one third have concomitant GSUI, making the *distinction difficult.* Most feel an urge to void immediately preceding the episode, but patients with neurologic disease may have no warning.

The *symptoms* include urgency, frequency, stress incontinence, and urge incontinence. Physical examination is usually normal unless detrusor hyperreflexia is present with associated neurologic abnormalities.

The diagnosis of motor urge incontinence is suggested by a *several second delay in urine loss during a urinary stress test.* The diagnosis is confirmed by cystometric evidence of involuntary detrusor contractions at rest, during bladder filling, or after provocative maneuvers. A smooth rise in pressure occurring simultaneously with visible urine leakage is typical. Urethrocystometry confirms that the involuntary contractions are preceded by a fall in urethral pressure. Urethroscopy and cystoscopy may reveal bladder trabeculation from hypertrophy of the detrusor muscle fascicles.

The *differential diagnosis* includes GSUI and sensory urge incontinence. In the latter, the patient can inhibit the leakage with strong encouragement, whereas motor urge incontinence cannot be inhibited. GSUI can be distinguished using provocative cystometry or simultaneous urethrocystometry.

Treatment

Behavior modification techniques using hypnosis, biofeedback, bladder retraining drills, and psychotherapy may be effective if neurologic disease is not responsible for the unstable bladder. *Bladder retraining* consists of having the patient void on schedule at intervals that are gradually lengthened in an attempt to regain cortical control over the voiding reflex. This may be effective in up to 80% but requires compulsive patient cooperation, and recurrence rates are high.

Medication will help in 50%–80% of patients and may affect a cure in 20%–30%. The most effective drugs are anticholinergic agents, but bladder analgesics, smooth muscle antispasmodics, calcium channel blockers, and prostaglandin synthetase inhibitors have been effective.

Surgery consisting of such procedures as denervation, cystoplasty, and urinary diversion usually are reserved for patients with severe permanent bladder instability from neurologic disease and when all other therapy fails.

Occasionally, indwelling catheters are used for patients who are severely incapacitated, but this adds the risk of chronic infection.

Prognosis

Recurrence rates are high, bladder retraining techniques require much time and effort, and medications have troublesome side effects. Hence, *motor urge incontinence is likely to be a long-term problem not easily resolved.* Theoretically, bladder retraining is ideal, since there are no side effects or surgery involved. If the patient responds initially, she is likely to respond to retraining should a recurrence develop.

SENSORY URGE INCONTINENCE

Sensory urge incontinence is diagnosed when incontinence occurs with a feeling of urgency in a stable bladder without marked descent of the urethra and bladder. The most common causes are *infection, diverticula, neoplasia, foreign body, and psychologic and neurologic factors.*

It is caused by either urethral relaxation or voluntary detrusor contraction. Normally, as the bladder fills, there is a reflex urge to urinate that is subconsciously inhibited until the bladder is full. Conditions that irritate the bladder or urethra (e.g., infection, trauma) over stimulate this reflex, resulting in intermittent urethral relaxation. This allows the *dribbling of small amounts of urine,* which further stimulates the bladder. If the patient fails to concentrate on maintaining continence, the detrusor may contract after urethral relaxation, resulting in a larger volume of urine lost.

Clinical findings typically include a *small bladder capacity* on cystometry that normalizes under anesthesia unless scarring is present. Urethral pressure profiles or simultaneous urethrocystometry reveals *urethral relaxation or marked variations in urethral pressure.* Cystometrograms show no detrusor activity as long as the patient *concentrates on not voiding.* Urethroscopy and cystoscopy are *essential* to avoid missing local treatable problems.

Treatment

Therapy is directed toward the direct cause if one is present. Treat infection (urinary or vaginal) with antibiotics. Chronic infection may have prolonged symptomatology due to the residual inflammation and edema long after bacteria have been destroyed. Urethral dilatation and instillation of anti-inflammatory agents into the bladder may provide relief. Neoplasia, diverticula, and calculi require surgery or lithotripsy. Estrogen deficiency may be responsible for sensory urge incontinence and is treated by estrogen replacement vaginally or orally.

The prognosis is good with cure of the underlying disorder. Chronic causes may result in recurrence or only partial relief.

OVERFLOW INCONTINENCE

Overflow incontinence is the result of urinary retention with subsequent overflow. Causes of retention are multiple. Neurogenic retention may be a result of a denervated bladder with diminished or absent detrusor contractions or from detrusor-sphincter dyssynergia, in which the urethra fails to relax with voiding attempts. Diabetes and lower motor neuron disorders are most commonly responsible. Also, obstruction of the urethra may occur postoperatively, with severe relaxation of pelvic supports, or from pelvic masses. Medications (e.g., ganglionic blockers, anticholinergic agents, alpha-adrenergic agonists, and spinal or epidural anesthesia) may cause overflow incontinence. Acute or chronic overdistention of the bladder results in myotonic decompensation and subsequent inability to contract. This may be idiopathic or psychogenic in origin.

Cystometric findings typically reveal a *large bladder capacity (as much as 1200 mL) with decreased sensation of the bladder and poor to absent detrusor contractility.*

Treatment

Treatment in cases of acute retention is directed toward *drainage to prevent myotonic decompensation, chronic retention, infection, and obstructive uropathy.* To reduce urethral closing pressure and increase detrusor contractility, alpha-adrenolytic agents (e.g., prazosin, phenoxybenzamine), striated muscle relaxants (e.g., diazepam, dantrolene), and cholinergic agents (e.g., bethanechol) are used. If the patient has chronic urinary retention, intermittent self-catheterization is helpful.

BYPASS INCONTINENCE

Urinary leakage will occur whenever the urethral sphincteric mechanism is bypassed. *Abnormalities, such as fistulas, ectopic ureters, and urethral diverticula, are the most common causes of bypass incontinence.* Both fistulas and diverticula may mimic GSUI, with exacerbation during stressful activity. The urinary diverticula may retain urine until the patient stands upright to walk or increases intraabdominal pressure, although the volume lost is usually less than with GSUI.

Treatment
Treatment is surgical with a good prognosis if successful. However, damage to the urethral sphincteric mechanism during surgery will result in incontinence.

PSYCHOGENIC INCONTINENCE

Stress incontinence, sensory urge incontinence, motor urge incontinence, and overflow incontinence may all have psychogenic origins. *Surgery is usually unsuccessful* in relieving psychogenic incontinence and *should be avoided if possible.* Psychiatric and medical therapy have the best chance of success as long as the patient's underlying psychologic conflicts are resolved.

INTERSTITIAL CYSTITIS

Interstitial cystitis is a *chronic inflammatory condition almost exclusively of women,* most of whom are perimenopausal. It may represent a defect in the protective glycosaminoglycan layer of the transitional epithelium (of uncertain origin) or an autoimmune disease.

Urinary frequency, urgency, suprapubic pain, discomfort with voiding, and dyspareunia strongly suggest urinary infection. When the *symptomatology persists despite treatment* for minimal urinary findings (including negative cultures), suspect interstitial cystitis. Interstitial cystitis is associated with stress or urge incontinence, which must be confirmed by urodynamic studies. Urethral syndrome is commonly a misdiagnosis for interstitial cystitis, but the latter may be noted in patients with hypersensitive bladders.

Chronicity of the urinary symptoms with suprapubic pain strongly suggests interstitial cystitis. Cystoscopy typically reveals a *pancystitis* and, occasionally, a localized *fibrotic scar(s)* or *ulceration (Hunner's ulcer).* Biopsies disclose *chronic inflammation* (including numerous mast cells) in the submucosa and muscularis, without evidence of cancer.

There is *no cure for interstitial cystitis.* Analgesics, bladder drill, or other feedback programs should relieve patients with slight to moderate interstitial cystitis. In severe cases, bladder distention under anesthesia or instillation of dimethyl sulfoxide or oxycholoresene sodium (Chlorpactin WCS-90) may give more lasting relief.

Resection or laser therapy of a Hunner ulcer may be helpful. Cystectomy or urinary diversion may be warranted in severe recalcitrant cases.

URETHRAL CARUNCLE

A small, *reddened, sensitive, fleshy excrescence at the urethral meatus is called a caruncle.* Most caruncles represent eversion (ectropion of the urethra) or infection at the urinary meatus or both; however, vascular anomalies or benign or malignant tumors also may cause caruncle formation. The vast majority of caruncles are benign, persistent lesions. Caruncles may occur at any age, but postmenopausal women are most commonly affected.

Caruncles appear as small, vividly red, sessile or flattened masses protruding from the urethral meatus. They may bleed, exude, or cause pain depending on the cause, size, and integrity. Dysuria, frequency, and urgency are uncommon. Laboratory tests are not diagnostic. If cancer is suspected, biopsy must be performed.

Estrogen therapy for postmenopausal women and avoidance of local irritation will probably *prevent and even heal caruncle* formation. Infections, including STDs, must be treated with appropriate antibiotics. Estrogen (vaginal suppositories of estradiol 0.5 mg every other night for 3 weeks) may be given before specific therapy in postmenopausal patients who have not been receiving estrogen.

If the caruncle is not markedly infected or malignant, light fulguration under local anesthesia, cryosurgery laser vaporization, or excision may be performed. If stenosis develops, the urethral meatus must be dilated. The prognosis is excellent in benign cases but guarded when malignant change has occurred.

URETHRAL DIVERTICULUM

Urethral diverticulum is a *sacculation caused by* (1) congenital cystic dilatation of paraurethral (wolffian) remnants; (2) infection of the paraurethral glands, with rupture to the urethra; or (3) urinary, obstetric, or gynecologic injury. Most patients are 40–50 years of age and multiparous.

The mid- or distal third of the urethra is the usual site. With congenital malformation, the cystic structure, usually 1–4 cm in diameter, may be an angled or multiloculated cavity. *Calculi* are present in the diverticulum in 10%–20% of patients.

Clinical Findings
Urinary urgency, frequency, nocturia, dribbling after urination, discharge of urinous or bloody, purulent fluid following stripping of

the urethra, vaginal pain, dyspareunia, urethral tenderness, pelvic discomfort, and vaginal fullness occur. There may be indefinite anterior vaginal fullness that is periodically painful.

Radiopaque contrast fluid studies generally will outline the diverticulum. Ultrasonography is not diagnostic. Insertion of a small urethral sound will demonstrate a slight stricture of the urethra and the diverticulum just beyond. Air cystoscopy or panendoscopy will reveal the *diverticular opening* in most cases.

Complications
Urethrovaginal fistula may follow unsuccessful diverticulectomy or spontaneous rupture (often during labor), erosion by stone, incisional drainage, or fulguration of the cystic abnormality. Transitional cell carcinoma or adenocarcinoma may develop in urethral diverticula. *Stricture of the urethra* may be a consequence of extensive or complicated surgery.

Differential Diagnosis
Urethritis is unassociated with postvoiding discharge or local fullness. Urethral abscess is a phase of diverticulum development. Urethrocele is not a swelling or herniation but a disengagement of the urethra from the points of attachment. Tumors may be primary or secondary and are firm, semifixed, and nontender.

Treatment
Transvaginal diverticulectomy with urethral catheter drainage for 10 days for patients with a symptomatic urethral cyst usually is curative.

URINARY TRACT INJURIES FOLLOWING OBSTETRIC AND GYNECOLOGIC SURGERY

Iatrogenic fistulas may occur in any part of the urinary tract and result from direct or indirect injury. Occlusions usually involve the *ureter* and occur as a *result of angulation or obstruction by a suture, scarring after injury, endometriosis or infection or as a complication of the treatment of pelvic cancer.* The kidney is rarely damaged directly during gynecologic surgery. The incidence of urinary tract injury in medical centers in the United States is about *0.8% following major gynecologic surgery and 0.08% following obstetric surgery.*

Postpartum fistulas of the bladder or urethra generally are caused by continued pressure of the presenting part or by instrumentation.

There is usually a history of prolonged labor (especially of the second stage) or complicated operative delivery.

CLINICAL FINDINGS

Symptoms and Signs

Unilateral ureteral injury usually causes flank pain, tenderness, and fever but does not alter the urinary volume. Ureteral injury may result in constriction of the ureter, fistula, or infection. Escape of urine from the abdominal or vaginal incision indicates ureteral or bladder fistulas or both. *Ileus often follows urinary obstruction or extravasation.* Urinary infection, especially with partial obstruction of the ureter, results in chills, fever, renal pain, and costovertebral and loin tenderness. *In the absence of preexisting bacteriuria, complete obstruction of one ureter usually is asymptomatic.* If urine leaks into the peritoneal cavity, there will be signs of free peritoneal fluid and peritoneal irritation. If leakage is retroperitoneal, regional pain and a fluid collection will develop.

Signs of perirenal or psoas inflammation are secondary to retroperitoneal extravasation or urine. *Anuria and uremia follow complete bilateral ureteral occlusion.* In acute cases, rule out dehydration, shock, lower nephron nephrosis, and congestive heart failure.

Laboratory Findings

- Passage of a *urethral catheter* should reveal obstruction.
- *Urethroscopy* will often expose blockage, perforating suture, or fistula.
- *Cystoscopy* will disclose large vesical fistulas, but small fistulas may escape detection.
- *Retrograde studies* of the urinary tract are especially useful to rule out ureteral injury. If the ureteral catheters pass readily to both renal pelves and clear urine is returned, ureteral injury is excluded, except perhaps in a case of a crushing injury or small perforation. If one of these complications seems likely, the catheter should be secured in the ureter for splinting and drainage for the 10–14 days necessary for healing.

URETERAL CONSTRICTION

Obtain *blood creatine and BUN tests* to identify renal impairment. *Ultrasonographic or x-ray findings* may disclose ureteral obstruction, fistula, or urinary extravasation. CT is the best radiographic modality for evaluating ureteral obstruction. It can also assess the degree of renal compromise, determine the site of a fistula or an obstruction, and determine the presence of extravasated urine.

Even the freshly *occluded kidney will not excrete the contrast agent on excretory urography*. Although the urogram can be used as a screening test, it is not as sensitive as CT for detecting extravasated urine. Moreover, the presence of intestinal gas will reduce the clarity of the roentgenogram.

Retrograde urography may be useful when a ureteral catheter is blocked by an occlusion. A radiopaque catheter should be used so that the level of the obstruction can be observed on the film. Injection of a contrast medium into a Braach bulb catheter may reveal a fistula above the bulb fixed in the most distal portion of the ureter.

Bladder Fistula and Extravasation

Obtain an anteroposterior scout film of the pelvis. Fill the bladder with 50 mL of suitable radiopaque medium in 200 mL of water, and take a second film. Drain the bladder, and obtain a third film at once. Slight extravasation, not visible in the second film, may be clearly seen in the third.

Complications

Peritonitis is the most serious complication of urinary tract injury. *Anuria or oliguria* may be associated with fatal uremia after bilateral ureteral occlusion. Other complications are *psoas or perirenal abscess or thrombophlebitis*. *Urinary tract infection* usually follows partial ureteral obstruction.

DIFFERENTIAL DIAGNOSIS

Clear, yellowish, odorless drainage from the abdominal wound may represent ascites or exudative peritoneal fluid, an antecedent of wound dehiscence. Thin, brownish discharge from an abdominal or vaginal suture line may be serum from a seroma or hematoma. In ureteral obstruction, oliguria or anuria may be due to shock, dehydration, or lower nephron nephrosis; abdominal distention may indicate dynamic ileus caused by intestinal obstruction or adynamic ileus due to peritonitis; fever may be due to an infected wound, peritonitis, or thrombophlebitis; and kidney pain and costovertebral or flank tenderness may be due to nephrolithiasis, ureterolithiasis, or pyelonephritis.

PREVENTION

Adequate *preliminary studies* of the urinary tract and *full knowledge* of the anatomy and pathologic processes involved are essential before surgery. The ureters should be catheterized and identified initially in all difficult cases, and the wire stylet should be left in the ureteral catheter for identification—to prevent the ureter from being cut or clamped by mistake.

All *structures must be identified* before clamping, incision, and ligation, and *care must be taken to prevent undue traction* and needless denudation of the ureter and base of the bladder. Only fine absorbable sutures should be used in or around the urinary tract. Multiple ligatures should not be used for hemorrhage. Instead, pressure should be applied and a single bleeding point secured. The integrity of the bladder and the course of the ureters must be traced at the completion of each abdominal operation if surgery was near the ureter.

The surgeon should personally remove ureteral catheters after surgery if it is decided not to leave them in place. A hang-up may indicate ureteral constriction.

TREATMENT

Emergency Measures
Treat shock, blood loss, and dehydration as indicated and catheterize the bladder. If oliguria or anuria is present, obtain creatine and BUN. Check the specific gravity of the urine.

Surgical Measures

Bilateral Ureteral Obstruction
If both ureters are obstructed and the patient is a poor surgical risk, nephrostomy or unilateral tube ureterostomy is preferred. Use the largest urethral catheter that will enter the ureter. The other kidney should not be left obstructed for more than a few days. As soon as the patient becomes a satisfactory operative risk, relieve the second blocked kidney by nephrostomy or tube ureterostomy. Deligation alone is not satisfactory unless it can be performed easily. If deligation is done, insert a splinting catheter through a longitudinal incision several centimeters above the point of obstruction, pass it to the kidney, bring it out from the urethra, and fix it to a Foley retention catheter for 10–14 days. Then remove both catheters. The retroperitoneal area must always be drained through a separate lower quadrant or flank stab wound.

A gallbladder T tube can be used in lieu of a catheter when the cross arm of the T is notched at the vertical segment; the ureter is incised longitudinally several centimeters about the defect; the tube is inserted so that its lower arm splints the point of injury; the upper arm of the tube is fixed in the proximal ureter, and the long arm is carried out retroperitoneally through a stab wound in the flank; a drain is placed in the retroperitoneal space underlying the T tube and allowed to remain until drainage ceases (about 1 week after removal of the tube).

Vesicoperitoneal Fistula

Perform laparotomy as soon as the diagnosis is established. With closure of the fistula in two layers using fine catgut, avoid the mucosa in suturing. Drain the bladder by cystostomy or with a Foley retention catheter, and use pelvic suction drainage for about 7 days.

Vesicovaginal Fistula

Treat local infection by removing old sutures and concretions and by giving systemic antibiotics. Repair is indicated as outlined for vesicoperitoneal fistula. In general, attempts at closure should be delayed until 4 months or more after injury, although the use of steroids and intensive antibiotics may allow more immediate repair. All but large, inaccessible, immobile vesicovaginal fistulas (85%–90% of the total) should be closed transvaginally.

Ureterovesicovaginal Fistula

Close the fistula abdominally using relatively few fine, absorbable, interrupted mattress sutures and avoiding the mucosa. Pursestring sutures should not be used.

Reimplantation of the severely damaged or severed ureter into the bladder (ureteroneocystostomy) is preferable to ureteroenterostomy on the same side. The bladder should be drained by cystostomy or with a Foley retention catheter, and suction drainage should be used for about 7 days.

Ligation of the damaged ureter and sacrifice of the kidney on the involved side are almost always contraindicated. The opposite kidney may be deficient or it may fail.

PROGNOSIS

Most *ureteral repairs are successful if performed carefully* and if urinary and extraperitoneal drainage is ensured. Very *small vesicovaginal fistulas often close spontaneously if the bladder can be kept collapsed and infection prevented. Urethral fistulas are notoriously resistant* to spontaneous closure if a urethral catheter is used. Many heal well, however, when simply repaired and when a *cystostomy* is used instead of a urethral catheter.

ANORECTAL PROBLEMS

Common lesions of the anal canal are shown in Figure 30-12.

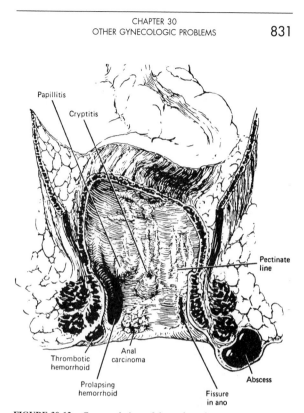

FIGURE 30-12. Common lesions of the anal canal.
(From J.L. Wilson, *Handbook of Surgery,* 5th ed. Lange, 1973.)

PROCTALGIA FUGAX

Proctalgia fugax, so-called *rectal spasm or rectal neuralgia, is a sudden cramping rectal pain of short duration.* It is *uncommon, and its cause is not known.* However, partial intussusception of redundant rectal mucosa is suspected. Cramping rectal pain begins without warning, ranges in intensity from marked to agonizing, and tends to recur. The discomfort starts low in the rectum and moves higher (perhaps combined with the urge to defecate). Pain is associated with sweating, agitation, and even collapse. It subsides gradually, leaving the patient weak and shaken.

Rectal examination readily differentiates proctalgia fugax from thrombosed hemorrhoids, fissure in ano, or abscess. The pain of factitial proctitis, which may follow intravaginal radium therapy or local treatment of acute rectal disease, is constant and is accompanied by rectal bleeding and ulceration. Sigmoidorectal obstruction causes extreme, unrelenting, progressive pain and is not likely to recur.

Ample sedation and filling of the rectum with 200–300 mL of air or warm fluid may give dramatic relief. Recurrent attacks may be treated by submucosal injections of a solution containing 4% phenol, 50% glycerine, and water. Injections of 1 mL each at four points 1 cm apart just below the rectosigmoid junction may be curative.

ANAL CONDYLOMAS

(See Condylomata Acuminata, p. 578)

HEMORRHOIDS

Hemorrhoids ("piles") are *anorectal varicosities* caused by lax pelvic veins and venous stasis. *Internal hemorrhoids* lie above the anorectal or mucocutaneous dentate line and are derived from the superior and middle hemorrhoidal veins. They usually are located in the right anterior and both posterior quadrants of the rectum. Internal hemorrhoids are covered by a thin rectal mucosa and are innervated by autonomic nerves. *External hemorrhoids* develop below the mucocutaneous line and may appear in any quadrant. They are covered by skin, are supplied by the inferior hemorrhoidal vein, and are innervated by cutaneous nerves. Combined external and internal hemorrhoids are uncommon, but they may be serious if they involve at least a third of the anorectal margin.

Hemorrhoids cause *itching, pain* (the most severe occurs with thrombosis), *protrusion, and bleeding.* Most women with hemorrhoids develop them during pregnancy or delivery. Never assume that hemorrhoids are the cause of bleeding from the bowel until careful and complete physical, proctologic, and laboratory studies have failed to reveal cancer, a benign tumor, or other local or systemic disease.

Prevention includes good bowel habits, avoidance of straining, and prompt treatment of diarrhea and anorectal disorders. No therapy is required for asymptomatic hemorrhoids. Stool softeners, laxatives, and fiber-rich foods together with ample fluids should be given.

Hemorrhoids causing *mild or infrequent symptoms* are treated with warm sitz baths, astringent ointments, or suppositories and oral analgesics. Avoid using sensitizing local anesthetics or antibiotics. Take measures to correct faulty bowel function.

Hemorrhoids with *moderate symptoms* (large or prolapsed hemorrhoids) should be treated as for mild symptoms. One hemorrhoid a week may be injected with 1 mL of 5% quinine and urea solution or 5% sodium morrhuate solution using a 22-gauge needle. Hemorrhoids with *severe symptoms* (large or strangulated hemorrhoids) are acutely painful. These and thrombosed external hemorrhoids should be *incised under local anesthesia* and the clot removed. For the first 24 h after clot formation, treat as for mild symptoms. Later, consider hemorrhoidectomy.

Symptomatic hemorrhoids during pregnancy should be treated for mild symptoms if possible. Hemorrhoidectomy should be deferred until after the puerperium.

Open radial hemorrhoidectomy (vascular ligation and excision) is the preferred surgical method. A cleansing enema should be administered before hemorrhoidectomy. Avoid packs or drains after surgery. Cover the incision with moist gel sponge. The patient should receive daily sitz baths, mild laxatives, and parenteral analgesics. Antibiotics may be given if needed. Perform gentle digital rectal dilation 5–7 days postoperatively and repeat two or three times every 5–7 days to prevent bridging and fistula formation.

Complications of hemorrhoidectomy include postoperative bleeding, perianal hematoma, infection, fecal impaction, delayed healing (with granulation tissue), rectal stenosis, and recurrence of hemorrhoids. Hemorrhoids are never precancerous, but cancer may coexist. Hemorrhoidectomy is curative. Hemorrhoids are unlikely to be permanently cured by injection therapy, but complications are uncommon.

FISSURE IN ANO

Anorectal mucosal lacerations occur frequently as a *result of sudden or marked distention* (e.g., during a difficult bowel movement). Acute fissures, although temporarily painful and perhaps associated with scant bleeding, generally heal rapidly. *Chronic fissures* may be persistent: either they fail to heal, or they heal and break down. Recurrent fissures may be associated with the eventual development of a sentinel pile, hypertrophic papillae, and anal spasm (especially painful on rectal examination).

Treatment of acute fissures is the same as that for hemorrhoids with mild symptoms. A single application of a mild styptic, such as 1% silver nitrate solution, may be beneficial.

For *chronic or recurrent fissures, surgical excision* of the sentinel pile or papilla and the fissure, preferably without suture closure, may be required. Postoperative care is similar to that after hemorrhoidectomy.

FISTULA IN ANO

Anal fistula (Fig. 30-13) is a chronically suppurating rectoperineal tract usually caused by pyogenic bacteria, often after obstetric trauma. A complete fistula has an internal (rectal) opening and one of more external (perianal) openings. An incomplete or blind fistula has an internal opening only.

Many others are associated with repair of a third-degree or fourth-degree perineal laceration. Anal fistulas also develop from an anal crypt, usually preceded by anal abscess.

Pain is reported when the fistula closes temporarily, suppuration develops, and drainage brings relief. *Periodic soiling* by fecal discharge is a common complaint. If the internal opening of a complete fistula is above the sphincter, *involuntary passage of flatus* is reported commonly.

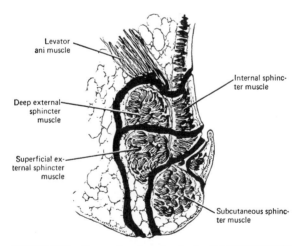

Levator ani muscle

Internal sphincter muscle

Deep external sphincter muscle

Superficial external sphincter muscle

Subcutaneous sphincter muscle

FIGURE 30-13.   Cross-section of muscles of anal wall showing usual paths of anal fistulas.

(From J.L. Wilson, *Handbook of Surgery,* 5th ed. Lange, 1973.)

Devious sinus tracts cause difficulty in identification of the internal opening. Injection of 1 part hydrogen peroxide and 2 parts methylene blue into the external openings releases oxygen by contact with the discharges. The blue dye is carried through the tract, and on anoscopic examination, the colored solution can be seen to bubble from the opening. For *x-ray studies,* injection of iodized oil (Lipiodol) may outline the fistulous tract.

Intestinal parasites should be identified by means of scrapings. Proper closure of an episiotomy or a complete perineal laceration usually will prevent fistula in ano. Prompt and adequate treatment of proctitis should prevent fistula in ano.

Chemotherapy should be used if parasites (e.g., *Eilistlytica*) are present. *Incision of the entire fistula with excision of all portions of the tract is the only curative treatment.* If the fistula is not totally exposed and removed, recurrence is likely.

ANAL INCONTINENCE

Anal incontinence follows obstetric lacerations, anorectal operations (especially fistulectomy), and neurologic disorders involving spinal nerves S2–4. When incontinence is the result of trauma or a complication of surgery, operative correction is indicated after the inflammation has subsided and initial healing is complete. Most serious lacerations due to childbirth injury should not be repaired until about 6 months after delivery.

ANAL CANCER

Anal cancer—almost always squamous cell type—represents only 1%–2% of all cancers of the colon, rectum, and anus. The cause is not known, but chronic granulomatous anal lesions are suspected.

Anal cancer appears as a slightly raised, firm, ulcerative, and slightly tender area. Anal cancer is frequently confused with chronic fissures in ano or bleeding hemorrhoids and is treated palliatively. It may be difficult to cure if the cancer extends upward into the sphincter and around the anus and metastasizes to the inguinal glands.

Biopsy of suspected or frankly tumorous anal lesions should be done under local anesthesia. Ample excision of very small anal cancers is feasible. Most lesions are large when they are first diagnosed accurately, however, and require abdominoperineal resection and radical groin resection. Radiation treatment, even for palliation, is unsatisfactory. The 5-year survival rate is only about 50%.

CHRONIC PELVIC PAIN

Acute pelvic pain and pain of <3 months duration are more likely to have identifiable causes, whereas it is unlikely to find the initiating etiology of most subacute (3–6 months duration) and chronic (>6 months duration) pain. Characteristically, the originating *event triggered pain* and the *pain led to affective responses* (suffering), which overtime, *led to pain behavior.* The cumulative adaptive changes collectively known as pain behavior may be functional or dysfunctional and are made based on the pain (that may no longer even be present). Chronic pain may be categorized as: *structural* (from ongoing diseases, e.g., cancer, osteoarthritis) *psychophysiologic* (e.g., muscle spasm leading to pain after the original insult has passed), and *somatic* (the internalization of stress which is expressed as pain). Some have labeled the latter two groups psychogenic or functional. Both tend to be chronic or recurrent. Women *25–45 years* of age are most susceptible. The reported incidence in gynecologic patients in the United States is *5%–25%,* depending on the interests and skills of the reporting physician.

Pain not attributable to physical causes may result from exaggeration of normal physiologic impulses, ignorance, fear, or tension, or from a lowered perceptual threshold to disturbing stimuli. Pain is associated with past or present environmental factors. The patient's complaint is often fixed on one anatomic area or organ system.

Before the pain is labeled psychogenic, there are four other alternatives to consider: the pain is from a disease process that is not yet detectable, the pain may be associated with vascular disorders where no disease process can be observed, the pain may be due to nongynecologic causes (e.g., gastrointestinal, genitourinary, or skeletal), and the psychogenic overlay is the result of chronic pain. A reasonable approach is to determine what organic problems are present and what psychologic factors are present and to treat both.

CLINICAL FINDINGS

SYMPTOMS AND SIGNS

Complaints are almost invariably multiple. In addition to pelvic pain, most patients also report dyspareunia, dysmenorrhea, abnormal menses, and other pelvic complaints. There may be numerous abdominal scars, indicating *polysurgery.* The patient insists that she is in great pain, but in at least 25% of cases, *no physical*

*abnormality can be found. In the rest, insignificant physical varia-
tions or minimal lesions may be present.*

The *historical investigation* should include a description and
timing of the pain (when, where, why, what relation to menses, relation to stress, degree, and character). It should be determined if
the patient has pain in other parts of the body (e.g., headache, backache, or genitourinary tract pain). A careful menstrual and sexual
history should be taken. Her work and leisure habits should be discussed. Inquiry should be made about pelvic and abdominal infections, previous operative procedures, and other gynecologic disorders (e.g., endometriosis, adenomyosis). A thoughtful social history
should be obtained, including marital status, children, stresses in
life (childhood, adolescent, and adult), and history of physical or
sexual abuse. Patients with chronic pelvic pain are more likely to
experience depression, substance abuse, sexual dysfunction, sleep
disorders, and somatization disorders. They are more likely to have
been sexually abused as a child or as an adult. Contributing factors
in the patient's life should be elicited, including physical or sexual
abuse, rape or incest, domestic discord, parental divorce, alcohol or
drug abuse, and so forth.

*A baseline general physical and neurologic examination is nec-
essary in every chronic pelvic pain case. Both the abdominal and
pelvic examinations should focus specific attention on pain reproduction.* Whereas laboratory evaluations are tailored to each patient
they often include CBC, ESR, VDRL, UA and culture, and cervical cytology.

SPECIAL EXAMINATIONS

Ruling Out Organic Disease
After appropriate initial evaluation, it may be necessary to rule out
organic disease by laparoscopy, ultrasound, CT scan, MRI, gastrointestinal endoscopy, and genitourinary studies. Psychologic testing should be performed by those expert in the field. Recall that
*minor abnormalities of the genitourinary system are frequently in-
appropriately blamed for chronic pelvic pain.*

COMPLICATIONS

*Psychoneurosis may progress to psychosis. A despondent patient
may commit suicide.* If unaffected uterus or ovaries are removed,
the symptoms may be transferred to the gastrointestinal or urinary
tract.

DIFFERENTIAL DIAGNOSIS

Psychogenic disease can be differentiated from organic disease by ruling out the latter or by recognition of psychoneurosis or psychosis while investigating organic pathology. Most patients with psychogenic pelvic pain have many characteristic features that make a direct diagnosis possible without extensive studies.

Chronic salpingitis or urinary tract infection, spastic and other types of colitis, and endometriosis must be ruled out, perhaps by laparoscopy. A comparison of organic and psychogenic pelvic pain may be helpful in diagnosis (Table 30-1).

TABLE 30-1
DIFFERENTIATION OF ORGANIC
AND PSYCHOGENIC PAIN

	Organic	Psychogenic
Type	Sharp, cramping, intermittent	Dull, continuous
Time of onset	Any time; may awaken patient	Usually begins well after waking, when social obligations are pressing
Localization	Localizes with typical point tenderness	Variable, shifting, generalized
Progress	Soon becomes either better or worse	Remains the same for weeks, months, or years
Provocative tests	Often reproduced or augmented by tests or manipulation, not mood	Not triggered or accentuated by examination but by interpersonal relationships

PREVENTION

Sex education, counseling, and early recognition and treatment of emotional illness are the best preventive measures.

TREATMENT

After examination and observation, the *patient should be reassured and given simple symptomatic therapy.* The physician must be *empathetic, unhurried, a good listener, and skilled in positive reinforcement and support.*

Once the diagnosis is established, the disorder must be explained to the patient in direct, convincing terms. The patient should be *given an acceptable escape.* A useful analogy may be that of tension headache. The physicians must gain the patient's cooperation, perhaps via reorientation and reeducation. A key is to *treat the patient promptly and continue on a regular basis.*

Simple analgesics are useful. Do not give sedatives, tranquilizers, amphetamines, or narcotics because these patients are prone to addiction. Sedatives may lead to depression and suicide. *Be prepared to spend a great deal of time talking to the patient. Do not perform operative procedures except on definite surgical indications. Psychotherapy or referral to a psychiatrist may be required. Every effort must be made to assist her to adjust socially.*

PROGNOSIS

These patients *often refuse psychotherapy, withdraw early from a treatment program, and change physicians frequently. The medical future is bleak unless the patient confronts the real problem.* Reassurance and symptomatic therapy result in temporary improvement in about three fourths of patients. Psychiatric treatment results in lasting improvement in many patients.

DYSPAREUNIA

Dyspareunia (painful coitus) may be functional (psychogenic), organic, or both. Functional dyspareunia occurs most frequently and is more difficult to treat. Either type may occur early (primary) or late (secondary) in the sexually active interval of life. The site of discomfort may be external (at the introitus) or internal (deep within the vagina or beyond), and some women describe both types of pain. Functional dyspareunia may be caused by psychosexual problems, a previous extremely negative experience (e.g., sexual molestation), fear of genital damage, fear of sexually transmittable disease, or fear of pregnancy.

Vaginismus, an involuntary spasm of the muscles of the introitus and levators when the thighs are abducted, *is an indication of extreme anxiety.* It may be due to psychologic factors or personal emotional problems, or it may occur in anticipation of or in response to pain.

External organic dyspareunia may be due to an occlusive or rigid hymen, vaginal contracture due to any cause, or inflammatory disorders. Traumatic or infectious processes are seen in younger patients and atrophic vulvovaginitis in postmenopausal women.

Organic causes of internal dyspareunia include vaginal disorders, severe cervicitis, marked fundal retroposition, uterine prolapse or neoplasm, tuboovarian disease, pelvic endometriosis, and severe disorders of the lower urinary tract or colon.

Psychiatric evaluation is indicated if complex psychosexual problems seem to be present. Specialized techniques of physical examination (e.g., cystoscopy, may be required to rule out organic disease).

Functional dyspareunia can be treated only by counseling and psychotherapy. Both partners should be interviewed. Information on contraception is often helpful. The importance of foreplay before sexual intercourse must be emphasized. An appropriate water-soluble vaginal gel may be useful. Adequate estrogen treatment often is required for postmenopausal women.

For functional dyspareunia, hymenal-vaginal dilations by the patient with a conical (Kelly) dilator or test tubes of graduated sizes may give confidence. Lubricants or anesthetic ointment applied to the introitus gives some relief but is of no permanent value.

The treatment of organic dyspareunia varies and depends on the basic underlying cause. Organic dyspareunia due to vaginal dryness may be treated with a water-soluble lubricant. Estrogen therapy is indicated for senile vulvovaginitis.

Hymenotomy, hymenectomy, perineotomy, and similar procedures should be performed only on *clear indications.* Obstructive lesions should be corrected. Treat symptomatic vaginitis or cervicitis appropriately. Few patients with functional dyspareunia are quickly and easily cured, even with psychotherapy. Organic dyspareunia subsides promptly after elimination of the cause.

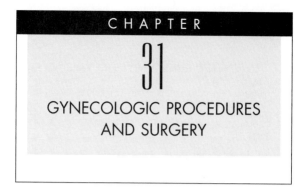

GYNECOLOGIC PROCEDURES

EXFOLIATIVE CERVICAL CYTOLOGIC STUDY (PAPANICOLAOU SMEAR)

Exfoliative cytologic examination of specimens from the lower genital tract (Pap smear) is a screening tool that has been so valuable in the detection of premalignant and malignant lesions that it has been almost universally adopted as the primary cancer screening method for cervical cancer, an integral part of the health care of women. This has resulted in a >50% reduction of invasive cancers of the cervix alone. Although cervical cytology may detect endometrial cancer (in 15%–50%), it does not carry the same reliability as a screening tool for endometrial neoplasia.

SCREENING GUIDELINES

- *Initial gynecologic screening* at age 18, or when the individual becomes sexually active.
- *Women whose initial smear is negative* (without significant atypia) *should have a second smear within 1 year* to rule out a false-negative smear.
- *High-risk women should be screened annually* (i.e., those with a history of early sexual activity or those with multiple sexual partners).
- *Low-risk women may be screened every 1–3 years* at the discretion of the physician. These are women with late exposure to coitus, those with only one sexual partner, and women after two successive negative annual smears. (Some authorities contend it is too difficult to ascertain low risk and simply recommend annual screening.)

- *Postmenopausal women* should receive annual screening.
- *Women after hysterectomy* should have an initial smear following surgery; if this is negative, cytology should be repeated every 3 years.

TECHNIQUE

Materials necessary for a Pap smear include a cervical spatula, shaped tongue depressor or cotton swab, glass slides and a means to identify the slide and patient, a speculum (warm, without lubricant), and a jar of fixative (97% ethanol) or spray fixative (e.g., Pro-Fixx or AquaNet) (Fig. 31-1).

The objective is to sample secretions from the endocervical canal, the transformation zone, and the vaginal pool. The last site is less productive and, therefore, of lesser priority. Sampling is accomplished by gently wiping away excess mucus and obtaining endocervical canal samples using the moist cotton swab or cervical spatula. This is smeared onto a glass slide and fixed. A spatula with an endocervical extension, or similar device is used to lightly scrape the entire transformation zone. In those with a small external os, a brush device may be helpful in guaranteeing that endocervical cells are sampled. This sample is spread on a slide and fixed immediately. Finally, the vaginal pool may be sampled by using the same spatula (again, fixing immediately). The reporting of cervical cytologic results is discussed on p. 524.

COLPOSCOPY

The colposcope is a binocular microscope of low magnification (10–40×) used for direct visualization of the cervix. Although colposcopy does not replace other methods of diagnosing cervical abnormalities, it is an important additional tool. *The patients who most benefit from colposcopy* are those with abnormal Pap smears. Colposcopy is also used to evaluate women who were exposed to DES in utero and in gynecologic cancer therapy follow-up.

Occult neoplasms in the upper cervical canal, where 10% –15% of cervical cancers develop, *cannot be detected by colposcopy.* Therefore, *endocervical curettage* should be performed in women who are being evaluated for abnormal cervical cytology.

Normally, columnar epithelium covers the ectocervix until adolescence, when it gradually changes to a squamous surface. The transformation zone can be inspected easily with the colposcope, and *dysplastic surface changes can be identified.* These include white epithelium (e.g., sheet of layered metaplastic cells), a mosaic pattern (e.g., sharply outlined cells and cell groups), punctation (e.g.,

Materials Needed:

One cervical spatula, cut tongue depressor, or cotton swab.

One glass slide (one end frosted). Identify by writing the patient's name on the frosted end with a lead pencil.

One speculum (warm but without lubricant).

One bottle of fixative (97% ethanol) or spray-on fixative, eg, Pro-Fixx or Aqua-Net.

1. Obtain vaginal pool material from the posterior fornix.

2. Place adequate drop 1 inch from end of slide, smear, fix, and dry.

3. Obtain cervical scraping from complete squamocolumnar junction by rotating spatula 360° around external os, high up in the endocervical canal.

4. Place the material 1 inch from end of slide, smear, fix, and dry.

FIGURE 31-1. Preparation of a Papanicolaou cytosmear.

vascular tufts between cell clusters), and leukoplakia (e.g., abnormal pale cell plaques).

Colposcopy allows recognition of cellular dysplasia and vascular or tissue abnormalities not otherwise visible. Colposcopy allows *selection of cancer-suspicious areas for biopsy.* A green filter accentuates the *vascular changes* (which frequently accompany pathologic alteration). Dilute (3%) acetic acid solution is used to remove mucus and to facilitate visualization. Other chemical agents and stains may also be used to improve visualization. A camera attached to the colposcope facilitates follow-up. Colposcope-directed biopsy decreases the number of false-negative reports and may eliminate the need for conization of the cervix, a cause of morbidity.

To perform colposcopy, proceed as follows.

- *Insert* a speculum and visualize the cervix.
- *Cleanse* the cervix with 3% acetic acid. This removes excess mucus, blanches the surface, and accentuates normal epithelium.
- *Focus* the colposcope on the cervix, beginning with low power (usually 13.5×). Inspect the squamocolumnar junction (transformation zone) carefully. A significantly abnormal area usually can be fully outlined.
- Take *biopsy* specimens with a Kevorkian or similar biopsy forceps, and record the sites most suggestive of cancer.
- *Consider* whether *endocervical curettage* should be performed.

Effective use of the colposcope requires thorough training and extensive experience.

EVALUATION OF PATIENT WITH ABNORMAL CERVICAL CYTOLOGY

In summary, a normal smear requires follow-up as noted previously. *Atypical squamous cells of undetermined significance* identifies cells that need *further studies to identify if they are reactive or neoplastic.* In these cases, if there is clinical infection, treatment against the offending agent with repeat cytology 6–8 weeks after the infection is eliminated and the tissue has healed may be all that is necessary. The more *ominous nature of atypical glandular cells of undetermined significance requires an evaluation for endocervical, endometrial, tubal, or ovarian pathology.*

Low-grade squamous intraepithelial lesions (LGSIL) include grade I cervical intraepithelial neoplasia (CIN), also termed mild dysplasia, and human papillomavirus lesions. Whereas *high-grade squamous intraepithelial lesion* (HGSIL) includes moderate and severe dysplasia (CIN II and III). Thus, when these reports are returned, prompt colposcopy is warranted. Any abnormal areas must be biopsied, and endocervical curettage must be performed. Possible invasive cancer requires immediate colposcopy and biopsy (including conization if necessary).

CULDOCENTESIS

(See Ectopic pregnancy, p. 311)

SOUNDING THE UTERUS

The *uterus may be sounded to* determine the patency of the cervical canal, the presence of cervical or uterine lesions that will bleed on contact, the size of the uterus, the position of the uterine fundus, and the direction of the uterine canal (before endometrial biopsy or other instrumentation). *Intrauterine pregnancy must be ruled out* before uterine sounding. Use a sterile, malleable, calibrated (in centimeters) instrument (e.g., Sims or Simpson uterine sound).

Visualize the external cervix with a speculum, and carefully *apply* an antiseptic solution (e.g., povidone-iodine). *Bend the sound* to the estimated curvature of the cervicouterine axis. After *warning the patient* of possible slight pain, *grasp the cervix* (on either anterior or posterior lip) by a double-toothed Braun or Allis clamp and exert gentle traction toward the introitus, using the nondominant hand. This immobilizes the cervix and straightens the endocervical canal.

Use the index finger and thumb of the dominant hand to *gently insert the sound in the cervicouterine axis* while pressing the third and fourth fingers against the vulva to brace the hand. A slight, transient resistance may be encountered at the level of the internal os. An obvious obstruction is encountered at the vault of the uterine cavity. Exert special care to *avoid perforation of the uterus* at the level of the cervicouterine junction (particularly in marked flexion) and at the top of the fundus. Note the length of the cervical canal, the direction of the axis, the depth of the uterine cavity, and any obstruction, distortion, or free bleeding.

In the absence of cervical stenosis and extreme flexion of the corpus, gentle traction and sounding of the uterus cause only a few slightly menstrual-like cramps. Careful patient preparation and analgesics, if necessary, make the procedure tolerable.

If sounding of the uterus is impossible with the usual instruments, it may be initiated using a fine, soft wire probe, followed by Hegar dilators (#5–10). The diagnosis of an abnormally wide internal cervical os (notably incompetent) is confirmed if #8 Hegar dilator passes without resistance.

BIOPSIES

VULVAR

(See p. 588)

CERVICAL

Multiple *cervical biopsies may be performed in the office* with little or no discomfort or danger, using Tischler, Schubert, Kevorkian, or similar punch biopsy forceps. Polypoid lesions may be removed by torsion or excision (Figs. 31-2 and 31-3). For microscopic analysis, do not crush the tissue. Anesthetics are not required because the *cervix is relatively insensitive* to this type of pain.

After *detailing the areas to be biopsied by colcoscopy,* immobilize the cervix using a tenaculum. First biopsy the posterior lip (so bleeding from more anterior biopsies will not obscure the field). The most frequent biopsy sites are at or *near the squamocolumnar junction.* Place the tissue in fixative (e.g., 10% formalin) immediately. Bleeding is variable and unpredictable. If necessary, *control bleeding* by pressure, Negatol, acetone, 5% silver nitrate solution, or fine catgut sutures.

ENDOCERVICAL CURETTAGE

This procedure is commonly used as an *adjunct to colposcopy in an effort to guarantee sampling of the entire endocervix.* Stabilize

FIGURE 31-2.   Multiple punch biopsy of cervix with Tischler.

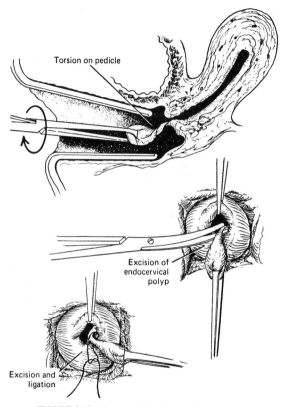

Torsion on pedicle

Excision of
endocervical
polyp

Excision and
ligation

FIGURE 31-3.   Three methods of cervical polypectomy.

the cervix using a tenaculum or Allis clamp, and curette the endocervix throughout its circumference by taking downward strokes
from the internal to the external os with a Kevorkian or other small
curet. Fix these strips of tissue immediately and submit them for
pathologic diagnosis. Anesthesia is rarely required, the procedure
generally is very short (<2 min), and bleeding is minimal. The principal complication is uterine perforation (usually at the cervicouterine junction).

ENDOMETRIAL BIOPSY

For *endometrial biopsy,* no anesthesia or only mild analgesia or paracervical block is required. *Contraindications* to endometrial biopsy include pregnancy; marked cervical stenosis; acute cervicitis; friable, bleeding cervical abnormalities; and profuse bleeding at the initiation of endometrial curettage.

The most common endometrial biopsy instrument currently used is a tubular plastic device for aspiration of strips of endometrium. After antiseptic preparation, sound the uterus. Next, direct the curet to the fundus and gently stroke downward against the uterine wall to the cervix while exerting gentle suction. Perform on both anterior and posterior uterine walls. Place the tissue obtained in fixative immediately.

INDUCED ABORTION

DEFINITION, INCIDENCE AND ASSOCIATIONS

In the United States, *elective abortion is persistently controversial.* Our purpose is to provide timely information, not to debate issues or enter into controversy. Therefore, in this summary there is no attempt to influence patients or health care providers for or against abortion, and none should be inferred. The statistical data in the following is summarized from the most authoritative source available at the time of writing, (i.e., Koonin LM, Strauss LT, Chrisman CE, Montalbano MA, Bartlett LA, Smith JC. Abortion Surveillance—United States, 1996, *Morbidity and Mortality Weekly Report,* July 30, 1999, 48:1–42).

The U.S. Centers for Disease Control and Prevention (CDC) defines legal induced abortion as *a procedure performed by a licensed physician or someone acting under the supervision of a licensed physician, that was intended to terminate a suspected or known intrauterine pregnancy and to produce a nonviable fetus at any gestational age.* Absolute numbers of abortions are not as sensitive an index of utilization by women in the reproductive years as are the *abortion ratio* (the number of abortions per 1000 live births per year in a given age group) and the abortion rate (the number of abortions per 1000 women in a given age group per year). Table 31-1 summarizes annual data for the United States.

U.S. legal abortion utilization has stabilized following the decline experienced earlier this decade. Whereas those <15 years have the highest ratio (723), older women (40–44 years) also have a

---

TABLE 31-1
NUMBER, RATIO AND RATE OF UNITED STATES
LEGAL ABORTIONS

Year	Number	Ratio	Rate
1970	193,491	52	5
1975	854,853	272	18
1980	1,297,606	359	25
1985	1,328,570	354	24
1990	1,429,577	345	24
1995	1,210,883	311	20
1996	1,221,585	314	20

higher ratio (376) of legal abortion. Ratios are lowest in women age 30–34 years (165). For over a decade, those with highest fertility rates (age 20–34 years) have had a stable abortion ratio. Rates are highest for women age 20–24 years (38%) and lowest at the reproductive extremes <15 years (2%) and 40–44 years (2%).

Associations with legal abortion utilization include age, race, and marital status. Women <25 years have >50% of legal abortions, and 32% are performed in the 20–24 year age group. White women comprise ~57% of women having legal abortions; but the white ratio of 202 is less than the ratio in black women (555), and women of other races (360). The legal abortion rate for black women (31%) is 2.6 times the rate for white women (12%). Unmarried women have 78% of legal abortions, more than 8-fold that of married women.

Most (54%) were obtaining a legal abortion for the first time, although 18% had at least two prior abortions. No previous live births had occurred in 43%, and ~87% of those having a legal abortion had ≤2 previous live births. More than one half of all abortions (55%) were performed at ≤8 weeks of gestation, and ~88% were performed before 13 weeks. Approximately 4% of abortions were obtained at 16–20 weeks, and 1.5% were obtained at ≥21 weeks. Younger women (i.e., women aged ≤24 years) were more likely to obtain abortions later in pregnancy than were older women.

Currently, nearly all (98%) of abortion are performed by curettage. Less than 0.5% are by intrauterine saline or prostaglandin administration. Complete data are available for 1992 when 10 women died as a result of complications from legal induced abortion (a case-fatality rate 0.7 abortion-related deaths per 100,000 legal induced abortions).

INDICATIONS

The most controversial abortions are totally elective (patient demand). *Social indications for interruption of pregnancy are probably the next most debated indications* and cover a broad spectrum: preservation of mental health, excessive family size, poverty, incest, and rape.

Perhaps the *least controversial are those termed "medically indicated."* Examples of medical diseases said to require interruption of pregnancy to preserve maternal life or vital functions include neuropsychiatric disorders (authorities disagree regarding qualifications), bilateral renal insufficiency, chronic resistant pyelonephritis, class III or IV cardiac disease (e.g., intractable atrial fibrillation, coronary occlusion), marked impairment of pulmonary ventilation (vital capacity of <1400 mL in the average-size person), progressive loss of vision or Kimmelstiel-Wilson syndrome in patients with diabetes mellitus, thromboembolic disorders, severe hemoglobinopathies, gammaglobulinopathies, clotting defects, severe ulcerative colitis, invasive cervical cancer, and advanced breast carcinoma.

Obstetric complications that seriously affect the fetus when abortion should be considered include rubella before 12–14 weeks gestation, severe isoimmunization, fetuses with known morphologic defects (e.g., anencephaly, acardius), and fetuses with known congenital disorders (e.g., Tay-Sachs disease, osteogenesis imperfecta, trisomy 13).

LABORATORY STUDIES

Ultrasound scanning both confirms the pregnancy and aids in determination of gestational age. If no fetal sac or fetal heartbeat is present, a qualitative hCG is performed, and if positive, a quantitative value obtained. *An hCG of ≥1750, in the absence of a fetal sac should alert the physician to the possibility of an ectopic pregnancy.*

COUNSELING

The provider has the responsibility to *explain the reputed advantages, disadvantages, and alternatives of elective abortion, just as with other procedures.* Additionally, the patient should be assured of *continued empathetic quality care whatever her decision.*

The patient must be informed about the nature of the procedure and its risks, including possible infertility or even continuation of pregnancy. All reasonable alternatives must be explored. The rights of the spouse, parents, or guardian vary considerably from state to state but must be considered. The patient's permission must be obtained. State or provincial laws must be obeyed, with special reference to patient age, residence, indications for abortion, duration of pregnancy, consent, and consultations required or advisable.

Protracted guilt feelings for the loss of the fetus and remorse may result from induced abortion, particularly when religious and social conflicts complicate the decision to abort. The reported incidence of *serious emotional sequelae following induced abortion is* <5%. Follow-up and special care for those adversely affected should be afforded the patient.

METHODS

Several trends are discernable in the techniques employed for legal abortion. There is increasing interest in, as well as utilization of, *nonsurgical abortion.* The percentage of *legal abortions performed by curettage (including D & E) has increased from 89% to 99%,* whereas *abortion by other surgical means has declined* (intrauterine instillation from 10% to 0.4%, and hysterectomy and hysterotomy from 0.6% to <0.01%). Some authorities recommend that all patient receive prophylactic antibiotics before the procedure.

Early Medical (Nonsurgical) Abortion

Mifepristone (RU486), which appears generally safe and effective ≤8 weeks gestation, is being utilized for early pregnancy termination elsewhere in the world and has just received FDA approval for use in the US. Additionally, there appears to be increasing use of methotrexate, misoprostol, and a combination of the two, to perform early medical abortions in the US.

Vaginal Evacuation

Two main techniques are used for vaginal evacuation of pregnancy, *suction curettage and D & C.* The *stated advantages of suction curettage* (compared to D & C using standard curets) are that suction curettage is more rapid (3 min average), less cervical dilation is necessary (thus, less likelihood of cervical tears and an incompetent cervix), fewer failed abortions result, less anesthesia and analgesia are required, blood loss is less, infection is less common, and there is less trauma to the uterus (protection of the basalis and muscularis layers makes traumatic amenorrhea and intrauterine adhesions less likely).

Very early abortion (first 3–4 weeks of gestation) by low-pressure suction curettage is accomplished using a 4–5 mm flexible plastic cannula without cervical dilatation or anesthesia. This is

FIGURE 31-4.   Suction method for therapeutic abortion.

termed *menstrual extraction or menstrual regulation.* This procedure has a relatively high rate of failed abortion and is contraindicated in women with acute cervicitis or possible salpingitis.

Suction curettage requires *cervical dilatation as well as some
form of anesthesia* (e.g., paracervical block) when performed at
6–12 weeks gestation (Fig. 31-4). However, cervical dilatation can
be accomplished using *osmotic dilators* (e.g., segments of Laminaria). When dry, osmotic dilators are small (2–3 mm diameter),
but the material is very hygroscopic and capable of expanding to
2–3 times its original diameter. The dilators must remain in the
cervix for at least 6–8 h to reach full size. Synthetic osmotic dilators also are available. The stated advantages of this method are less
pain (compared to mechanical dilatation) and fewer cervical lacerations. A disadvantage is that the dilators must be placed in the
cervix some hours before the procedure.

After 12–13 weeks of pregnancy, suction curettage is usually
performed on an outpatient basis in an operating suite. These later
terminations (generally up to 20 weeks—called dilatation and evacuation, D & E) require several osmotic dilators or graduated mechanical dilators, a larger suction cannula, and forceps to complete

evacuation. Although this technique has fewer complications than the various methods for induction of uterine contractions and is more rapid than induction of contractions, it requires greater technical expertise. The long-term effects (primarily of possible cervical trauma) remain unknown.

IV sedation, as well as a NSAID, is commonly used in office settings where the procedures are performed under paracervical block. In surgicenters, terminations are more often performed with general anesthesia. As noted previously, most patients receive preoperative antibiotics and that generally is continued for 3 doses postoperative. Methergine 0.2 mg po Q 6 h for 6 does is used to assist in uterine involution.

INDUCTION OF UTERINE CONTRACTIONS

With Live Fetus

The *various techniques* of second trimester abortion by induction of contractions include intraamniotic saline infusion (100–200 mL 20% solution), intraamniotic infusion of prostaglandin ($PGF_{2\alpha}$, 40 mg), intravaginal prostaglandin vaginal suppositories (E_2, 20 mg), and intramuscular 15-methyl $PGF_{2\alpha}$. The coagulation system is altered temporarily by injection of hypertonic saline (decreased fibrinogen and platelets, increased fibrin degradation products) and the patient's fluids and electrolytes must be monitored carefully.

The *noninvasive techniques* (using prostaglandins) require less technical expertise and have a lower morbidity. However, prostaglandins should not be used in patients with asthma or in those who have had prior uterine surgery. The prostaglandins usually cause marked gastrointestinal side effects (nausea, vomiting, and diarrhea), which require appropriate premedication. However, the success rate is >95%.

With Dead Fetus in Second or Third Trimester

PGE_2 suppositories are most successful for use after spontaneous fetal death when it occurs in the second or third trimester. As with the other prostaglandins, PGE_2 suppositories must be repeated, result in a rapid abortion (8–12 h), and include all the side effects noted above, plus chills and fever.

Hysterotomy and Hysterectomy

Abdominal or vaginal hysterotomy, major surgery, has the disadvantage of much higher morbidity and *should be avoided if possible*.

Hysterectomy, feasible up to 23 weeks gestation, may be warranted for patients requiring hysterectomy for other reasons.

FOLLOW-UP OF PATIENTS AFTER INDUCED ABORTION

Rh$_o$ immune globulin prophylaxis (e.g., RhoGAM) should be administered <72 h after abortion if the patient is Rh negative (except when the father is Rh negative). For the first trimester abortion, the recommended dose of Rh immune globulin is 50 μg IM, and for second trimester abortion, the dose is 300 μg IM. As with term gestations, if there is evidence of fetal–maternal hemorrhage, additional Rh immune globulin should be given.

The patient should take her temperature daily and avoid coitus, douching, and use of vaginal tampons until her follow-up visit (usually ~2 weeks). Effective contraception should be made available according to the patient's needs and desires. She should report fever, unusual bleeding, or flulike symptoms at once. She should be offered counseling and support similar to that following term pregnancy and delivery. Follow-up care should include pelvic examination to rule out continued pregnancy, endometritis, parametritis, salpingitis, or failure of involution.

COMPLICATIONS

The major complications of induced abortion include uterine perforation, pelvic infection, hemorrhage, and embolism. *The mortality rate for legal abortions in the United States is 0.7/100,000 (v. ~9/100,000 for delivery).* The longer the duration of gestation, the greater the threat to the woman's life.

USE OF VAGINAL PESSARIES

The vaginal pessary is a *rubber or plastic prosthesis,* often with a metal band or spring frame. The usual widely accepted indications for pessaries include *poor-risk patients or those who refuse surgery* for uterine prolapse or other vaginal hernias, *aiding preoperative healing of cervical stasis ulcerations* associated with cervical prolapse, *nonoperative reduction* of cystocele or rectocele, and to *facilitate the evaluation and performance of hysteropexy* (by holding the uterus in position). A vaginal pessary is probably most useful for the support of a prolapsed uterus or cervical stump.

Gehrung   Gellhorn   Lucite ring

Ball   Hodge

Doughnut   Napier cup and stem
with waistband

Inflatable
Ball valve

FIGURE 31-5. Types of pessaries.

Pessaries are *contraindicated* in patients with acute genital tract infections and in those with adherent uterine retroposition. In most cases, adequate anterior support and a reasonably good perineal body are required. Otherwise, the pessary may slip from behind the symphysis to be extruded from the vagina.

The various useful types of pessaries are shown in Figures 31-5 and 31-6. The Hodge pessary (Smith-Hodge, or Smith and other

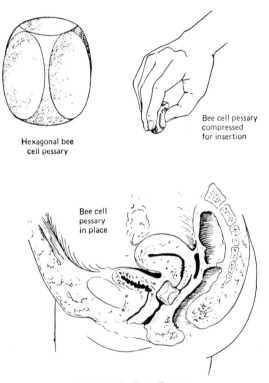

Hexagonal bee
cell pessary

Bee cell pessary
compressed
for insertion

Bee cell
pessary
in place

FIGURE 31-6. Bee cell pessary.

variations) is an elongated curved ovoid that supports the uterus after repositioning. The Gellhorn and Menge pessaries are for correction of marked prolapse when the perineal body is adequate. The Gehrung pessary rests in the vagina, cradling the cervix between the long arms, while it arches to the anterior vaginal wall to reduce a cystocele. Hard or soft ring pessaries (as well as the hollow plastic ball or sponge rubber bee cell) distend the vagina, elevate the cervix, and reduce cystocele and rectocele by direct pressure. Inflatable pessaries function similarly. If the perineum is inadequate, these pessaries may require a perineal belt and pad for support. The Napier pessary has a cup–stem arrangement supported by a belt and affords uterine support for a prolapsed cervix or uterus when the perineum is incompetent.

Pessaries are never curative, but they may be useful for months or years of palliation. Nonetheless, their use should be *properly supervised.* A neglected pessary may encourage genital infection(s) and may even cause fistulas. If the pessary is displaced, becomes uncomfortable, or requires cleaning, it must be removed. The frequency of removal varies depending on the pessary and the patient's status. To preserve the vaginal mucosa, a bee cell or inflatable pessary should be removed and cleaned nightly. Other pessaries may be left in longer. Acetic acid douches help to maintain hygiene while wearing a vaginal pessary.

When *pessaries are fitted,* the patient should be *shown how to insert, remove, and clean it.* Patients should be *warned of difficulties* (e.g., pessaries may cause infection, pressure necrosis, and ulceration or fistulas). Patients should be closely supervised. If not contraindicated, estrogen cream will assist in preserving the vaginal mucosa.

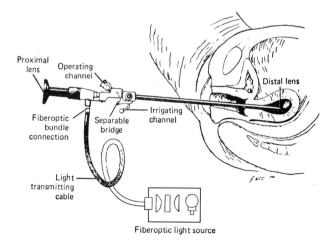

FIGURE 31-7.   Diagrammatic representation of hysteroscope in use.
(From R.F. Valle and J.J. Sciarra, *Minn Med* 1974;57:892.)

HYSTEROSCOPY

Hysteroscopy is visual examination of the uterine cavity with a small fiberoptic endoscope (Fig. 31-7). Paracervical anesthesia or analgesia is generally required, although general anesthesia may be necessary. After appropriate preparation with an antiseptic solution, the uterus is gently sounded and the cervix is dilated sightly to accept the hysteroscope. Intrauterine instillation of 35% dextran, dextran and saline, or CO_2 is used to slightly distend the uterus.

This *technique is useful* for removal of a foreign body (e.g., a intrauterine device), diagnosis of abnormal uterine bleeding (a polyp or other small tumor not discovered by other techniques), biopsy of specific sites (e.g., D & C may miss areas of endometrial cancer), lysis of intrauterine synechiae (i.e., Asherman's syndrome), some infertility investigations, removal of polypoid leiomyomas, and in operative management of a subseptate uterus.

Contraindications to hysteroscopy include pregnancy, acute cervicitis or salpingitis, the presence of STDs, and hemorrhage.

GYNECOLOGIC SURGERY

DILATATION AND CURETTAGE (D & C)

Dilatation of the cervix and curettage of the endometrium (D & C) is the most common gynecologic surgical procedure. If D & C is being performed for suspected endometrial or cervical cancer, specimens must be taken first from the endocervix (before sounding and dilatation) and submitted separately from those of the endometrium. This is fractional curettage. Because even more information may be acquired by hysteroscopy and endocervical curettage, that procedure is increasingly utilized. The indications for D & C are summarized in Table 31-2.

D & C is almost always accomplished in office or outpatient surgical settings. For D & C, the patient is placed in the dorsal lithotomy position. Although local anesthetics (e.g., paracervical blocks) are most commonly used, sedation, or general anesthetic occasionally will be necessary.

The *usual steps* in a D & C are as follows. Repeat the pelvic examination. Cleanse the vagina and perineum with an antiseptic and place the drapes. Insert a weighted speculum into the posterior vagina. Visualize, then grasp the cervix with a tenaculum or Allis clamp. Curette the endocervical canal with a Kevorkian or similar curette. Sound the uterus. Dilate the cervix using progressive

TABLE 31-2
INDICATIONS FOR DILATATION AND CURETTAGE

Diagnostic	Therapeutic
Irregular menstrual bleeding	Endometrial hyperplasia
Heavy menstrual bleeding	Endometrial polyps
Postmenopausal bleeding	Pedunculated submucous myomas
	Retained products of conception following abortion
	Missed abortion

dilators (e.g., Hegar) to 8 mm (Figs. 31-8 and 31-9). Introduce a polyp forceps and gently rotate before closing (in an attempt to grasp any polyps present). Introduce a standard sharp curette and begin the curettage by taking strokes across the fundus. Next, start at a given point and proceed around the entire uterus by bringing the curette from the fundus to the endocervix. Remove the curette after each stroke. This facilitates obtaining strips of tissue, all of which are submitted for analysis. Proceed until a gritty sensation (myometrium) is noted. *The most common complications of D & C are hemorrhage, infection, uterine perforation, and cervical laceration.*

CERVICAL CONIZATION

Cervical conization may be used to diagnose possible cancer or to excise CIN or other abnormal (on colposcopy) tissue extending beyond the field of vision up the cervical canal (10%–15% of cervical cancers develop in the upper cervical canal).

Most cervical conizations are performed as outpatient surgical procedures. Paracervical or general anesthesia may be required. Antiseptic solutions may be used, but care is taken not to touch the external cervical os. Suspicious areas that should be biopsied have generally previously been mapped by colposcopy. Conization is most commonly accomplished by *LEEP, scalpel (cold conization)* (Fig. 31-10), *or laser* and involves removing a thin circular portion of the cervix exterior to the squamocolumnar junction and extending variably up the endocervical canal. Rarely should the excision

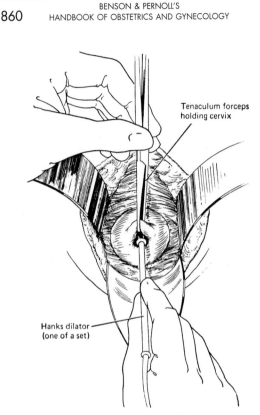

Tenaculum forceps
holding cervix

Hanks dilator
(one of a set)

FIGURE 31-8. Cervical dilatation.

extend to the level of the internal os. Scalpel cervical conization may be facilitated by introduction of a uterine sound to or just beyond the internal os so the tip of the blade approximates the sound. Generally, the tissue removed exceeds 0.3 cm in thickness. A suture usually is inserted at the top of the cone to aid the pathologist in tissue orientation for histology.

A major *problem of conization is damage to the internal cervical os.* Moreover, the majority of lesions occur at the squamocolumnar junction and during the reproductive years, the squamocolumnar junction is located on the portio of the cervix. Therefore, to avoid the potential of internal os injury many authorities currently

FIGURE 31-9. Curettage.

recommend taking the specimen in a "doughnut" configuration without an extended endocervical portion. The endocervix is then curetted and the tissue submitted for analysis.

If the cervix is deeply lacerated, segmental excision of tissue may be required to constitute a complete sample. Each fragment must be identified, and a diagram to aid the pathologist facilitates accurate analysis.

FIGURE 31-10.   Conization of the cervix.

Bleeding is generally less using the LEEP procedure and is easily controlled using that device, whereas sutures may be necessary with scalpel conization. *Hemorrhage* necessitates vaginal packing or deeply placed sutures or both. *Secondary hemorrhage* (related to infection of the surgical site) *occurs in 10% of cases and may occur as late as 7–14 d.* It is treated with antibiotics and vaginal packing but occasionally requires suturing. *Another late complication of conization is incompetent cervix* (from taking the specimen too far up the endocervical canal).

Conization of the cervix during pregnancy is fraught with hemorrhage and pregnancy wastage. Therefore, it has largely been replaced by colposcopically directed biopsies.

LAPAROSCOPY

Laparoscopy (Fig. 31-11) is a transperitoneal endoscopic technique for visualization of the abdominal and pelvic contents. It is an intraabdominal operation performed through a small subumbilical or intraumbilical incision, and it provides excellent visualization of the pelvic structures, permitting diagnosis of many gynecologic abnormalities and surgery without laparotomy. Considerable experience is required to achieve facility with the instrumentation, but in capable hands, laparoscopy is a well-tolerated surgical method that

FIGURE 31-11. Pelvic laparoscopy with patient in Trendelenburg position. (From A.E. Long, *Current Obstetric & Gynecologic Diagnosis & Treatment,* 4th ed. R.C. Benson, ed. Lange, 1982.)

can supplant laparotomy for diagnosis or treatment of many intraabdominal problems.

Laparoscopy is almost always a same-day surgery (i.e., the procedure is performed under anesthesia in an operating room, but the patient recovers and goes home the same day) procedure. *Fiberoptic illumination and carbon dioxide pneumoperitoneum* are used. *General anesthesia with endotracheal intubation* is employed. With the patient in the supine position, the abdomen is prepared, and sterile drapes are applied. Then, a Veress needle is inserted near the projected site of surgery, and the abdomen is insufflated with CO_2. Once it is certain the pneumoperitoneum is sufficient to displace the bowel, a trochar bearing the laparoscope sleeve is inserted. Next, the laparoscope is inserted, and pneumoperitoneum is maintained by continued smaller amounts of CO_2.

In addition to the equipment used for observation, a variety of accessories for *biopsy, coagulation, aspiration, and manipulation* can be passed through a separate cannula (second puncture technique) or inserted through the same cannula as the laparoscope.

There are numerous indications for laparoscopy.

- *Diagnosis.* Examples are uterine anomaly, endometriosis, biopsy of ovarian tumors, omentum, spleen, or liver, and differentiation between ectopic pregnancy and salpingitis or between psychogenic and organic pelvic pain.
- *Evaluation.* Examples include investigation of infertility (e.g., tubal patency test) and assessment of response to treatment in women with ovarian or other pelvic cancer.
- *Therapy.* Tubal sterilization by fulguration, application of Silastic rings, or metal clips.
- *Lysis of adhesions.*
- *Elimination of a disorder* (e.g., vaporization or fulguration of endometriosis).
- *Removal of foreign body* (e.g., an extruded intrauterine device).

Absolute contraindications to laparoscopy are intestinal obstruction and general peritonitis. Severe cardiac or pulmonary disease is a relative contraindication.

Complications depend on the problem, the status of the patient, and the expertise of the person performing the laparoscopy. Minor problems (e.g., abdominal or shoulder pain) are common but rarely serious. Indeed, the shoulder pain may be expected, for it represents diaphragmatic irritation from nitrogen replacement of the residual intraperitoneal carbon dioxide. Severe complications include perforation of a viscus, thermal burn of the bowel, severe bleeding (vascular injury), or cardiac arrest (rare but often critical). If not noted at the time of surgery, thermal bowel injuries do not generally become apparent until several days later, when peritonitis occurs. The incidence of major complications (mostly with bipolar instruments) in the United States is $<5\%$. The overall mortality rate in laparoscopic sterilization is $<2/100,000$.

Other complications of laparoscopy include insufflation of the abdominal wall from improper placement of the Veress needle and hypercarbia from improper anesthetic management of CO_2 insufflation.

STERILIZATION

Sterilization is the permanent prevention of pregnancy. There are as many reasons for sterilization as there are for contraception. Nonetheless, *elective sterilization is rapidly becoming the most used method of limiting family size in developed countries.* Little controversy surrounds voluntary sterilization in the United States,

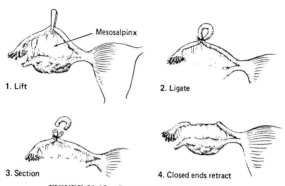

FIGURE 31-12. Pomeroy method of sterilization.

and it is legal in all states. Sterilization is used as a contraceptive means by about *one third of all married couples in the United States.* It is most commonly used when no more children are desired, the woman is >30 years of age, or the marriage is of >10 years duration.

METHODS

Tubal obstruction is the most commonly used sterilization procedure. This may be accomplished by ligation, diversion, or excision. Ligation may be done with segmental resection (Pomeroy, Fig. 31-12) or with crushing and ligation (Madlener). Excision may be effected by salpingectomy, removal of the infundibular portion of the tube, resection of the isthmic portion of the tube (cornual resection), burial of the proximal extremity of the tube beneath the visceral or parietal peritoneum (Irving, Fig. 31-13, or Uchida, Fig. 31-14), or cauterization-occlusion of the uterotubal ostia through the uterine cavity.

Most tubal sterilizations in the United States are done by laparoscopy on an outpatient basis. The tubes are either fulgurated in their midportion, occluded by clips of various material or by Silastic rings, or closed by a combination of techniques. The *methodology* and *complications* of laparoscopy are noted on pages 863–864. Because unipolar coagulation is safer and has a higher reanastomosis success rate, it is the fulguration method of choice. The total *complication* rate of laparoscopic tubal fulguration is 1%–6%,

1. Uterine tube lifted and cut.

2. Double ligation with gut; one tie left long for traction (special traction suture). Mesosalpinx stripped back.

3. Special traction suture inserted in tunnel in anterior uterine wall.

Figure-of-eight fixation suture

4. Implantation of the proximal tubal limb into a tunnel in the anterior uterine wall.

5. Traction suture tied and proximal tube sutured in tunnel.

FIGURE 31-13. Irving method of sterilization.

with major problems (hemorrhage or bowel injury) occurring in 0.6% of cases.

Minilaparotomy, a limited celiotomy procedure for tubal sterilization, can be performed on an outpatient basis. This procedure requires a small (usually transverse, suprapubic) skin incision with

1. Saline with epinephrine injected below serosa, which becomes inflated locally. Muscular tube, and even blood vessels, can be separated from serosa, which is then cut open.

2. Muscular tube emerges through opening or is pulled out to form a U shape.

3. Fimbriated end is untouched, while the end leading to the uterus is stripped of serosa. This can usually be done without damaging blood vessels.

4. About 5 cm of muscular tube is cut away; the end is buried automatically in serosa. Fimbriated end and serosa opening are closed and tied together.

5. Blood supply continues normally between ovary and uterus. Hydrosalpinx or adhesion has not been noted.

FIGURE 31-14.   Uchida method of sterilization.

dissection into the peritoneal cavity. This operation is often performed under analgesia and local anesthesia.

The uterus is elevated (by a uterine sound inserted before surgery or by use of a small intraabdominal retractor), and adequate visualization is afforded by small angular retractors. Both the ovary and the fimbriated end of the tube should be inspected to differentiate the tube from the round ligament. Tubal ligation may be carried out by any of the techniques noted previously.

Minilaparotomy is contraindicated when the patient is obese or has an enlarged or immobile uterus or when adnexal disease or endometriosis is suspected. Nonetheless, in some circumstances, minilaparotomy is simpler, safer, and less costly than laparoscopy for sterilization.

COUNSELING

All forms of sterilization have reported failures (occasional pregnancies occur). Abdominal and tubal pregnancies have been reported (rarely) even after total hysterectomy. Contemporay failure rates for the various procedures are shown in Table 31-3.

About 1% of sterilized women request reversal. Pregnancy rates following microsurgical tubal reanastomosis are at least 50%, depending on the method used for tubal ligation. The laparoscopic band techniques afford the best reversal rates (75%) and should be considered in the younger patient.

It is useful to have more than one counsellor when sterilization is requested by any woman <25 years of age and in a nulliparous woman <40 years old without children. The health care provider usually explains that with tubal interruption alone, no organ is removed. Tubal sterilization merely prevents conception. The benefits and risks of the operative procedure must be explained. The operation is not desexing and will not reduce libido or alter her appearance. There is usually no adverse change in sexual function following tubal sterilization. On the contrary, many women who feared pregnancy before the operation report increased satisfaction in sexual intercourse and are pleased with the operative result. However, *5%–10% report less frequent orgasm and regret the procedure.*

STERILIZATION IN THE MALE

Male sterilization by vas ligation (an office procedure) is far less dangerous than female sterilization. This alternative should be offered to the couple who desire limitation of childbearing, particularly when the woman is not an appropriate candidate for surgery.

TABLE 31-3
FAILURE RATES OF MINILAPAROTOMY AND
LAPAROSCOPY STERILIZATION PROCEDURES

Procedure	Failure Rate (%)
Minilaparotomy procedure	
Uchida	<0.1
Fimbriectomy	<0.1
Irving	<0.1
Pomeroy	<0.4
Salpingectomy	<1.9
Madlener	0.3–2
Simple ligation	20
Laparoscopy procedure	
Coagulation and excision	<0.6
Coagulation and division	0.1–2
Coagulation (only)	1–2
Silastic (Falope) rings	0.23
Spring loader (Hulka) clips	0.2–0.6

Data from Department of Medical and Public Affairs, George
Washington University Medical Center. *Popul Rep* (May) 1976;
Series C, No. 7.

Impotence does not result. Sterility cannot be assumed until ejaculates are found to be completely free of sperm (1–2 months or 15–20 ejaculations).

Disadvantages of vasectomy include occasional and unlikely spontaneous recanalization (<1%), the occasional development of a spermatocele, and the possible development of antisperm antibodies. Hematoma formation, epididymitis, and psychologic problems are occasional complications. Atrophy of the testes may result if the vasculature is inadvertently ligated.

In the United States, *6% –7% of men who have had vasectomy request reversal.* Reanastomosis of vasectomy results in 45%–60% pregnancy rates.

HYSTERECTOMY

Hysterectomy may be the third or fourth most common operation in the United States. Critics have charged that hysterectomy is too often employed for otherwise correctable menstrual problems or for sterilization. In any event, with recent advances, hysterectomy is performed increasingly for conditions refractory to other therapy.

A number of modifiers are used to more accurately describe hysterectomy. *Hysterectomy* is used interchangeably with total hysterectomy, both meaning *complete removal of the uterus, including the cervix*. *Subtotal hysterectomy* is the removal of the uterine corpus only. *Abdominal hysterectomy* is removal of the uterine corpus and cervix through an abdominal incision. *Vaginal hysterectomy* is removal of the cervix and corpus through the vagina. *Extrafascial hysterectomy* is removal of the uterus and cervix together with the outer fascial layer of the cervix (endopelvic fascia). *Intrafascial hysterectomy* is the removal of the uterus and cervix from within the cervical endopelvic fascia. *Radical hysterectomy* involves dissection and isolation of each ureter as well as the uterine artery and vein, followed by the en bloc removal of the uterine corpus, uterine cervix, a portion of the upper vagina, parametrial tissue, and uterosacral ligaments. Radical hysterectomy is usually combined with adnexectomy and pelvic lymphadenectomy.

INDICATIONS

The indications for hysterectomy are summarized in Table 31-4.

TABLE 31-4
INDICATIONS FOR HYSTERECTOMY

Gynecologic malignancy
Cervical
Uterine
Ovarian
Tubal
Benign gynecologic diseases (refractory to other therapy)
Uterine leiomyoma
Symptomatic adenomyosis
Symptomatic endometriosis
Symptomatic pelvic relaxation syndromes
Chronic incapacitating central pelvic pain
Severe pelvic inflammatory disease or pelvic abscess
Intractable uterine bleeding
Obstetric complications
Uncontrollable uterine bleeding
Molar gestation

PREOPERATIVE EVALUATION

Cervical cytology (to detect occult cancer) should be performed within 3 months of planned hysterectomy, and any abnormalities should be evaluated. Endometrial assessment (hysteroscopically directed biopsies, D & C) is recommended to detect occult cancer before hysterectomy in any woman >35 years of age who is experiencing abnormal uterine bleeding.

Preoperative workup should include CBC, UA, coagulation profile, chest x-ray, and ECG for those ≥45 years, and a stool guaiac determination. Uncomplicated hysterectomy rarely requires transfusion. Hence, type and screen for possible transfusion is often used in many institutions, as opposed to the more costly and time-consuming type and crossmatch procedures. The vagina should be prepared with povidone-iodine douches or a similar antiseptic the night before or the morning of surgery.

TECHNIQUE

Abdominal Hysterectomy

The patient is placed in the supine position, and a Foley catheter is placed in the bladder. The abdomen is prepared using an antiseptic solution (e.g., povidone-iodine), and sterile drapes are applied. Although the skin incision depends on the nature of the problem, for most benign conditions a low transverse (Pfannenstiel) incision may be used. For malignancy or complicated cases, a lower midline (symphysis pubis to umbilicus) incision affords better exposure and potential for extension.

With a *transverse incision,* the fascia is incised transversely, laterally curving superiorly to avoid the inguinal area. The pyramidalis muscles are separated together with the rectus muscles. Then, the posterior rectus sheath and peritoneum are entered carefully. The peritoneum is generally incised vertically.

The cecum and appendix are *visualized,* and the *upper abdomen* (kidneys, liver, gallbladder, stomach, proximal small bowel, and pancreas) *is explored.* The bowel is packed gently into the upper abdomen. This is facilitated by placing the patient in a slight Trendelenburg position. The *round ligaments* are suture ligated and cut. By sharp dissection, an incision is carried along the anterior broad ligament, allowing the leaves of the broad ligament to separate and the retroperitoneal space to be opened. This incision passes just superior to the uterovesical fold. By sharp and then blunt dissection, the *bladder* is separated from the cervix. At this point, with minimal additional blunt dissection, the pelvic vessels and ureters may be identified. The midline dissection is extended toward the vagina until the *anterior lip of the cervix* is palpated. At that point, blunt dissection is carried out laterally to remove the ureters from the uterine vessels.

If *oophorectomy* is to be performed, the posterior peritoneum is incised vertically just lateral to the infundibulopelvic ligament for 1 cm. Once it is ascertained that the ureter is clear, the *infundibulopelvic ligament* is doubly ligated. The posterior broad ligament is incised under direct visualization from the ovary and tube until near the uterus, when the incision is directed toward the *uterosacral ligament* insertion into the uterus. The ovaries are brought medial. If the adnexa are to remain, each *uteroovarian ligament* is clamped and ligated at its uterine insertion in a pedicle including the *fallopian tube,* and the posterior peritoneum is incised toward the uterosacral ligament insertion.

The *pelvic vessels* are identified and isolated at the level of the internal os. The *artery and vein* are clamped and doubly ligated. The *cardinal ligament* is clamped (usually by sliding the clamps off the cervix), incised, and ligated in several segments on each side. When the *uterosacral ligaments* are encountered, they are clamped, ligated, and incised. At this point, the cervix may be palpated, and the *vagina* is entered (usually anteriorly) by sharp dissection. A circumferential incision is carried out, and the specimen is removed. *Both uterosacral and cardinal ligaments are sutured to the angles of the vagina* to ensure vaginal support, and the vagina is closed with sutures. The vaginal closure may be mucosa to mucosa by suturing the vagina closed (anterior to posterior), or the vaginal lumen may be left open (generally for drainage) by simply suturing about the vagina. In both cases, absorbable sutures are used. The pelvic peritoneum is often closed, but recent studies indicate that this may not always be necessary.

Following a correct count of all sponges, needles, and instruments, the parietal peritoneum is closed and the fascia reapproximated with sutures. The subcutaneous tissue is closed, and the skin is closed with sutures or clips. A dry dressing is applied to end the procedure.

Vaginal Hysterectomy

Vaginal hysterectomy should be undertaken with caution if the uterus is >10 weeks gestation size or if there are numerous adhesions from pelvic inflammatory disease, endometriosis, or previous surgery (especially cesarean section). The procedure is facilitated if there is uterine prolapse.

The patient is placed in the dorsal lithotomy position, and the vagina and pudendum are prepared with an antiseptic solution. Sterile drapes are applied, and a posterior weighted speculum is placed in the vagina. The *cervix* is grasped, and mobility is reconfirmed. A circumferential incision is made to the *fascia* at the cervicovaginal junction, and the *cul-de-sac* is entered. Once it is ascertained that the *cul-de-sac* is clear, the *uterosacral ligaments* are identified, clamped, incised, and ligated. At this point, it is advisable to suture the posterior vaginal mucosa to the peritoneum to arrest bleeding from this area.

If the anatomy allows, modified sharp and blunt dissection is used to free the *bladder from the cervix* to incise the *anterior peritoneum.* If this is difficult, one or more segments of the *cardinal ligaments* may be clamped, incised, and ligated. Once the anterior peritoneum is entered, blunt dissection is carried laterally to retract the ureters from the uterine vessels, whereupon a retractor is placed to elevate and retain the bladder. The *uterine vessels* are identified, clamped, ligated, and incised bilaterally. Following clamping, ligating, and incising the *broad ligaments* bilaterally, *uteroovarian ligaments, fallopian tubes, and round ligaments* are clamped, incised, and ligated in one pedicle. The *ovaries* are inspected, and hemostasis is secured. The *peritoneum* is closed using a pursestring suture so that all pedicles are extraperitoneal. The lowermost segment of the cardinal ligament and the uterosacral ligaments are sutured to the superior vaginal angle, and generally, the uterosacral ligaments are sutured together in the midline. Finally, the vaginal cuff is closed with absorbable sutures.

Laparoscopic-assisted vaginal hysterectomy recently has begun to be widely applied. In this procedure, the infundibulopelvic ligament (if the ovaries are to be removed) or ovarian ligament and fallopian tube (if the ovaries are not to be removed), round ligament, and often, the uterine vessels are hemostatically transacted through the laparoscope. The hysterectomy is completed by vaginally resecting the uterosacral ligaments and lower portion of the cardinal ligaments. Vaginal closure techniques similar to those for vaginal hysterectomy are used.

COMPLICATIONS

The most common complications of hysterectomy include *bleeding, atelectasis, wound sepsis or disruption, urinary tract injury or infection, thrombophlebitis, and pulmonary embolism* (see p. 826 for urinary complications).

Bleeding is the most common intraoperative complication of either vaginal or abdominal hysterectomy. This is most commonly from the infundibulopelvic pedicle, the uteroovarian pedicle, the uterine pedicle, or an angle of the vagina. The only site of bleeding accessible for ligation without reoperation is the angle of the vagina. Nonetheless, if bleeding is persistent or sufficient to cause tachycardia, hypotension, or other signs of serious compromise, reoperation may be necessary.

Wound infection may occur about 3–5 days postoperatively and is associated with fever, pain, redness, swelling, and increased warmth about the wound. Treatment includes systemic antibiotics, opening the incision, local debridement, and proper wound care.

Wound disruption may occur 4–8 days postoperatively as a result of infection but is most often a combination of sutures or suture technique, infection, and altered healing. Wound dehiscence is heralded by an obvious serous discharge from the wound. When evisceration is suspected, the patient should be taken to the operating room, and the incision should be explored. Usually, only retention sutures must be placed in the incision.

Ureteral compromise may occur by sutures, crushing injury, or actual division. Ureteral injury may be the most serious complication of hysterectomy. The most common site of ureteral injury is just lateral to the cervix, and the second most common site is at the pelvic brim beneath the infundibulopelvic ligament.

Common symptomatology of ureteral compromise includes fever, flank pain, and a ureterovaginal or ureteroperitoneal fistula. Fistulas occur 5–21 days postoperatively (see p. 826 for a discussion of this and other urinary complications of hysterectomy).

ANTERIOR COLPORRHAPHY

Anterior colporrhaphy is used for repair of cystocele. With a large cystocele, however, care must be taken not to overcorrect (i.e., reduce the cystocele so completely that incontinence results). Anterior colporrhaphy is less useful for treatment of stress incontinence.

Anterior colporrhaphy is performed with the patient in the dorsal lithotomy position. General or spinal, epidural anesthesia is required. After preparation and draping, the vagina mucosa is incised in the midline from the superior extent of the defect to the urethra. Then, the *pubocervical fascia* is separated from the vaginal mucosa by blunt and sharp dissection. Particular attention must be given to the urethrovesical junction. Often a Foley catheter will identify the area where sutures must be placed.

A *plicating suture* (e.g., 2-0 polyglycolic) is placed on either side of the junction. This may be followed by an additional suture to reinforce the urethrovesical junction. Bladder plication is performed by placing sutures in the *paravaginal tissues*. After the vaginal mucosa is sutured, the procedure is terminated.

Complications of the technique include hemorrhage, infection, vesicovaginal or urethrovaginal fistula, incontinence of urine, and failure of repair (recurrence of cystocele).

POSTERIOR COLPORRHAPHY

Rectocele repair is accomplished by posterior colporrhaphy. The preparation for surgery is similar to that for anterior colporrhaphy. The vaginal mucosa is incised at the introitus, and the vaginal mucosa is freed from the endopelvic fascia and perineal muscles *to the level of the uterosacral ligaments.* If the uterosacral ligaments have not been *plicated,* they are sutured together.

Starting at the height of the vaginal apex (just below the uterosacral ligaments), the endopelvic fascia (and in some cases the perineal muscles) are reapproximated in the midline using slowly absorbed sutures (e.g., polyglycolic). Care should be taken not to perforate the rectum and not to markedly reduce the vaginal diameter. The lower portion of the repair is similar to that of an episiotomy closure. *Care must be taken to properly reconstitute the introitus and perineal body.*

Complications include bleeding, hematoma, infection, rectovaginal fistula, and excessive narrowing or shortening of the vagina.

REPAIR OF AN ENTEROCELE

Enterocele is *primary* (developmental) or *secondary,* as after inadequate closure of the cul-de-sac or after an abdominal or vaginal hysterectomy. Enterocele correction follows the principles of hernia repair. Repair of enterocele may be accomplished vaginally or abdominally. The *sac contents are reduced* (adherent contents complicate the repair). The *peritoneal pouch must be obliterated* and the *opening closed.* Then, the defect is reinforced by approximating stronger tissues over the defect. In enterocele, the tissues available for closure are the *peritoneum, the uterosacral ligaments, and the levator ani fascia and muscles.* In both, the uterosacral ligaments are brought together and plicated in the midline. Some surgeons use nonabsorbable suture for this. If the uterosacral ligaments cannot be identified, the cul-de-sac may be obliterated by concentric sutures in the endopelvic fascia. If the procedure is accomplished abdominally, the status of the posterior vagina should be investigated because a posterior colporrhaphy may be necessary for a lasting repair.

In addition to the usual surgical complications, enterocele repair may damage the ureters, rectum, or sigmoid colon.

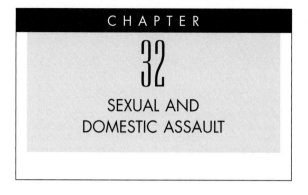

CHAPTER

32

SEXUAL AND DOMESTIC ASSAULT

SEXUAL ASSAULT (RAPE)

The legal definition of rape varies from state to state, but for medical purposes, *rape is physical assault or penetration of the genital, oral, or anal cavities by the assailant's body or foreign object with force or without consent of the victim.* Thus, in medical environments, *rape is better termed sexual assault.* Sexual assault is perpetrated primarily against women or children. Far fewer rape victims are males. Rape is increasing, especially the number of elderly victims. Although it is a felony and the *perpetrator is known to the victim in 80% of cases, only 20% of rapes are reported* to the police. The relative lifetime risk that a woman will be raped is over *15%.* Most rapes occur in the victim's home (50%) or neighborhood (80%).

Rape is perpetrated by men <25 years old in 45% of cases. Many rapists have serious psychologic or sociologic problems and rape to terrify, humiliate, and degrade rather than to achieve sexual gratification (as evidenced by the high rate of nonejaculation). The average rapist has committed many rapes before being apprehended. Rape can be divided into *three categories:* power rape (>50%), anger rape (40%), and sadistic rape (5%).

Power rape is usually premeditated. Included in this category are *multiple assailant rapes and date rape.* The latter may involve the use of alcohol or the drug flunitrazepam (Rohypnol). Rohypnol is readily available as a "street drug" and affects the woman's ability to anticipate or ward off an attack. Additionally, there is some amnestic effect. The perpetrator is often a young male who wants to show his dominance over the victim, occasionally resorting to kidnap and multiple assaults. Serious physical injury of the victim is not typical, but is more likely with multiple assailant rapes.

Anger rape is not usually premeditated and is often on impulse, but the victim is more likely to be injured than in power rape. The victim is subject to the assailant's rage and may receive threats of death if the crime is reported.

Sadistic rape frequently results in death or serious injury. The crime is most often premeditated, and torture or mutilation may ensue. Sadistic rape assailants are more likely to be psychotic than other rapists and often have a history of abuse of a wife or child.

The victim's most common response during the attack is to survive. Many do not fight for fear of being killed or seriously injured. Lack of resistance may lead to later *guilt feelings* because they did not try to protect themselves. *Disorientation, isolation, anguish, and fear of a later attack* are common reactions of victims. During medical evaluation and treatment, the victim may be reluctant to talk and try to *establish self-control* by appearing detached and calm.

DIAGNOSIS

Because the examining physician is a potential trial witness, the chart should include "findings consistent with the history obtained" or "alleged assault" rather than "rape," which is a legal conclusion. Legally and medically, it is crucial to *record the site, type, and extent of the assault; the degree of physical injury; the risk of pregnancy and possible acquisition of STD; and the treatment administered.* Emotional aspects of the assault must be addressed because emotional trauma can be devastating, regardless of the degree of physical injury.

Be *empathetic.* Begin with a statement such as, "This is a terrible thing that has happened to you. I want to help." Medical personnel should carefully avoid further emotional trauma to the rape victim. Show *respect, support, and concern.* Be aware of the impact of talking to co-workers. If the victim hears herself referred to as "the rape case in treatment room 1," she will feel even more degraded and shamed.

HISTORY AND PHYSICAL EXAMINATION

A *brief gynecologic history, as well as full details of the assault, should be recorded.* Activities between the assault and examination should be noted (e.g., bathing, douching, defecation, voiding, drinking, and eating).

Because a meticulous pelvic examination is required, anesthesia may be required to enable patient cooperation. With *witnesses present* (and named in the records), inspect the perineum and vulva for abrasions, ecchymoses, and lacerations. *Over 90% of victims will have trauma at one or more of four locations: posterior fourchette, labia minora, hymen, and fossa navicularis.* Tears occur most frequently on the posterior fourchette and fossa. The labia most often evidence abrasions and ecchymoses are most often seen on the hymen.

Ideally, *photographs* of all external injuries should be taken, accompanied by a written description and location of each. An *ultraviolet or Wood's lamp (fluorescence)* should be used to check the patient and her clothing for semen. Positive areas should be blotted with saline-moistened filter paper, labeled, and packaged separately. *Pubic hair* should be combed, and both the comb and material obtained should be packaged together. Pubic hair cuttings should be obtained, as well as *scrapings from under the fingernails.*

Each specimen should be packaged separately and labeled with source, patient's name, and date. All assembled items should be sealed individually, then sealed in a large container to verify that they were unaltered during transfer to the law enforcement agency. The person who accepts the evidence should sign for the material, and this transfer should become part of the chart. In brief, *the record should reflect the chain of evidence.*

The *vaginal speculum should be moistened with saline* only, and careful inspection of the vagina should be performed. Saline-moistened cotton swabs may be used to obtain fluid from the vaginal pool and the endocervix and placed in labeled, corked sterile glass tubes for culture for *Neisseria gonorrhoeae.* The same fluid should be applied to glass slides and air-dried but not fixed. Next, deposit 2 mL of saline in the vaginal vault, and with aspiration, *search for motile sperm* (often motile even 4–6 h after ejaculation). A cytologic (Pap) smear should be performed to show sperm if present.

If the mouth or anus was invaded, similar cultures should be obtained. Blood should be drawn for VDRL and blood type. HIV, as well as hepatitis (B,C) testing at this time and later should be offered. A pregnancy test is advisable if the patient may have become pregnant during the assault. Proper labeling of all samples is essential.

TREATMENT

Treatment centers on treatment of *physical injuries and prevention of STDs and pregnancy, together with the psychologic problems of the patient.*

Physical injuries should be treated as indicated. For prophylaxis against STD (gonorrhea, syphilis, *Trichomonas, Candida,* and bacterial vaginosis), follow standard treatment protocols. Tetanus prophylaxis is suggested for possibly contaminated external injury.

Prevention of pregnancy should be discussed if pertinent. *Endocrine postcoital pregnancy prophylaxis* is effective if administered <72 h after the assault, but before hormonal therapy is initiated, one must determine whether or not the woman is pregnant. Several hormonal regimens are effective (i.e., ethinyl estradiol 50 μg and norgestrel 0.5 μg, 2 tablets at examination and 2 tablets 12 h later, is effective and has few side effects). Ethinyl estradiol 5 mg PO daily for 5 days also is effective, but antiemetics should be given also because 80%–90% will be significantly nauseated.

Initiate follow-up emotional counseling and support of the victim.

PROGNOSIS

Physical recovery almost always precedes emotional recovery. Some women and children never fully recover emotionally.

The *acute phase reaction* lasting days or weeks includes initial agitation or surprising calmness, followed by *somatic complaints* of sleep disturbances, nightmares, nausea, headache, or musculoskeletal pain (from tension). *Emotional lability* is common, fluctuating from fear and guilt to anger and desire for revenge. Inability to concentrate and easy startle and fear reactions are frequent. Because a rape affects the attitude of friends and family as well as the victim, unexpected changes in interpersonal relationships are not unusual.

The *long-term reaction* may be a permanent behavior modification of the victim. Changing jobs, home, telephone number, and city is typical. Some victims will fear isolation, and others will fear men or crowds. Sleep disturbances may persist. *Reestablishing normal sexual responses is difficult for 50% of victims.* This negative effect is more pronounced in women who have never been sexually active. Victims of sexual assault have an increased likelihood of substance abuse, suicide, neurosis, and psychosis.

CHILD SEXUAL ABUSE

In the case of children who are suspected of being victims of sexual abuse, written informed consent (witnessed) must be obtained from the child's legal guardian, giving permission for examination, collection of evidentiary samples, photographs, release of information to the appropriate authorities, and treatment.

The history should be obtained from the child, if possible, and *recorded in the child's own words.* Note the type of injury sustained and who is the alleged perpetrator. The *child's behavior* should be carefully detailed, as well as composure, mental state, and his or her responses.

The examination should follow the techniques outlined in Chapter 18, with the addition of an ultraviolet (Wood's lamp) examination for semen on the skin and clothing. Collection of foreign materials (e.g., hair, sand, grass) is essential with proper labeling as to site of removal. Fingernail scrapings should be obtained. Semen stains should be sampled in the same manner as with adult victims. Vaginal fluid should be obtained using sterile moistened cotton swabs for culture, wet preparation, cytology, and acid phosphatase determination. Cultures of the pharynx, anus, vagina, and urethra should be taken regardless of history. All specimens must be individually labeled, sealed, and stored in the same meticulous manner as with adult sexual assault to ensure a proper chain of evidence admissible in court.

In suspected child sexual abuse, the *local child advocacy or protection agency should be contacted* for temporary placement when a parent is suspected of sexual molestation until further investigation can be effected.

DOMESTIC VIOLENCE

Violence against women affects at least 2–4 million women per year in the United States. This incidence of domestic violence is higher than the combined injuries from vehicular accidents, muggings, and rapes (by unknown assailants). One in ten women seen in emergency rooms (for any cause) are a victim of domestic abuse. Twenty-five percent of women who attempt suicide have a history of domestic violence. *Spousal/partner abuse is defined as intentional violent or controlling behavior by someone who has been intimate with the victim* and may or may not reside in the same home. *Coercive behaviors* take many forms and often include more than one of the following: sexual assault, physical assault, threatened physical assault, forced social isolation, psychological abuse (e.g., intimidation), threats or privilege removal, economic manipulation, and using children to manipulate.

The abused woman may go through several phases. Initially, she may respond to abuse by increasing efforts to make the relationship work and to prevent future abuse. Different strategies are often *attempted to appease* her partner, but eventually the futility of these efforts becomes apparent. At that point, she may begin to *tolerate* the abuse, feeling partially responsible and grasping at the positive aspects of the relationship. The woman may cautiously seek outside assistance, but does not want to affect her partner's social status, fearing for her safety or even simply feeling ashamed or humiliated that she is in this situation. Eventually, the woman *realizes that she truly does not deserve the abuse* she is receiving. Concomitantly, she often realizes that she is in *danger.* This phase is often marked by her *leaving and the returning* to her partner several times. She may consider *suicide or death of the abuser.* At this time, she may be most receptive to proposed assistance. To recover, she must eventually maintain her separation from the abuser.

Men who batter women may have been abused themselves as children or had male role models who were hostile to women. They may have not been raised in a loving or nurturing environment and possibly were exposed to alcoholism, racism, and oppressive behaviors as the norm. Most abusers blame the victim for making them angry enough to abuse. It is not unusual for the abuser to be *contrite* immediately after the violent episode and promise that it will not happen again. Unfortunately, the promise is rarely kept and the time periods of loving and nonviolence are ever more compressed between escalating episodes of abuse. *Partners of alcoholics have almost a 50% risk of abuse.*

The astute health care provider looks for clinical clues of domestic violence in all female patients. *One in seven women seen for general medical care in office practices have an abuse history.* Often *complaints are very vague* and include: chronic pain, sleep and appetite disturbances, chronic headaches, fatigue, abdominal complaints, gynecological complaints (i.e., frequent vaginal and urinary infections, dyspareunia, and pelvic pain), panic or anxiety attacks, depression, and requests for tranquilizers or pain medication. *Physical clues* include multiple bruises in various stages of healing, repeated injuries, numerous injuries at multiple sites, contusions, abrasions, sprains, lacerations, and fractures. The extent of the injury often seems implausible given the woman's explanation of how the injury occurred. *The pregnant woman may be at increased risk for abuse.* Commonly, the breasts, abdomen, and genital area are injured. Late or sporadic prenatal care may be a clue as well as "spontaneous" abortions and preterm labor. Short intervals between pregnancy and unintended or unwanted pregnancy increase the risk of domestic violence. *Clues to domestic violence may also come from the woman's partner.* For example, suspicion should occur if the woman's partner insists upon being present for the clinical visit, answers the questions directed at her, and minimizes any injuries seen. The patient may be reluctant to speak in front of her partner or blame herself for his outbursts of violence.

Although medical providers for women should be in the best position to recognize signs of domestic abuse, they often fail to make inquiries or intervene on behalf of their patient. Simply asking the question about domestic abuse causes discomfort for several reasons: fear of offending the patient, feeling powerless to help, frustration when the patient does not accept recommendations and change her situation, the fear that it will take up too much office time to address the issues fully, and the mistaken belief that it is not a common problem.

The following series of questions from Salber and Taliaferro's *The Physicians Guide to Domestic Violence* can be incorporated into a written health assessment.

SCREENING QUESTIONS FOR DOMESTIC VIOLENCE

- Are you in a relationship in which you have been physically hurt?
- Have you ever been physically hurt in an intimate relationship?
- Are you (have you ever been) in a relationship in which you felt you were treated badly? In what ways?
- Has your partner ever threatened to harm you or someone you love?
- Have you ever been forced to have sex when you did not want it?
- Have you ever been forced to participate in sexual practices that you didn't want to do?

If the patient answers "yes" to any of the above questions, the danger to the patient may be assessed by asking the following questions.

ASSESSMENT QUESTIONS FOR DOMESTIC VIOLENCE

- Has he ever threatened you with a weapon?
- Has he ever used a weapon? Is there a gun in the house?
- Has he ever tried to choke you? Has he ever threatened to kill you? Have you ever been afraid you might die while he was attacking you?
- Does he use "upper" drugs such as amphetamines (speed), angel dust (PCP), cocaine, or crack cocaine?

- Does he get drunk every day or almost every day?
- Does he control your daily activities, such as where you can go, who you can be with, or how much money you can have?
- Were you ever beaten by him when you've been pregnant?
- Is he violent and constantly jealous of you?
- Has he ever used threats or tried to commit suicide in order to get you to do what he wants?
- Have you ever threatened or attempted suicide because of problems in the relationship?
- Are you thinking of killing yourself now? Do you have a plan? A weapon?
- Is he violent toward your children?
- Is he violent outside of your home?

When a woman seeks medical attention for domestic violence, *meticulous medical documentation is crucial.* It should include dates and times, names of accompanying persons, description of the event in the patient's words if possible, abuser's name, description of the injuries (include photographs if applicable), names of treating personnel, and the name and badge number of any law enforcement officer involved. The patient should be aware that her medical record can be used by her and only with her permission as evidence if legal action is undertaken.

The health care provider should understand that *simply giving information about domestic violence to victims is actually a therapeutic intervention* in and of itself. If the health care provider does not indicate how serious the situation truly is, the victim may believe that the provider tacitly approves, or accepts the abuse. She must be respected in her attempts to make her own decisions, even when they seem inordinately delayed. Couple counseling is contraindicated because the partners must be assessed and treated separately. It is vital to offer her help in developing a safety plan before she leaves the current setting, even if that includes referral to another person or organization with expertise in domestic violence.

SAMPLE SAFETY PLAN

- If an argument seems unavoidable, try to have it in a room or area that has *access to an exit* and not in the bathroom, kitchen, or anywhere near weapons.
- *Practice how to get out of your home safely.* Identify which doors, windows, elevator, or stairwell would be best.
- *Identify a neighbor* that you can tell about the violence and ask that they call the police if they hear a disturbance coming from your home.

- *Devise a code word* to use with your children family, friends, and neighbors when you need the police.
- *Use your own instincts and judgment.* If the situation is very dangerous, consider giving the abuser what he wants to calm him down. You don't deserve to be hit or threatened. You have the right to protect yourself until you are out of danger.
- *Prepare a plan to leave* even if you don't think you will do it.
- Locate someone you trust that will *shelter* you (and your children) temporarily if you must leave in a hurry. If they cannot shelter you, ask them to *safeguard your important items* for pick up when needed.
- If there is no one available to provide shelter, locate and visit the nearest *women's shelter.* It may be listed in the Yellow Pages under Crisis Intervention Services. Keep their number and sufficient change or a telephone card on you at all times.
- *Pack a bag* with a few clothes for you and the children, a spare set of keys to the car and house, as well as copies of important documents (e.g. birth certificates, driver's license, green card, passport, social security card, immunization/medical records, school records, welfare identification cards, and bank books), medications with dosing instructions, and money (in the form of traveler's checks). Leave it with a person you trust.
- *List the appropriate legal advocate* to contact to receive a restraining/protective order and other legal advice, especially for child custody and divorce. Keep the protective order with you at all times. Make sure that family and friends know that you have the protective order.
- *Notify security at your place of work* regarding your situation. Have someone escort you to your car, bus, or train, if possible.
- If you are considering returning to a potentially abusive situation, discuss an *alternative plan* with someone you trust.
- To support yourself emotionally, attend a women's or victim's *support group* for a minimum of 2 weeks.

The Massachusetts Medical Society has devised an acronym (RADAR) to help physicians improve their response to victims of domestic violence.

- **Remember** to ask routinely about partner violence in your own practice.

- **Ask** directly about violence with such questions as, "At any time has a partner hit, kicked or otherwise hurt or frightened you?" Interview your patient in private at all times.
- **Document** your findings. Information about "suspected domestic violence" or "partner violence" in the patient's chart can serve as a valuable function in court should the woman decide to seek legal redress. A physician's documentation validates the woman's position.
- **Assess** your patient's safety. Is it safe for her to return home? Find out if any weapons are kept in the house, if the children are in danger, and if the violence is escalating.
- **Review** options with your patient. Know about the types of referral options (e.g., shelters, support groups, and legal advocates).

INDEX

NOTES

NOTES

NOTES

NOTES

NOTES

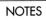
NOTES

NOTES

NOTES